Minimally Invasive
Spine Surgery

Minimally Invasive Spine Surgeons of India

Minimally Invasive Spine Surgery

Editor

Arvind G Kulkarni

MBBS, MS (Orthopedics), Diploma (SICOT), Diploma (Orthopedics)

Consultant Spine Surgeon

Mumbai Spine Scoliosis and Disc Replacement Centre

Bombay Hospital and Medical Research Centre

Mumbai, Maharashtra, India

Joint Secretary

MISSI

Associate Editor

Vishwanath Patil

MS Orth, FMISS

Consultant Spine Surgeon

Assistant Professor

Department of Orthopaedics

SDM College of Medical Sciences

Dharwad, Karnataka, India

Forewords

Shrinivas M Rohidas

Arvind Jaiswal

Amit Jhala

S Rajasekaran

Kevin T Foley

Jean Destandau

Jin-Sung Kim

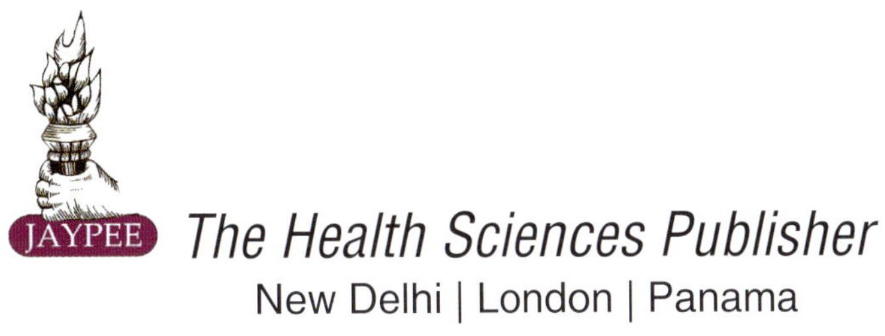

New Delhi | London | Panama

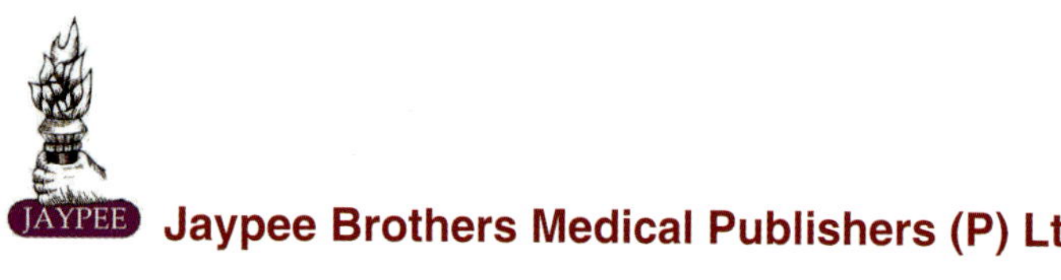

Jaypee Brothers Medical Publishers (P) Ltd

Headquarters

Jaypee Brothers Medical Publishers (P) Ltd
4838/24, Ansari Road, Daryaganj
New Delhi 110 002, India
Phone: +91-11-43574357
Fax: +91-11-43574314
Email: jaypee@jaypeebrothers.com

Overseas Offices

J.P. Medical Ltd
83 Victoria Street, London
SW1H 0HW (UK)
Phone: +44 20 3170 8910
Fax: +44 (0)20 3008 6180
Email: info@jpmedpub.com

Jaypee Brothers Medical Publishers (P) Ltd
17/1-B Babar Road, Block-B, Shaymali
Mohammadpur, Dhaka-1207
Bangladesh
Mobile: +08801912003485
Email: jaypeedhaka@gmail.com

Jaypee-Highlights Medical Publishers Inc
City of Knowledge, Bld. 235, 2nd Floor, Clayton
Panama City, Panama
Phone: +1 507-301-0496
Fax: +1 507-301-0499
Email: cservice@jphmedical.com

Jaypee Brothers Medical Publishers (P) Ltd
Bhotahity, Kathmandu
Nepal
Phone: +977-9741283608
Email: kathmandu@jaypeebrothers.com

Website: www.jaypeebrothers.com
Website: www.jaypeedigital.com

Inquiries for bulk sales may be solicited at: jaypee@jaypeebrothers.com

Minimally Invasive Spine Surgery

First Edition: **2018**

ISBN: 978-93-5270-054-7

Printed at: Ajanta Offset & Packagings Ltd., Faridabad, Haryana.

Dedicated to

All the Students of Minimally Invasive Spine Surgery

CONTRIBUTORS

Aaron J Clark MD, PhD
Department of Neurological Surgery
University of California
San Francisco, California, USA

Abhay Nene
Wockhardt Hospital
Mumbai, Maharashtra, India

Abhilash Dhruv
DNB (Orthopaedics)
Dip. (Orthopaedics); FASSI
Consultant Spine Surgeon

Aditya P Panda

Ajoy P Shetty MS(Ortho), DNB(Ortho)
Senior Consultant
Spine and Orthopaedic Surgeon
Ganga Hospital, Coimbatore, Tamil Nadu, India

Alok Ranjan MBBS, MS General Surgery, MCh (Neuro Surgery)
Senior Consultant Neurosurgeon
Apollo Health City Hospital
Jubilee Hills, Hyderabad
Andhra Pradesh, India

Amandeep Gujral MBBS, D Ortho, DNB(Ortho)
Senior Consultant
Nanavati Institute of Spine Surgery
Mumbai, Maharashtra, India

Amit Jhala MS, DNB
Consultant Spine Surgeon
Chirayu Hospital
Ahmedabad, Gujarat, India

Ankit Patel

Arun Bhanot
Chief of Spine Services
Paras Hospital, Gurugram
Haryana, India

Arvind Bhave MS (Ortho), IPTM, FICOE, Fellow
Spinal Injury Centre, Fukuoka, Japan, Hokkoido University, Sapporo, Japan, Fellow MISS, Korea
Professor in Orthopedics
Bharati Vidyapeeth Medical College
Pune, Maharashtra, India
Spine and MISS Surgeon, Deenanth Mangeshkar Hospital, Pune, Maharashtra, India

Arvind G Kulkarni MBBS MS (Orthopedics) Diploma(SICOT) Diploma (Orthopedics)
Consultant Spine Surgeon
Mumbai Spine, Scoliosis and Disc Replacement Centre
Bombay Hospital and Medical Research Centre
Mumbai, Maharashtra, India
Joint Secretary, MISSI

Benjamin Kuhns MD
Research Coordinator
Department of Orthopedic Surgery, Rush University Medical Center, 1611 W. Harrison St. Suite #300, Chicago, IL USA

Benjamin Mayo BA
Research Coordinator
Department of Orthopedic Surgery, Rush University Medical Center, 1611 W. Harrison St. Suite #300
Chicago, USA

CE Deopujari MB, MS, MCh, MSc
Consultant Neurosurgeon
Bombay Hospital
Mumbai, Maharashtra, India

Christopher D Witiw MD
Resident
Division of Neurosurgery, Department of Surgery
University of Toronto
Toronto, Ontario, Canada

Dhruv Patel
Clinical Spine Fellow
Chirayu Hospital, Ahmedabad
Gujarat, India

Doshi Preeti P MD, FRCA, FIPP
Consultant and In-Charge of Pain Clinic
Jaslok hospital and Research Centre
Mumbai, Maharashtra, India

Dustin Massel BS
Research Coordinator
Department of Orthopedic Surgery, Rush University Medical Center, 1611 W. Harrison St. Suite #300, Chicago, USA

DK Baheti MD
Consultant Pain Physician and Anesthesiologist
Bombay, Lilavati, Raheja and Shushrusha Hospitals,
Mumbai, Maharashtra, India

G Balamurali MBBS, MRCS(Ed), MD(UK), FRCS (Neurosurgery)
Head of Spine Surgery
Kauvery Advanced Spine Centre
Kauvery Hospital
Chennai, Tamil Nadu, India

Hussain Bohra MS Ortho
Fellow in Minimally Invasive Spine Surgery
Fortis Hospital, Mulund
Mumbai, Maharashtra, India

Jain Vikas
Spine Fellow
Mumbai, Maharashtra, India

John E O'Toole MD
Rush University Medical Center
Chicago, IL, USA

Junyoung Ahn MD
Resident Physician
Department of Orthopedic Surgery, Rush University Medical Center, 1611 W. Harrison St. Suite #300, Chicago, IL, USA

Kern Singh MD
Professor, Attending Physician
Department of Orthopedic Surgery, Rush University Medical Center, 1611 W. Harrison St. Suite #300, Chicago, IL, USA

Kevin T Foley MD
Department of Neurosurgery, University of Tennessee Health Science Center
Memphis, Tennessee, USA

Krishna Modi BS
Research Assistant
Department of Orthopedic Surgery, Rush University Medical Center, 1611 W. Harrison St. Suite #300, Chicago, IL, USA

Kshitij Chaudhary MS Orth, DNB Orth
Consultant Spine Surgeon
Sir HN Reliance Foundation Hospital and Research Centre
Mumbai, Maharastra, India

Kumar Shetty
Consultant Spine Surgeon
Fortis Hospital
Mumbai, Maharastra, India

Kunal Shah MBBS, MS
Fellowship in Spinal Surgery, Spine Surgeon
Spine Clinic
Mumbai, Maharastra, India

Kurt M Eichholz MD
St Louis Minimally Invasive Spine Center
St Louis, MO, USA

Laura A Snyder MD
Barrow Neurologic Institute
Phoenix, AZ, USA
Maharastra, India

Manish Kothari
Fellow in Spine Surgery
Hinduja Hospital
Mumbai, Maharastra, India

Matthew T Brown MD
Department of Neurosurgery, University of Tennessee Health Science Center
Memphis, Tennessee, USA
Michigan Head and Spine Institute

Mehta Satyen MS Ortho, MRCS (Glasg)
Consultant Spine Surgeon
Spine Specialist Clinic
Mumbai, Maharastra, India

Mick J Perez-Cruet MD
Michigan Head and Spine Institute
Southdield, MI

Mihir R Bapat MS, DNB
Director
Nanavati Institute of Spine Surgery
Mumbai, Maharastra, India

Mohinder Kaushal MBBS, DNB (Ortho), MNAMS, FMISS (France)
Chairman and Managing Director
Trinity Hospital and Medical Research Institute
Zirakpur, Punjab, India
Arthroscopy and Spinal Endoscopy Centre

Navin Mewara MS(Ortho)
Fellow Spine Surgery
Mumbai Spine Scoliosis and Disk Replacement Center
Bombay Hospital and Medical Research Centre
Mumbai, Maharashtra, India
Fortis Hospital, Mulund
Mumbai, Maharashtra, India

Neeraj Gupta MBBS, DNB(Ortho), FNB, DTB, MRCS, MNAMS
Consultant Spine Surgeon
Indian Spinal Injuries Centre
New Delhi, India

Nitin Garg MBBS, MS(Gen Surgery), MCh(Neuro Surgery
Neurosurgeon and Spine Surgeon
Bansal Hospital, Bhopal, MP, India

Pradyumna Pai Raiturkar
MS DNB Fellowship trained Spine Surgeon
Deenanath Mangeshkar Hospital
Sai Shree Hospital
Pune, Maharashtra, India

Pramod K Sudarshan MBBS, MS
Fellow in Spine Surgery
Consultant Spine Surgeon, People Tree Hospitals
Bengaluru, Karnataka, India

Pramod Saini MBBS, MS, DNB(Ortho), FNB
Spine Surgeon
Jaypee Hospital
Noida, Uttar Pradesh, India

Rahul Lath MBBS, MCh(Neurosurgery), DNB(Neurosurgery)
Neurosurgeon
Apollo Health City
Jubilee hills
Hyderabad, Telangana, India

Rajkumar Deshpande MBBS, MCh(Neurosurgery)
Fellowship in Skull Base Surgery
Director, Department of Neurosurgery
Fortis Hospital
Bengaluru, Karnataka, India

Ravish Patel
Spine Fellow, Bombay Hospital, Mumbai
Maharashtra, India

Richard G Fessler MD, PhD
Professor, Department of Neurosurgery
Rush University Medical Center
1725 W. Harrison St. Suite 855
Chicago, IL, USA

Rishi Aggarwal MBBS, MS, DNB, FCPS, MCh, MRCSEd
Senior Registrar in Orthopedics
Seth GS Medical College and KEM Hospital
Mumbai, Maharashtra, India

Rishi M Kanna MS, MRCS, FNB Spine Surgery
Associate Consultant
Ganga Hospital
Coimbatore, Tamil Nadu, India

Sachin Patil
Spine Surgeon, MVP Medical College
Nashik, Maharashtra, India

Sajan K Hegde MS
Fellowship in Spine Surgery
Consultant Spine Surgeon
Apollo Hospitals
Chennai, Tamil Nadu, India

Sambhav Shah MBBS
Consultant Spine Surgeon
Saifee Hospital, Bhatia Hospital
Mumbai, Maharashtra, India

Sameer Ruparel

Samir Dalvie MS, D Ortho, FCPS, DNBE
Neuro-spinal Fellowship(UK)
Pediatric Spine and Deformity Fellowship (UK)
Adult Reconstructive Spine Surgery (UK)
Consultant Orthopedic and Spine Surgeon
PD Hinduja Hospital, Breach Candy Hospital,
Mumbai, Maharashtra, India

Sandeep Diwan MD, DA (Anesthesia)
Consultant Anesthesiologist and Pain Physician
Sancheti Hospital
Pune, Maharashtra, India

Satishchandra Gore MS Orth Fabmiss
Consultant Spine Endoscopy
Mission Spine

Satish Rudrappa MCh(Neurosurgery), FASS(US)
Senior Consultant—Neurosurgery
Head—Spine Surgery
Director—Skull Base Surgery, Sakra World Hospital
Brain and Spine Clinic
Bengaluru, Karnataka, India

Shumayou Dutta MBBS, MS(Orth), FASSI
Clinical Spine Fellow
Bombay Hospital
Mumbai, Maharashtra, India

SM Rohidas MS(General Surgery), MCh(Neurosurgery)
Neurosurgeon
Dr Rohidas's Centre for Minimally Invasive Spine and Neurosurgery
Kolhapur, Maharashtra, India

S Rajasekaran MS, DNB, FRCS(Ed), MCh(Liv), FACS, FRCS(Eng), PhD
Clinical Director and Head of Department of Spine
Ganga Hospital
Coimbatore, Tamil Nadu, India
President, SICOT

Sreeharsha MS (Ortho), DNB, FNB (Spine Surgery)
Consultant Spine Surgeon
Sree Sharada Health Care
Mysuru, Karnataka, India

Subir N Jhaveri
Jhaveri Spine Hospital
Ahmedabad, Gujarat, India

Susmit Naskar
Spine Fellow
Mumbai, Maharashtra, India

Tarun Dushad
Associate Spine Surgeon
Mumbai Institute of Spine Surgery, Bombay Hospital
Mumbai, Maharashtra, India

T Ganesh Keshav
Spine Fellow, Kauvery Hospital
Chennai, Tamil Nadu, India

Umesh Srikantha MBBS, MCh (Neuro, NIMHANS), FMISS (S Korea)
Consultant Neurosurgeon
Head of Spine services
Center of Excellence: Brain and Spine
Aster CMI
Bengaluru, Karnataka, India

Vignesh Pushparaj
Associate Spine Surgeon
Kauvery Advanced Spine Centre
Kauvery Hospital
Chennai, Tamil Nadu, India

Vikas Gupte
Fortis Hosptial, Mumbai
Maharashtra, India

Vishal Kundnani MBBS, MS
Consultant Orthopedics and Spine Surgery
Bombay Hospital
Mumbai, Maharashtra, India

Vishwanath Patil MS Orth, FMISS
Consultant Spine Surgeon
Assistant Professor
Department of Orthopaedics
SDM College of Medical Sciences
Dharwad, Karnataka, India

William Long BA
Research Assistant
Department of Orthopedic Surgery, Rush University Medical Center, 1611 W. Harrison St. Suite #300, Chicago, IL, USA

FOREWORD

This book *Minimally Invasive Spine Surgery* by Dr Arvind G Kulkarni is a detailed accounting of minimalism in spine surgery.

There has been always a constant pressure from the patients for less painful techniques with improved results. Similarly, nowadays, every surgeon also wants to assure the patient that he or she is undergoing less painful surgery, i.e. minimally invasive surgery to decrease approach-related pain in postoperative period. The progress and comparable results in laparoscopic and gynecological surgery compelled other specialties to think of adopting less painful surgeries. Minimalism in spine surgery started with percutaneous techniques, progressing to development of various retracting systems. Minimalism in spine surgery has progressed in last few years with the help of improvements in endoscopes, developments in camera, single chip to three chip to HD camera and the upcoming of 3D endoscope with camera. This has helped in minimizing the criticism related to the quality of the image of endoscope.

This book *Minimally Invasive Spine Surgery* attempts to provide reader with details of minimally invasive spine surgery techniques, for treating common conditions of cervical, thoracic and lumbar spine by percutaneous, tubular retractors with associated instrumentations techniques. Furthermore, it provides the reader a synopsis of basics of endoscopic spine surgery, tubular retractors in spine surgery with various instrumentation stabilization techniques, along with indications, appropriate patient selection and clinical outcome. I strongly believe that this new text will motivate, especially the younger spine surgeons to become more interested in endoscopic spine surgery which will help them in getting their own identity in this more competitive future in medicine.

Special features of this book are in the form of very clear, informative photographs—well planned and organized, simplified smooth flow of excellent pictorial description, imaging, and very good endoscopic photographs with illustrations—with tricks and pitfalls. This book especially by Indian minimally invasive spine surgeons will encourage Indian spine surgeons to opt for these techniques with steep learning curve.

This book gives opportunity to younger surgeons to compare various techniques of endoscopic diskectomy, endoscopic canal decompression and minimally invasive fixation techniques. This helps them in developing their own concepts of minimalism in spine surgery and also helps them in overcoming the myths related to difficulties, results of these various techniques.

I strongly recommend this brilliant book as must have and read for all neuro/ortho/spine surgeons and to be found on shelves of all the departments, colleges, institutions and hospitals imparting training or practising minimalism in spine surgery.

Shrinivas M Rohidas
MS (General Surgery), MCh (Neurosurgery)
Neurosurgeon Dr Rohidas's
Centre for Minimally Invasive Spine and Neurosurgery
Kolhapur, Maharashtra, India

FOREWORD

This is the "Age of Renaissance" for spine surgery as, in this era, the art and science of spine surgery has been in constant evolution. A giant leap in the field has occurred after the advent of better imaging, improved diagnostic methods, and surgical care. In the past 15 years, a greater understanding of spine anatomy and the development of more sophisticated radiological imaging and instrumentation have further illuminated what is possible in spine care. This book has a collection of chapters that define why a minimally invasive approach should be chosen and how to perform such a procedure, written by authors who have established themselves as experts in the field.

The authors describe the pearls and wisdom that only come by practising spine surgery over an extensive period of time. This type of information is invaluable, for it is not necessarily presented at many academic meetings that spine surgeons attend. This book is unique in that the authors present an authoritative text with a focus on evaluative questions to make a strong determination as to which approach would be best for the patient. Experienced neurosurgeons, orthopedic surgeons, and spine surgeons will find this book a useful resource when considering the option of minimally invasive surgery, whereas residents and spine fellows who have a growing interest in the specialty will look to this as an invaluable guide in acquiring and refining new skills. This book will aid in making their spine surgical practice safer and more efficient with lesser complications.

For a surgeon like me who has been one of the pioneers of minimally invasive surgery, I am reassured by the enthusiasm, dedication and seriousness of the surgeons whose work is outlined in the book. Having been known as a minimally invasive spine surgeon, I am firmly convinced that minimally invasive spine surgery is here to stay and will advance in leaps and bounds in the coming times. This text goes a long way in supporting this thesis. This book should become a vade mecum for minimally invasive spine surgeons in this decade.

Arvind Jaiswal
Orthopaedic Surgeon and Head
Department of Spine Surgery
Primus Super Speciality Hospital, New Delhi, India
Ex-Chief of Spine
All India Institute of Medical Sciences
New Delhi, India

FOREWORD

Minimally invasive spine surgery has been gradually evolving for over 20 years. Recently, for the past 5 years, there has been a sudden surge in various procedures and techniques along with the tremendous advances in the technology. MISS which initially started with a procedure limited to lumbar spine and diskectomies has grown leaps and bounds and crossed all the boundaries and is applied at all the levels of spine with expanding indications. This has made mandatory for surgeons treating spine pathologies to become well versed with different techniques and procedures. To bring all the techniques under one roof and propagate and train surgeons interested in developing the skills of minimally invasive spine surgery, the pioneers of the MISS formed a formal organization of "Minimally Invasive Spine Surgeons of India". As a part of this endeavor, the organization felt the need of a handy book, which encompasses all the minimally invasive techniques, and of a must-read book for those interested in developing the skills of minimally invasive spine surgery. The leaders in the techniques have contributed each chapter of the book with lots of individual experience behind them. All the chapters have been concisely written with clear anatomical and technical points and figures so that book will be a perfect technical guide. The philosophy, scope and outcomes of minimally invasive spine surgery give insight to the reader regarding how the philosophy of MIS can increase the width to which MIS can be applied and the long-term results of the procedure. All in all, it is a worth book on minimally invasive spine surgery. It deserves lots of praise for the effort from Dr Arvind G Kulkarni and his team.

Amit Jhala MS, DNB
Consultant Spine Surgeon
Chirayu Hospital
Ahmedabad, Gujarat, India

FOREWORD

It is my privilege to write a foreword for this valuable and dedicated book on minimally invasive spine surgery.

Minimally invasive surgery for spine problems is a useful development that has brought tremendous advantages to the surgeon and the patient. To the patient, it means smaller incisions, lesser pain, preservation of anatomy, less destruction of functional structures, and early mobilization. To the surgeon, the uses of the microscope, endoscope and special retractor have allowed good visualization, illumination, magnification and access to internal structures with minimal destruction of normal anatomy. On the economic front, it means shorter hospital stay and better utilization of resources.

Minimally invasive spine surgery is thus becoming very popular amongst patients and surgeons alike, and the time is not too far away before it replaces standard open access surgeries. This book will undoubtedly become a standard and preferred source of reference, because of its well-structured format. The 41 chapters cover the entire spectrum of minimally invasive spine surgery without leaving any gaps. Although it has multiple authors, each chapter is very comprehensive and has an excellent coverage of the subject that includes indications, preoperative planning, appropriate imaging, intra-operative techniques, postoperative care and possible complications. It is also well illustrated with appropriate figures and has an easy narration that makes reading easy and clearly understandable.

The book is a must for any surgeon who is interested in minimally invasive spine surgery and will easily finds its place of pride into the library of all spine surgeons from the beginners to the well experienced. My congratulations to the editor and all the authors for their excellent endeavor.

S Rajasekaran
MS, DNB, FRCS (Edin), FRCS (Lon), MCh, PhD
Chairman, Department of Orthopaedics and Spine Surgery
Ganga Hospital, Coimbatore, Tamil Nadu, India
President, SICOT
Chair, International Research Commission, AO Spine
Past President, ASSI and IOA

FOREWORD

It is my great pleasure, as one of the fathers of minimally invasive spine surgery, to provide this foreword to the Minimally Invasive Spine Surgeons of India (MISSI) textbook *Minimally Invasive Spine Surgery*. It was my honor to address the MISSI Society during its inaugural meeting in Ahmedabad in 2014. As you will see, the MISSI textbook provides a broad overview of minimally invasive spine surgery and adds a distinctive Indian flair and point of view regarding this broad field. All of us who are dedicated to minimally invasive spine surgery are motivated to improve patient outcomes and lessen the morbidity of traditional open spinal surgeries. My colleagues in India have helped to advance minimally invasive spine surgery and have added their surgical skills and expertise to this effort. I applaud the members of MISSI for their exemplary accomplishments and look forward to their future advancements in the field.

Kevin T Foley MD FACS
Professor
Neurosurgery, Orthopedic Surgery and
Biomedical Engineering
University of Tennessee Health Science Center
Memphis, TN, USA

FOREWORD

It is clear that invasive surgery and specially endoscopic techniques are becoming the standards in surgery, and of course, it includes spine surgery.

This excellent book edited by Dr Arvind G Kulkarni gives a wide review of what can be done today in spine surgery. From simple decompression with microscopic or endoscopic control to minimally invasive percutaneous fusion, all the different techniques are described by the experts, giving a realistic opinion with a good description of the surgical steps, the advantages and the complications.

The interest of different tools as ultrasonic bone dissector to prevent damage of nervous structures or navigation to reduce the irradiation of the patients are presented.

I recommand this book to any spine surgeons and to residents who are learning spine surgery as they will find in it the answers of most of their questions.

Jean Destandau
Endoscopic Spine Neurosurgeon
Bordeaux, France

FOREWORD

With the remarkable advances in technology and related surgical techniques, minimally invasive spine surgery (MISS) like other surgical fields is replacing conventional surgery and has become the mainstream of spinal surgery.

In keeping with the times, it seems very appropriate that Dr Arvind G Kulkarni published this book and provided excellent guidelines for the spine surgeons.

The book I mention today, entitled *Minimally Invasive Spine Surgery*, will be a standard model of its kind in terms of evidence-based basic knowledge and the techniques of each surgical procedure. The perspective that this textbook offers will surely help each and every spine surgeons to get a better understanding and grasping of the techniques of MISS and follow worldwide trends of spine surgery that compose it. If readers use this book well, I am sure that it will be a valuable chance to increase the quality of spine surgery in their clinical fields and to help them resolve thirst for MISS.

I also extend my deepest appreciation to Dr Arvind G Kulkarni, for he is an awesome pedagogue, and an heir, as my many colleagues said, to the minimally invasive spine surgery in India.

This textbook, *Minimally Invasive Spine Surgery* will be, therefore, a key reference not only for conventional spine surgeons but also for beginners who are willing to be an expert in the field of MISS.

Jin-Sung Kim
MD, PhD
Professor
Spine Center, Department of Neurosurgery, Seoul St. Mary's Hospital
College of Medicine, The Catholic University of Korea

PREFACE

This textbook is a powerhouse of knowledge for the reader who is keen to understand and learn the state-of-art techniques in minimally invasive spine surgery (MISS). Not leaving any stone unturned, almost every pathology at any remotest anatomical corner, which can be dealt with utilizing minimally invasive techniques, has been described in this book by masters in the field. The authors realize that there is no match or comparison for hands-on experience and none of the masters who are the authors here would subscribe to performance of surgery by just reading this book. However, the reader would find that the methodical way in which procedures and techniques are described here, performance would be just a step away. Such is the thrilling curiosity, interest and confidence that this textbook will generate. India and the international sphere have been witness to the ever-rising interest and enthusiasm in MISS. Similarly, once MISS became an integral part of our practice and indications for MISS extended in terms of pathologies addressed as well as locations and regions accessed, an idea ignited to capture our experience in words. Dearth of MISS specific textbooks and literature, especially from the subcontinent gave further stimulus to this endeavor. The birth of Minimally Invasive Spine Surgeons of India (MISSI) was a booster to this literary effort. Regular interaction with MIS-experts was an eye-opener to the wonderful and exemplary path-breaking work that our colleagues in various streams or MIS-gharanas (music gurukuls of different genres as Dr Arvind Jaiswal [founder president of MISSI] described) were performing. Infrastructure and technology form the foundation of MISS, and the authors have represented the paraphernalia specific to each technique extensively in this book. This book comprehensively and systematically describes the basic philosophy, applied anatomy, indications and procedural techniques, including pain management techniques by authorities in the field. While the readers would track and read the procedural topics specific to their gharana (stream), the authors would recommend each and every chapter. This would enhance basic understanding of the rationale and applied anatomy of other streams and probably lead to evolution of newer ideas and techniques. Considerable time, energy, patience and effort are ingredients of a successful venture. In this respect, the contribution of each and every international and national author is highly appreciated. This book is a milestone for MISSI and will serve as a teacher for the beginner, reference book for the seasoned spine surgeon and will open up novel ideas to innovate for the accomplished MIS surgeons.

Arvind G Kulkarni

ACKNOWLEDGMENTS

Dr Vishwanath Patil (Spine Surgeon, SDM Medical College and Hospital, Dharwad, Karnataka, India) deserves an applause for being extremely pursuant and persistent in integrating and organizing the textbook. Mr Sabarish Menon from M/s Jaypee Brothers Medical Publishers (Mumbai Branch) has been one of the supporting pillars without whom the textbook would not have seen the light of the day.

CONTENTS

SECTION 1 Fundamentals

SECTION 2 MIS in Cervical Spine

SECTION 3 MIS in Lumbar Spine—Non-instrumented

SECTION 4 MIS in Lumbar Spine—Instrumented

SECTION 5 Tumors, Infections and Osteoporosis

SECTION 6 Pain Management

1

SECTION

Fundamentals

Section Outline

1

CHAPTER

Introduction and Scope of Minimally Invasive Spine Surgery

Christopher D Witiw, Richard G Fessler

ABSTRACT

Within 20 years minimally invasive spine surgery has evolved from an interesting peculiarity to mainstream surgical technique. Initially limited to simple procedures, such as lumbar diskectomy, it is now used for decompression of stenosis, fusion, tumors, deformity, and trauma. As its applicability expanded, and the magnitude and complexity of procedure is for which it was used increased, its advantages became increasingly more apparent. Not only are pain, recovery, blood loss, and infections, to name only a few, decreased, but these are achieved while decreasing cost. This chapter will review the rationale and scope of applicability of minimally invasive spine surgery procedures.

INTRODUCTION

Surgeons and patients alike share a predilection toward less invasive surgical procedures. This has compelled the development of approaches through small corridors to surgically treat a myriad of pathologic processes across a wide range of specialties. In the field of spinal surgery, reports of minimally invasive procedures date back to the early 20th century.[1] However, the movement toward widespread adaptation of less invasive techniques only began gaining substantial momentum in the mid-1990s. This was spurred on by the development of innovative retractor systems and supported by improvements in endoscopic and fluoroscopic technologies. These early landmark developments were founded upon the primary tenet that disruption of the normal osteoligamentous anatomy of the spinal column and surrounding muscles should be minimized during the surgical exposure while still maintaining sufficient access to address the underlying pathological process in a safe and effective manner.

Minimally invasive spine surgery (MISS) gained its foothold in the specialty as a means to treat degenerative pathology of the lumbar spine but remarkable innovations in surgical techniques, augmented by parallel advances in technology have spurred the reinvention of a multitude of spinal surgical procedures. This a had led to advancements in the range of spinal pathologies that may be treated with MISS and over the last 2 decades we have seen a dramatic shift from the traditional standard practice of open spinal surgery to a movement toward widespread adaptation of MISS.

The aim of this chapter is to provide a concise introduction to the field of MISS. We will reviews the rationale for MISS and the evidence supporting it. This will be followed by an overview of the scope of MISS, organized by pathology. The majority of the focus will be on degenerative pathology, where many important early advances were made but the discussion will be extended to include more recent inroads into the effective treatment of spinal treatment of trauma, malignancy and deformity by minimally invasive techniques. This is not meant to be a comprehensive review but instead set the stage for detailed descriptions of specific procedures and indications in the subsequent chapters of the text.

THE RATIONALE

In this modern era of evidence-based medicine, it is insufficient to claim a procedure is better simply by its less invasive nature. Novel developments must withstand the rigors of preclinical and clinical investigation and demonstrate safety and efficacy. This section will focus on the evidence that has mounted to support the adaptation of minimally invasive techniques for spinal surgery.

Biological Support

Traditional open surgical approaches require extensive muscular dissection and disruption of the patient's native anatomy. Histological and biochemical evidences of injury to the back muscles have been shown with traditional open surgical approaches.[2] Patients undergoing minimally invasive approaches have lower serum levels of inflammatory cytokines when compared with their counterparts undergoing open approaches, suggesting less physiological stress.[3] Progressive muscular dilation with the use of tubular retractors in MISS have been shown to exert significantly less pressure on the surrounding soft tissues that those used for open procedures, and this is associated with less postoperative muscular edema, suggesting less damage.[4] Experimental studies have shown positive correlations between trunk muscle activity and the reduction of the cross-sectional muscle area following posterior spinal surgery.[5] The muscular protective effects of MISS have been further substantiated by clinical studies revealing that percutaneous pedicle screw fixation is associated with less change in the cross-sectional paraspinal muscle area and greater postoperative trunk muscle function than open techniques.[6]

Concerns about anatomic disruption with open exposures extend beyond the muscular injury to include the bony and ligamentous anatomy. Disruption of the posterior spinal elements in traditional open laminectomy results in increased flexion-extension and axial rotation at the surgical site. This has the potential to lead to segmental instability in cases where fusion is not performed. Minimally invasive approaches afford relative preservation of these elements and less postoperative motion, conferring theoretical protection against the development of untoward postoperative instability.[7]

Clinical Outcome Support

Biological studies suggest many advantages of MISS over open approaches, but some of the most compelling evidence is found in clinical outcome studies. Overall MISS matches open spinal surgical procedures in terms of long-term outcome metrics, such as pain, disability and rates of fusion; however, the less invasive approaches frequently outperform their open counterparts in many important measures of approach related morbidity with significant reductions in operative blood loss, length of stay and postoperative pain.[8-11] Improvements in all of these metrics are thought to be associated with less tissue disruption during the exposure stages of the surgery. One of the most notable improvements afforded by MISS is a reduction in the rate of surgical site infections (SSIs) which may be attributable to less exposure, protection of the surgical site from the skin edge by tubular retractors and reduced dead-space after tissue closure.[12,13]

Economic Support

Spinal surgical interventions are among some of the most costly; individual procedure costs are on the rise and these increases are mirrored by the trend in the number of operations performed.[14] As assessments of value in health care become a priority, it is imperative that costs are factored into the assessment of new surgical innovations.[15] Studies of MISS utilizing value-based metrics have demonstrated promise for reducing costs on already overburdened healthcare systems.[16]

Numerous studies have demonstrated decreased direct hospital costs, often attributed to the aforementioned improvements in perioperative clinical outcomes, such as shortened lengths of stay, less postoperative analgesic requirement and reduced incidence of SSIs.[17,18] Equally important are indict personal costs and costs to society as a whole which have too been shown to be significantly reduced through the incorporation of minimally invasive techniques.[19] Furthermore, economic support is conferred by the favorable performance of MISS in cost–utility studies. In a recent comparison, it was shown that MISS lumbar decompression was superior to both open laminectomy and epidural steroid injection in cost–utility outcomes.[20]

SCOPE

The foundations of MISS are in the realm of degenerative pathology of the lumbar spine. Some of the most notable technical advances have been made in methods of muscular dilatation through novel tubular retractors and percutaneous instrumented spinal fixation. This section will focus on the advancement of MISS techniques for the treatment of degenerative pathology and will then extend to more recent advancements in the field that have allowed for the application of minimally invasive techniques to a wide array of progressively more complex spinal pathologies, including trauma, malignancy and deformity correction.

Degenerative Spinal Pathology

Some of the earliest attempts at minimizing tissue destruction during intervention for degenerative spinal pathology involved percutaneous treatment of lumbar disk herniations. Chemonucleolysis was first described in the 1960s and heralded as a means to reduce the compressive effects of an intervertebral disk herniation by the percutaneous injection of a proteolytic enzyme.[21] This was followed, in the 1970s, by the first percutaneous nucleotomy, where a cannula was inserted from a posterolateral percutaneous approach and used to fenestrate the annulus fibrosis and partially resect the nucleus pulposus of the intervertebral disk to reduce the mass effect on the adjacent nerve root.[22] In the following decade, interest developed in the utilization of the application of laser energy delivered percutaneously through a cannula to the intervertebral disk to evaporate water and encourage a herniated disk to recede.[23] These percutaneous techniques were met with variable degrees of success. Active study in these realms continues, but none have attained widespread acceptance and are generally regarded as experimental.[24]

While percutaneous techniques afford minimal disruption of the normal anatomy, they are greatly limited by the visualization that is afforded by a traditional open microdiskectomy. One of the major advances in the field of MISS is the concept of minimizing tissue trauma through progressive muscular dilation and the ensuing development of tubular muscle retractors. This was coupled with advances in technology for endoscopic visualization and led to the first description of the microendoscopic diskectomy (MED) in 1997.[25] The combination of familiar lumbar microsurgical techniques with endoscopy allows surgeons to address free-fragment disk herniations as well as lateral recess stenosis. The associated safety, efficacy and improvements in approach-related morbidity have lead to widespread adaptation.[26,27] The tubular retractor systems have expanded in versatility and also accommodate the more familiar operative microscope and the scope of degenerative pathologies that could be addressed has expanded rapidly. A major advance was the recognition that the tubular retractor systems allow for effective bilateral lumbar decompression via a unilateral approach for lumbar stenosis.[28] Furthermore, these minimally invasive techniques can be used to treat far lateral lumbar disk herniations, synovial cysts and have gained acceptance for a posterior approaches to nerve root decompression in the cervical spine.[11,29-31] Parallel gains have been made in anterior approaches for treatment of intervertebral disk herniations. The development and optimization of laparoscoic and thoracoscopic technologies and techniques in other specialties such as general surgery and urology have been used to minimize the morbidities associated with open thoracotomy and laparotomy. This sets the stage for the development of less invasive anterior and lateral approaches to thoracic and lumbar disk pathology, which are now well described.[32-34]

While decompression of degenerative pathology is often sufficient there are many cases where segmental fusion is needed. Traditional open posterior exposures allow for the identification of anatomic boney landmarks to guide the insertion of spinal instrumentation from a posterior approach; however, this obviates the advantages of minimally invasive exposures for decompression. Percutaneous insertion of pedicle screws greatly reduces the degree of tissue disruption required, but early attempts in the 1990s were limited by a need for temporary external longitudinal fixation and the associated patient discomfort and infection risk.[35] The technology was advanced to a great extent and at the turn of the century when a system was described to allow wholly percutaneous insertion of pedicle screws and adjoining rods for posterior instrumented fixation.[36] This allowed for a combination of minimally invasive access through tubular retractors for posterior decompression with percutaneous insertion of instrumentation for fixation. Soon thereafter reports of minimally invasive posterior lumbar interbody fusion (PLIF) and minimally invasive TLIFs emerged and have since gained widespread acceptance.[37-40] Applications of 3-dimentional stereotactic navigation technology have allowed for computer assisted real-time determination of transverse width, longitudinal depth and angle of trajectory and have improved accuracy of percutaneous pedicle screw placement.[41]

Traditional open anterior lumbar interbody fusions (ALIF) have been modified to minimize tissue trauma during surgical approach with the use of mini-open and laparoscopic techniques.[42,43] However, these approaches do carry risks of large vessel injury, sexual dysfunction and visceral damage. In order to address this, a novel minimally invasive means of access to the lumbar spine through a lateral retroperitoneal transpsoas approach was described.[44] Termed the extreme lateral lumbar interbody fusion (XLIF) this approach uses dilators and tubular retractors passed through the psoas muscle after dissection through the retroperitoneal fat plane. This permits access for diskectomy and interbody fusion at the desired level **(Figures 1A to D)**.

Trauma

Trauma represents an area of spinal surgery that holds great potential for the application of minimally invasive techniques. Often, patients with spinal trauma have numerous concurrent injuries and the tenuous nature of their clinical status may preclude open interventions to address the traumatic disruption of their spinal anatomy. Percutaneous pedicle screw fixations have been shown to be effective for the treatment of unstable thoracolumbar fractures.[45,46] The less invasive approaches hold promise to shorten critical care and hospital stays, reduce need for mechanical ventilation and minimize blood transfusions in these patients.[47,48] Further study is needed to define the most appropriate injuries and techniques for the incorporation of MISS techniques in spine trauma, but it is likely that this area will see rapid expansion in the coming years.

Malignancy

Advances in minimally invasive techniques have allowed for the treatment of both intradural and extradural tumors. The spinal column is a common site of metastatic tumor spread, and this is often associated with pain and neurological

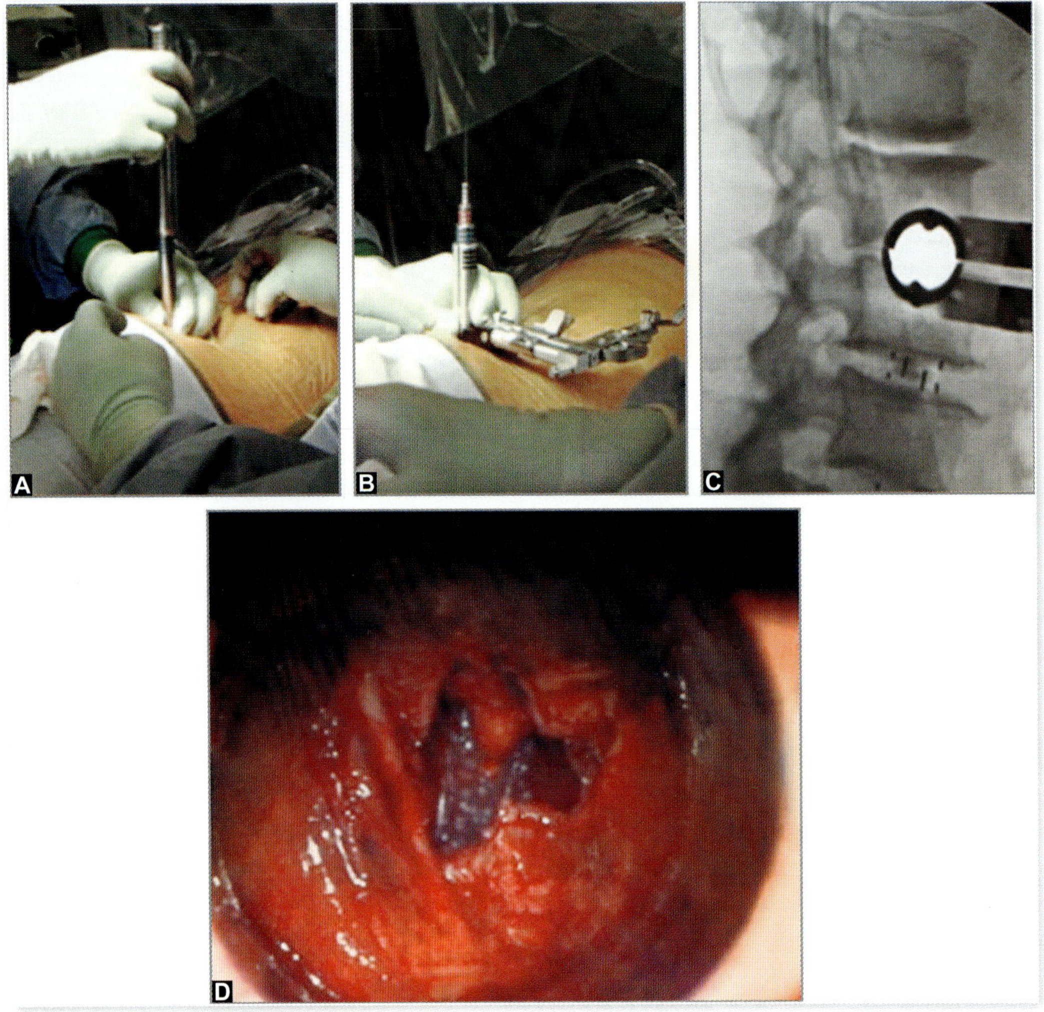

Figures 1A to D: Extreme lateral lumbar interbody fusion. (A and B) Insertion of graded dilatation tubes through the psoas muscle via a lateral retroperitoneal approach; (C) Fluoroscopic confirmation of exposure of the intervertebral disk space; (D) Intraoperative visualization through the tubular retractor system

deficits from compression. Surgical interventions for decompression and stabilization have been associated with improved outcomes.[49] Unfortunately, the burden of medical comorbidities and decreased life expectancy represent major limiting factors in surgical candidacy of patients with metastatic spinal tumors. Minimally invasive approaches with decreased perioperative morbidity are attractive options for these patients as a means to maximize the quality of life remaining. Minimally invasive techniques have been developed for corpectomy and cage reconstruction of the vertebral column **(Figures 2A to D)**. This can be accomplished using a anterior (thoracoscopic), anterolateral (retropleural), posterolateral (extracavitary) or posterior (transpedicular) approaches providing neural decompression and reconstruction.[50] As these techniques continue to develop and surgeons gain greater experience, the indications should continue to expand and reduce the overall morbidity associated with open surgical decompression in patients with spinal metastases and hopefully broaden the range of patients who are considered surgical candidates.

MISS has also demonstrated safety and feasibility for resection of intradural tumors.[51,52] These approaches are associated with limited postoperative spinal column instability.[53,54] Most commonly the tumors removed are extramedullary such as meningiomas and schwannomas but some intramedullary tumors are amenable to minimally invasive resection. As surgeon familiarity with these approaches continue to mature it is likely that more and more intradural spinal tumors will be addressed through minimally invasive means.

Deformity Surgery

Correction of spinal deformity through traditional open surgical approaches often requires long posterior exposures for multisegment instrumented fixation. These long

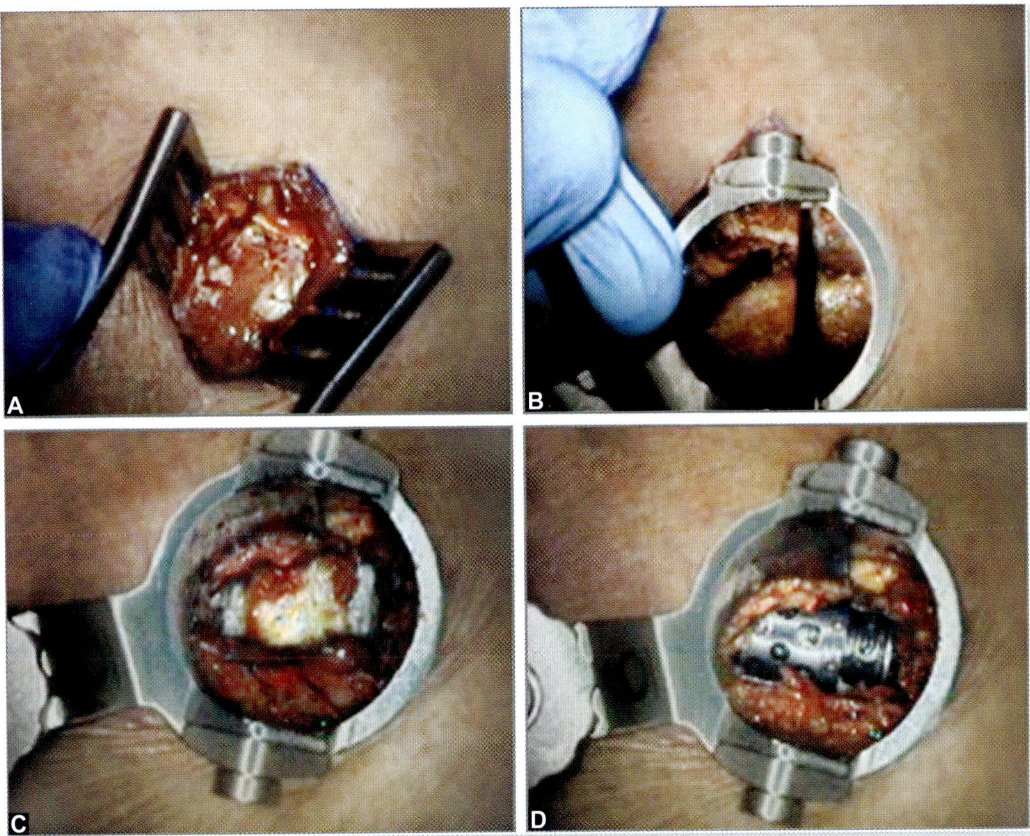

Figures 2A to D: Minimally invasive thoracic corpectomy through a posterolateral approach. (A) Small posterolateral skin incision; (B) dissection through a tubular retractor; (C) visualization of the involved vertebral body; (D) vertebral column cage reconstruction following vertebrectomy

and technically demanding surgeries are associated with substantial perioperative morbidity.[55] Complete minimally invasive treatment of adult spinal deformity has been recently developed and is now well described. This incorporates lateral access techniques for multisegmental interbody fusions allowing for mobilization and correction of the deformity followed by posterior percutaneous pedicle screw instrumentation. Hybrid techniques that incorporate minimally invasive techniques and open oseotomies have also been described for instances where the surgeon feels coronal or sagittal imbalance can not be fully corrected with a complete minimally invasive approach.[56] These techniques have been shown to provide significant improvements in pain and disability with good radiographic correction of the deformity.[57] These techniques hold great promise for minimizing the perioperative complications which has been demonstrated in initial comparisons with open techniques.[58]

CONCLUSION

Over the past 20 years, the filed of spinal surgery has witnessed a remarkable expansion of the scope of indications for MISS. The techniques developed for the treatment of lumbar degenerative pathology have been rapidly adapted for utilization in a broad spectrum of spinal conditions. No longer are minimally invasive approaches regarded as emerging. MISS is now firmly established, and we are now moving in a direction toward universal acceptance. Surgeon's proclivity for innovation has been paced stride for stride with developments in technology. With no reason to suspect that this will change, it is likely that the field of minimally invasive spine surgery will continue to evolve leading to less complications and better outcomes for a myriad of spinal pathologies.

REFERENCES

1. Pool J. DIrect visualization of dorsal nerve roots of the cauda equina by means of a myeloscope. Archives of Neurology & Psychiatry. 1938;39:1308-12.
2. Kawaguchi Y, Matsui H, Tsuji H. Back muscle injury after posterior lumbar spine surgery. A histologic and enzymatic analysis. Spine (Phila Pa 1976) 1996;21:941-4.

3. Huang TJ, Hsu RW, Li YY, et al. Less systemic cytokine response in patients following microendoscopic versus open lumbar diskectomy. J Orthop Res 2005;23:406-11.
4. Stevens KJ, Spenciner DB, Griffiths KL, et al. Comparison of minimally invasive and conventional open posterolateral lumbar fusion using magnetic resonance imaging and retraction pressure studies. J Spinal Disord Tech. 2006;19:77-86.
5. Bresnahan L, Fessler RG, Natarajan RN. Evaluation of change in muscle activity as a result of posterior lumbar spine surgery using a dynamic modeling system. Spine (Phila Pa 1976). 2010; 35:E761-7.
6. Kim DY, Lee SH, Chung SK, et al. Comparison of multifidus muscle atrophy and trunk extension muscle strength: percutaneous versus open pedicle screw fixation. Spine (Phila Pa 1976). 2005;30:123-9.
7. Bresnahan L, Ogden AT, Natarajan RN, et al. A biomechanical evaluation of graded posterior element removal for treatment of lumbar stenosis: comparison of a minimally invasive approach with two standard laminectomy techniques. Spine (Phila Pa 1976). 2009;34:17-23.
8. Asgarzadie F, Khoo LT. Minimally invasive operative management for lumbar spinal stenosis: overview of early and long-term outcomes. Clinics No Am. 2007;38:387-99; abstract vi-vii.
9. Rahman M, Summers LE, Richter B, et al. Comparison of techniques for decompressive lumbar laminectomy: the minimally invasive versus the "classic" open approach. Minim Invasive Neurosurg. 2008;51:100-5.
10. Khoo LT, Fessler RG. Microendoscopic decompressive laminotomy for the treatment of lumbar stenosis. Neurosurgery. 2002;51:S146-54.
11. Fessler RG, Khoo LT. Minimally invasive cervical microendoscopic foraminotomy: an initial clinical experience. Neurosurgery 2002;51:S37-45.
12. Parker SL, Adogwa O, Witham TF, et al. Post-operative infection after minimally invasive versus open transforaminal lumbar interbody fusion (TLIF): literature review and cost analysis. Minim Invasive Neurosurg. 2011;54:33-7.
13. Phan K, Rao PJ, Kam AC, et al. Minimally invasive versus open transforaminal lumbar interbody fusion for treatment of degenerative lumbar disease: systematic review and meta-analysis. European spine journal : official publication of the European Spine Society, the European Spinal Deformity Society, and the European Section of the Cervical Spine Research Society 2015;24:1017-30.
14. Rajaee SS, Bae HW, Kanim LE, et al. Spinal fusion in the United States: analysis of trends from 1998 to 2008. Spine (Phila Pa. 1976) 2012;37:67-76.
15. Witiw CD, Nathan V, Bernstein M. Economics, innovation, and quality improvement in neurosurgery. Neurosurg Clin N Am. 2015;26:197-205, viii.
16. Al-Khouja LT, Baron EM, Johnson JP, et al. Cost-effectiveness analysis in minimally invasive spine surgery. Neurosurgical focus 2014;36:E4.
17. Mansfield HE, Canar WJ, Gerard CS, et al. Single-level anterior cervical diskectomy and fusion versus minimally invasive posterior cervical foraminotomy for patients with cervical radiculopathy: a cost analysis. Neurosurgical Focus. 2014;37:E9.
18. Uddin OM, Haque R, Sugrue PA, et al. Cost minimization in treatment of adult degenerative scoliosis. Neurosurg: Spine. 2005;23(6):798-806.
19. Parker SL, Mendenhall SK, Shau DN, et al. Minimally invasive versus open transforaminal lumbar interbody fusion for degenerative spondylolisthesis: comparative effectiveness and cost-utility analysis. World Neurosurg. 2014;82(1-2):230-8. Epub 2013;Jan 12.
20. Udeh BL, Costandi S, Dalton JE, et al. The 2-year cost-effectiveness of 3 options to treat lumbar spinal stenosis patients. Pain practice. 2015;15:107-16.
21. Smith L. Enzyme dissolution of the nucleus pulposus in humans. JAMA : the journal of the American Medical Association 1964;187:137-40.
22. Hijikata S. Percutaneous nucleotomy. A new concept technique and 12 years' experience. Clinical Orthopaedics and Related Research. 1989:9-23.
23. Choy DS, Case RB, Fielding W, et al. Percutaneous laser nucleolysis of lumbar disks. The New England journal of medicine 1987;317:771-2.
24. Gibson JN, Waddell G. Surgical interventions for lumbar disk prolapse: updated Cochrane Review. Spine (Phila Pa 1976). 2007;32:1735-47.
25. MM FKTS. Microendoscopic diskectomy techniques in Neurosurgery. 1997;3:301-7.
26. Ryang YM, Oertel MF, Mayfrank L, et al. Standard open microdiscectomy versus minimal access trocar microdiscectomy: results of a prospective randomized study. Neurosurgery. 2008;62:174-81; diskussion 81-2.
27. Righesso O, Falavigna A, Avanzi O. Comparison of open diskectomy with microendoscopic diskectomy in lumbar disk herniations: results of a randomized controlled trial. Neurosurgery. 2007;61:545-9; discussion 9.
28. Guiot BH, Khoo LT, Fessler RG. A minimally invasive technique for decompression of the lumbar spine. Spine (Phila Pa 1976). 2002;27:432-8.
29. Foley KT, Smith MM, Rampersaud YR. Microendoscopic approach to far-lateral lumbar disk herniation. Neurosurgical Focus. 1999;7:e5.
30. Sandhu FA, Santiago P, Fessler RG, et al. Minimally invasive surgical treatment of lumbar synovial cysts. Neurosurgery. 2004;54:107-11; discussion 11-2.
31. O'Toole JE, Eichholz KM, Fessler RG. Minimally invasive far lateral microendoscopic diskectomy for extraforaminal disk herniation at the lumbosacral junction: cadaveric dissection and technical case report. The spine journal : official journal of the North American Spine Society. 2007;7:414-21.
32. Obenchain TG, Cloyd D. Laparoscopic lumbar diskectomy: description of transperitoneal and retroperitoneal techniques. Neurosurg Clin N Am 1996;7:77-85.

33. Dezawa A, Yamane T, Mikami H, et al. Retroperitoneal laparoscopic lateral approach to the lumbar spine: a new approach, technique, and clinical trial. J Spinal Disord 2000;13:138-43.
34. Sasani M, Fahir Ozer A, Oktenoglu T, et al. Thoracoscopic surgery for thoracic disk herniation. J Neurosurg Sci. 2011;55:391-5.
35. Leu HF, Hauser RK. Percutaneous endoscopic lumbar spine fusion. Neurosurg Clin N Am. 1996;7:107-17.
36. Foley KT, Gupta SK, Justis JR, et al. Percutaneous pedicle screw fixation of the lumbar spine. Neurosurgical focus. 2001;10:E10.
37. Foley KT, Lefkowitz MA. Advances in minimally invasive spine surgery. Clin Neurosurg. 2002;49:499-517.
38. Foley KT, Holly LT, Schwender JD. Minimally invasive lumbar fusion. Spine (Phila Pa 1976) 2003;28:S26-35.
39. Holly LT, Schwender JD, Rouben DP, et al. Minimally invasive transforaminal lumbar interbody fusion: indications, technique, and complications. Neurosurgical Focus. 2006;20:E6.
40. Khoo LT, Palmer S, Laich DT, et al. Minimally invasive percutaneous posterior lumbar interbody fusion. Neurosurgery. 2002; 51:S166-1.
41. Bourgeois AC, Faulkner AR, Bradley YC, et al. Improved Accuracy of Minimally Invasive Transpedicular Screw Placement in the Lumbar Spine with Three-dimensional Stereotactic Image Guidance: A Comparative Meta-analysis. J Spinal Disord Tech. 2014.
42. Lieberman IH, Willsher PC, Litwin DE, et al. Transperitoneal laparoscopic exposure for lumbar interbody fusion. Spine (Phila Pa 1976). 2000;25:509-14; discussion 15.
43. Zdeblick TA, David SM. A prospective comparison of surgical approach for anterior L4-L5 fusion: laparoscopic versus mini anterior lumbar interbody fusion. Spine (Phila Pa 1976). 2000; 25:2682-7.
44. Ozgur BM, Aryan HE, Pimenta L, et al. Extreme Lateral Interbody Fusion (XLIF): a novel surgical technique for anterior lumbar interbody fusion. The spine journal : official journal of the North American Spine Society 2006;6:435-43.
45. Yue JJ, Sossan A, Selgrath C, et al. The treatment of unstable thoracic spine fractures with transpedicular screw instrumentation: a 3-year consecutive series. Spine (Phila Pa 1976). 2002;27:2782-7.
46. Vanek P, Bradac O, Konopkova R, et al. Treatment of thoracolumbar trauma by short-segment percutaneous transpedicular screw instrumentation: prospective comparative study with a minimum 2-year follow-up. Journal of neurosurgery. Spine. 2014;20:150-6.
47. Scaramuzzo L, Tamburrelli FC, Piervincenzi E, et al. Percutaneous pedicle screw fixation in polytrauma patients. European spine journal : official publication of the European Spine Society, the European Spinal Deformity Society, and the European Section of the Cervical Spine Research Society. 2013;22 Suppl 6:S933-8.
48. Giorgi H, Blondel B, Adetchessi T, et al. Early percutaneous fixation of spinal thoracolumbar fractures in polytrauma patients. Orthop Traumatol Surg Res. 2014;100:449-54.
49. Patchell RA, Tibbs PA, Regine WF, et al. Direct decompressive surgical resection in the treatment of spinal cord compression caused by metastatic cancer: a randomised trial. Lancet. 2005;366:643-8.
50. Lall RR, Smith ZA, Wong AP, et al. Minimally invasive thoracic corpectomy: surgical strategies for malignancy, trauma, and complex spinal pathologies. Minim Invasive Surg. 2012; 2012:213791.
51. Tredway TL, Santiago P, Hrubes MR, et al. Minimally invasive resection of intradural-extramedullary spinal neoplasms. Neurosurgery. 2006;58:ONS52-8; discussion ONS-8.
52. O'Toole JE, Eichholz KM, Fessler RG. Minimally invasive approaches to vertebral column and spinal cord tumors. Neurosurg Clin N Am. 2006;17:491-506.
53. Ogden AT, Bresnahan L, Smith JS, et al. Biomechanical comparison of traditional and minimally invasive intradural tumor exposures using finite element analysis. Clin Biomech (Bristol, Avon) 2009;24:143-7.
54. Xie T, Qian J, Lu Y, et al. Biomechanical comparison of laminectomy, hemilaminectomy and a new minimally invasive approach in the surgical treatment of multilevel cervical intradural tumour: a finite element analysis. European spine journal : official publication of the European Spine Society, the European Spinal Deformity Society, and the European Section of the Cervical Spine Research Society. 2013;22:2719-30.
55. Baron EM, Albert TJ. Medical complications of surgical treatment of adult spinal deformity and how to avoid them. Spine (Phila Pa 1976). 2006;31:S106-18.
56. Park P, La Marca F. Combined "hybrid" open and minimally invasive surgical correction of adult thoracolumbar scoliosis: a retrospective cohort study. Neurosurgery. 2013;72:151-8; discussion 8-9.
57. Park P, Wang MY, Lafage V, et al. Comparison of two minimally invasive surgery strategies to treat adult spinal deformity. Journal of neurosurgery. Spine. 2015;22:374-80.
58. Uribe JS, Deukmedjian AR, Mummaneni PV, et al. Complications in adult spinal deformity surgery: an analysis of minimally invasive, hybrid, and open surgical techniques. Neurosurgical focus. 2014;36:E15.

2

CHAPTER

Development of Minimally Invasive Spine Surgery

Laura A Snyder, John E O'Toole, Kurt M Eichholz, Mick J Perez-Cruet, Richard G Fessler

ABSTRACT

The modern era of minimally invasive spine surgery has its roots in percutaneous techniques developed in the mid-twentieth century. However, the widespread application of minimally invasive techniques seen today is predicated upon technological developments of only the last 10 years. This chapter reviews the development of minimally invasive spinal surgery as it has evolved for the cervical, thoracic, and lumbar spine. Each new development has sought to equal or improve upon the effectiveness demonstrated by comparable open surgical techniques while reducing iatrogenic tissue trauma and resultant postoperative pain and disability to produce overall better outcomes for patients.

INTRODUCTION

Minimally invasive spinal surgery is one of the recent developments in the long history of our intellectual and technological evolution in understanding and treating spinal disease. The earliest appreciations of spine pathology were found in Egyptian mummies dated 2900 BC and further elucidated in the Edwin Smith papyrus written circa 1550 BC. In fact, the first description of the spinal column was offered by the Egyptians in the djed symbol used for the god Osiris to represent stability, duration, and durability.[1] Hippocrates has been credited as the father of spine surgery, as evidenced by his seminal teachings and writings, underlined by his principles of sound reasoning and accurate observation.[2] However, the first concrete delineation of operative treatment of the spinal column was proposed by Paulus of Aegina in the seventh century.[3] He advocated and conducted direct removal of osseous tissue at the site of pathology. Since then, various approaches and techniques for operative treatment of the spine have been developed and evolved to address numerous conditions. In this chapter, we will review the evolution of minimally invasive techniques in the spine. Although the developments of specific techniques applicable to the cervical, thoracic, or lumbar spine often developed simultaneously and frequently were interdependent, a spinal "level" approach has been adopted in this chapter to enhance readability. Although this artificially imposes an apparent anatomic "logic" to development of minimally invasive spinal surgery (which, in fact, did not exist) it does highlight the importance of specific innovations to our surgical techniques within each individual region.

Cervical Spine

Endoscopic-assisted Transoral Surgery

Fang and Ong[4] published the first series of patient to undergo transoral decompression for irreducible atlantoaxial abnormalities in 1962. However, undue morbidity and mortality led to limited acceptance of this approach. Subsequent advancements in imaging techniques and the availability of the operative microscope have significantly improved procedural safety and efficacy. Pathology approached via this technique, however, may require extended exposures including palatal resection, mandibular splitting, or maxillotomy for decompression of clival abnormalities. These result in increased surgical time and complexity, prolonged recovery, and increased patient morbidity.[5] One of the disadvantages of using the microscope is that the lens is located at some distance from the working field, and in transoral surgery, the view is limited by the narrow dimensions of the oral cavity. Frempong-Boadu et al.[5] demonstrated the efficacy of endoscopic-assisted transoral surgery in limiting these extended approaches in a series of seven patients. With the endoscope, the optics and illumination are within the surgical field immediately adjacent to the pathological target. Thus bypassing the limiting walls of the oral cavity, one can visualize even clival abnormalities, without the extended exposures otherwise necessary.[5]

Cervical Microendoscopic Laminectomy/Discectomy

Scoville and Whitcomb[6] introduced the concept of posterior cervical disk surgery. Although the anterior approach to the cervical spine has become more popular, the posterior approach is an effective procedure in selected cases of laterally herniated disk fragments, isolated foraminal narrowing, multilevel foraminal narrowing without central stenosis, continued root symptoms after anterior cervical discectomy and fusion, and cases in which anterior approaches are contraindicated. However, it is usually necessary to use moderately-sized incisions and significant paraspinous muscle dissection in these operations. Postoperative wound pain and muscle spasms can therefore be significant, and postoperative recovery is often relatively slow.

The microendoscopic discectomy (MED) system was developed to minimize the tissue trauma and postoperative discomfort seen with open procedures (see lumbar microendoscopic discectomy below). It provides equally good exposure of the involved segment compared to an open microdiscectomy. In cadaveric studies, Roh et al.[7] performed posterior cervical foraminotomies using either the MED system or conventional open technique. Their results demonstrated that nerve root decompression and percentage of facet removed using the MED technique were equal to or greater than that achieved with open technique. The transmuscular dilation with an endoscopic tubular working channel can minimize postsurgical pain and provide rapid postoperative recovery. Excellent results in early clinical series were reported by Adamson[8] and Fessler and Khoo.[9] Minimally invasive application of posterior cervical instrumentation was first described by Wang et al.[10] and remains in current development.

Thoracic Spine

Thoracoscopic Spine Surgery

Jacobaeus, a professor of internal medicine in Stockholm, Sweden, is credited with performing the first thoracoscopic procedure in 1910.[11] As an internist, he was involved in the diagnosis and treatment of pulmonary tuberculosis, and he thought that the ability to observe the pleural space was crucial. After his initial diagnostic procedure, Jacobaeus described the technique of lysis of tuberculous pleural adhesions, which was performed with a cystoscope and a heated platinum loop.[12] In 1990, with the introduction of video imaging to standard endoscopy, the modern era of thoracoscopy began. Mack et al.[13] in the United States and Rosenthal et al[14] in Europe first reported the technique of video-assisted thoracoscopic surgery (VATS) in 1993 and 1994. Thoracoscopic spine procedures were initially implemented for disk herniations, sympathectomies, pathologies of the vertebral body, abscess drainage, and tumor biopsies. In the ensuing years, it has been implemented for scoliosis correction, anterior interbody fusion, osteotomies and bone grafting, corpectomies, and vertebral instrumentation in the treatment of tumors and fractures.

Posterior/Posterolateral Endoscopic Diskectomy

In a further attempt to reduce tissue trauma and enhance postoperative outcome, a thoracic microendoscopic diskectomy approach has been developed to treat thoracic disk herniations from a direct posterior or posterolateral endoscopic approach. Jho[15] described the technique of endoscopic transpedicular thoracic diskectomy with 0- and 70-degree 4 mm endoscopes, requiring relatively small 1.5 to 2 mm incisions and minimal tissue dissection. This approach avoids the need for separate skin incisions in the chest wall (required for thoracoscopic approaches) and the need for postoperative chest drainage. Chiu and Clifford[16] demonstrated the safety and efficacy of posterolateral endoscopic thoracic discectomy followed by low-energy nonablative laser for shrinkage and tightening of the disk (laser thermodiskoplasty) using a 4 mm 0-degree endoscope. Thoracic discectomy using the METRx system (Medtronic Sofamor Danek, Memphis, TN) has been described by Isaacs et al.[17] in cadavers and clinically by Perez-Cruet et al.[18] More recently, thoracic corpectomy and reconstruction using minimally invasive technique has also been developed in cadavers and used clinically for trauma and tumor (see chapter by O'Toole et al. "Minimally Invasive Approaches to Vertebral Column and Spinal Cord Tumors," in this volume). Recently, minimally invasive techniques have also been utilized to remove intradural, extramedullary tumors at all levels of the spine.[9]

Lumbar Spine

Chemonucleolysis

In 1941, Jansen and Balls[20] first isolated chymopapain, a proteolytic enzyme extracted from papaya latex. In 1956, Thomas[21] administered intravenous injections of crude papain to rabbits and noticed that their ears drooped. Intrigued by Thomas' article, Lyman Smith postulated the therapeutic use of papain to treat chondroblastic tumors. In 1963, Smith et al[22] were the first to inject chymopapain into a herniated nucleus pulposus for the treatment of sciatica. This process, aptly called chemonucleolysis, alters the characteristics of the nucleus pulposus by liberation of chondroitin sulfate and keratin sulfate through hydrolysis of noncollagenous mucopolysaccharide proteins leading ultimately to polymerization of the nucleus pulposus. Nordby and Javid[23] published the results of a 14-year study of 3000 patients treated with chemonucleolysis, with an 82% success rate for the first 1000 patients and an overall success rate of 87.2%.

Percutaneous Arthroscopic Discectomy

Ottolenghi[24] in Argentina in 1955 and Craig[25] in 1956 described posterolateral biopsy of the spine. In 1975, Hijikata et al.[26] demonstrated a percutaneous nucleotomy by utilizing intradiscal arthroscopic techniques for disk removal in the treatment of posterior or posterolateral lumbar disk herniations under local anesthesia. After discography using Evans blue dye, specifically designed instruments were placed in a 5 mm cannula and inserted against the lateral annulus. A circular incision was made in the annulus, and the blue-stained nucleus pulposus was removed with pituitary forceps. Refinements to the technique involved the use of an automated system.

In 1983, Kambin and Gellman[27] performed a discectomy by inserting a Craig cannula and a small forceps into the disk space after an open laminectomy to evacuate the nucleus pulposus and observed the effects on the surrounding anatomic features. In 1985, Onik et al.[28] reported the development of a 2 mm blunt-tipped suction-cutting probe for automated percutaneous diskectomy at L4–L5 or higher levels. Their reported outcomes indicate an overall success rate of 75%, with a complication rate of 1%.

Subsequent developments led to the design of a 2.7 mm glass arthroscope combined with a videodiscoscope with a single working portal.[29] This development enabled observation of periannular structures, including the foramen and the spinal nerve. Arthroscopic disk surgery allows removal of herniated disks via a posterolateral approach. This is accomplished with biportal access via triangulation into the intravertebral disk with inline irrigation and suction.[29]

Numerous studies on the efficacy of arthroscopic disc surgery have been published. Kambin and colleagues[27,30] reported an 88% excellent or good outcome rate with arthroscopic microdiscectomy, and others have reported similar success. In a prospective randomized study evaluating the efficacy of microscopic disk surgery compared with endoscopic disk extraction, Mayer and Brock[31] achieved favorable outcomes with minimal complications using the percutaneous arthroscopic technique.

Percutaneous Laser Discectomy

Ascher and Heppner[32] were the first to use the technique of percutaneous laser discectomy to treat lumbar disk disease. Their technique involved measuring the intradiscal pressure before and after laser discectomy using a saline manometer. They postulated that the removal of even a small volume of tissue from the disk caused a corresponding decrease in intradiscal pressure.[33]

The results of percutaneous laser disk decompression in cases involving back and leg pain with disk protrusions are still unclear. No controlled prospective studies have been performed to evaluate the results of percutaneous laser discectomy. The largest experience in the literature was reported by Choy et al.[34] They reported an 87.4% excellent result rate in a study of 333 patients, with a mean follow-up of 26 months. Early experience with the KTP/532 laser device was reported by Davis,[35] who achieved an 85% success rate. Yeung[36] reported good to excellent results in 86.4% with the KTP/532 device.

Percutaneous Intradiscal Radiofrequency Thermocoagulation

Intradiscal electrical thermocoagulation (IDET) has been used to treat primary discogenic back pain. This therapeutic innovation is specifically designed to treat pain derived from internal disk disruption and annular tears. In 2000, Saal and Saal[37] reported on 62 patients with low back pain treated with IDET and showed that 71% of patients experienced a mean improvement of 3 points in their VAS back pain score.

Spinal Endoscopy

In 1931, Burman[38] introduced the concept of myeloscopy for direct spinal cord observation. In 1934, Mixter and Barr[39] reported an open hemilaminectomy with intraoperative discotomy for treatment of intervertebral disk rupture into the spinal canal. In 1938, Pool[40] expanded on Burman's work and reported myeloscopic inspection of the dorsal nerve roots of the cauda equina. In 1942, Pool[41] introduced the concept of intrathecal endoscopy and reported the results of more than 400 myeloscopic procedures.

Myeloscopy fell out of favor for a time because of the morbidity associated with insertion of a large-bore scope into the dural cavity. The state of spinal endoscopy remained essentially the same until Ooi et al.[42] used an endoscope to examine the intrathecal space before surgery. Using improved technology, Ooi et al.[43] were able to describe pathological features in greater detail, including chronic arachnoiditis and nerve root excursion during claudication associated with lumbar spinal stenosis.

Lumbar Microendoscopic Discectomy

Microscopic lumbar disk resection through a tubular retractor was first reported by Faubert and Caspar.[44] Friedman described a similar procedure using a large bore chest tube.[45] Utilizing advances in endoscopic technology, microendoscopic discectomy (MED) through tubular retraction was first reported by Foley and Smith.[46]

MED combines standard lumbar microsurgical techniques with endoscopy, enabling surgeons to successfully address free-fragment disc herniations as well as lateral recess stenosis. The endoscopic approach allows smaller incisions and less tissue trauma compared with standard open microdiscectomy. Routine outpatient application reduces hospital stays and costs.

Muramatsu et al.[47] reported on a series of 70 patients who underwent MED and 15 patients for whom Love's method was used to treat lumbar disk disease. MED resulted in less blood loss (mean 12.1 mL) than Love's method (mean 59.1 mL); analgesics (suppositories) were required by 52.0% of the MED-treated patients after surgery, whereas all of the patients treated with Love's procedure required analgesics; and MED reduced the mean number of days before the patients became ambulatory (MED, 1.0 day; Love's method, 4.9 days).

Guiot et al.[48] demonstrated the technical feasibility of percutaneous microendoscopic bilateral decompression of lumbar stenosis via a unilateral approach in a human cadaveric study, and successful clinical application of this technique has been reported by Khoo and Fessler.[49] MED technique has also been applied in treating far lateral disc herniation,[50] synovial cysts,[51] and recurrent disk herniations.[52]

Endoscopic Pedicle Screw Fixation of Lumbar Spine

The video-assisted posterolateral approach was developed by Boden and associates.[53] Posterior keyhole approaches for endoscopic placement of pedicle screws has been performed using multiple portals or a single portal between the two pedicles.

Muller et al.[54] described the use of multiple portals in a cadaveric study to identify bony landmarks and to test the feasibility of performing endoscopic pedicle screw fixation. These investigators performed a transmuscular insertion of a pedicle screw-rod fixation device using a rigid operating sheath. The sheath (Thoracoport, AutoSuture Co., Norwalk, CT) measured 1.5 cm in diameter and 5 cm in length, and was used with a disposable trocar system consisting of a blunt-tipped obturator, a threaded sleeve, and a shroud to secure the system. The surgical field was illuminated by an endoscope (Hopkins 11, Karl Storz GmbH & Co., Tuttlingen, Germany) with a diameter of 4 mm, a length of 18 cm, and angles of 0, 30, and 70 degrees. The Diapason pedicle probe (Stryker Instruments, Kalamazoo, MI) with a blunt tip was used to discover whether the pedicle walls were intact. The system has pedicle screws that have a U-shaped screw head.[54] The connecting rods are fixed in the screw heads via a ball-ring interface and are locked with locking screws. The pedicle screws are placed using an inclinometer, which provides the surgeon with instant feedback during screw placement.

MacMillan et al.[55] described a fluoroscopically-directed, "arc" based percutaneous trans-sacral fusion of L5-S1 in which transgluteal dilators were used to reach the iliac wings adjacent to the ala. Drilling through the iliac wing at the ala then provided access to the L5-S1 disk and L5 vertebral body.

Percutaneous posterior fusion and instrumentation using a mechanically directed rod system was described by Foley and Gupta.[56] Minimally invasive transforaminal lumbar interbody fusion with percutaneous posterior instrumentation was described by Khoo et al.[57]

Laparoscopic Lumbar Spine Surgery

The modern era of laparoscopy began in the 1980s when Kurt Semm performed the first appendectomy in Germany.[58] Semm, a physician and an engineer, developed many tools that are still in use. The first human laparoscopic cholecystectomy was performed in 1987 by DuBois et al.[59] With the advantages of laparoscopic exposure being championed by urological, gynecological, and general surgeons, it is natural that spine surgeons would consider extending these technologies to the anterior lumbar spine. The advantages of transperitoneal laparoscopic spinal surgery include improved observation of surgical anatomic features, marked reductions in postoperative pain, early hospital discharges, and reduced incidence of postoperative ileus. In 1991, Obenchain[60] reported the first use of a laparoscopic approach to the lumbar spine for a discectomy (Fig. 1.12). Regan et al[61] described the technique and reported preliminary results for laparoscopic anterior lumbar fusion.

Gaur[62] was the first to describe an endoscopic retroperitoneal approach for urological procedures, which was later applied to fusion of the lumbar spine by McAfee et al.[63]

ADDITIONAL MINIMALLY INVASIVE DEVELOPMENTS

Application of Image-guidance Systems in the Spine

Image-guidance systems are widely used in intracranial surgery and have been adapted to assist with screw placement since the mid-1990s. The use of image-guidance systems for pedicle screw placement has improved overall accuracy. These systems typically rely upon precise localization of the bony anatomy with preoperative computed tomography (CT). In this way, the transverse width, longitudinal depth, and trajectory angle can be easily measured (Fig. 1.13) on a computer-assisted work station.

Nolte et al.[64] described the principles of computer-assisted pedicle screw fixation. The overall accuracy of their system was 1.74 mm, using CT scans with 2 mm slice increments. Intraoperative surgical exposure of the posterior vertebral elements was performed using standard surgical techniques. An infrared camera (Optotrak; Northern Digital, Waterloo, Ontario, Canada) tracked specific instruments (i.e., pedicle probe, awl, and space pointer) equipped with light-emitting diodes. The dynamic reference was fixed to the spinous process of the vertebra to be instrumented. Normal bony landmarks and their correlations with the images confirmed the calibration accuracy. Using that computerized system, they reported a pedicle screw misplacement rate of 4.3% under clinical conditions.

Choi et al.[65] reported the use of computer-assisted fluoroscopic targeting for pedicle screw fixation. They described a system in which the pedicle entry site and the depth of insertion were determined by intraoperative anteroposterior and lateral fluoroscopic scans. Those authors compared the accuracy of placement with the fluoroscopy-guided system versus the CT-guided system and observed no significant differences.

Vertebroplasty

The spine is composed of a rich trabecular lattice of cancellous bone encased in a hard cortical shell. Moreover, the spine is exposed to degrees of compressive loads and tensile stresses that are in symbiotic biomechanical play with the inner and outer matrices of the vertebral bodies. Osteoporotic bone loss or neoplastic invasion of the vertebral bodies results in erosion of the cancellous network and development of vertebral compression fractures (VCFs), which can contribute to debilitating pain, neurological deficit, gross spinal instability, and resultant deformity. Surgical management involves considerable risk because of the high prevalence of significant comorbidities in these patients. Surgical decompression and reconstruction involves internal fixation using screws, plates, wires, cages, or rods and requires extensive surgical exposure. The time required for recuperation from open fixation procedures can be lengthy. Obtaining satisfactory fixation in osteoporotic bone can be technically difficult, and the failure rate for spinal arthrodesis is significant.

In an attempt to reduce such invasive operative treatment, percutaneous vertebroplasty (PVP) was developed in 1984 by Galibert and Deramond[66] in France as a minimally invasive outpatient procedure to offer immediate pain relief by the injection of polymethylmethacrylate (PMMA) bone cement into the vertebral body through a transpedicular approach. Although rapidly popularized in Europe, PVP was not adopted in the United States until 1994.[67]

Kyphoplasty

In an effort to reduce the high incidence of cement extravasation and detrimental sequelae such as infection, cement toxicity, and adjacent fracture development due to altered sagittal balance, kyphoplasty was developed in the mid-1990s by Dr Mark Reiley.[68] Kyphoplasty implements inflatable bone tamps inserted via a bilateral percutaneous transpedicular approach. Balloon inflation ultimately both decreases intravertebral pressure by creating a cavity which is filled with PMMA and also distracts the vertebral endplates to restore vertebral height.[69]

CONCLUSION

Minimally invasive spine surgery has evolved rapidly over the last decade. However, its basis lies in ideas and techniques that date back much longer than that, in some cases nearly 100 years. Recent advances in areas such as optics, miniaturizations, arc-based guides (Sextant), fluoroscopic visualization, and image guidance have provided the technology necessary to enable rapid creation and evolution of surgical techniques. Fluoroscopy and the isolation of chymopapain first enabled the approach to the lumbar disk through minimal incisions and percutaneous passage through the spinal musculature. However, the inability to directly visualize the operative field and early complications from the enzyme limited widespread use of this procedure. Improvements in endoscopic optic technologies then enabled more direct manipulation of the disk. Nevertheless, small uniportal access limited both visual acuity and the working size of instruments.

Simultaneously, however, these improved endoscopic optics were applied to "thoracoscopic" and "laparoscopic" spinal techniques. Combined with modifications of surgical instruments and anesthetic technique, it became obvious that much larger spinal surgical procedures could be performed through minimally invasive technique than had previously been imagined. However, the technical difficulties of these procedures limited their widespread adoption.

Combining the "tubular dilator" approach with an endoscope (and later a microscope) switched the minimally invasive focus back to the posterior spine, and thus provided the technology needed to rapidly develop minimally invasive techniques for most spinal pathologies within a surgical field of view familiar to most spinal surgeons. The most common applications of these techniques are now being widely adopted. It is anticipated that with continued improvements in optics, image guidance, neuromonitoring, and biological and/or genetic therapies, most spinal surgery will ultimately be performed using minimally invasive technique.

REFERENCES

1. Lang JK, Kolenda H. First appearance and sense of the term "spinal column" in ancient Egypt. Historical vignette. J Neurosurg. 2002;97(1 Suppl):152-155.
2. Marketos SG, Skiadas P. Hippocrates. The father of spine surgery. Spine. 1999;24(13):1381-7.
3. Knoeller SM, Seifried C. Historical perspective: history of spinal surgery. Spine. 2000;25(21):2838-43.
4. Fang HSY, Ong GB. Direct anterior approach to the upper cervical spine. J Bone Joint Surg Am. 1962;44A:1588-1604.
5. Frempong-Boadu AK, Faunce WA, Fessler RG. Endoscopically assisted transoral-transpharyngeal approach to the craniovertebral junction. Neurosurgery. 2002;51(5 Suppl): S60-66.
6. Scoville WB, Whitcomb BB. Lateral rupture of cervical intervertebral disks. Postgrad Med. 1966;39(2):174-80.
7. Roh SW, Kim DH, Cardoso AC, Fessler RG. Endoscopic foraminotomy using MED system in cadaveric specimens. Spine. 2000;25(2):260-4.
8. Adamson TE. Microendoscopic posterior cervical laminoforaminotomy for unilateral radiculopathy: results of a new technique in 100 cases. J Neurosurg. 2001;95(1 Suppl):51-7.
9. Fessler RG, Khoo LT. Minimally invasive cervical microendoscopic foraminotomy: an initial clinical experience. Neurosurgery. 2002;51(5 Suppl):S37-45.
10. Wang MY, Prusmack CJ, Green BA, Gruen JP, Levi AD. Minimally invasive lateral mass screws in the treatment of cervical facet dislocations: technical note. Neurosurgery. 2003;52(2):444-7; discussion 447-8.
11. Jacobeus HC. Possibility of the use of the cystoscope for investigation of serous cavities. Munch Med Wochenschr. 1910;57:2090-2.
12. Jacobeus HC. The practical importance of thoracoscopy in surgery of the chest. Surg Gynecol Obstet. 1921;32:493-500.
13. Mack MJ, Regan JJ, Bobechko WP, Acuff TE. Application of thoracoscopy for diseases of the spine. Ann Thorac Surg. 1993;56(3):736-738.
14. Rosenthal D, Rosenthal R, de Simone A. Removal of a protruded thoracic disc using microsurgical endoscopy. A new technique. Spine. 1994;19(9):1087-91.
15. Jho HD. Endoscopic microscopic transpedicular thoracic discectomy. Technical note. J Neurosurg. 1997;87(1):125-9.
16. Chiu J, Clifford T. Microdecompressive percutaneous discectomy: spinal discectomy with new laser thermodiskoplasty for nonextruded herniated nucleus pulposus. Surg Technol Int. 1999;8:343-51.
17. Isaacs RE, Podichetty VK, Sandhu FA, et al. Thoracic microendoscopic discectomy: a human cadaver study. Spine. 2005;30(10):1226-31.
18. Perez-Cruet MJ, Kim BS, Sandhu F, Samartzis D, Fessler RG. Thoracic microendoscopic discectomy. J Neurosurg Spine. 2004;1(1):58-63.
19. Tredway TL, Santiago P, Hrubes MR, Song JK, Christie SD, Fessler RG. Minimally invasive resection of intradural-extramedullary spinal neoplasms. Neurosurgery. 2006;58(1 Suppl):ONS52-58; discussion ONS52-58.
20. Jansen EF, Balls AK. Chymopapain: a new crystalline proteinase from papaya latex. J Biol Chem. 1941;137:459-60.
21. Thomas L. Reversible collapse of rabbit ears after intravenous papain, and prevention of recovery by cortisone. J Exp Med. 1956;104(2):245-52.
22. Smith L, Garvin PJ, Gesler RM, Jennings RB. Enzyme dissolution of the nucleus pulposus. Nature. 1963;198:1311-2.
23. Nordby EJ, Javid MJ. Continuing experience with chemonucleolysis. Mt Sinai J Med. 2000;67(4):311-3.
24. Ottolenghi CE. Diagnosis of orthopaedic lesions by aspiration biopsy; results of 1,061 punctures. J Bone Joint Surg Am. 1955; 37-A(3):443-64.
25. Craig FS. Vertebral-body biopsy. J Bone Joint Surg Am. 1956;38-A(1):93-102.
26. Hijikata S, Yamagishi M, Nakayama T, Oomori K. Percutaneous diskectomy: a new treatment method for lumbar disc herniation. J Toden Hosp. 1975;39:5-13.
27. Kambin P, Gellman H. Percutaneous lateral discectomy of the lumbar spine: a preliminary report. Clin Orthop. 1983;174:1 27-32.
28. Onik G, Helms CA, Ginsburg L, Hoaglund FT, Morris J. Percutaneous lumbar diskectomy using a new aspiration probe. AJR Am J Roentgenol. 1985;144(6):1137-40.
29. Kambin P. Arthroscopic microdiscectomy. Arthroscopy. 1992;8(3):287-95.
30. Kambin P, Sampson S. Posterolateral percutaneous suction-excision of herniated lumbar intervertebral discs. Report of interim results. Clin Orthop Relat Res. 1986(207):37-43.
31. Mayer HM, Brock M. Percutaneous endoscopic discectomy: surgical technique and preliminary results compared to microsurgical discectomy. J Neurosurg. 1993;78(2):216-25.
32. Ascher PW, Heppner F. CO2-Laser in neurosurgery. Neurosurg Rev. 1984;7(2-3):123-33.
33. Ascher PW. Status quo and new horizons of laser therapy in neurosurgery. Lasers Surg Med. 1985;5(5):499-506.
34. Choy DS, Ascher PW, Ranu HS, et al. Percutaneous laser disc decompression. A new therapeutic modality. Spine. 1992;17(8):949-56.
35. Davis JK. Early experience with laser disc decompression: a percutaneous method. J Fla Med Assoc. 1992;79:37-9.
36. Yeung AT. The evolution of percutaneous spinal endoscopy and discectomy: state of the art. Mt Sinai J Med. 2000;67(4):327-32.

37. Saal JA, Saal JS. Intradiscal electrothermal treatment for chronic discogenic low back pain: a prospective outcome study with minimum 1-year follow-up. Spine. 2000;25(20):2622-7.
38. Burman MS. Myeloscopy or the direct visualization of the spinal cord and its contents. J Bone Joint Surg. 1931;13:695-6.
39. Mixter WJ, Barr JS. Rupture of intervertebral disc with involvement of spinal cord. N Engl J Med. 1934;211:210-15.
40. Pool JL. Direct visualization of dorsal nerve roots of the cauda equina by means of a myeloscope. Arch Neurol Psychiatr. 1938;39:1308-12.
41. Pool JL. Myeloscopy: intraspinal endoscopy. Surgery. 1942;11:169-82.
42. Ooi Y, Sato Y, Morisaki N. Myeloscopy: the possibility of observing the lumbar intrathecal space by use of an endoscope. Endoscopy. 1973;5:901-6.
43. Ooi Y, Sato Y, Mikanagi K, Morisaki N. [Myeloscopy]. No To Shinkei. 1977;29(5):569-74.
44. Faubert C, Caspar W. Lumbar percutaneous discectomy. Initial experience in 28 cases. Neuroradiology. 1991;33(5):407-10.
45. Friedman WA. Percutaneous discectomy: an alternative to chemonucleolysis? Neurosurgery. 1983;13(5):542-7.
46. Foley KT, Smith MM. Microendoscopic discectomy. Tech Neurosurg. 1997;3:301-7.
47. Muramatsu K, Hachiya Y, Morita C. Postoperative magnetic resonance imaging of lumbar disc herniation: comparison of microendoscopic discectomy and Love's method. Spine. 2001;26(14):1599-1605.
48. Guiot BH, Khoo LT, Fessler RG. A minimally invasive technique for decompression of the lumbar spine. Spine. 2002;27(4):432-8.
49. Khoo LT, Fessler RG. Microendoscopic decompressive laminotomy for the treatment of lumbar stenosis. Neurosurgery. 2002;51(5 Suppl):S146-54.
50. Cervellini P, De Luca GP, Mazzetto M, Colombo F. Micro-endoscopic-discectomy (MED) for far lateral disc herniation in the lumbar spine. Technical note. Acta Neurochir Suppl. 2005;92:99-101.
51. Sandhu FA, Santiago P, Fessler RG, Palmer S. Minimally invasive surgical treatment of lumbar synovial cysts. Neurosurgery. 2004;54(1):107-111; discussion 111-102.
52. Le H, Sandhu FA, Fessler RG. Clinical outcomes after minimal-access surgery for recurrent lumbar disc herniation. Neurosurg Focus. 2003;15(3):E12.
53. Boden SD, Moskovitz PA, Morone MA, Toribitake Y. Video-assisted lateral intertransverse process arthrodesis. Validation of a new minimally invasive lumbar spinal fusion technique in the rabbit and nonhuman primate (rhesus) models. Spine. 1996;21(22):2689-97.
54. Muller A, Gall C, Marz U, Reulen HJ. A keyhole approach for endoscopically assisted pedicle screw fixation in lumbar spine instability. Neurosurgery. 2000;47(1):85-95; discussion 95-86.
55. MacMillan M, Fessler RG, Gillespy M, Montgomery WJ. Percutaneous lumbosacral fixation and fusion: anatomic study and two-year experience with a new method. Neurosurg Clin N Am. 1996;7(1):99-106.
56. Foley KT, Gupta SK. Percutaneous pedicle screw fixation of the lumbar spine: preliminary clinical results. J Neurosurg. 2002;97(1 Suppl):7-12.
57. Khoo LT, Palmer S, Laich DT, Fessler RG. Minimally invasive percutaneous posterior lumbar interbody fusion. Neurosurgery. 2002;51(5 Suppl):S166-161.
58. Semm K. Endoscopic appendectomy. Endoscopy. 1983;15(2):59-64.
59. Dubois F, Icard P, Berthelot G, Levard H. Coelioscopic cholecystectomy. Preliminary report of 36 cases. Ann Surg. 1990;211(1):60-2.
60. Obenchain TG. Laparoscopic lumbar discectomy: case report. J Laparoendosc Surg. 1991;1(3):145-9.
61. Regan JJ, McAfee PC, Guyer RD, Aronoff RJ. Laparoscopic fusion of the lumbar spine in a multicenter series of the first 34 consecutive patients. Surg Laparosc Endosc. 1996;6(6):459-68.
62. Gaur DD. Laparoscopic operative retroperitoneoscopy: use of a new device. J Urol. 1992;148(4):1137-9.
63. McAfee PC, Regan JJ, Geis WP, Fedder IL. Minimally invasive anterior retroperitoneal approach to the lumbar spine. Emphasis on the lateral BAK. Spine. 1998;23(13):1476-84.
64. Nolte LP, Zamorano LJ, Jiang Z, Wang Q, Langlotz F, Berlemann U. Image-guided insertion of transpedicular screws. A laboratory set-up. Spine. 1995;20(4):497-500.
65. Choi WW, Green BA, Levi AD. Computer-assisted fluoroscopic targeting system for pedicle screw insertion. Neurosurgery. 2000;47(4):872-8.
66. Galibert P, Deramond H. [Percutaneous acrylic vertebroplasty as a treatment of vertebral angioma as well as painful and debilitating diseases]. Chirurgie. 1990;116(3):326-34; discussion 335.
67. Barr JD, Barr MS, Lemley TJ, McCann RM. Percutaneous vertebroplasty for pain relief and spinal stabilization. Spine. 2000;25(8):923-8.
68. Garfin SR, Yuan HA, Reiley MA. New technologies in spine: kyphoplasty and vertebroplasty for the treatment of painful osteoporotic compression fractures. Spine. 2001;26(14):1511-5.
69. Dudeney S, Lieberman IH, Reinhardt MK, Hussein M. Kyphoplasty in the treatment of osteolytic vertebral compression fractures as a result of multiple myeloma. J Clin Oncol. 2002;20(9):2382-7.

CHAPTER

Concept of Tubes in Minimally Invasive Spine Surgeries

Arvind G Kulkarni, Abhilash Dhruv

ABSTRACT

The concept of minimally invasive spine techniques in the field of spine surgery has revolutionized the basic approach in handling spine pathologies. The use of Tubular Retractors in the last decade in India has given new dimensions for an effective and value based spine care. Initially, it was used for simpler procedures like diskectomy, till recently it is also used for canal stenosis, tumor, trauma and deformity corrective surgeries. This chapter focuses on the evolution of tubes in India and gives an overview of its Indications and uses.

INTRODUCTION

A basic tenet of surgery is to effectively treat pathology leaving "the smallest footprint." This is accomplished by designing procedures that require smaller incisions, resulting in less soft-tissue disruption, and involving limited surgical corridors. The development of these procedures has been implemented through technological advances in illumination, magnification, and instrumentation.

Tubular access to the lumbar disk was first reported by Faubert and Caspart in 1991 and this led to the way for development of tubular retractor systems and low profile instruments. The first report of the microendoscopic discectomy (MED) procedure came from Foley and Smith in 1997. The initial system utilized an endoscope, so was quickly adapted by the orthopedic surgeons due to their familiarity with arthroscopes. With the adaptation of the microscope to the use of tubular retractors in 2003, the METRx system (Medtronic, Inc.), more neurosurgeons implemented these techniques.

This chapter focuses on "tubular retractor", the work-horse of MISS. Many Tubular retractor systems are available in the market, but the basis of all systems is the same. The system consists of a series of concentric dilators and thin-walled tubular retractors of variable length. The spine is accessed via serial dilation of the cleavage plane between the muscle fascicles. The tubular retractors create a temporary, collapsible channel to gain access to the pathology, while leaving the the midline supporting musculoligamentous structures intact.

Due to familiarity with the instrumentation, we shall describe the METRx system.

METRX SYSTEM

The system consists of a series of metal dilators, a flexible arm assembly, the final tube and the source of illumination and magnification (endoscope or a microscope).

The metallic dilators range from 5.3 mm diameter (the first dilator) to 24.8 mm diameter (for the METRx X-Tube system). Each dilator has four concentric rings with a different colour-code at the superficial end **(Figure 1)**.Each dilator has markings on it to indicate the depth which in turn helps decide the length of the tube to be used. The first dilator (5.3 mm) needs to be threaded over a blunt tipped guidewire which is inserted under fluoroscopic guidance. Once the dilator is on the bone, the guide-wire is withdrawn. The dilator is then used as a Cobb elevator to sweep the soft-tissues off the bone, along with palpating the anatomical landmarks in both coronal and sagittal planes. Once the satisfactory position is achieved, serial dilatation with increasing diameter dilators is performed. It is important to

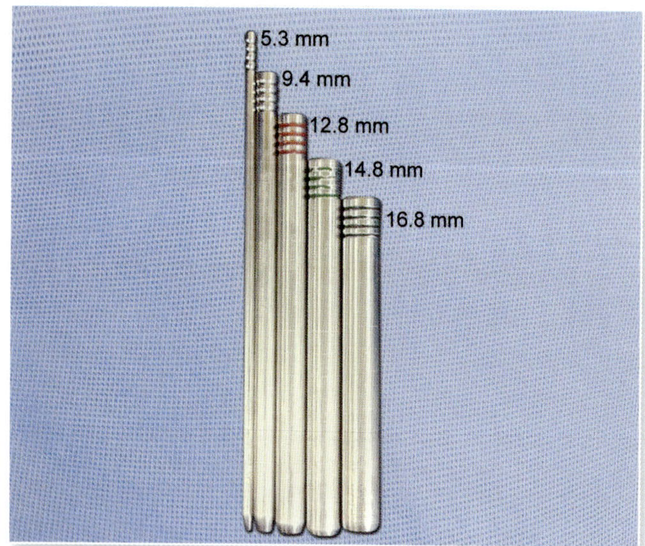

Figure 1: Different dilator sizes with color-coding

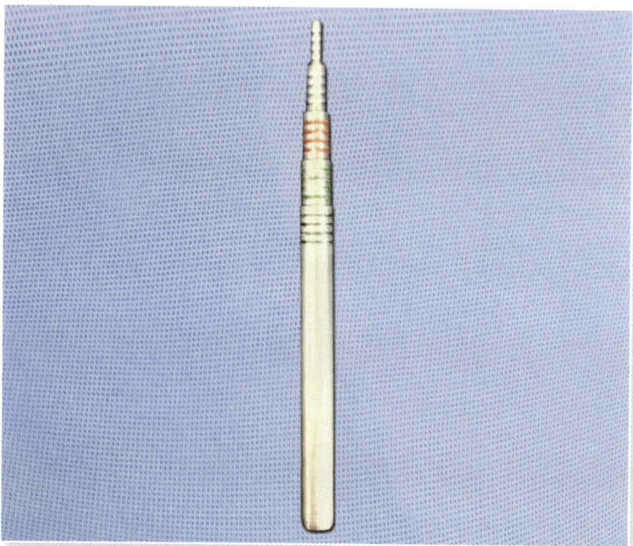

Figure 2: Arrangement of tubes. Note that all four rings are seen on each successive dilator

see all four rings of each dilator as the successive dilator is threaded over the previous one, to ensure proper entry and seating on the bone **(Figure 2)**. The dilators are introduced in gentle screwing motion.The calibrations on the final dilator are then used to determine the length of the final tube. Depending on the size of the tube being used the final dilator may be 12.8 mm (for 14 mm tube), 14.8 (for 16 mm tube), 16.8 mm (for 18 mm tube) or 20.8 mm (for 22 mm tube) **(Figure 3).**

We tend to use the 16 mm tube for diskectomies and 18 mm for lumbar canal stenosis decompression. It is advisable to use 18 mm tube for discectomy till requisite expertise is achieved. A 22 mm tube may be used for a TLIF or a PLIF

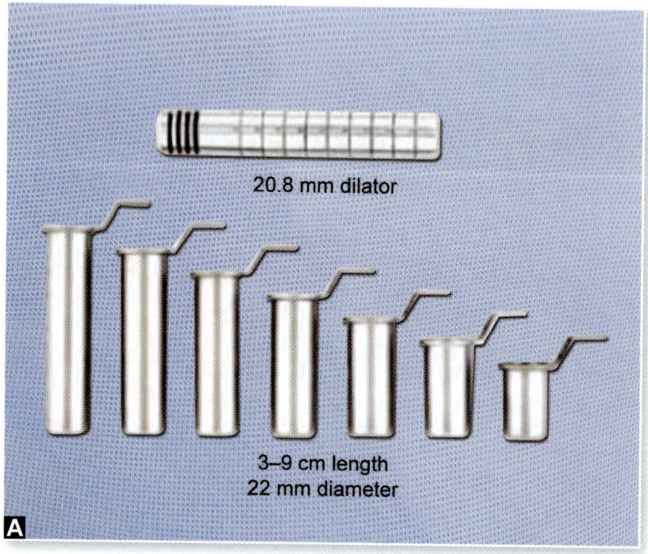

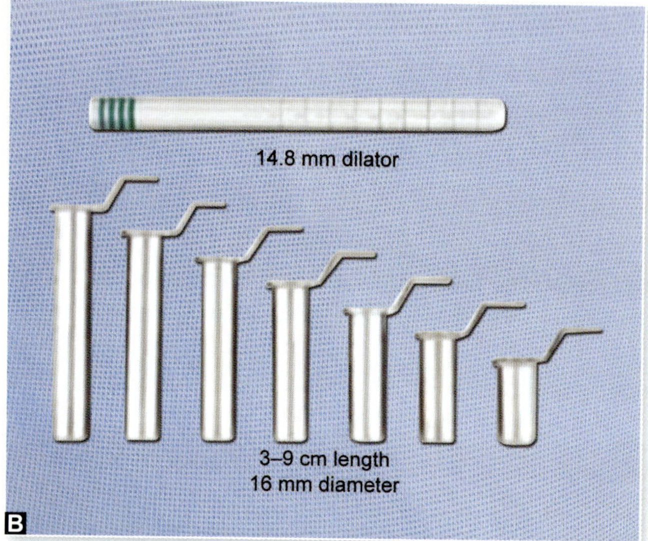

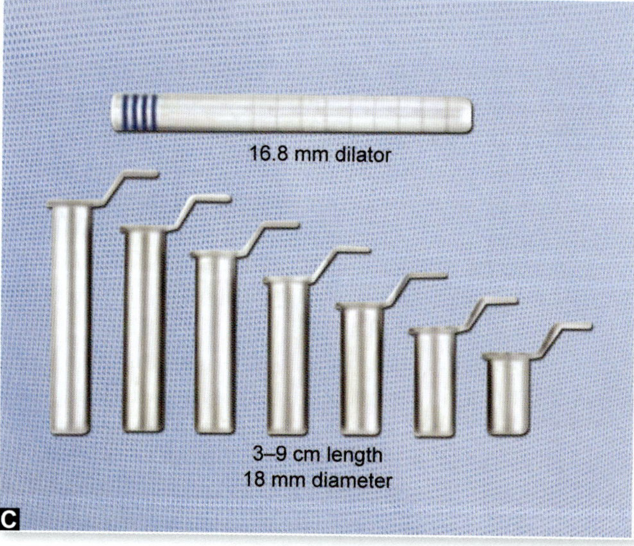

Figures 3A to C: Different sizes of final dilators and tubes. Note different lengths of the final tube available in each diameter

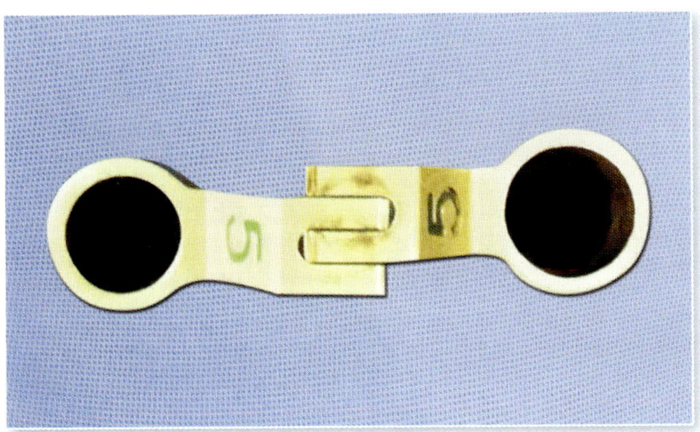

Figure 4: 16 mm tube (left) and the 18 mm tube (right). Note the number indicating the depth of the tube

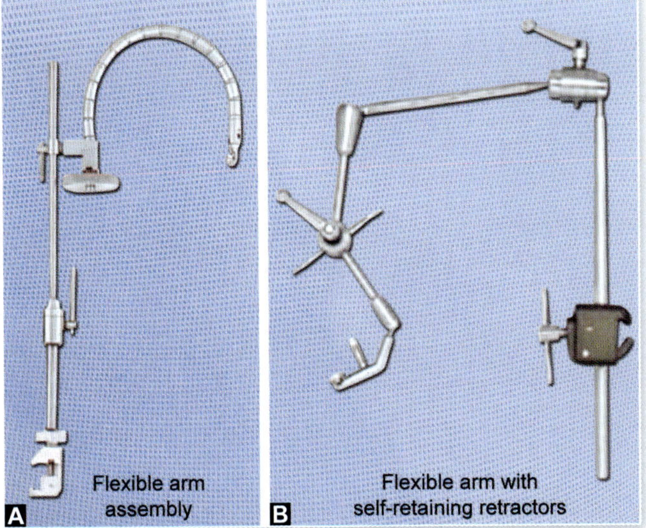

Figures 5A and B: The two variants of the Flexible Arm Assembly

procedure, depending on the surgeons' experience. The final tube has a number etched on it which indicates the tube depth **(Figure 4)**. The tubes are available in a variety of depths from 3 cm to 9 cm, and a variety of diameters as discussed above.

Once the final depth of the tube is selected, the tube is threaded and attached to the Flexible Arm Assembly. This component is a post and a flexible arm with steel links or articulations **(Figures 5A and B)**. The assembly attaches to the operating table. The final tube is attached to the post by the arm and the connection is tightened to hold the tube firmly in position.

It is desirable to visualize the final seating of the tube in the lateral and/or the anteroposterior fluoroscopy image. Any final adjustments are made at this point. The dilators are then sequentially removed and the endoscope or the microscope is then used to visualize the anatomy.

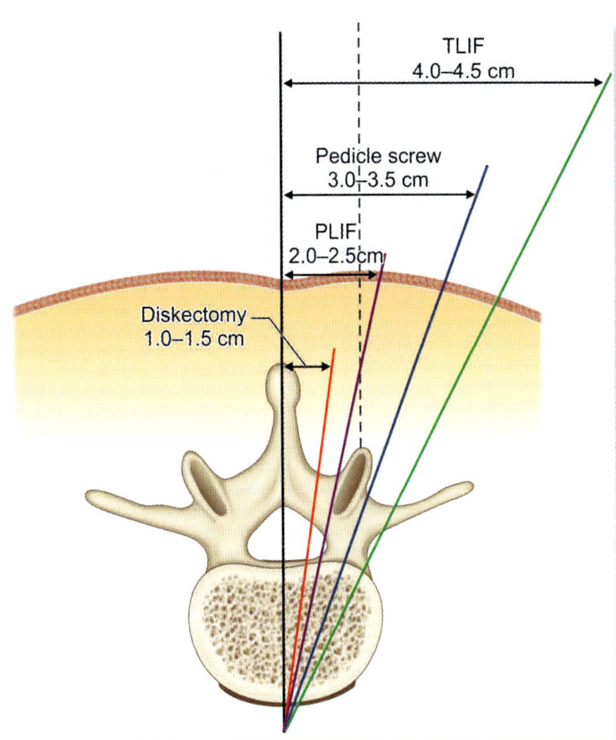

Figure 6: Recommended docking points

The system may utilize an endoscope or a microscope for the purpose of visualization, and illumination. The endoscope uses a television monitor for the visualization and the surgical field is visualized as a two-dimensional image. The endoscope is prone to fogging and requires frequent cleaning during the procedure. The microscope helps in direct visualization with a three dimensional effect and avoids the problems associated with fogging. The surgeon may utilize a powerful head-lamp and loupes to achieve the same effect, but loupes require constant adjustment of the neck to focus, each time the surgeons head moves. This can be quite cumbersome. There are different systems available for minimally invasive TLIF procedures which utilize illumination through the fiber-optic cables through a channel in the tube, and the surgeon uses the loupes for magnification.

The docking point of the tube varies with the procedure being performed. Our preferred docking points are as shown in the **Figure 6**.

ADVANTAGES OF THE TUBES

Apart from the obvious advantages of the minimal disruption of the softtissues, the tube is a very maneuverable device. The tube can be used for contralateral decompression from an ipsilateral entry or two adjacent level pathologies

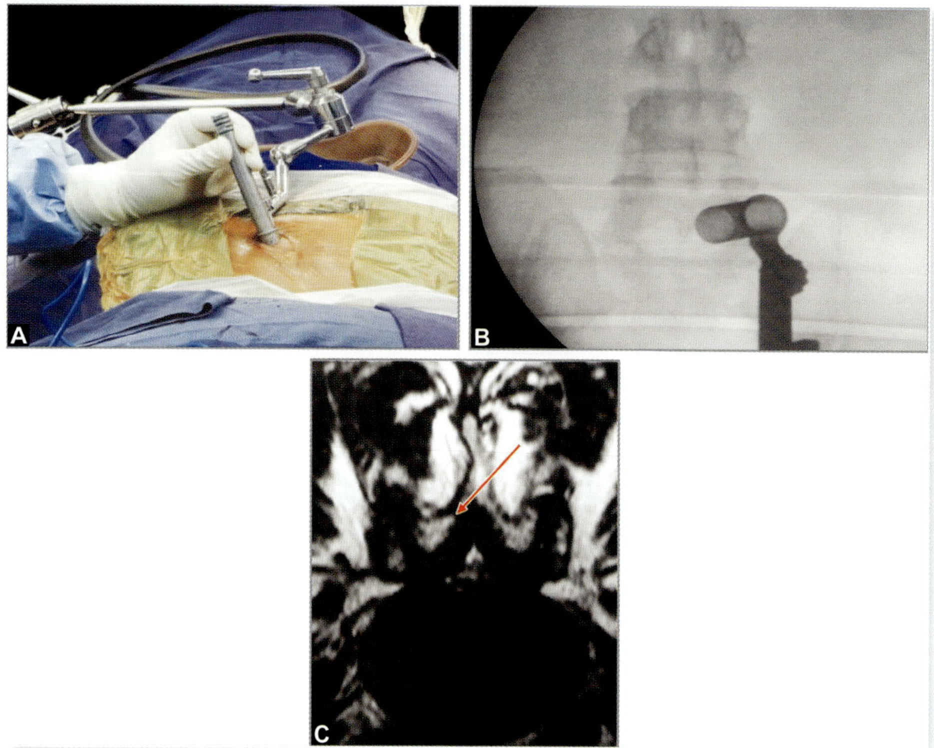

Figures 7A to C: Tube directed medially across the midline for contralateral decompression

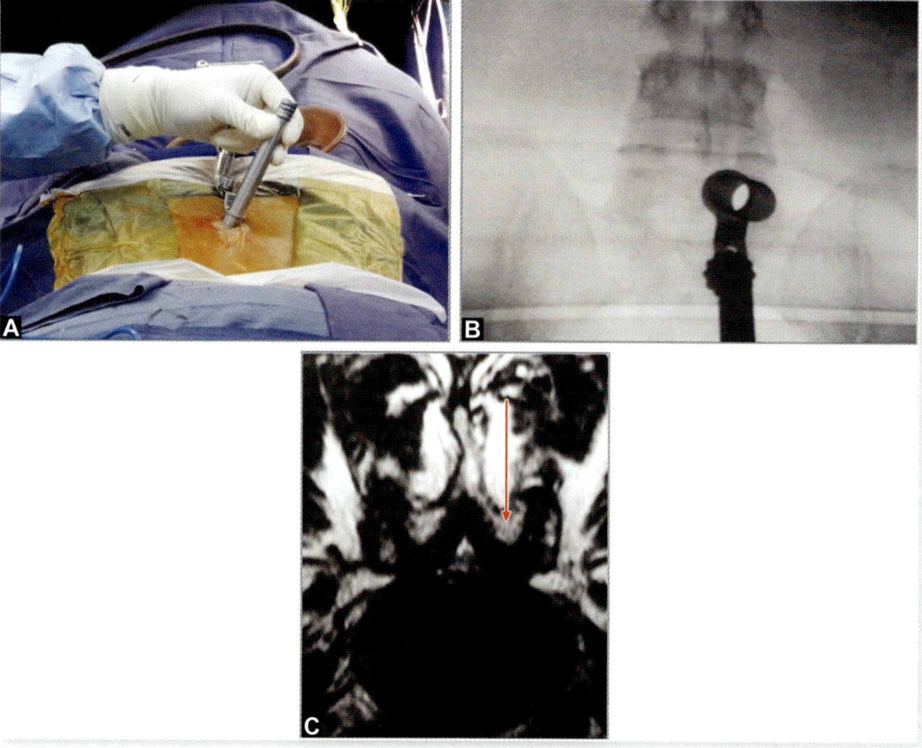

Figures 8A to C: Tube directed laterally for ipsilateral decompression

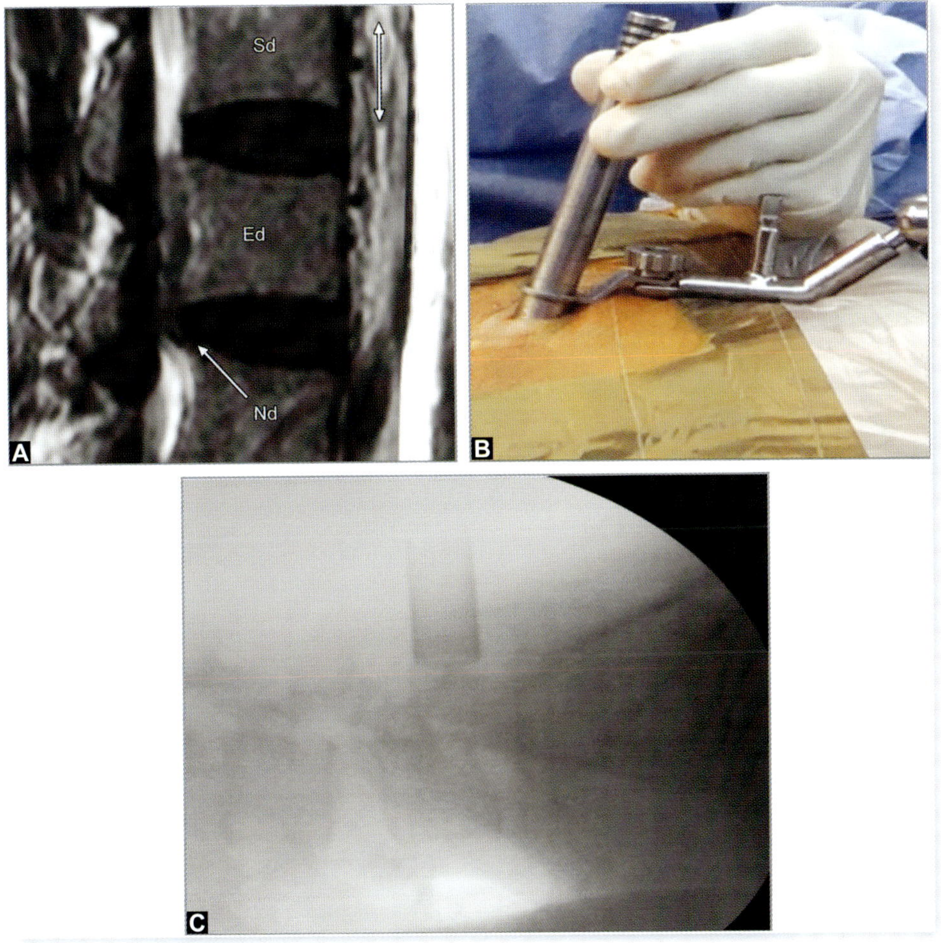

Figures 9A to C: Tube tilted cranially for a superiorly migrated disk

through a single port. This can be achieved by a technique called "wanding".

When performing contralateral decompression, the flexible arm assembly and the tube connection is loosened and the tube tilted to ipsilateral side so that the contralateral side can be visualized **(Figures 7A to C)**. In this process, the patient is tilted to the opposite side to aid in the visualization. Similarly an opposite maneuver can be carried out for ipsilateral lateral recess decompression **(Figures 8A to C)**.

The tube can be used to tackle pathology like a disk herniation or canal stenosis at two adjacent levels through the same port of entry especially if the pathology is at L4–5 and L5–S1 levels. This is achieved by manipulating the tube in the sagittal plane to visualize cranially or caudally **(Figures 9A to C and 10A to C)**.

The vision through the tube is thus not limited but substantial due to the maneuverability. This allows the surgeon to perform targeted decompressions over a wider area with minimal exposure **(Figure 11)**.

There is a steep learning curve associated with the tubular retractor assisted systems, but gaining expertise in the systems would widen the applications of this system to a variety of conditions. The tubular retractors are widely used for lumbar diskectomies, lumbar canal stenosis decompressions, minimally invasive TLIF/PLIF, posterior cervical foraminotomies, tumors and trauma. This allows a spine surgeon to deal with a majority of degenerative conditions through a minimally invasive approach. The various applications will be discussed elsewhere in this book.

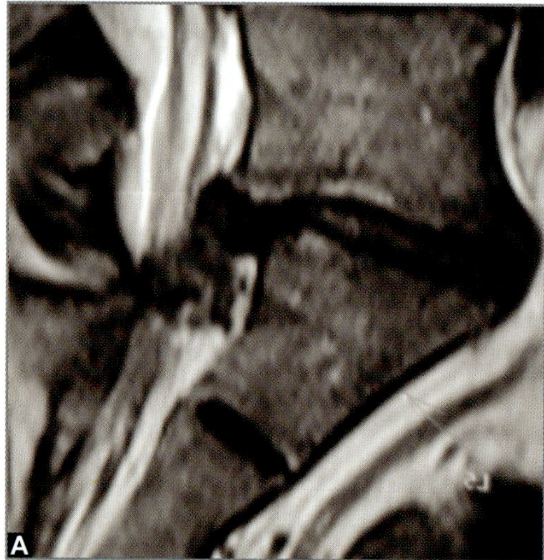
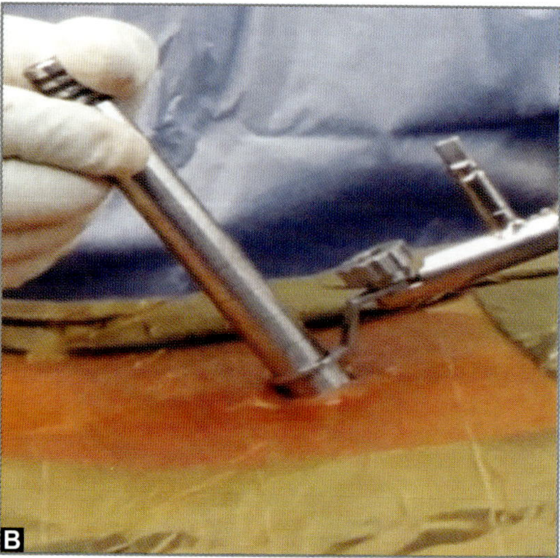
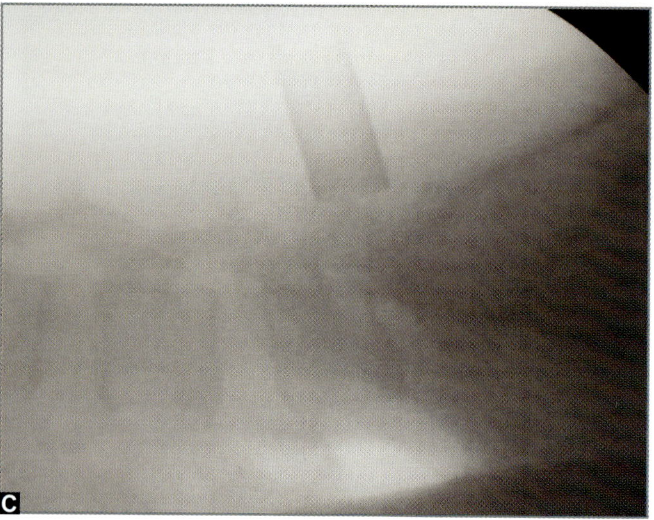

Figures 10A to C: Tube tilted caudally for an inferiorly migrated disk

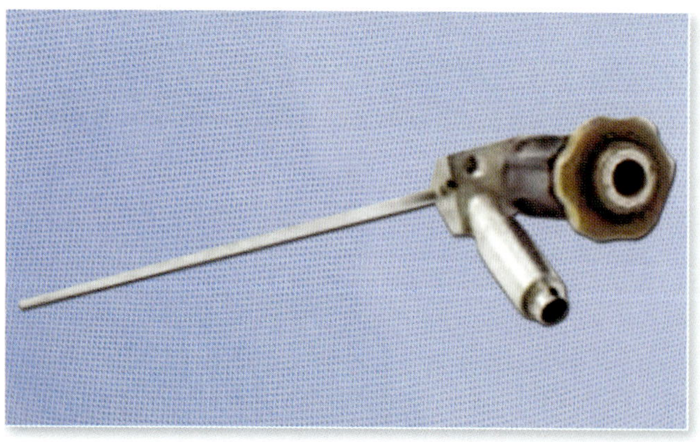

Figure 11: METRx MED system reusable endoscope

BIBLIOGRAPHY

1. Faubert C, Caspar W. Lumbar percutaneous discectomy. Initial experience in 28 cases. Neuroradiology. 1991;33:407-10.
2. Foley KT, Smith MM: Microendoscopic discectomy. Tech Neurosurg. 1997;3:301-7.
3. METRx® Surgical Procedure Technique Manual, Medtronic Sofamor Danek downloaded from http://www.rch.org.au/uploadedFiles/Main/Content/ortho/19742_METRx_ST-NMB-OUS.pdf
4. Oppenheimer JH, DeCastro Igor, McDonell DE: Minimally invasive spine technology and minimally invasive spine surgery: a historical review. Neurosurg Focus. 2009;27(3)E9.

4

CHAPTER

Applied Anatomy and Surgical Approaches in MISS Surgeries

Rishi Aggarwal, Kshitij Chaudhary

ABSTRACT

The approach to the minimally Invasive spine surgeries (MIS) have evolved over a period of time with the aim of achieving excellent outcomes with minimal damage to soft tissues. The main advantages of MIS surgeries is less morbidity and helps in faster rehabilitation, early recovery which is the need of hour in the present day practice. The breakthrough invention of tubes, good understanding of the anatomy has helped in the evolution of the current approaches in spine surgeries.

Intricate understanding surgical anatomy has been the key to performing successful surgery since the times of Andreas Vesalius. The focus of this chapter is on applied anatomy of the most commonly performed minimally invasive surgical approaches. The description of the surgical approach is mentioned briefly. However, a detailed description for each surgery can be found in their respective chapters.

PARASPINAL LUMBAR APPROACH

Minimally invasive paraspinal lumbar approach can be used to treat variety of pathologies. This is a muscle sparing approach through which decompression as well as instrumented fusion can be performed.

Indications

- Lumbar canal stenosis with neurogenic claudication
- Degenerative spondylolisthesis with spinal stenosis
- Adult isthmic spondylolisthesis
- Disc herniation including far-lateral disc herniations **(Figure 1)**
- Revision spinal decompression
- Foraminal stenosis
- Facet cyst
- Spondylolysis repair

Relative Contraindications

- Morbid obesity is a relative contraindication is it decreases the working length available and also increases the depth of surgical field.

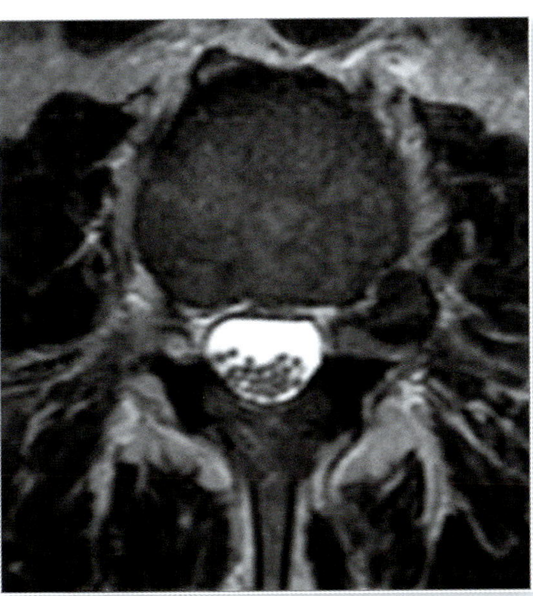

Figure 1: Far Lateral disk herniation

- Revision surgery
- Multilevel decompression and fusion
- High grade spondylolisthesis
- Congenital spinal stenosis at multiple levels.

Advantages

- Small skin incision, muscle sparing
- Bilateral decompression can be performed with unilateral approach
- Preservation of midline structures and reduced damage to facet joints.
- Extent of decompression that can be achieved is comparable to open approach
- Reduced blood loss
- Early mobilization and quicker rehabilitation
- Long term results comparable with open surgery

Disadvantages

- Multiple level surgery, especially fusion is technically demanding
- Limited visualization outside the target area
- Learning curve has to be overcome to become efficient

Surgical Approach

Meticulous preoperative planning is a must using X-rays, MRI and/or CT scan. General anesthesia with complete muscle relaxation is preferred. Muscle tightness can interfere with positioning and manipulation of the tubular retractor. Kyphotic positioning on a Wilson frame is helpful for decompressive surgeries. As with any minimally invasive surgery, preoperative localization of the intended level is performed using a spinal needle. An 18- 20 mm incision is taken 1 cm lateral to the midline on the side of the intended decompression. For fusion surgery the incision should be around 4 cm from the midline, in line with pedicles on AP view. The initial dilator is used as a dissector as well as a palpating device. Subsequent dilators split the muscle fibres and establish a surgical corridor. Finally, an appropriate size tubular retractor is slid down the dilators and yoked to the table securely. Pedicular screws may be passed if instrumented fusion is planned **(Figure 2)**. The decompression now can be performed in a similar manner as with open surgery, however, this does require magnification and illumination using either a microscope or headlights with loupe. Over-the-top decompression (contralateral decompression) can be performed by "wanding" the tubular retractor and excising the base of the spinous process to gain assess to the contralateral lateral recess.[1]

Similar approach can be used for extraforaminal disc herniations. The tubular retractor is dock over the inter-

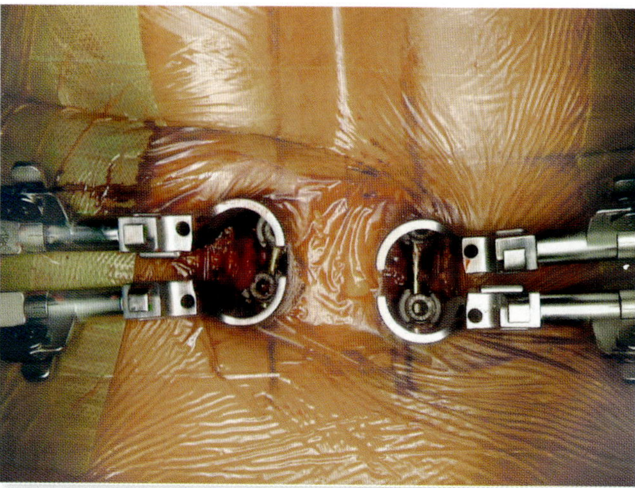

Figure 2: Pedicular screws passed through the tubes

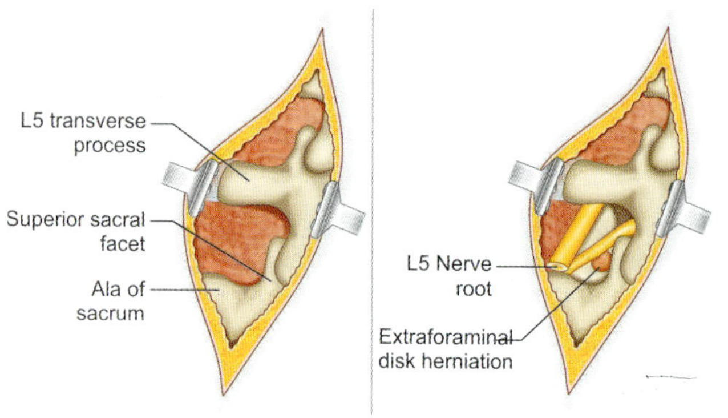

Figure 3: Exposure of root through the superior facet of superior vertebra

transverse area. The intertransverse ligament is detached from its attachment to the transverse process. The lateral part of superior facet of the caudal vertebra can be removed using burr. This exposes the disc herniation which is usually medial to the exiting nerve **(Figure 3)**.

APPLIED ANATOMY

The paraspinal region is made up of predominantly two groups of muscles: the erector spinae and spino-transverse group.[2,3] The erector spinae group is made up of spinalis, longissimus and iliocostalis. The spinotransverse group is made up of rotatores, multifidus and semispinalis. The erector spinae group is innervated by lateral branches of the dorsal rami of the spinal nerves while the spino-transverse group is innervated by the medial branches of the dorsal rami of the appropriate spinal nerves. Longissimus and multifidus are the two muscle most frequently encountered during the paraspinal approach.

Longissimus is the central component of erector spinae. It assumes a series of attachments at sites that are homologous to the junction of the transverse and costal elements of the segment. At lumbar level, these are represented by the accessory process and medial half of the transverse process respectively. The fascicles pass inferiorly and laterally. Those from the first four lumbar vertebrae converge on to a common flat tendon that covers the lateral surface of the muscle and separates it from the lumbar fibres of iliocostalis, for which reason it is called the lumbar intermuscular aponeurosis.

Multifidus lies lateral to the spinous processes and covers the laminae of the underlying vertebrae. At the lumbosacral junction, it expands to cover the posterior surface of the sacrum. It arises from the caudal edge of the lateral surface of the spinous process and from the caudal end of its tip. It inserts into the transverse processes of the vertebra 2 - 5 levels below.

Wiltse et al. first described the paraspinal approach in 1968.[4] They utilized the natural cleavage between multifidus and longissimus to approach the posterolateral surface of the lumbar spine and lumbosacral junction. A recent study demonstrated that the cleavage between multifidus and longissimus was well-visualized in patients.[5] This plane can be seen on MRI also **(Figure 4)**. This cleavage plane has fat and blood vessels in most patients. A cadaveric study by Vialle et al showed that the distance of this cleavage plane from the midline is variable.[6] The mean distance of this cleavage plane from the midline is 4.04 cm with majority values ranging from 3.5 to 4.5 cm. They also noticed that the cleavage plane is well defined below L4 and gradually disappeared above the L4 transverse process.

TRANS-PSOAS APPROACH

The trans-psoas approach for the interbody fusion, also known as extreme lateral lumbar interbody fusion (XLIF) or lateral lumbar interbody fusion (LLIF), is a popular, minimally invasive alternative to anterior lumbar interbody fusion (ALIF). The approach utilizes a direct lateral, retroperitoneal access to the disc space through the substance of the psoas muscle.

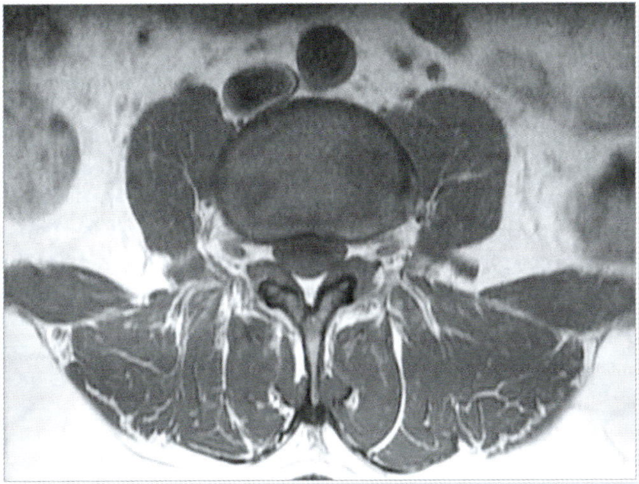

Figure 4: Intermuscular plane visualized on MRI

Advantages

- Minimally invasive, with limited tissue disruption and peritoneal handling leading to shorter recovery time.
- Aorta or vena cava mobilization is not required and "access" surgeon is not needed.
- Can be performed in obese patients without increase in morbidity.
- Inherent stabilizers of the spine such as the anterior and posterior longitudinal ligament are preserved leading to superior construct strength.
- Large footprint implant is used that spans the ring apophysis which is the strongest load bearing area of the endplate. This leads to better deformity correction and prevents subsidence of implant.
- Large surface area is available for fusion.

Disadvantages

- Direct decompression cannot be performed as epidural space cannot be visualized.
- Extensive vertebral body lesions cannot be addressed.
- Lumbar plexus is at risk for injury especially at L4–5. Femoral nerve injury is a dreaded complication.
- Iliac crest prevents access to the L5–S1 disk.
- L4–5 occasionally cannot be accessed either due to high iliac crest or variations in the neural anatomy of the lumbar plexus.
- Numbness along distribution of Genito-femoral nerve.[7]
- Transient hip flexion weakness.[8]

Indications

This approach can be used to treat variety of degenerative disorders such as disk disease with instability, adjacent segment disc degeneration, low grade degenerative and adult isthmus spondylolisthesis and degenerative scoliosis.[9] Restoration of disc height can lead to indirect decompression of foramina and preclude a formal posterior decompression.[10]

It can also be employed for revision surgeries such as pseudarthrosis, recurrent disc herniation or stenosis, revision of failed total disc replacement device.[11] The approach can also provide access for thorough debridement in patients with discitis.

Limitations and Contraindications

The iliac crest prevents access to the L5–S1 disk space via this approach. Some have advocated partial removal of the iliac crest to gain access, but generally this is not recommended.[12]

In some cases, due to variations in anatomy, there is a definite risk of injury to the lumbar plexus that resides within the substance of the psoas muscle. This is especially true for L4–5 level.[13] High grade spondylolisthesis is also not suitable for treatment with this approach as the anterior migrated lumbar roots from the listhetic segment preclude a safe placement of the retractor. Patients with transitional anatomy, such as lumbarization of sacral segment with L5-6 level as the functional L4–5 level may also present with a challenge due to anterior migration of the psoas as well as the lumbar plexus ("rising psoas sign")[14]

Previous retroperitoneal surgery is a contraindication for this approach due to scarring and potential for injury to abdominal viscera or vasculature.[15] Variations in vascular anatomy may interfere with a direct lateral approach and preoperative MRI should be studied, especially in patients with scoliosis.

Surgical Approach

Positioning is critical for success of this operation. The patient is positioned securely in the lateral decubitus position. The right lateral decubitus with left side up may be preferred as this reduces the risk of injury to vascular structures.[16] The hips are flexed to relax the femoral nerve. Mild lateral flexion by breaking the table between the greater trochanter and the iliac crest reduces the overhang of the iliac crest over the L4–5 level. Excessive lateral flexion should be avoided as it not only increases tension in the psoas muscle but also translates the lumbar plexus ventrally. In general, a left sided access is preferred, however regional vascular and neural anatomy and spinal deformity may alter the surgeon's choice. The positioning should allow for perfect orthogonal fluoroscopy. Without true AP and lateral views of the disc space, the safe zones for surgical access cannot be accurately determined. The table, not the C-arm, has to be adjusted such that the disc space is perpendicular to the or floor and parallel to the or wall.

The approach to the retroperitoneal area can be performed using single or double incision technique. The double incision technique involves gaining access to the retroperitoneal area just lateral to the erector spinae muscle. With blunt dissection through the muscle layers, the retroperitoneal fat layer is reached. The peritoneal is dissected off anteriorly with finger. This second incision is made anterior to the second incision direct over the intended disc space and a dilator is introduced with the surgeon's finger in place to prevent injury to the peritoneum. Alternatively, a direct approach can be employed using a single incision. The three abdominal layers, external oblique, internal oblique and transversus abdomenus are sequentially split in the direction of their fibers while avoiding any neural structures (subcostal, iliohypogastric and the ilioinguinal nerve) that course between these layers. Injury to these nerves can result in abdominal hernia and pain and dysesthetic sensations. The peritoneum is the gently dissected off the inner wall of the abdomen to reach the psoas muscle. The retroperitoneal dissection has to be gentle to prevent injury to these nerves as they travel along the inner wall over the quadratus lumborum muscle. The psoas muscle is then visualized and a dilator is placed over it, its location verified under fluoroscopy.

Understanding the lumbar plexus anatomy in relation to the lateral aspect of the lumbar spine is essential to safely navigate through the psoas muscle. Orthogonal views of the spine with neuromonitoring is essential to establish a safe corridor. The safe zones for docking the dilator is the midpoint of Zone III at L1–2, L2–3 and L3–4 level and the junction of Zone III and IV at the L4–5 level.[17] Zone II at L2–3 and Zone I at L3–4 and L4–5 are not safe due to the presence of the genitofemoral nerve. Triggered EMG is used to identify proximity of the nerves. Genitofemoral nerve is difficult to monitor using this technique unless cremaster muscle is monitored. It is best to avoid these zones or to dock the dilators under vision to make sure that the genitofemoral nerve is not injured.

Sequential dilators are used and finally a specialized retractor is secured to the table. The posterior retractor blade position (posteriorly lies the lumbar plexus) is kept constant and the anterior blades are expanded **(Figure 5)**. The disk is visualized and diskectomy and endplate preparation can then be performed in the usual manner.

APPLIED ANATOMY

Retroperitoneal space is an anatomical space located in the abdominal cavity behind the parietal peritoneum containing

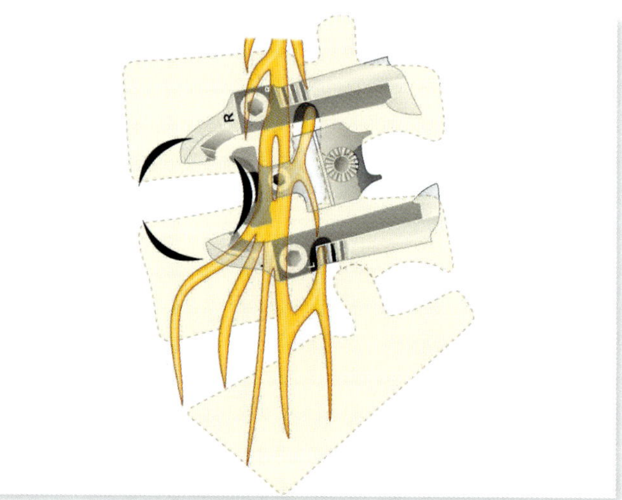

Figure 5: Anterior plates are enlarged to visualize the disk

variable amount of fatty connective tissue. This potential space is exploited during the trans-psoas approach. The space is bound by the peritoneum and abdominal structures anteriorly, quadratus lumborum and iliopsoas muscle posteriorly, superiorly by the diaphragm and inferiorly by the retroperitoneal pelvic space. The ilioinguinal, iliohypogastric and lateral cutaneous nerves emerge from the lateral border of the psoas and course downwards in this space, over the quadratus lumborum to reach the anterior iliac crest after piercing the lateral abdominal wall.

From superficial to deep, the lateral abdominal wall muscles include external oblique, internal oblique and transverses abdominis. The iliohypogastric and ilioinguinal nerves run between these muscles can can be encountered during this approach.

The psoas major muscle is divided into superficial and deep parts. The deep part originates from the transverse processes of L1–L4. The superficial part originates from the lateral surfaces of the last thoracic and first 4 lumbar vertebrae and the their adjoining discs. The lumbar plexus lies within the substance of the psoas muscle between these two layers.

Lumbar plexus originates from the anterior primary rami of L1–L4. The nerve of the lumbar plexus emerge from the lateral border of the psoas muscle, except for the genitofemoral nerve that emerges on the anterior surface and the obturator nerve that emerges medial to the psoas tendon **(Table 1)** enumerates the nerves of the lumbar plexus with their corresponding innervations.

Table 1

Nerves of the lumbar plexus

Nerve	*Roots*	*Motor innervation*
Iliohypogastric N	T12–L1	Transversus Abdominis Internal oblique
Ilioinguinal N	L1	
Genitofemoral N	L1–2	Cremaster
Lateral femoral cutaneous N	L2–3	
Obturator N	L2–4	Adductor longus Adductor magnus gracilis Pectineus Obturator externus
Femoral N	L2–4	Quadriceps Sartorius Pectineus Iliopsoas
Direct muscular branches	T12–L4	Psoas Major Quadratus Lumborum Iliac Lumbar inter transverse

Several cadaver and imaging studies have described the relationship of the lumbar plexus with the lateral aspect of the lumbar spine by dividing the vertebral body into four equal zones (zone 1 to IV) **(Figures 6 and 7)**.[17,18] The psoas muscle is thin at L1–2 level and progressively increases in size as one goes caudally. At L1–2 level, the the nerves (iliohypogastric, ilioinguinal and genitofemoral) are found in zone IV and posterior. At the L2–3 level, the genitofemoral nerve is found to cross posterior to anterior in Zone II and the L2 root is found in zone IV. At the L3–4 level, majority of neural structures are found in zone IV (L2 division of lumbar plexus, L3 nerve root, and lateral femoral cutaneous nerve). Here, the genitofemoral nerve is found in zone I. The the

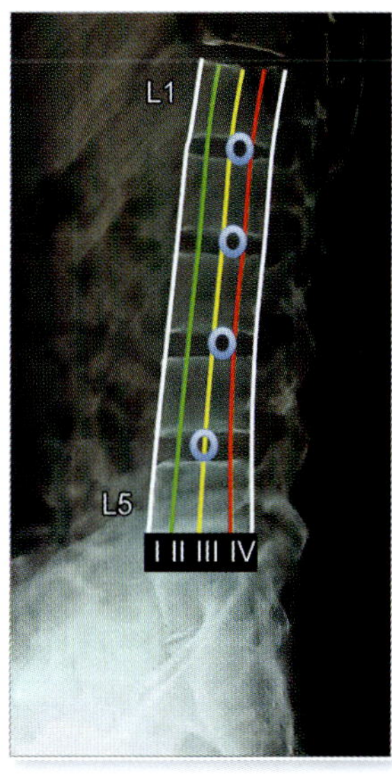

Figure 6: The division of zones in lateral approach to lumbar spine

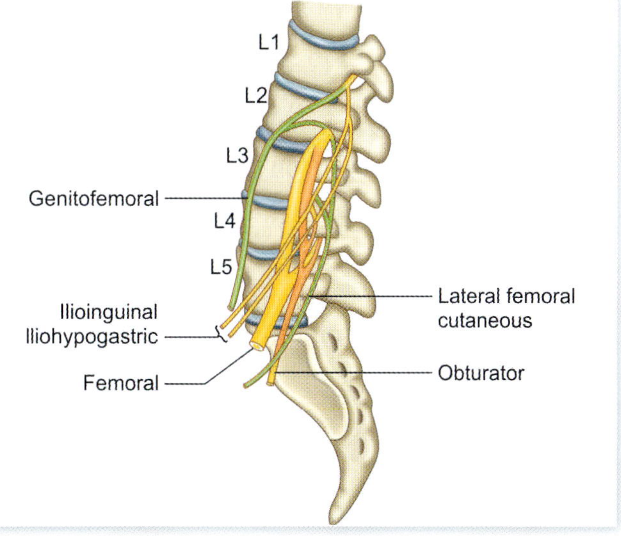

Figure 7: Relation of nerves to the lumbar vertebra

L4–5 level the neural structures are more anterior placed in zone III and IV (femoral nerve, L4 contribution to the sciatic nerve and the obturator nerve). The genitofemoral nerve is in zone I at this level on the anterior surface of the psoas muscle. Thus the genitofemoral nerve is found on the anterior surface of the psoas in zone I at L3–4 and L4–5 level and zone II at L2–3 level. The most posterior zone, zone IV, contains neural structures at all levels. However, variations in anatomy exist especially at the L4–5 level. The position of the lumbar plexus may vary from right to left in the same patient.

Bifurcation of the aorta and vena cava into the common iliac vessels usually occurs at the L4–5 disk space. At each segment, a pair of lumbar segmental vessels cross the lateral aspect of the mid vertebral body. There are no vascular structures over the lateral aspect of the disk space.

MINIMALLY INVASIVE ANTERIOR MIDLINE APPROACH TO LUMBOSACRAL SPINE (MINI ALIF)

Minimally invasive anterior midline approach to lumbosacral spine (also known as mini-open ALIF) is a modification of the standard anterior midline approach. This was first described by Mayer in 1997 as an alternative to laparoscopic lumbar interbody fusion.[19] This minimally invasive approach can be performed either transperitoneally or retroperitoneally, however the later is preferred to avoid to inherent potential problems associated with intraperitoneal surgery. This approach uses microsurgical technique using microscopes (or head-lights with loupes) and specialized retractors to gain assess to the lumbar spine (L2 to S1). Laparoscopically-assisted mini ALIF, is not routinely performed because it is fraught extremely limited access, very steep learning curve, long operative time.[20,21]

Indications (Similar to Those for ALIF)

- Degenerative disc disease with or without instability
- Degenerative or isthmus spondylolisthesis
- Lumbosacral fusion caudal to a long fusion construct in adult deformity
- Recurrent disc herniation or stenosis
- Pseudoarthrosis or revision of TLIF/PLIF
- Infective spondylodiskitis
- Disc replacement[22]

Contraindications

- Previous abdominal surgery and scarring limits mobilization of vascular and visceral structures. This is more so a contraindication for the MIS approach compared to the open approach.
- Multi-level fusion
- Vascular anomaly or variation preventing access to the disc space, especially at L4–5 level.
- Morbid obesity

Advantages

- Minimal peritoneal handling, thus reducing the degree of postoperative ileus.
- Shorter recovery times and earlier rehabilitation
- Reduced surgical blood loss
- Can be converted to an extensile approach if required
- Better cosmesis
- Both interbody grafting and total disk replacement can be performed via this approach

Disadvantages

- Limited visualization and degree of freedom for manipulation of instruments
- Multi-level procedure is not possible. One or two levels can be safely performed
- Injury to vascular and viscera structures is a possibility
- Learning curve

Surgical Approach

The patient is positioned supine with slight extension of the lumbosacral area using a gel pad. The incision is planned after plotting the trajectory of intended disc space as projected on the midline using lateral fluoroscopy. Position of the pubic symphysis relative to the L5–S1 trajectory is important to consider while planning the incision for L5–S1 level. A transverse skin incision (4–5 cm long) is made as per level **(Figure 8)**. Inferior epigastric vessels are superolateral to the incision. The anterior rectus sheath is open transversely and the rectus muscle is retracted laterally away from midline. The transversalis fascia is incised to enter the preperitoneal area as identified by presence of adipose tissue. The blunt dissection proceeds retroperitoneal to reach the lumbosacral area. The bifurcation is identified and vascular structures on either side are retracted to expose the disc space using specialized retractor frames that fix to the operating table (SynFrame, Synthes). The middle sacral vessels are ligated to expose the L5–S1 disk. Electrocautery is avoided to prevent injury to the superior hypogastric plexus, which can result in retrograde ejaculation. Exposure of L4–5 disk requires ligation of the iliolumbar vein before mobilization of the vessels across the anterior aspect of disk. Discectomy, endplate preparation, implantation is performed using standard instruments. Closure of transversalis fascia is optional. Anterior rectus sheath is closed followed by subcutaneous tissue and skin.

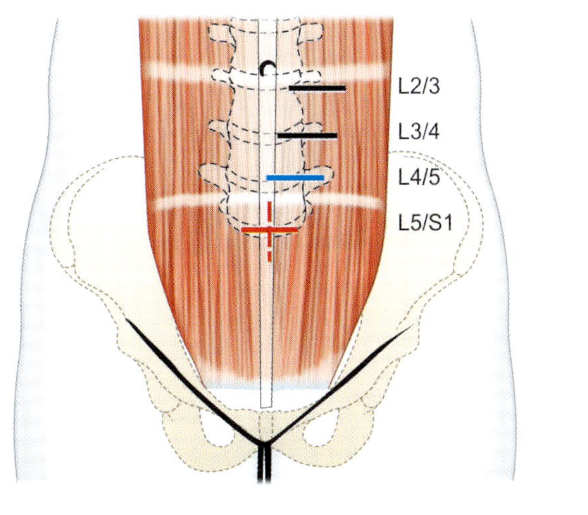

Figure 8: Incision sites depending on the level

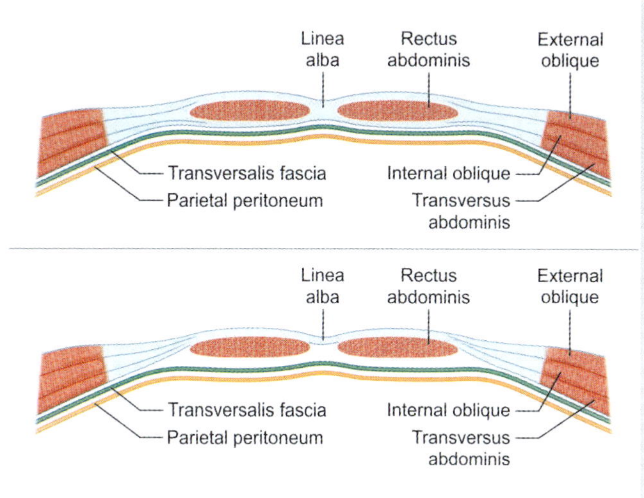

Figure 10: Anatomy of rectus sheath

Applied Anatomy

The subcutaneous layer of the anterior abdominal wall below the umbilicus consists of two layers: the superficial fatty layer (Camper's fascia) and the deep membranous layer (Scarpa's fascia) **(Figure 9)**. The muscles of the abdominal wall are three lateral muscles (external oblique, internal oblique and the transversus abdominis from superficial to deep) and two vertical muscles (rectus abdominis and pyramidalis). Deep to these muscle is the transversalis fascia and the peritoneum **(Figure 9)**.

The lateral muscles begin posterolaterally, travel anteriorly and are replaced by aponeurosis that eventually forms the rectus sheath. The rectus sheath completely encloses the upper three-quarters of the rectus abdominis muscle and covers only the anterior surface of the muscle in the lower quarter **(Figure 10)**. The point at which this transition occurs—roughly midway between the umbilicus and the pubic symphysis)—is marked by a line called as the arcuate line. Below this line the rectus muscle is in direct contact with the transversalis fascia. The nerve and blood supply to the rectus muscle is from its lateral border, hence the muscle is retracted laterally during exposure to preserve this segmental innervation. The midline condensation of fascia between the right and left rectus muscle is called the linea alba and becomes less distinct below the umbilicus.

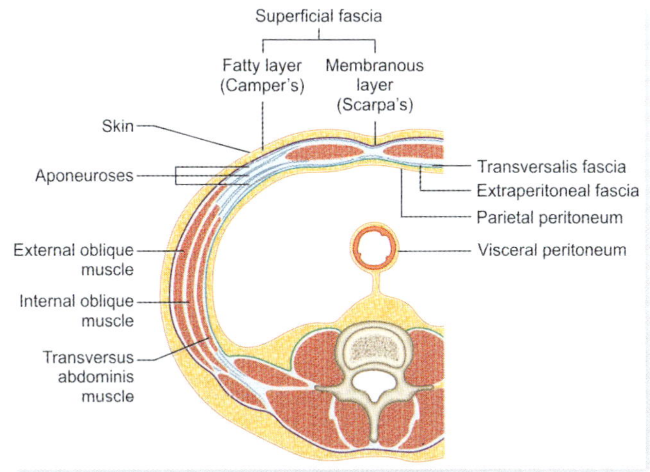

Figure 9: Anterior exposure to lumbar spine

The inferior epigastric vessels arise from the external iliac artery and travel along the posterior surface of the rectus muscle from lateral to medial. They are vulnerable to injury if more lateral approach is taken to enter the retroperitoneal area.

The ureters are generally retracted along with the peritoneum as one proceeds with retroperitoneal exposure of the lumbosacral area. They are encountered running anterior to the bifurcation of common iliac vessels. Excessive dissection around the ureter can devascularize or injure them and should be avoided.

It is extremely crucial to be intimate with the vascular anatomy in this region and be cognizant that there is considerable variability in anatomy, especially concerning relationship of vessels with L4–5 and L5–S1 discs. The L5–S1 disc is typically exposed between the bifurcation **(Figure 11)**. The L4–5 disk is exposed lateral to the vessels, typically from the left side as it is easier to handle an artery. In a large radiographic study, the aortic bifurcation was found at L3–4 disc level in 21.9%, L4 body level in 63.7% and L4–5 disk level in 14.4% of patients.[23] The iliocaval confluence was found at L4 body level in 13.7%, L4–5 disk level in 38.4%, L5 body level in 43.8% and L5–S1 disk level in 4.1% of patients. The L5–S1 disk space was limited by right iliac artery and left iliac vein in 65.1%, limited by right iliac vein and left iliac vein in

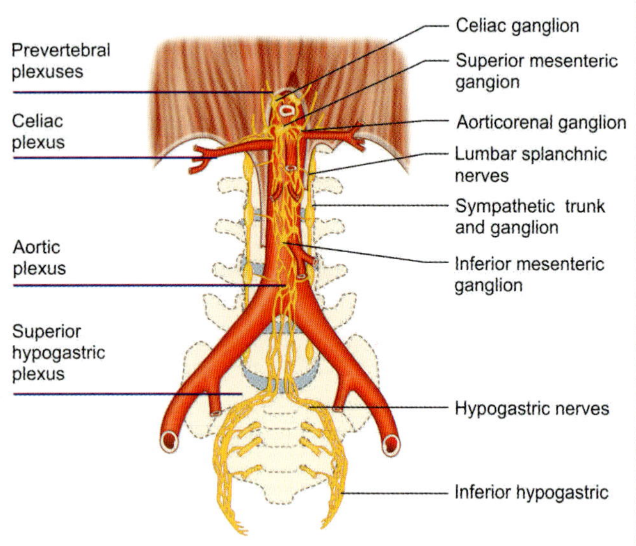

Figure 11: Relationship of L5–S1 disk to the bifurcation of major vessel

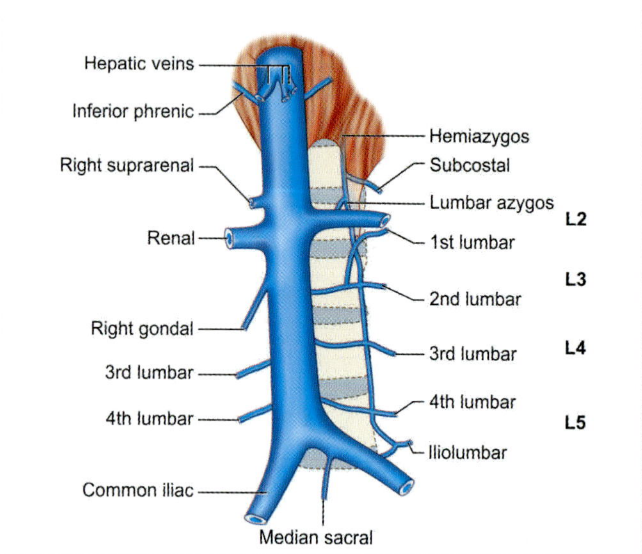

Figure 12: Relationship of iliolumbar vein to L4–5 disk

30.1%, and limited by right iliac artery and left iliac artery in 4.8% of patients. The vascular window was defined by the distance between the most medial iliac vessels at the L5-S1 disc level and the distance between the iliocaval vein and the lateral border of the L4-5 disk at the L4-5 disk level. At L5-1 level, the vascular window was found to be less than 25mm in 25% of patients. At L4-5 level, the vascular window was larger than 25 mm in only 33% patients.[23] Smaller the vascular window, greater the need for mobilization of the vessels and more is the risk of vein injury. Venovertebral veins, present in approximately in 74% patients, drain into the posterior margin of the left common iliac vein from L5 vertebral body. These can be injured by mobilization of the left iliac vein.[24] The iliolumbar vein—the first segmental off the common iliac vein—needs to be isolated and ligated before the retraction of the major vessels to gain access to L4-5 disk **(Figure 12)**. Failure to address this vein may lead to its avulsion off the posterior aspect of the common iliac vein leading to torrential and potentially life-threatening bleeding. One has to keep in mind that multiple iliolumbar veins may be present in upto 25.8 % of patients. Multiple ILVs if present must be ligated prior to discectomy.[25] Similarly, the median sacral vessels have to be ligated to expose the L5-S1 disk. Rarely, variations in vascular anatomy will preclude a safe access to the lumbosacral area and alternative means of fusion should be planned.[26]

Injury to the superior hypogastric plexus can cause retrograde ejaculation and sterility.[27] It is located anterior to the L5 vertebral body level **(Figure 11)**. From the plexus, sympathetic fibers travel along the hypogastric nerves to reach the inferior hypogastric plexus which innervates the pelvic viscera. Over the lumbosacral area the plexus is situated predominantly over the left side, hence, in transperitoneal approach a slightly right sided incision should be made to avoid the plexus.[28] Anatomical studies have found that the plexus lies in a distinct fascia in the retroperitoneum, called the autonomic nerve fascia and can be lifted off the aorta and lumbosacral junction as long as one remains in the correct surgical plane during the retroperitoneal approach.[28] Bone morphogenetic protein-2 (BMP-2) has been used in spinal fusions and has been associated with inflammatory and neuroinflammatory adverse reactions, which may contribute to RE development after anterior lumbar surgery.[29]

PRESACRAL APPROACH TO L5–S1 (AXIALIF)

The presacral approach to the lumbosacral spine to achieve trans-sacral fusion has been in vogue since recent years. The technique involves percutaneous trajectory via the presacral space to achieve fusion across the L5-S1 and possibly L4-5 disc spaces. Minimally invasive presacral approach was first described by Cragg et al. in 2004.[30]

Indications

- Indications are similar to those for other methods of interbody fusion
- Degenerative disk disease
- Low-grade spondylolisthesis
- Recurrent stenosis or disk herniations
- Pseudoarthrosis at L5-S1
- Lumbosacral fusion caudal to long fusion constructs in patients with degenerative scoliosis

Contraindications

- Previous rectal or colon surgery
- History of infection or inflammatory bowel condition such as diverticulitis or pelvic/rectal abscess in the past
- Prior radiation to pelvic viscera
- Variations in local anatomy that prevent safe execution of trajectory. Suitable trajectory cannot be achieved in excessively kyphotic or straight sacrum.

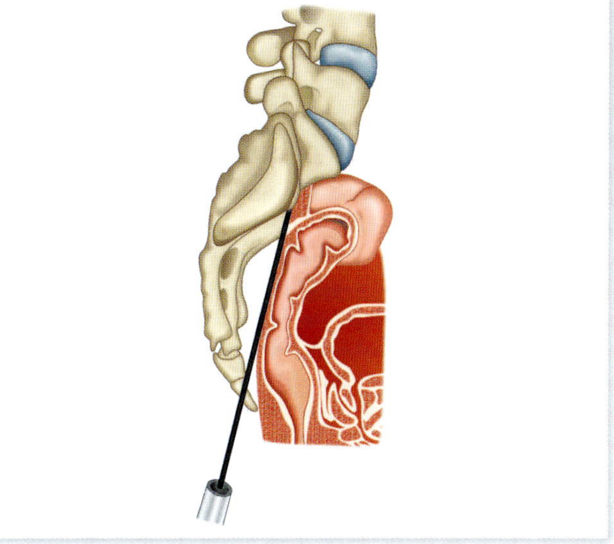

Figure 13: Passing of blunt probe anterior to sacrum

Advantages

- Percutaneous approach. Spares muscles and posterior elements.
- No "access" surgeon required
- Quick recovery
- Annulus and other ligamentous structures are not sacrificed.

Disadvantages

- There is an ever-present risk of injury to the rectum or vascular structures.
- Risk of infection due to proximity of incision to the anus.
- Limited to L5–S1. In some cases can be extended to two-levels up to L4–5. But isolated L4–5 fusion is not possible.
- Restoration of disc height and local lordosis is variable is not guaranteed
- Cannot provide coronal deformity correction
- Direct decompression is not possible. Indirect decompression via restoration of foraminal height is also variable. Patient with predominant symptoms due to foraminal or central stenosis are best treated using alternative methods.
- Limited ability to prepare endplate may compromise fusion potential
- May require to be backed up with posterior instrumentation.

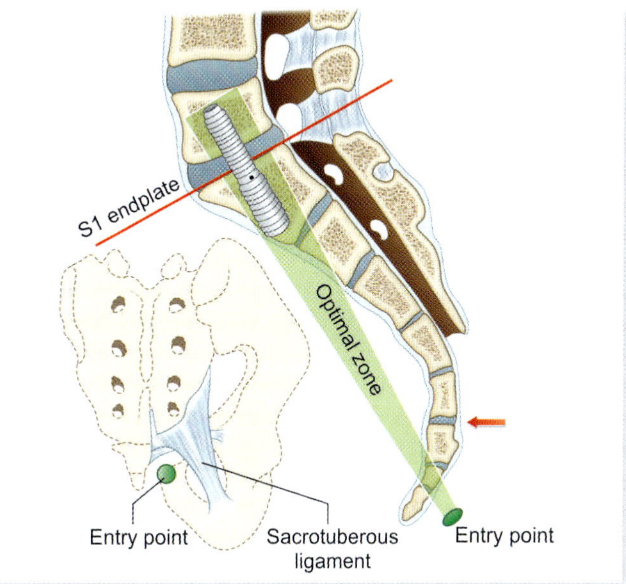

Figure 14: Entry point and trajectory of AXIlif implant

Surgical Approach

Standard bowel preparation as done for colonic surgeries is performed the night before surgery. Patient is placed prone with the hips flexed. Preoperative antibiotics that cover for abdominal flora are administered. The area is prepped thoroughly. The incision is approximately 2 cm lateral to the coccyx. Blunt dissection is used to locate the anterior surface of the sacrum. A blunt dissecting tool or probe is advanced on the anterior surface of the sacrum in the midline under biplanar fluoroscopic control **(Figure 13)**. Docking is usually at the S1-2 level. This probe is now replaced with a K-wire that is introduced into S1 vertebral body across the L5–S1 disk. A series of dilators are used for placement of a working channel through which a path is drilled from the S1 to the L5 vertebral body. Specialized instruments are used through this path to perform diskectomy and prepare the endplates. The disc space is filled with graft and an appropriate length AxiaLIF implant is screwed in place transfixing the L5–S1 segment **(Figure 14)**. Working channel and the K-wire is removed and the wound is irrigated and closed. Optionally, posterior instrumentation can be added via minimally invasive techniques.

Applied Anatomy

The area between the sacrum and the rectum is called the mesorectum, and it contains fatty tissue with lymph nodes and blood vessels. It is bound anteriorly by the fascia propria of the rectum and posteriorly by the presacral fascia (Waldeyer's fascia) overlying the sacrum.[31] This is the space (known as presacral space) that is exploited in this approach. Although one might think that this is a safe area, there are many important structures at risk here.

To understand the regional anatomy one has to recognize the importance of presacral fascial structures. They are divided into 5 layers: the periosteum over the sacrum, the presacral fascia, the rectosacral fascia, the autonomic nerve fascia (also known as prehypogastric nerve fascia), and the fascia propria of the rectum **(Figure 15)**.[32]

The presacral fascia covers the median and lateral sacral artery, presacral venous plexus and the sympathetic trunk. The presacral venous plexus is formed from two lateral sacral veins, median sacral vein. Horizontally placed communicating veins connect these two longitudinal venous systems forming a stair-like pattern.[32,33] "Coronal safe zone" was defined by Yuan et al. as the distance (6–6.9 cm) between medial margins of right and left internal iliac vessels.[34] Sacral nerves as they exit bilaterally from the neural foramina can be avoided if the approach remains strictly midline under biplanar fluoroscopy. However, no area in this "coronal safe zone" is safe if presacral fascia is breached during dissection. This can injure the valveless, presacral venous plexus and cause torrential, uncontrollable bleeding.[32]

The existence of rectosacral fascia is controversial and some consider it as an artefact of fascial adhesions as it has been shown to be highly variable in thickness. This fascia divides the presacral space into inferior and superior portions.[35] The surgical plane for the trajectory lies between the rectosacral fascia and the presacral fascia in lower presacral space and between autonomic nerve fascia and presacral fascia in the upper presacral space.

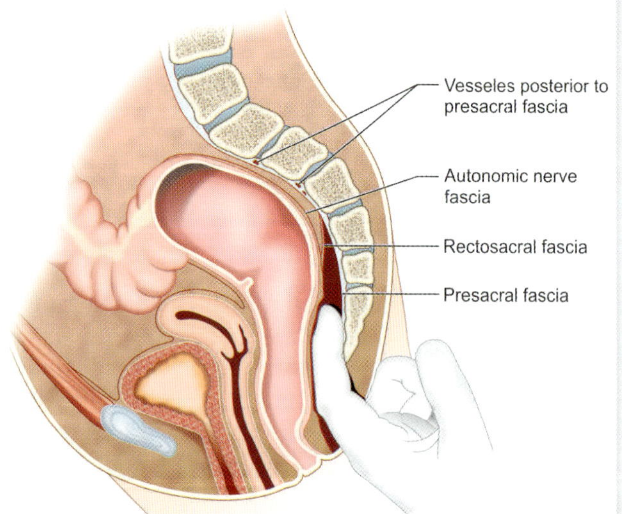

Figure 15: Anatomy of presacral fascial structures

The autonomic nerve fascia covers the inferior hypogastric plexus that is a paired structure closely adherent to either side of the rectum.[28] Contributions to this plexus include: the hypogastric nerve from the superior hypogastric plexus, sacral splanchnic nerves and the pelvic splanchnic nerves. Branches of the inferior hypogastric plexus innervate the pelvic viscera. The sacral splanchnic nerves (sympathetic) stimulate contraction of smooth muscles in the internal urethral sphincter in men, and internal anal sphincter in men and women. They also influence smooth muscle contraction in the reproductive tract and their accessory glands. Contractions in the epididymis and other glands move secretions into the urethra to form semen during ejaculation. The pelvic splanchnic nerves or nervi erigentes (parasympathetic) originate from the anterior branches of S2–S4 and pierce the presacral fascia and join the inferior hypogastric plexus that is in close proximity to the rectum. They regulate emptying of the bladder, stimulate erection and influence motility of the rectum.

Yuan et al. and Guvencer et al. described the "sagittal safe zone" as the distance between the anterior sacral margin and the rectum (width of the mesorectum) with the hope that enough distance as measured on MRI would prevent rectal injury.[34,36] However, wider presacral space on MRI may not necessarily be safe, as it may be an indicator of some rectal disorder.[37] The sagittal safe zone is probably the maximum allowable anterior mobilization of the rectum that dissection in the presacral space allows. Cadaveric study by Li et al. found that the pelvic splanchnic nerves are the main structures that limit the anterior mobilization of the rectum.[32] Excessive anterior mobilization of the rectum can result in stretch injury of the pelvic splanchnic nerves and result in sexual and urinary dysfunction.

VIDEO-ASSISTED THORACOSCOPIC APPROACH

Thoracoscopy involves using a 30° endoscope inserted into the thoracic cavity for magnified visualization and illumination. This technique utilizes small portals (keyhole incisions) for the endoscope as well as the working channels for specialized instruments. Mack et al. was the first surgeon to use VATS for spinal disorders.[38] Since then, VATS has been used for treatment of a variety of spinal disorders.

Indications

- Herniated thoracic disk[39]
- Anterior release and instrumented correction of thoracic scoliosis[40]

- Tuberculosis of thoracic spine.[41]
- Thoracic sympathectomies.[42]
- Fracture of thoracic vertebra.[43]
- Resection of tumors of the thoracic spine.[44]

Contraindications

- A calcified thoracic disk herniation is a relative contraindication
- Patients who are unable to tolerate one lung ventilation, such as patients with severe cardiopulmonary compromise or acute lung injury.
- Three column injury or spinal dislocation.

Advantages

- Keyhole access and hence truly minimally invasive
- Direct vision of the pathology. 30º scope provides an extended vision.
- Multi-segmental pathologies can be addressed without extending or widening the surgical approach.
- Less disruption of anatomy. Access is gained without sacrificing the rib.
- Less postoperative pain, less blood loss, and quicker rehabilitation
- Cosmetic scars result in higher patient satisfaction.

Disadvantages

- Technically demanding procedure that requires thoracoscopic training.
- Challenging learning curve and a long time is required to achieve proficiency.
- Trauma to surrounding viscera and vascular structures can result in serious, life-threatening injury.
- Depth perception and manipulation of instrumentation is difficult as endoscope provides a 2D view of the chest cavity.
- Single lung ventilation requires special medical and anesthetic care during surgery.

Surgical Approach (Video-assisted Thoracoscopic approach)

Preoperative imaging includes X-rays, MRI and if required a CT scan. Imaging is mandatory to study the vascular and visceral anatomy in relation to the lesion being treated. Pulmonary function test is used to assess whether the patient can tolerate single-lung ventilation. The patient is positioned in a lateral decubitus position under general anesthesia and is securely taped down to prevent motion during surgery. The side of approach usually is dependent on the position of the great vessels in relation to the lesion and as to be decided on preoperative imaging. The surgeon usually stands on the abdominal side with the assistant standing on the dorsal side of the patient. The equipment around the patient is arranged as per the figure. Image intensifier is used to accurately identify the lesion. Orthogonal X-rays need to be obtained so that any parallax in imaging in eliminated. The correct placement of the portals is extremely crucial.

The first portal is the optical (endoscope portal) **(Figures 16 and 17)**. A small 15 mm incision is made in the posterior axillary line, two to three intercostal spaces cranial to the targeted lesion. If the lesion is in the upper thoracic spine then the optical portal is placed caudal to the lesion. The muscles are split in the direction of their fibres and a hemostat is used to enter the thoracic cavity. A flexible trocar of appropriate size is inserted, followed by the 30º endoscope. A visual inspection of the thoracic cavity is made. The subsequent portals are placed under direct vision of the endoscope. The working portal is centered over the targeted lesion **(Figures 16 and 17)**. The suction/irrigation portal is placed 5–10 cm anterior to the optical and working portal (near the anterior axillary line). If required, a fourth portal for a fan retractor to retract the lung or diaphragm can similarly be placed **(Figure 17)**.

Further steps are similar to an open approach. However, to achieve this requires deft manipulation of specialized instruments. The principle is to never perform a step blind, without adequate visualization using an endoscope. Controlling the segmental vessels using vascular clips is the key to a clean, blood-less operative field **(Figure 18)**. Diaphragm may need to be opened for access below the T12 level. Care must be taken to suture it back to prevent herniation of abdominal contents. After the procedure, the lung is inflated and a chest tube is placed under endoscopic guidance.

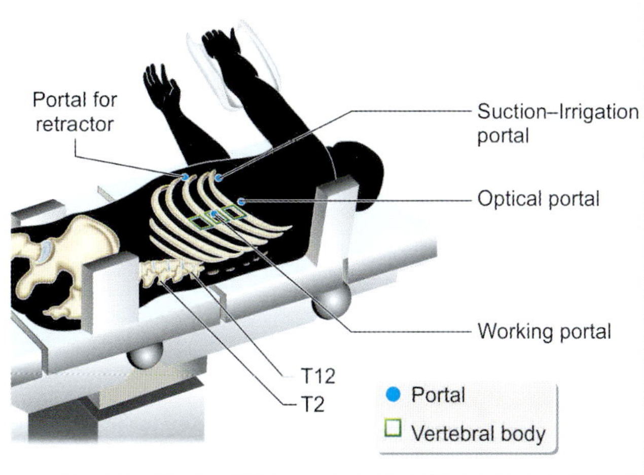

Figure 16: Positioning and portals in VATS

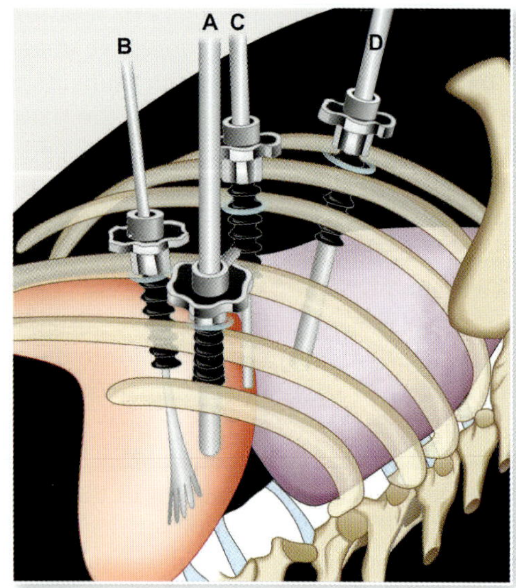

Figure 17: Centering of portals over targeted area

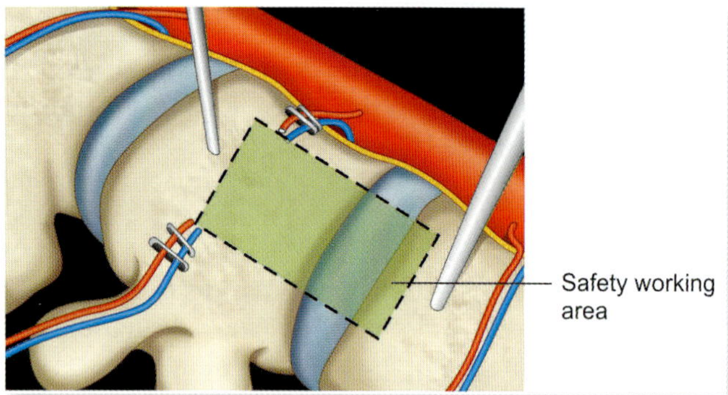

Figure 18: Working area

EXTREME LATERAL MINITHORACOTOMY APPROACH

Minithoracotomy is an approach that uses the same principles as the lateral transpsoas approach to achieve exposure of the anterior thoracic spine. A direct access is achieved using sequential dilators and a table-mounted retractor system that is similar to XLIF or DLIF approach.

Indications are similar to open thoracotomy approaches for lesion from T4 to T12/L1.

Contraindications

- Previous thoracotomy in the area
- Preexisting lung condition that compromises pulmonary function
- Large, obese patients are relative contraindication as the working depth is increased substantially.

Advantages

- Reduce collateral damage to normal anatomy and early recovery.
- Single-lung ventilation is not mandatory.
- 3D, direct vision of the pathological anatomy. A microscope provides excellent illumination and magnification
- Injury to intercostal nerves is less likely.
- Usually no rib resection is required. If require it can be limited to a small length of the rib.[45]
- Reduced risk of post thoracotomy intercostalgia.[45]

Disadvantages

- Multilevel access may require multiple intercostal approaches unlike thoracoscopic surgery
- As compared to open thoracotomy, a direct lateral approach involves a deep working field, making manipulation of instruments tricky.
- The retractor blades can injure surrounding viscera or vascular structures.
- Learning is steep, although does not require adjustment to triangulation as needed in thoracoscopic surgery.

SURGICAL APPROACH (EXTREME LATERAL MINITHORACOTOMY)

As in the VATS approach, preoperative imaging is crucial to determine the relative anatomy of the vessels and viscera with respect the intended line of approach. The patient is secured to the operative table in a 90° lateral decubitus position. Upper thoracic lesions (T6 and above) a right sided approach may be preferable due to the presence of arch of aorta on the left side. For mid and lower thoracic lesions, left sided approach may be easier because it is easier to handle aorta than the thin-walled vena cava. However, the exact location and side of the pathology finally decides the surgical approach.

Perfect orthogonal X-rays (end-on view of endplates and spinous process in the midline) are mandatory to plan the surgical incision. The incision is made directly over the targeted lesion. Rib resection is optional. Pleural is open gently without injuring the underlying lung. Blunt finger dissection is carried out to break any adhesions if present. Long hand-held retractors can be used to retract the lung or diaphragm. The lateral aspect of the thoracic spine is visualized directly. K wires should not be used in the thoracic spine because they can cause serious injury. Instead the smallest dilator is placed directly over the targeted disc space. Sequential dilators are used, followed by placement of the retractor. Radiographic confirmation of the level is mandatory at all stages of establishing a surgical corridor. The lung may tend to creep between the blades of the retractor and can be packed away using tagged sponges for easy retrieval. Special shims are available that can extend the width of the retractor blades to achieve similar retraction. The surgery can be performed using a microscope or head-light with loupes. Henceforth, the surgical steps are similar to open thoracotomy. Bayonetted instruments can be used to execute these steps. Closure of the thoracotomy after placement of an intercostal drain.

APPLIED ANATOMY OF THE THORACIC CAVITY

A thorough knowledge of thoracic cavity is essential to perform the thoracoscopic and mini thoracotomy approach.

The muscles of the chest wall are broadly divided into two groups. The intrinsic muscles (e.g. intercostals, serratus posterior, etc.) originate and insert on the chest wall. The extrinsic muscles (e.g. trapezius, latissimus dorsi, pectorales major, etc.) connect the upper limb with the chest wall.

The anterior and posterior axillary lines are guidelines for trocar placement in thoracoscopic surgery. The anterior axillary line is formed by the lateral border of the pectoralis major, whereas the posterior axillary line is formed by the lateral border of the latissimus dorsi. The serratus anterior muscle forms the medial wall of the axilla.

The parietal pleura covers the inner walls of the chest cavity as well as the great vessels, trachea, esophagus, and the spinal column. External to the pleura is a thin layer of loose connective tissue, the endothoracic fascia, analogous to the transversalis fascia of the abdominal wall. Due to this, the parietal pleural can be easily separated from the chest wall by blunt dissection.

The visceral pleura encases the lung and cannot be distinguished from the lung. It also continues into the fissures between lobes of lung. The right lung is composed of three lobes and the left lung has two lobes. There are one to two fissures within the lobes as well.

Mediastinum is bounded laterally by the lungs, anteriorly by sternum and posteriorly by thoracic vertebral column. A pericardial sac envelops the heart. The thoracic aorta can be divided into the ascending aorta, arch of aorta and the descending aorta. Only the arch of aorta is in the superior mediastinum. Hence, right side is preferred for high thoracic spine approaches. The relationship of the descending aorta with the spinal column can vary and sometimes it is quite laterally placed interfering with the exposure of the spine.

The diaphragm is a musculotendinous dome that separates thoracic and abdominal cavities. The diaphragm has three parts: sternal, costal and lumbar. The sternal part arises from posterior aspect of xiphoid process. The costal part arises from inner surface of lower six costal cartilage and adjoining ribs. The lumbar part arises from two

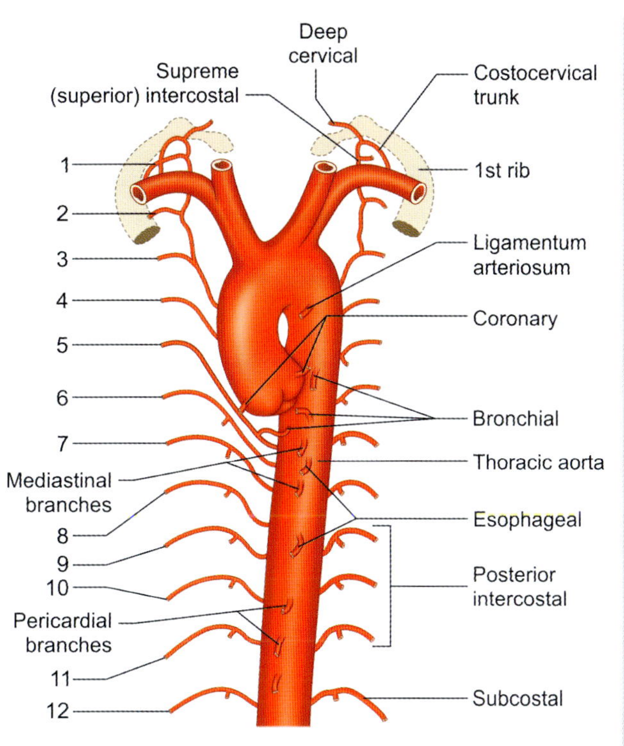

Figure 19: Anatomy of intercostal arteries

aponeurotic arches (medial and lateral arcuate ligaments) and upper lumbar vertebral bodies via two crura. All these muscle fibres converge towards a central tendon. There are three large openings, for the aorta, esophagus and inferior vena cava. The aortic hiatus formed by the median arcuate ligament is located at T12. During expiration the diaphragm can rise up to 4-5th rib. This should be considered during trocar placement to avoid perforating the diaphragm.

There are eleven pairs of posterior intercostal arteries **(Figures 19 and 20)**. The first two arise from the superior intercostal artery which is a branch of costocervical trunk. The other nine arise directly from the aorta. The intercostal vessels are found running across the middle of the vertebral body. Then they travel along the intercostal groove that is on the inner inferior border of the rib. Each artery has a vein above and a nerve below except in the upper spaces where nerve lies above the artery.

The posterior intercostal veins accompany the arteries along their course. The first posterior intercostal veins on both sides ascends near the neck of the first rib and arches above the pleural dome to drain into the brachiocephalic vein **(Figure 21)**. The second and third (sometimes fourth) posterior intercostal vein joins to form the superior intercostal vein. The left superior intercostal vein ascends across the left side aortic arch, lateral to the vagus and medial to the phrenic nerve and drains into the left brachiocephalic vein. The right superior intercostal vein

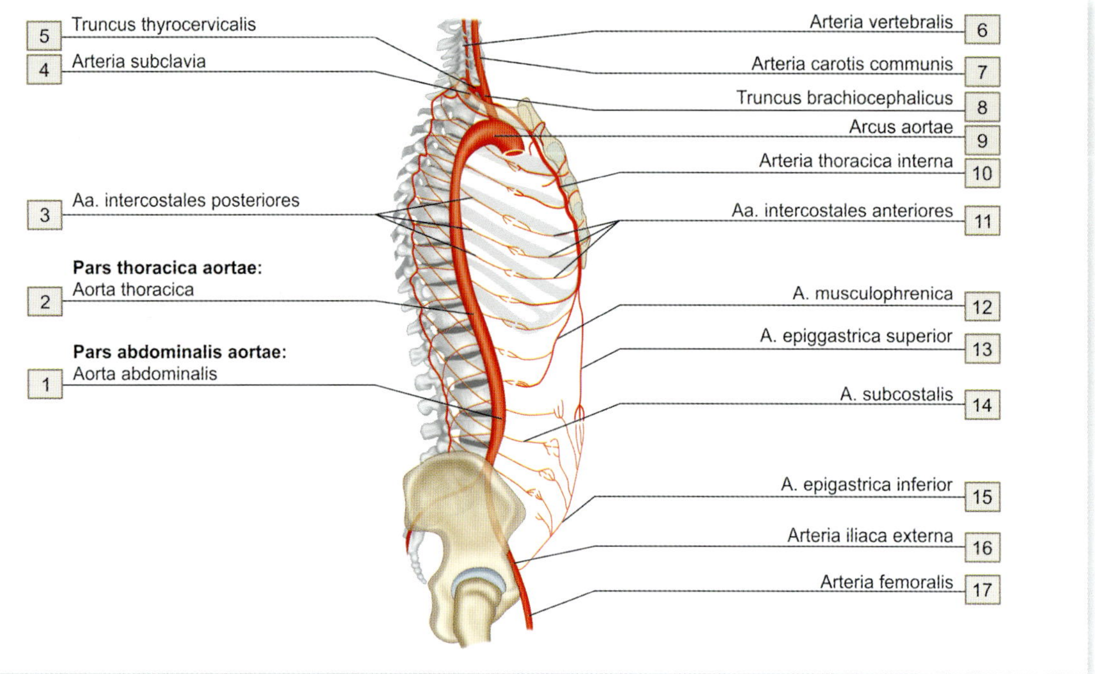

Figure 20: The anatomy of major arterial trunk

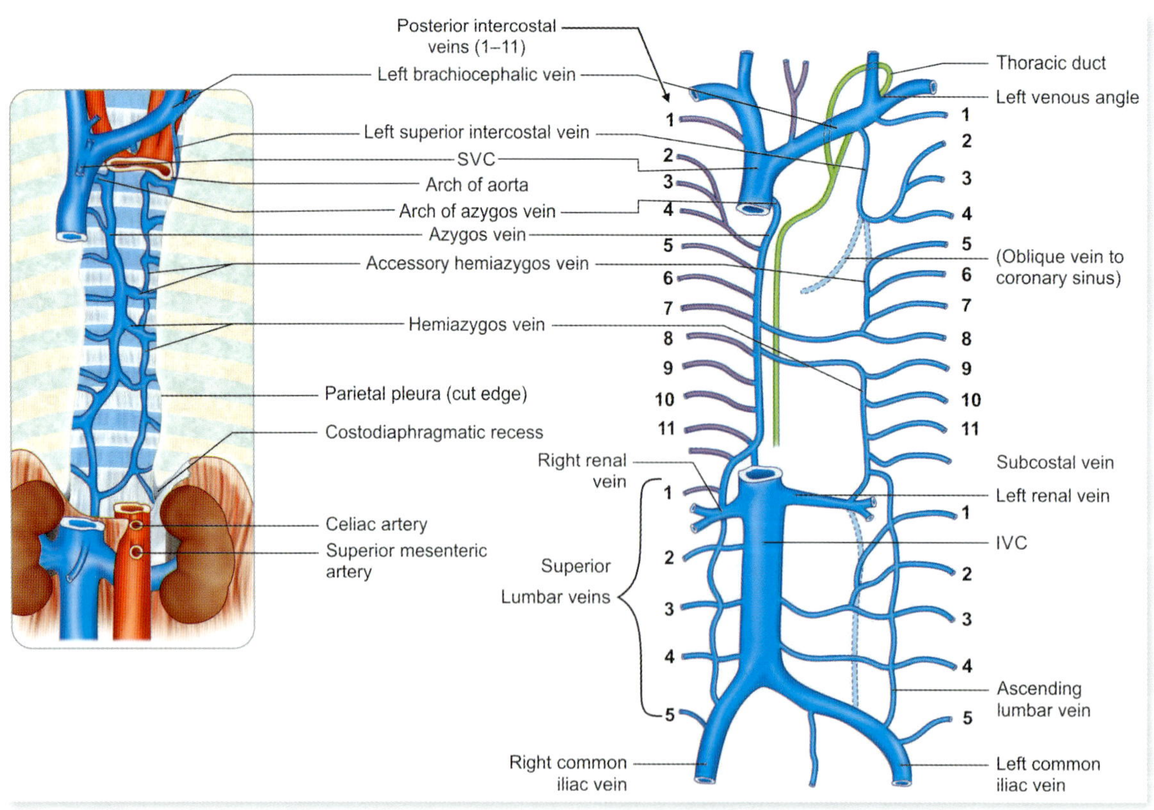

Figure 21: The anatomy of major veins and branches

joins the arch of azygos vein. The remaining right posterior intercostal veins drain directly into the azygos vein. The left posterior intercostal veins from fourth or fifth to eighth intercostal spaces drain in the accessory hemiazygos vein, and veins from the ninth to the eleventh intercostal spaces drain into the hemiazygos vein. The accessory hemiazygos vein joins the azygos vein behind the esophagus at the level of T8. The hemiazygos vein joins the azygos vein behind the oesophagus at the level of T9.

The thoracic sympathetic chain contains 11–12 ganglia (rarely 10 or 13).[46] Except for the second and lowest two or three, the thoracic ganglia lie against the rib heads, posterior to the parietal pleura. The second thoracic sympathetic ganglion is commonly located in the second intercostal space, and the lowest two or three ganglia lie lateral to the bodies of the corresponding vertebrae. The sympathetic trunk is a fundamental part of the sympathetic nervous system, part of the autonomic nervous system.

The phrenic nerve is a mixed nerve. It is the sole motor supply to the diaphragm. It carries sensations from mediastinal pleura and pericardium. Within the thorax, the phrenic nerve descends anterior to the pulmonary hilum between the fibrous pericardium and mediastinal pleura.

There are 12 thoracic vertebrae that articulate with corresponding ribs. A typical thoracic vertebra has three sites for articulation with the ribs. A rib articulates with the transverse process costal facet and the superior demifacet of the corresponding vertebra and the inferior demifacet of the caudal vertebra. This the rib head straddles the thoracic disk. The 1st, 10th, 11th and 12th ribs articulate with a single vertebra and the 11th and 12th rib do not have costotransverse articulation. Radiate ligament hold the rib head firmly to the adjacent vertebral body and the annulus. The pedicle lies deep to the rib and can be visualized once the rib head is excised. This is an important landmark to be identified to gain access to the spinal canal.

Anterior Cervical Foraminotomy

Anterior cervical foraminotomy is a minimally invasive approach that utilizes either a microscope or an endoscope to decompress the nerve via unilateral resection of the the uncovertebral joint without damaging the adjacent disk. It still lacks universal appeal, as literature is limited to few retrospective case series.

Indications

- Unilateral radiculopathy secondary to one or two level lesion that has failed conservative therapy.
- Radiographic evidence of intraforaminal compression either due to a disc fragment or spondylotic spurs.

Contraindications

- Cervical myelopathy
- Bilateral radiculopathy
- Predominant neck pain syndrome
- Radiographic central canal stenosis or segmental instability
- Dorsal cause of foraminal nerve root compression e.g. facet arthropathy.

Advantages

- Minimally invasive approach with shorter operative times and quicker recovery
- Motion preserving surgery
- Avoid fusion and graft-related complications (implant failure, nonunions and adjacent segment disease)
- Direct removal of compression with least handling of nerve root compared to posterior foraminotomy approach.

Disadvantages

- Risk if injury to the vertebral artery. Preoperative vertebral artery evaluation is mandatory using MRI/CT. Risk is maximum while removal of C6-7 disk.[47] Risk is higher if variations of course of vertebral artery occur. If the vertebral artery enters the transverse foramen through C4 or C5 instead of C6, it may be injured while lateral exposure of the cervical spine.[48] Thus, knowing the course preoperatively helps in avoiding such complications.
- Technically demanding and involves a learning curve especially if endoscope is used.
- Bilateral decompression and multilevel decompression is not possible.
- Concomitant central stenosis cannot be addressed.
- Spinal instability and collapse of the neural foramen due to excessive removal of uncinate process.
- Risk of Horner's syndrome.[49]

Surgical Procedure

First described by Jho et al. and later modified bi saringer and Jho himself.[47,50-52] Preoperative imaging involves AP, lateral and oblique X-rays to evaluate the foramen. MRI scan and occasionally CT scan is required to study the local anatomy. The patient is positioned supine, similar to conventional ACDF approach. The side of the foraminotomy decides the side of the surgical approach. It is important to localize the skin incision using lateral fluoroscopy. The surgical approach, too is similar to the

ACDF approach. A transverse 3 cm incision is made just medial the sternocleidomastoid and platysma a cut in line with the incision. The layer beneath the platysma is undermined. The deep investing layer of fascia is dissected bluntly and a surgical plane between the medial visceral structures (trachea and esophagus) and lateral vascular structures (carotid sheath) is entered. Dissection is limited to the mid portion of the vertebral body. The longus colli is exposed and is transversely cut at the level of the intended foraminotomy after reconfirming the level radiographically. A special retractor system is used that uses a medial screw anchor in the vertebral body and a lateral blade to retract the longus colli laterally. The vertebral artery is not intentionally exposed. The uncovertebral joint is now exposed **(Figure 22)**. The uncus is burred down using a 2 mm burr keeping the lateral wall of the uncus intact to protect the vertebral artery. The posterior cortical bone and posterior part of the lateral wall of the uncus is remove using a diamond burr. Spondylotic spurs and soft tissue overlying the nerve can be removed using a 2-mm Kerrison rongeur. Foraminal disk herniation, if present, can be removed using a microhook. The disk fragment is found in the axilla of the nerve root. Epidural bleeding may be encountered while removal of the disk fragment and is controlled by combination of gelfoam and bipolar cauterization. Nerve root should be now completely visualized from its origin to its exit out of the foramen. The retractor is removed, platysma and skin are closed in layers.

Applied Anatomy

Knowledge of fascial anatomy of the neck is important to understand the anterior cervical approach. The fascia of the neck is divided into superficial layer and four deep layers. The superficial layer consists of the subcutaneous fat and the platysma muscle. The superficial layer of the deep cervical fascia is the investing layer that envelopes the sternocleidomastoid anteriorly. The middle cervical fascia envelopes the strap muscles and the pretracheal fascia, the thyroid gland. The carotid sheath encloses the carotid artery, internal jugular vein and the vagus nerve. The deepest layer is the prevertebral fascia that covers the anterior longitudinal ligament, longus colli and the scaleni muscles.

The platysma is a thin subcutaneous muscle that depresses the lower jaw and the lip. The sternocleidomastoid originates from the medial clavicle and the manubrium and inserts on the mastoid process. The strap muscles mainly function to control the movement of the hyoid and the larynx. The longus colli originates from the anterior aspect of the vertebral bodies from C1 to T3 and inserts to the anterior tubercles of the transverse processes of C3–6. The longus capitis originates from the basilar portion of the occipital bone to be inserted onto the anterior tubercles of the transverse processes of C3–6.

The inferior surface of the vertebral body is convex in the coronal plane and concave in the sagittal plane and the reverse is true for its superior surface. Thus, two projections are created on either side of the superior surface called the uncus. These uncal processes project upward and articulate with the inferolateral border of the cephalad vertebra from the joint of Luschka.

At transverse process of the subaxial cervical vertebrae have a foramen called the foramen transversarium. The vertebral artery and vein passes through this foramen, except at the C7 level where the vertebral artery passes from outside the foramen. The anterior tubercle of the C6 is called the Chassaignac tubercle and is easily palpable.

The neural foramina are bounded by the uncovertebral joints and the adjacent disk anteriorly and by the facet joint posteriorly. Superior and inferiorly it is bound by the pedicles.

The relationship of the vertebral artery with the uncus is crucial in this approach **(Figure 23)**. The vertebral artery lies just lateral to the uncinate process, just anterior to the nerve root. It is in line with the middle third of the vertebral body. At the C7, it lies outside the foramen transversarium

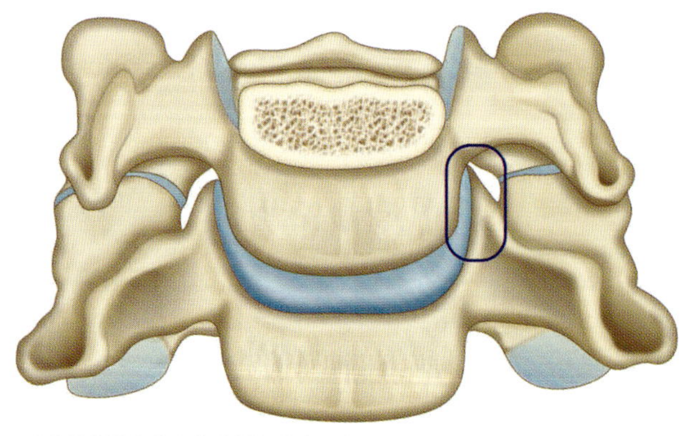

Figure 22: Uncovertebral joint

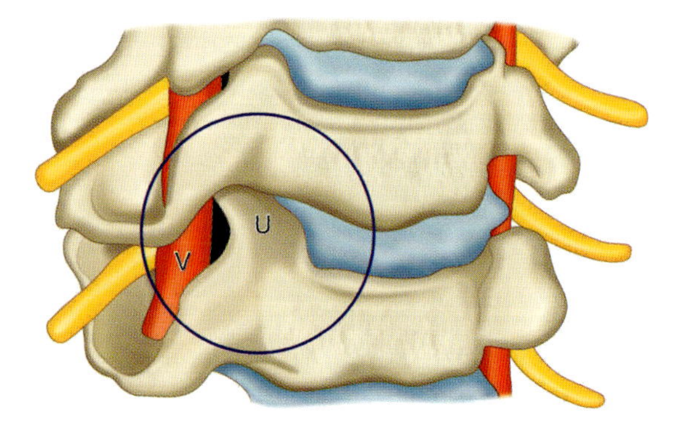

Figure 23: Relationship of vertebral artery with uncus

and is prone to injury here esp while removal of C6–7 disk. In 2%, the artery may enter at C7. The artery may also enter above C6 in 8% of the patients. It may enter at C5 (5%), C4 (2%) and C3 (1%).[53]

Posterior Cervical Foraminotomy

Minimally invasive posterior cervical foraminotomy utilizes microscopic or microendoscopic access via tubular retractor systems. Adamson et al. first described this approach in 2001 using the endoscope.[54] Holly et al. and Hilton in 2007 used the microscope through tubular retractors for posterior cervical foraminotomy.[55,56]

Indications

- Cervical radiculopathy unresponsive to conservative care with foraminal stenosis or foraminal disk herniation as the cause of the radiculopathy
- One or two level, unilateral disease is the best indication; however, multilevel and bilateral pathologies can also be potentially treated with this technique.

Contraindication

- Spinal cord compression with or without symptomatic myelopathy
- Central disc herniation
- Spondylolisthesis or segmental instability

Advantages

- Minimally invasive approach that preserves the posterior musculature of the cervical spine
- Reduced morbidity and early recovery.[57]
- Motion preserving as compared to anterior cervical fusion. Also avoid complications related to anterior cervical approach.
- Outcome comparable to open surgery.[58]

Disadvantages

- Multilevel and bilateral pathologies cannot be easily access and are technically demanding
- Postoperative exacerbation of neck pain is a possibility
- Cannot address patient with concomitant spinal cord compression or myelopathy.

Surgical Procedure

MRI and/or CT scan is used to study the foraminal anatomy. Dynamic radiographs are used to assess instability. The patient is position prone using a Mayfield skull clamp. The neck should be slightly flexed to ease the exposure and decompression. The correct level is determined using lateral fluoroscopy using spinal needle. A paramedian incision is made and the smallest dilator is advanced to the intended level under image guidance. The dilators should not be advanced on K wires in the cervical spine as inadvertent migration can occur. Sequential dilators are used followed by a tubular retractor that is usually 16–18 mm in diameter. Head light with loupe magnification or microscope is required. The view through the retractor should include the medial half of the facet joint along with the adjacent interlaminar space **(Figure 24)**.

A burr is used to remove the medial part of the inferior facet along with some portion of the hemilamina. Care should be taken not to remove more than 50% of the facet joint. This exposes the superior facet and this is thinned down to its inner cortex. The inner cortex is then removed with either a 1mm Kerrison or a small curette. This completes the foraminotomy **(Figure 25)**. The pedicles of both vertebrae are now palpated. The nerve root is exposed. The nerve root can be retracted cranially to identify and excise the herniated portion of the disc **(Figure 26)**. Hemostasis is achieved using bipolar cautery. Closure is performed in layers.

Applied Anatomy

Posterior cervical musculature is can be anatomically divided into three groups: superficial, intermediate and deep. Trapezius is part of the superficial group is responsible for the movement of the shoulder girdle. The intermediate layer is formed by the splenius capitis and splenius cervicis. These originate from the spinous processes of cervicothoracic vertebra and insert into the transverse

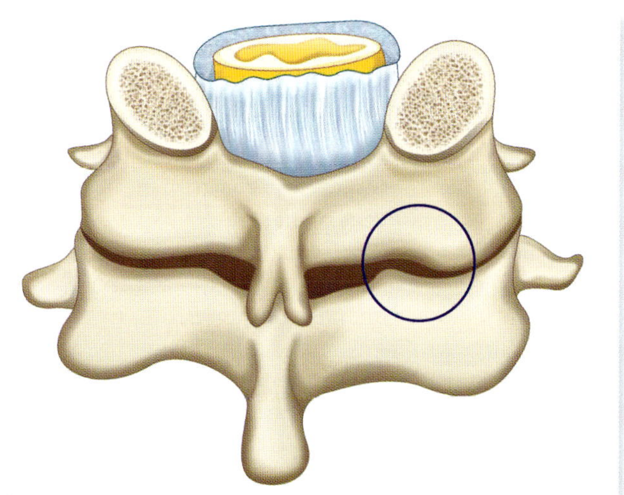

Figure 24: Exposure through the tubular retractor

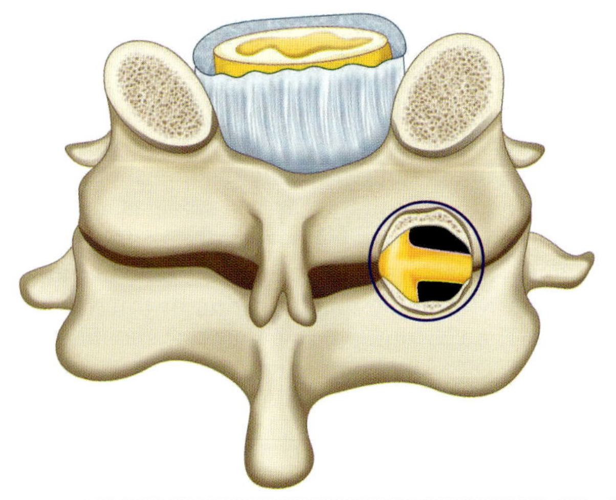

Figure 25: Foraminotomy window

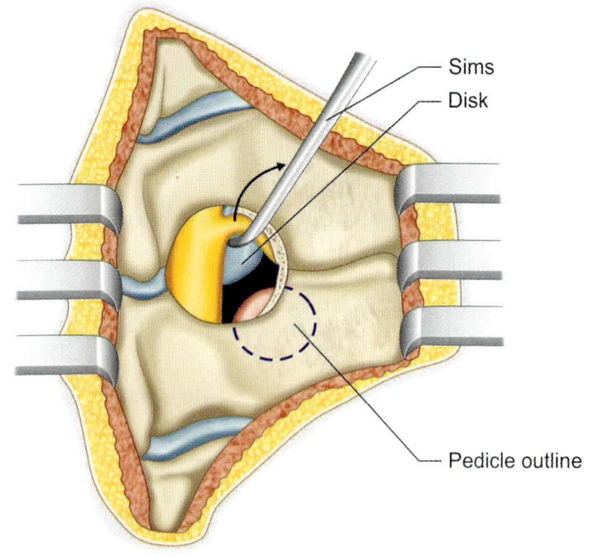

Figure 26: Root retracted cranially and disk excised

processes of upper cervical vertebrae and the occipital base. Deep layer contains the superficial and deep erector spinae group of muscles. These muscles along with the ligamentum nuchae form a strong tension band and are very important to maintain the lordotic cervical spine alignment.

The cervical nerve roots exit the spinal canal through the intervertebral foramen. As the nerve roots exit, they are situated in a grove that extended from the medial border of the pedicle to the lateral border of the transverse process where it is bound by the anterior and posterior tubercles. This groove can be divided into three zones: medial zone (pedicle), middle zone (vertebral artery) and the lateral zone. In the medial zone, the nerve root lies superior to the pedicle of the caudal vertebra, posterolateral to the uncinate process and anterolateral to the medial part of the superior articular process. In the middle zone, the nerve root is posterior to the vertebral artery as it passes through the foramen transversarii and anterior to the lateral part of the superior articular process. In the lateral zone it lies between the anterior and posterior tubercle of the transverse process.[59]

The shape of the intervertebral foramen (medial zone) is like a funnel with the narrow end medial, while the radicular dural sheath is conical with a wider medial part (origin from the dural sac). Hence, nerve root compression mostly occurs in the entrance zone of the intervertebral foramen.[60]

The medial zone of the groove corresponds to the intervertebral foramen and is clinically most important as pathological processes that cause nerve root compression are found here. Nerve root compression from the anterior aspect can be caused by protruded disks and uncovertebral osteophytes. Superior articular process arthrosis and ligamentum flavum hypertrophy can caused nerve root compression from the posterior aspect. Posterior cervical foraminotomy involves removing the portion of the superior articular process and the adjacent ligamentum flavum to de-roof the intervertebral foramen up to the lateral border of the pedicle. Therefore, if one can pass a small probe and can feel the lateral border of the pedicle then the decompression is sufficient and further facet resection is not need. In fact facet resection beyond this point can result in instability.

REFERENCES

1. D. Greg Anderson, Chadi Tannoury. Patient Selection for Minimally Invasive Spinal Surgery. In: A. Vaccaro, C. Bono. Minimally Invasive Spine Surgery. New york: Informa Healthcare; 2007. p 25-32.
2. Bustami FM. A new description of the lumbar erector spinae muscle in man. J Anat. Wiley-Blackwell; 1986;144:81-91.
3. Macintosh JE, Bogduk N. 1987 Volvo award in basic science. The morphology of the lumbar erector spinae. Spine. 1987;12(7):658-68.
4. Wiltse LL, Bateman JG, Hutchinson RH, Nelson WE. The paraspinal sacrospinalis-splitting approach to the lumbar spine. Journal of Bone and Joint Surgery. 1968;50(5):919-26.
5. Palmer DK, Allen JL, Williams PA, Voss AE, Jadhav V, Wu DS, et al. Multilevel magnetic resonance imaging analysis of multifidus-longissimus cleavage planes in the lumbar spine and potential clinical applications to Wiltse's paraspinal approach. Spine. 2011;36(16):1263-7.
6. Vialle R, Court C, Khouri N, Olivier E, Miladi L, Tassin JL, et al. Anatomical study of the paraspinal approach to the lumbar spine. Eur Spine J. 2004;14(4):366-71.
7. Berjano P, Balsano M, Buric J, Petruzzi M, Lamartina C. Direct lateral access lumbar and thoracolumbar fusion: preliminary results. Eur Spine J. Springer-Verlag; 2012;21(S1):37-42.

8. Ozgur BM, Agarwal V, Nail E, Pimenta L. Two-year clinical and radiographic success of minimally invasive lateral transpsoas approach for the treatment of degenerative lumbar conditions. SAS Journal. 2010;4(2):41-6.
9. Castro C, Oliveira L, Amaral R, Marchi L, Pimenta L. Is the lateral transpsoas approach feasible for the treatment of adult degenerative scoliosis? Clin Orthop Relat Res. 2014;472(6):1776-83.
10. Kepler CK, Sharma AK, Huang RC, Meredith DS, Girardi FP, Cammisa FP, et al. Indirect foraminal decompression after lateral transpsoas interbody fusion. Journal of Neurosurgery: Spine. American Association of Neurological Surgeons; 2012;16(4):329-33.
11. Leary SP, Regan JJ, Lanman TH, Wagner WH. Revision and explantation strategies involving the CHARITE lumbar artificial disc replacement. Spine. 2007;32(9):1001-11.
12. Bergey DL, Villavicencio AT, Goldstein T, Regan JJ. Endoscopic lateral transpsoas approach to the lumbar spine. Spine. 2004;29(15):1681-8.
13. Benglis DM, Vanni S, Levi AD. An anatomical study of the lumbosacral plexus as related to the minimally invasive transpsoas approach to the lumbar spine. Journal of Neurosurgery: Spine. American Association of Neurological Surgeons; 2009;10(2):139-44.
14. Voyadzis J-M, Felbaum D, Rhee J. The rising psoas sign: an analysis of preoperative imaging characteristics of aborted minimally invasive lateral interbody fusions at L4-5. Journal of Neurosurgery: Spine. American Association of Neurological Surgeons; 2014;20(5):531-7.
15. Glassman SD, Carreon LY, Djurasovic M, Dimar JR, Johnson JR, Puno RM, et al. Lumbar fusion outcomes stratified by specific diagnostic indication. Spine J. Elsevier; 2009;9(1):13-21.
16. Kepler CK, Bogner EA, Herzog RJ, Huang RC. Anatomy of the psoas muscle and lumbar plexus with respect to the surgical approach for lateral transpsoas interbody fusion. Eur Spine J. 2011;20(4):550-6.
17. Uribe JS, Arredondo N, Dakwar E, Vale FL. Defining the safe working zones using the minimally invasive lateral retroperitoneal transpsoas approach: an anatomical study. Journal of Neurosurgery: Spine. American Association of Neurological Surgeons. 2010;13(2):260-6.
18. Moro T, Kikuchi S-I, Konno S-I, Yaginuma H. An anatomic study of the lumbar plexus with respect to retroperitoneal endoscopic surgery. Spine. 2003;28(5):423-8–discussion 427-8.
19. Mayer HM. A new microsurgical technique for minimally invasive anterior lumbar interbody fusion. Spine. 1997;22(6):691-9 discussion 700.
20. Liu JC, Ondra SL, Angelos P, Ganju A, Landers ML. Is laparoscopic anterior lumbar interbody fusion a useful minimally invasive procedure? Neurosurgery. 2002;51(5 Suppl):S155-8.
21. Zdeblick TA, David SM. A prospective comparison of surgical approach for anterior L4-L5 fusion: laparoscopic versus mini anterior lumbar interbody fusion. Spine. 2000;25(20):2682-7.
22. Aryan HE, Acosta FL, Ames CP. The Charité Artificial Disc: insertion technique. Neurosurgery Clinics of North America. 2005;16(4):637-50–vii.
23. Barrey C, Ene B, Louis-Tisserand G, Montagna P, Perrin G, Simon E. Vascular anatomy in the lumbar spine investigated by three-dimensional computed tomography angiography: the concept of vascular window. World Neurosurgery. Elsevier; 2013;79(5-6):784-91.
24. Maeng DH, Kim S-Y, Lee S-H, Jang J-S. Venovertebral vein: morphometric analysis and significance for the transabdominal spine surgeon. Journal of Spinal Disorders and Techniques. 2007;20(8):582-5.
25. Nalbandian MM, Hoashi JS, Errico TJ. Variations in the iliolumbar vein during the anterior approach for spinal procedures. Spine. 2013;38(8):E445-50.
26. Garg J, Woo K, Hirsch J, Bruffey JD, Dilley RB. Vascular complications of exposure for anterior lumbar interbody fusion. J Vasc Surg. Elsevier; 2010;51(4):946-50 discussion 950.
27. Zaitouna M, Alsaid B, Diallo D, Benoit G, Bessede T. Identification of the origin of adrenergic and cholinergic nerve fibers within the superior hypogastric plexus of the human fetus. J Anat. 2013;223(1):14-21.
28. Lu S, Xu Y-Q, Chang S, Zhang Y-Z, Shi J-H, Ding Z-H, et al. Clinical anatomy study of autonomic nerve with respective to the anterior approach lumbar surgery. Surg Radiol Anat. Springer-Verlag; 2009;31(6):425-30.
29. Comer GC, Smith MW, Hurwitz EL, Mitsunaga KA, Kessler R, Carragee EJ. Retrograde ejaculation after anterior lumbar interbody fusion with and without bone morphogenetic protein-2 augmentation: a 10-year cohort controlled study. Spine J. Elsevier; 2012;12(10):881-90.
30. Cragg A, Carl A, Casteneda F, Dickman C, Guterman L, Oliveira C. New percutaneous access method for minimally invasive anterior lumbosacral surgery. Journal of Spinal Disorders and Techniques. 2004;17(1):21-8.
31. Kaiser AM, Ortega AE. Anorectal anatomy. Surg Clin North Am. 2002;82(6):1125-38–v.
32. Li X, Zhang Y, Hou Z, Wu T, Ding Z. The Relevant Anatomy of the Approach for Axial Lumbar Interbody Fusion. Spine. 2012;37(4):266-71.
33. Baqué P, Karimdjee B, Iannelli A, Benizri E, Rahili A, Benchimol D, et al. Anatomy of the presacral venous plexus: implications for rectal surgery. Surg Radiol Anat. 2004;26(5):355-8.
34. Yuan PS, Day TF, Albert TJ, Morrison WB, Pimenta L, Cragg A, et al. Anatomy of the percutaneous presacral space for a novel fusion technique. Journal of Spinal Disorders and Techniques. 2006;19(4):237-41.
35. García-Armengol J, García-Botello S, Martinez-Soriano F, Roig JV, Lledó S. Review of the anatomic concepts in relation to the retrorectal space and endopelvic fascia: Waldeyer's fascia and the rectosacral fascia. Colorectal Dis. Blackwell Publishing Ltd; 2008;10(3):298-302.
36. Güvençer M, Dalbayrak S, Tayefi H, Tetik S, Yılmaz M, Erginoğlu U, et al. Surgical anatomy of the presacral area. Surg Radiol Anat. 2008;31(4):251-7.

37. Oto A, Peynircioglu B, Eryilmaz M, Besim A, Sürücü HS, Celik HH. Determination of the width of the presacral space on magnetic resonance imaging. Clin Anat. Wiley Subscription Services, Inc., A Wiley Company; 2004;17(1):14-6.
38. Mack MJ, Regan JJ, Bobechko WP, Acuff TE. Application of thoracoscopy for diseases of the spine. Ann Thorac Surg. 1993;56(3):736-8.
39. Connelly CS, Manges PA. Video-assisted thoracoscopic discectomy and fusion. AORN J. 1998;67(5):940-5 –947–8–950 passimquiz 953–6.
40. Lonner BS, Kondrachov D, Siddiqi F, Hayes V, Scharf C. Thoracoscopic spinal fusion compared with posterior spinal fusion for the treatment of thoracic adolescent idiopathic scoliosis. Surgical technique. Journal of Bone and Joint Surgery. The American Orthopedic Association; 2007;89 Suppl 2 Pt.1(2_suppl_1):142-56.
41. Huang TJ, Hsu RW, Chen SH, Liu HP. Video-assisted thoracoscopic surgery in managing tuberculous spondylitis. Clin Orthop Relat Res. 2000;(379):143-53.
42. Han PP, Kenny K, Dickman CA. Thoracoscopic approaches to the thoracic spine: experience with 241 surgical procedures. Neurosurgery. 2002;51(5 Suppl):S88-95.
43. Dickman CA, Rosenthal D, Karahalios DG, Paramore CG, Mican CA, Apostolides PJ, et al. Thoracic vertebrectomy and reconstruction using a microsurgical thoracoscopic approach. Neurosurgery. 1996;38(2):279-93.
44. Konno S, Yabuki S, Kinoshita T, Kikuchi S. Combined laminectomy and thoracoscopic resection of dumbbell-type thoracic cord tumor. Spine. 2001;26(6):E130-4.
45. Uribe JS, Smith WD, Pimenta L, Härtl R, Dakwar E, Modhia UM, et al. Minimally invasive lateral approach for symptomatic thoracic disc herniation: initial multicenter clinical experience. Journal of Neurosurgery: Spine. American Association of Neurological Surgeons; 2012;16(3):264-79.
46. Zhang B, Li Z, Yang X, Li G, Wang Y, Cheng J, et al. Anatomical variations of the upper thoracic sympathetic chain. Clin Anat. Wiley Subscription Services, Inc., A Wiley Company; 2009;22(5):595-600.
47. Jho H-D, Kim M-H, Kim W-K. Anterior cervical microforaminotomy for spondylotic cervical myelopathy: part 2. Neurosurgery. 2002;51(5 Suppl):S54-9.
48. David H. Jho, Hae-Dong Jho. Anterior Cervical Foraminotomy. In: Burak Ozgur, Edward Benzel, Steven Garfin. Minimally Invasive Spine Surgery. A Practical Guide to Anatomy and Techniques. London: Springer. 2011. p 23-32.
49. Koç RK, Menkü A, Tucer B, Göçmez C, Akdemir H. Anterior cervical foraminotomy for unilateral spondylotic radiculopathy. Minim Invasive Neurosurg. © Georg Thieme Verlag Stuttgart · New York; 2004;47(3):186-9.
50. Jho HD. Microsurgical anterior cervical foraminotomy for radiculopathy: a new approach to cervical disc herniation. J Neurosurg. Journal of Neurosurgery Publishing Group; 1996;84(2):155-60.
51. Jho H-D, Kim W-K, Kim M-H. Anterior microforaminotomy for treatment of cervical radiculopathy: part 1--disc-preserving "functional cervical disc surgery". Neurosurgery. 2002;51(5 Suppl):S46-53.
52. Saringer W, Nöbauer I, Reddy M, Tschabitscher M, Horaczek A. Microsurgical anterior cervical foraminotomy (uncoforaminotomy) for unilateral radiculopathy: clinical results of a new technique. Acta Neurochir (Wien). Springer-Verlag; 2002;144(7):685-94.
53. Susan Standring. Gray's Anatomy: The Anatomical Basis of Clinical Practice. London: Elsevier. 2015.
54. Adamson TE. Microendoscopic posterior cervical laminoforaminotomy for unilateral radiculopathy: results of a new technique in 100 cases. J Neurosurg. 2001;95(1 Suppl):51-7.
55. Holly LT, Moftakhar P, Khoo LT, Wang JC, Shamie N. Minimally invasive 2-level posterior cervical foraminotomy: preliminary clinical results. Journal of Spinal Disorders and Techniques. 2007;20(1):20-4.
56. Hilton DL. Minimally invasive tubular access for posterior cervical foraminotomy with three-dimensional microscopic visualization and localization with anterior/posterior imaging. The Spine Journal. Elsevier; 2007;7(2):154-8.
57. Tumialán LM, Ponton RP, Gluf WM. Management of unilateral cervical radiculopathy in the military: the cost effectiveness of posterior cervical foraminotomy compared with anterior cervical discectomy and fusion. Neurosurg Focus. American Association of Neurological Surgeons; 2010;28(5):E17.
58. Winder MJ, Thomas KC. Minimally invasive versus open approach for cervical laminoforaminotomy. Can J Neurol Sci. 2011;38(2):262-7.
59. Ebraheim NA, Xu R, Yeasting RA. The location of the vertebral artery foramen and its relation to posterior lateral mass screw fixation. Spine. 1996;21(11):1291-5.
60. Tanaka N, Fujimoto Y, An HS, Ikuta Y, Yasuda M. The anatomic relation among the nerve roots, intervertebral foramina, and intervertebral discs of the cervical spine. Spine. 2000;25(3):286-91.

CHAPTER

Ultrasonic Bone Dissectors in Minimally Invasive Spine Surgery

SM Rohidas

ABSTRACT

The techniques of minimally invasive spine surgery has evolved over a period of time from conventional open methods to small incision endospine procedures. The inherent advantages of the minimally invasive techniques are lesser tissue trauma and early return to today activities. Ultrasonic bone dissectors have helped in endospine techniques of spine surgery. This chapter focuses on its Indications, advantages and complications associated with Ultrasonic bone dissectors in endospine surgeries.

INTRODUCTION

In the past two decades, spinal surgery has advanced greatly with the help of operating microscope, high speed drills and endoscope with HD camera vision. Spine surgery is entering into new era of minimalism in spine surgery with the help of endoscope and HD camera vision. With the help of angulation property of endoscope, it is easy to access the narrow corridors of the opposite side inside the spinal canal. However, when the endoscopic drill is used adjacent to the soft tissues in narrow corridors, such as dura, nerve roots, the cord, and vessels, there is always some risks of damaging these important tissues by drilling, even under endoscopic magnified high definition camera vision. These risks are high during removal of masses with hard consistency near delicate tissues. In addition, cooling fluid is required to protect soft tissues from heat injury, and while using endoscope, surgery may have to be interrupted frequently for irrigation and suction to clean the debris over lens and fogging of lens of an endoscope. The protection of the surrounding soft tissue using cotton is not recommended because of the risk of cotton tangling with the high speed drill. The kicking movement is dangerous, particularly in deep corridors with delicate structures.

Ultrasonic aspirators have been effectively used to debulk large brain tumors and some spinal tumors for several decades.[1-3] Now ultrasonic bone currettes are available for skull base surgery and spinal surgery.[4,5] We discuss the clinical application of ultrasonic bone dissectors in Minimally invasive spine surgery using Endospine—the Destandau's technique has been discussed in this chapter. Also discussed are its advantages and disadvantages in comparison with drills.

CLINICAL MATERIAL AND METHODS

From August 2009 to June 2013, we have used ultrasonic bone dissector/rasp/cutter, Sonoca 300, for spinal degenerative disorders with endospine. The surgical device comprises a power supply unit with irrigation and suction, foot switch, handpieceswith various tips. The handpiece is bayonet shaped, with irrigation and aspiration channels **(Figures 1A and B)**.

The dissector handpiece weighs 81 g, with working length of 100 mm, tip width is 4.5 mm, and height is 3.5 mm, irrigation is from outside through a sheath and aspiration is through the central channel, with frequency of 35 kHz.

Ultrasonic Rasp (Figures 2A to E)

The bone cutting handpiece is with working length of 100 mm, frequency of 35 kHz, cutting tip diameter is 3 mm, cutting is 7 mm, cutting width is 0.9 mm, irrigation is outside with no aspiration. The rasp is of frequency of 35 kHz, with working length of 100 mm, cutting width of 2 mm, irrigation from inside

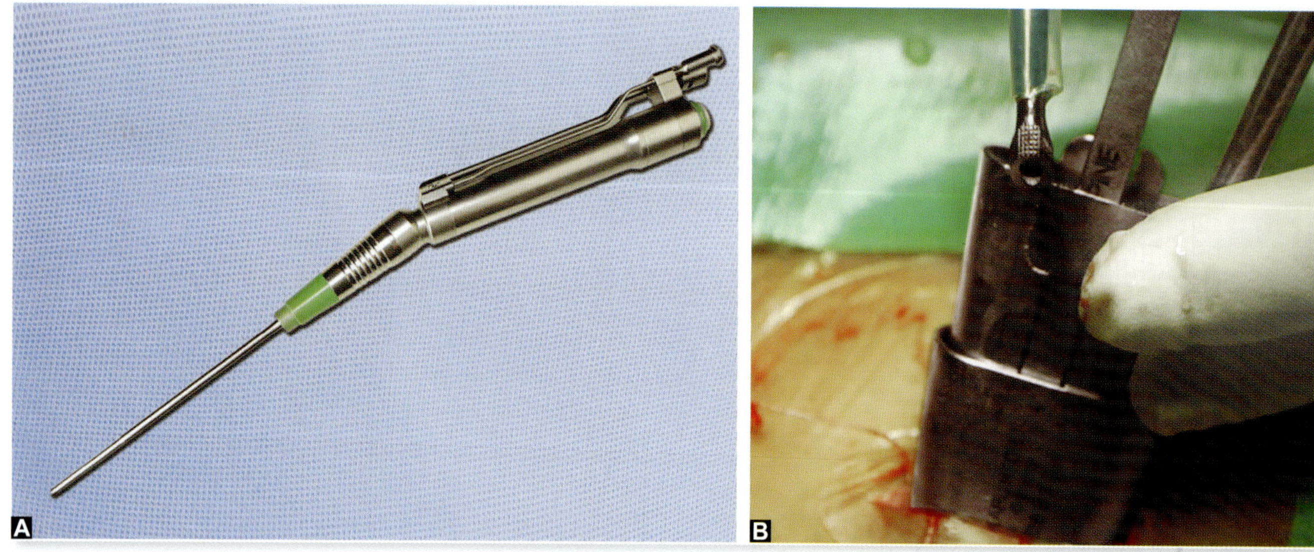

Figures 1A and B: (A) Bayonetted handpiece; (B) Surgical device with irrigation and aspiration details

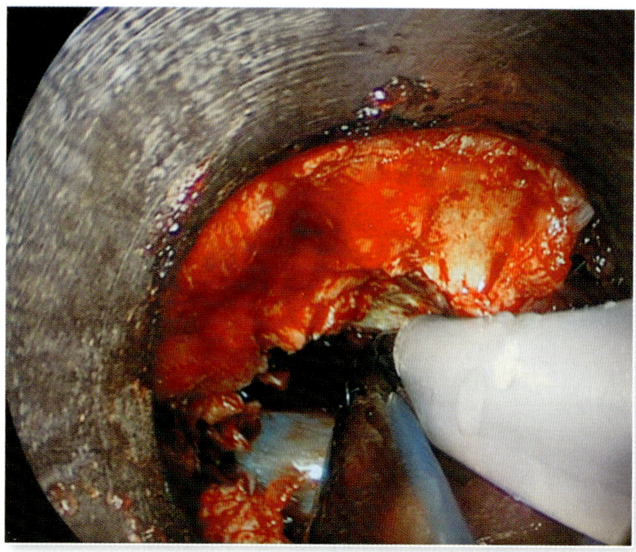

Figure 2A: Ultrasonic dissector

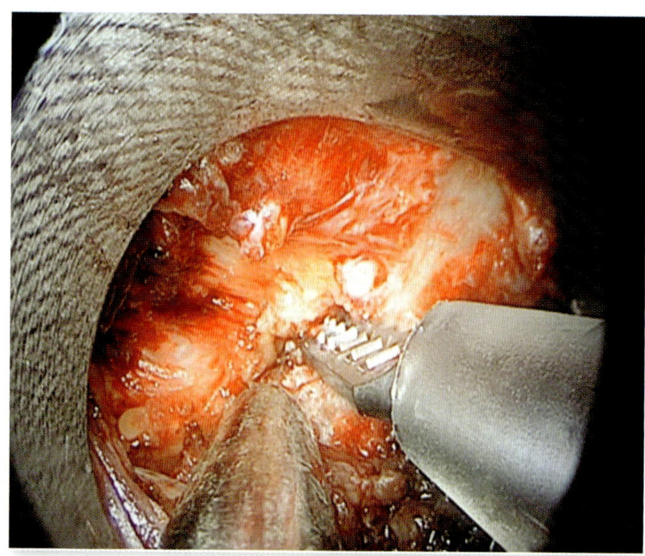

Figure 2B: Ultrasonic cutter/loop

and outside and no aspiration. The dissector handpiece is reusable as it can be autoclaved. But the rasp and cutter tips are not reusable as the tips become blunt after use on bone.

Ultrasonic bone dissector/rasp/cutter (loop), is used to remove bone near dura, nerve root, blood vessel in following procedures—endoscopic bilateral decompression using unilateral approach in lumbar spine, posterior cervical diskectomy and canal decompression, for stenosis, and endoscopic anterior cervical diskectomy.

Ultrasonic Basics (Figures 3A and B)

Ultrasonic movement is measured in Hertz. For example 25 kHz is 25000, Hz equal to 25000 cycles per second. One cycle is one Hz.

Less than 20 Hz is infrasound, 20 Hz to 20 kHz is audible spectrum of sound. Ultrasound is 20 kHz to 20 MHz. Frequencies suitable for ultrasonic dissecton are from 20 kHz to 60 kHz.

The generator converts the mains voltage into electric energy of desired frequency. Then the converter transforms this electric energy into mechanical energy. The stack of piezoelectric quartzes transforms the electric energy of generator into longitudinal, deformational, mechanical vibration of the sonotrode tip. The sonotrode is designed such that the entire system—converter, final mass, sonotrode is in resonance. The stroke at distal tip is 120 micrometer. The deformation movement is around 10 micrometers **(Figure 4)**.

Three physical effects are used—(1) Cavitation, (2) Mechanical abrasion, and (3) Thermal effect.

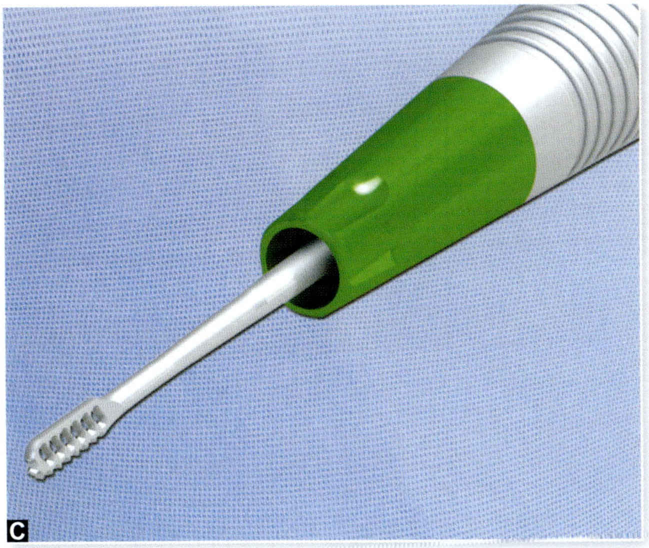

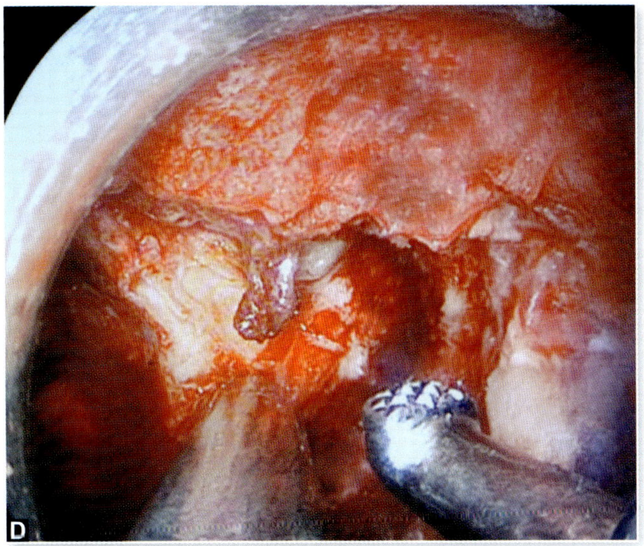

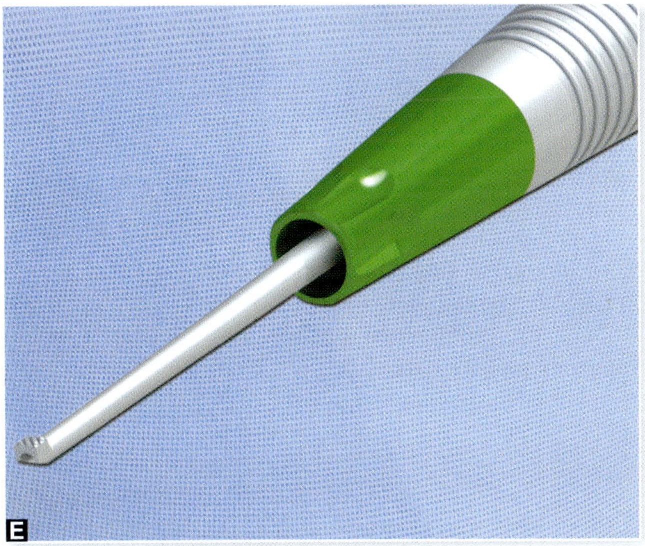

Figures 2C to E: Ultrasonic Rasp

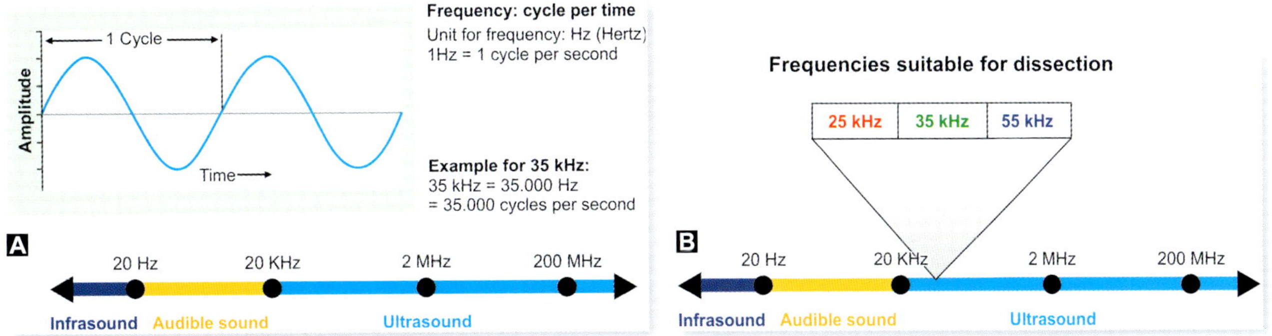

Figures 3A and B: Ultrasonic basics

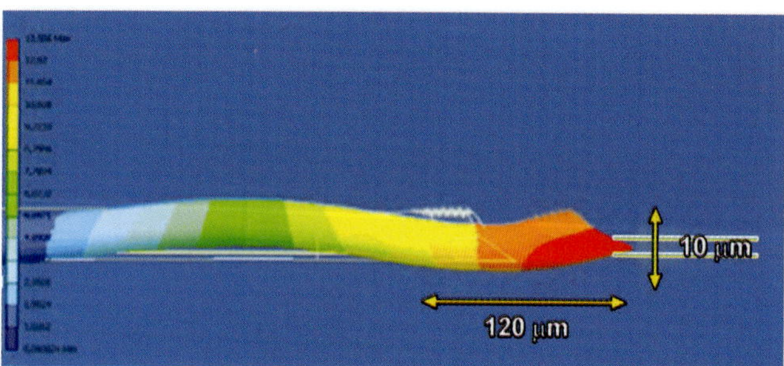

Figure 4: Physical effects

Cavitation

The pressure fluctuations are caused by the vibrating sonotrode. The forward movement of the sonotrode tip displaces the surrounding liquid while the backward movement forces the liquid to return back. The pressure of the surrounding liquid changes rapidly between high and low values. Due to the high speed and mass inertia of the surrounding medium, the volume cannot be fully compensated by returning liquid. During the backward movement, the pressure drops so much that the liquid evaporates and small bubbles are formed. During the forward movement, the pressure rises, and bubbles collapse. The imploding bubbles transmit high energy pulses into immediate vicinity.

So the cascade of events is as follows - 1. Small gas bubbles are formed. 2. These gas bubbles grow because the surrounding liquid evaporates. 3. The bubbles then reach maximum volume. 4. Then implosion starts by unilateral inversion. 5. The liquid perforates the bubble wall and generate a shockwave **(Figure 5)**.

Abrasion

On hard, rigid, firm surface, the oscillating movement of sonotrode acts like a file. Bone tissue incapable of following the vibrating sonotrode is pulverized by friction and abrasion on edges and tips. On soft tissue no abrasion occurs as soft tissue is pushed away from the sonotrode tip because of its elasticity. This is the basic principle of Ultrasonic bone dissectors.

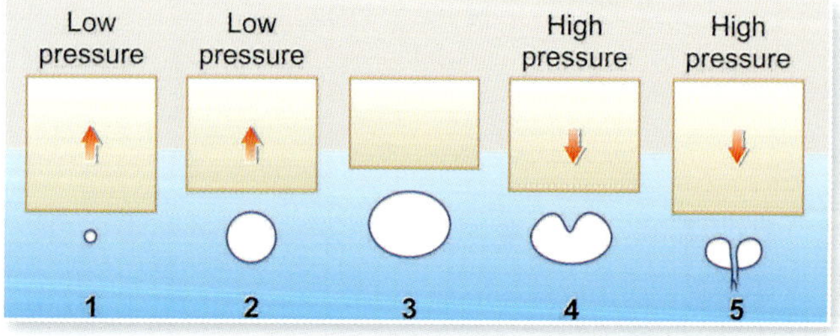

Figure 5: Pressure fluctuations at low and high pressures

Thermal Effect

The vibrating sonotrode generates friction heat in the liquid but also directly on the tissue concerned. The benefit of heat is coagulation effect on soft tissue. But for the bone tissue local overheating is prevented by continuous irrigation of the tip.

SURGICAL TECHNIQUES AND RESULTS

Endoscopic Bilateral Lumbar Canal Decompression with Unilateral Approach (Figures 6 and 7)

Endospine is used for endoscopic bilateral canal decompression with unilateral approach in degenerative lumbar canal stenosis. Angulation of endospine is used to approach the contralateral lateral recess. Here, the endoscope, and the working instrument is inside the spinal canal underneath the base of spinous process in a narrow lateral recess. In degenerative canal and lateral recess stenosis due to severe medial facet hypertrophy the lateral recess is still compromised with edematous compressed nerve root. To use drill in this narrow corridor is difficult. Slipping of drill or kicking back of drill may traumatize the nerve root. We use ultrasonic bone dissector/rasp to undercut the opposite lamina and medial facet. The tip of dissector/rasp is kept near the bone and then foot switch is on. Scraping movement of tip side to side and to and fro will remove bone. Irrigation is used around 5 - 7 mL/min with aspiration for dissector at 80 Torr. The endoscope lens gets fogged due to irrigation fluid and bone dust. During the use ultrasonic tip is withdrawn a little bit so that the irrigating fluid cleans the lens. Again we can continue with dissection. This maneuver helps in cleaning the lens tip and also cleans the operating area. This also helps in decreasing the heat generated during use.

From August 2009 till June 2013, out of ---- lumbar endoscopic cases we used ultrasonic bone dissector / rasp in -- -- cases. Ultrasonic bone dissector / rasp is used to shave off thick osteophyte stretching the nerve root, undercut the opposite lamina, undercut medial facet. Also in transforaminal approach we enlarge the neural foramen at the isthmus so as to decompress the exiting nerve root. Ultrasonic bone cutter is used to undercut thick base of spinous process at higher lumbar level. In lumbar region the interlaminar distance and interpedicular distance becomes narrow as we go cranial from the lowermost level that is L5/S1. Because of this, the base of spinous process also becomes thick. We use cutter to cut the base of spinous process at higher lumbar level so as to reach the opposite lateral recess and spinal canal.

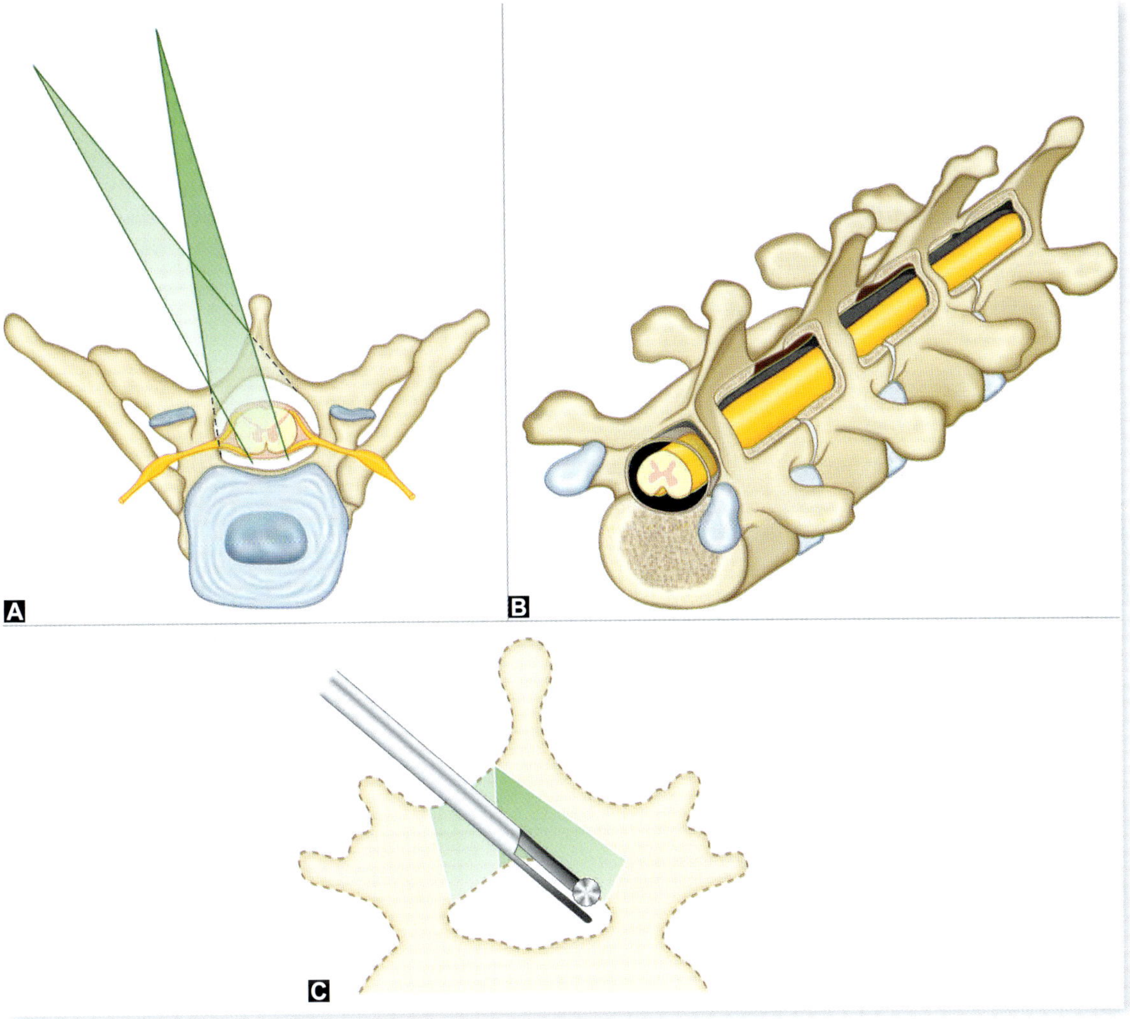

Figure 6: Multiple foraminotomies: Opposite canal decompression with drill

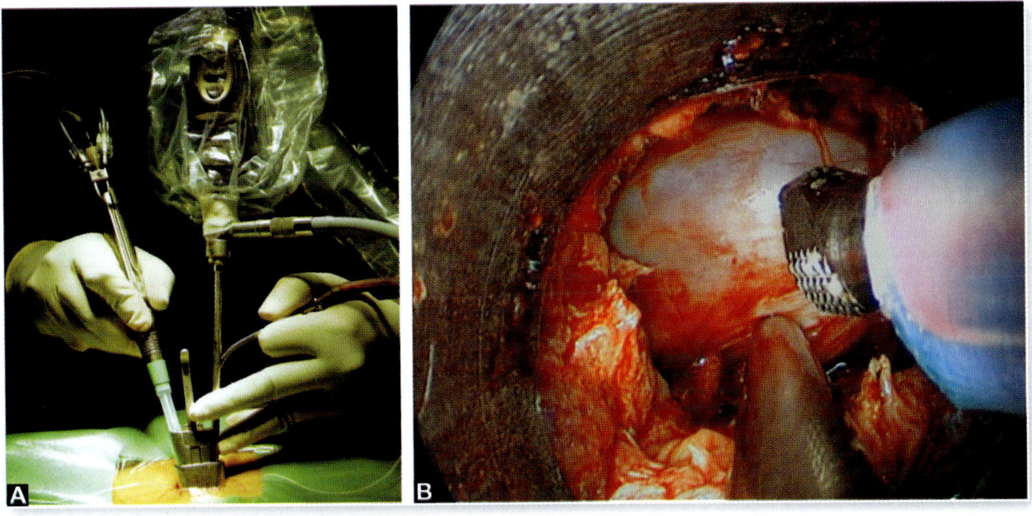

Figures 7A and B: Endospine and ultrasonic bone dissector

Endoscopic Posterior Cervical Diskectomy and Canal Decompression

We use endospine in posterior cervical approach to perform foraminotomy and opposite canal decompression using unilateral approach. Neural foramen is widened with ultrasonic dissector/rasp to decompress the nerve root. Cervical canal decompression is achieved with undercutting of the base of spinal process and opposite lamina **(Figures 8A and B)**. The endoscope and working instrument is inside the spinal canal. In cervical region there is very little space and cervical cord cannot be pushed with cotton wool as unlike in lumbar region where the dural tube can be pushed to create some more space. Slipping or kicking of drill over slippery lamina in this narrow corridor can have serious complications like cord injury leading to quadriplegia. Ultrasonic bone dissector / rasp is used over a cotton wool without pushing the cervical cord. The cotton wool will help in preventing the heat transfer along with irrigating fluid. Out of 35 posterior cervical cases we used ultrasonic dissector/ rasp in 25 cases.

Endoscopic Anterior Cervical Diskectomy and Canal Decompression (Figures 9A and B)

We use endospine to approach disk hernia through transuncal approach. In this approach the operating window is around 8–10 mm. The nerve root length from the dural sleeve to medial border of vertebral artery is around 6 mm. Ultrasonic bone dissector is used to remove bone over medial border of vertebral artery. This helps in protecting vertebral artery and the venous plexus around it. For canal decompression with this approach through this small window we have to use suction and working instrument. While using working instrument one cannot put pressure over cord. Here we use rasp with up cutting edge to undercut bone of cranial and caudal vertebral bodies **(Figure 10)**. It is very safe to use rasp as the cutting edge is always away from the cord. Out of 36 cases of anterior cervical endoscopic discectomy we have used ultrasonic dissector/rasp in 25 cases.

RESULTS

There was no major procedure-related intraoperative complication, such as cord injury, nerve root injury or vertebral artery injury. Postoperative cerebrospinal fluid leakage did not occur. Intraoperative dural injury, wound infection did not occur in any case where ultrasonic bone dissector was used.

DISCUSSION

Complications related to spinal surgery are reported to occur with a frequency of 8.6% (1569/18334).[6] These include general complications, neurological and meningeal complications, vascular complications, infections, bone graft failure, mechanical problems. Among these, complications related to drilling procedure include spinal cord and nerve root injury, esophageal perforation, vascular injury,

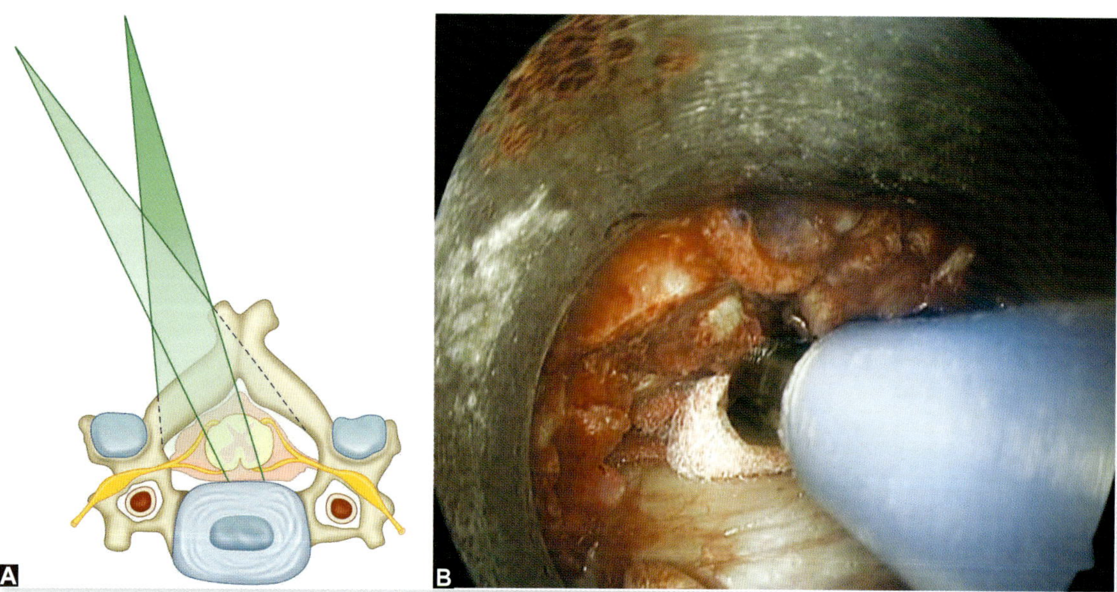

Figures 8A and B: Cervical cord opposite lamina undercutting C3-4 level Lt. to Rt

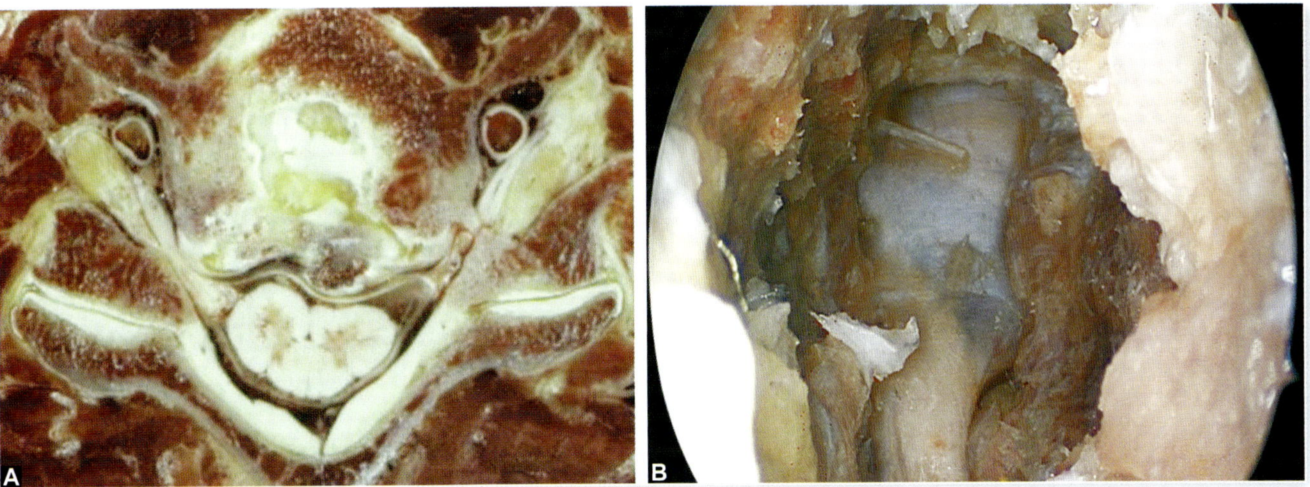

Figures 9A and B: Axial view cervical cord and root transuncal view

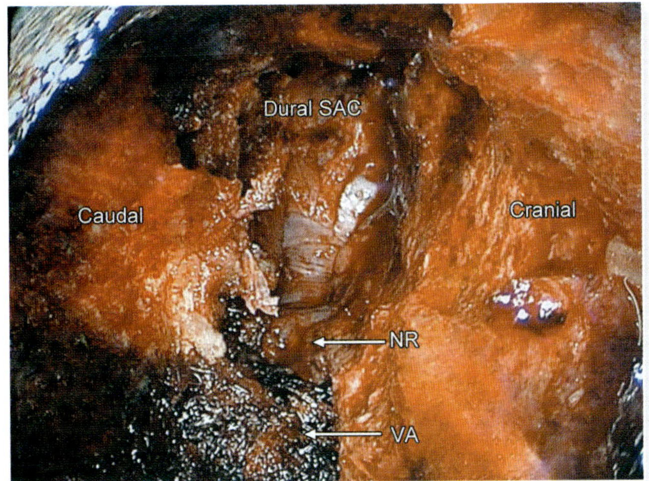

Figure 10: Relationship with cranial and caudal vertebra with nerve root

cerebrospinal fluid leak. The iatrogenic complications are relatively rare but, are sometimes life threatening like cord injury, vascular injury, pharyngeal injury in anterior cervical spine surgery. When one minimizes incision in minimally invasive spine surgery the operative corridor becomes narrow. To use endoscopic drill in such narrow corridor needs skill and training. The use of ultrasonic bone dissector mentioned in various procedures will reduce the surgical complication rate.

The ultrasonic aspirator was first developed in 1947 for removal of dental plaque.[7] Flamm et al. tested the ultrasonic aspirator in 1978, in studies on animal brains to access its efficacy and safety. He applied ultrasonic aspirator first to remove meningiomas and schwannomas same year.[8]

We always have some risk of injury to the dura, neural tissue, and vessels while using high speed drills in spine surgery, and minimally invasive spine surgery is not immune to it in spite of very good vision in narrow corridors due to HD image. In way to avoid drill related complications, surgeon has to use both hands to hold drill in spine surgery. While using Endospine we hold the drill shaft like a pencil and support over the working channel so that it should not drop inside and surgeon can use drill sideways rather than to and fro. The drill tip is always at an angle of 12 degrees from suction and endoscope. But it is difficult to maintain the angle of drill away from cottonoid. It is difficult to use cottonoid in narrow corridor at depth. Due to fear of iatrogenic injuries while drilling, training of young endoscopic spine surgeons is a very challenging task.

The handpiece is very light weight 80 g. It helps reduce operator fatigue while using it for long period. To prevent direct thermal damage of delicate neural tissues we use continuous irrigation. For more safety we recommend intermittent usage to avoid thermal damage. Also where ever it is possible we use cottonoid over nerve root and cord to prevent direct mechanical injurydue to slippage or kicking back of handpiece. There is no chance of gripping of cottonoid unlike mechanical drill. The endoscope lens becomes dirty due to bone dust and the irrigating fluid during use. A simple trick of pulling out the ultrasonic handpiece while in use will clean the endoscope lens to get good endoscopic image, contrary to need of taking out of drill to clean it up. This is possible with rasp and cutting tip. But with the dissector tip which has aspiration channel inside sometimes large bone fragment can block the aspiration channel. In this situation surgeon has to take out the handpiece and remove the block. This may be time consuming.

The ultrasonic bone dissector//rasp/cutter(loop), cannot replace the routine endoscopic drill. It is very time consuming to remove large amount of bone away from neural structures. Hence it has to be used specifically to remove bone near a nerve, over cord, or near blood vessels so as to reduce operative time.

The ultrasonic bone dissector/rasp/cutter(loop), technique used for mentioned procedures is the same as with other routine instruments like drill and Kerrison punch. In lumbar canal stenosis to achieve bilateral canal decompression through unilateral approach opposite lateral recess decompression is difficult due to hypertrophied medial facet compressing oedematous traversing root. It is difficult because of the depth, narrow space, and lack of control over the tip of instrument. The ultrasonic bone dissector/rasp cutting edge is always away from the nerve and dura. The angle of the hypertrophied facet and cutting edge of dissector/rasp helps in minimizing trauma to neural structures along with basic ultrasonic safety. The same is true for cervical posterior canal decompression and anterior cervical discectomy with cord decompression. Here, also the cutting edge of ultrasonic instrument is away from neural structures. In posterior cervical approach to use Kerrison punch is not possible as there is no space to maneuver the punch over cord. To use drill is also difficult because of slippery edges of lamina and flavum. Ultrasonic dissector/rasp is more safe as even if it accidently slips over lamina it does not have effect on dura, cord, nerve root. There is not possibility of tangling of cottonoid with tip.

In these endoscopic spine approaches, the use of Ultrasonic bone dissector/rasp/cutter(loop), is obviously helpful, safe, and reduce complications. The use of this new technology involves a learning curve.

REFERENCES

1. Flamn ES, Ransoff J, Wuuchinich D, et al. Preliminary experience with ultrasonic aspiration in neurosurgery, Neurosurgery. 1978;2(3):240-5.
2. Inoue T, Ikezaki K, Sato Y, Ultrasonic surgical system(Sonapet), for microsurgical removal of brain tumours, Neuro Res. 2000;22(5):490-4.
3. Sawamura Y, Fukushima T, Terasaka S, et al, Development of a handpiece and probes for microsurgical ultrasonic aspirator instrumentation and application . Neurosurgery. 1999;45(5):1192-7.
4. Hadeishi H, Suzuki A, Yasui N, et al. Anterior clinoidectomy and opening of internal auditory canal using an ultrasonic bone currete Neurosurgery. 2003;52:867-71.
5. Inoue H, Nishi H, Shimizu T, et al. Microsurgical ligamentectomy for patients with central lumbar stenosis a unilateral approach using an ultrasonic bone scalpel. Spinal surgery 17(2).
6. Yamamoto H, Nation wide survey for spine surgery, Japan spine research society, a committee report. Spine surgery. 1999;10(2);332-9.
7. Sawamura Y, Fukushima T, Terasaka S, Sugai T. Development of a handpiece and probes for a microsurgical ultrasonic aspirator, instrumentation and application. Neurosurgery. 1999;45(5): 1192-6.
8. Epstein F. Thecavitron ultrasonic aspirator in tumor surgery. Clin. Neurosurger. 1984;31:487-505.

CHAPTER

Hazards of Radiation in Minimally Invasive Spine Surgery

Subir N Jhaveri

ABSTRACT

The world has witnessed the devastating effects of radiation, time and again, since 1945, with the twin nuclear bombing of Hiroshima and Nagasaki, to the more recent Chernobyl nuclear mishap in 1986 and the Fukushima nuclear spill in 2011 in Japan. Thousands of innocent lives were lost, and entire generations remained affected, with reproductive deficits as well as enhanced risk of a variety of malignancies.

INTRODUCTION

We, as citizens of this earth, are constantly exposed to natural radiation, emanating from the galaxy as well as from naturally occurring radioactive materials found in soil, water and air. Radon, a naturally occurring gas, emanates from rock and soil and is the main source of natural radiation. However, owing to the very low levels, background radiation does not produce any perceptible damage. On the other hand, pilots, aircrew and astronauts are constantly exposed to cosmic radiation. Cosmic radiation can potentially accelerate neurodegenerative processes and produce Alzheimer's type of disease, based on a mice model study conducted by NASA.[1] The major concern lays in exposure to harmful radiation from human made sources, such as nuclear power generation and medical use of radiation in diagnosis as well as treatment.

The advent of the image intesifying television (IITV) (C-arm) into orthopedic theaters changed the way things were practiced, and the most open surgeries, were gradually converted into closed, minimal invasive surgeries. The same was true for spine surgery. After the development of the microendoscopic diskectomy (MED) system, using a series of tubular dilators in 1994, spine surgery became gradually less invasive than before. However, one of the most crucial aspects of minimal invasive spine surgery is the ability to visualize the spine using the C-arm. It is these emissions from the C-arm, which are harmful to the human body, and if not checked, can lead to disastrous consequences for the patient, as well as the health worker himself.

HOW IS RADIATION MEASURED?

Exposure describes the amount of radiation traveling through the air. Many radiation monitors measure exposure. The units for exposure are the roentgen (R) and coulomb/kilogram (C/kg).[2]

The radiation dose absorbed by a person, i.e., the amount of energy deposited in human tissue by radiation, is measured using the conventional unit 'rad' or the SI unit 'gray' (Gy).[2]

The biological risk of exposure to radiation is measured using the conventional unit 'rem' or the SI unit 'sievert' (Sv). (1 Sv = 100 rem or 1mSv = 100 mrem) For beta and gamma radiation, the dose equivalent is the same as the absorbed dose. By contrast, the dose equivalent is larger than the absorbed dose for alpha and neutron radiation, because these types of radiation are more damaging to the human body.[2]

For all practical purposes, exposure to a radiation of 1 R dose, leads to an absorpition of 1 rad dosage by the body, which has a dose equivalent of 1 rem = 1000 mrem (10 mSv).[2]

EFFECTS OF IONIZING RADIATION

The harmful effects of ionizing radiation are observed depending on the dose received by the patient, as well as the duration of exposure. Acute exposure to a large dose of radiation causes more damage; however; the same degree of radiation exposure may produce less effects if it occurs over a prolonged period. Different tissues have different thresholds, so effect on a specific organ system varies with the degree of exposure.

Acute effects of radiation include skin redness, hair loss, radiation burns and is known as acute radiation syndrome. The dose threshold for acute radiation syndrome is about 1 Sv (1000 mSv).

If the dose is low or delivered over a prolonged period, the damaged cells may heal themselves but may incorporate errors, which are then transferred further during cell division. In general, exposure to 100 mSv or less is not associated with any significant side effect, nor any detectable increase in risk of cancer. Exposures greater than 500 mSv may cause opacification of the lens of the eye, and even induce posterior subcapsular cataracts. Full body exposure of the same dose may lead to reduction of peripheral blood lymphocytes. Partial exposure of dosages higher than 3000 mSv lead to skin redness, hair loss and even permanent damage to the reproductive organs leading to infertility. Full body exposure to such dosages leads to death of almost 50% of exposed personnel within one month, and death of all personnel occurs at 7000–10000 mSv exposure, within few days **(Figure 1).**

RADIATION EMITTED IN ROUTINE RADIOLOGICAL PROCEDURES

A single chest X-ray, causes exposure to only 0.1 mSv, while a single mammogram can cause emission of up to 3 mSv of radiation **(Figure 2)**. Exposure to radiation varies with the type of CT scan and the Institute where it is done. A head CT scan can cause emission of 2 mSv, which is equivalent to 442 chest X-rays or 74 mammograms; whereas, a multiphasic abdomen and pelvis CT can emit from 2 mSv to 31 mSv.[3] A coronary CT Angiography can emit radiation equivalent to 771 chest X-rays or 15 mammograms.[3] The major concern is the radiation emitted by the fluoroscopy machines, and it has been estimated that **1 minute of fluoroscopic exposure emits radiation equivalent to 150 chest X-rays**. This risk is doubled in case of children and adolescents; multiplied by 10 times for fetuses; and is halved in the elderly. Prenatal exposure to ionizing radiation causes brain damage during the 8–25 weeks of pregnancy, and cancer risks are similar to childhood exposure. According to a study by Brenner et al, 600,000 abdominal and head CT scans are performed in children less than 15 years, annually in the USA, and 500 of these children will die from cancer due to this CT radiation.[4]

RADIATION AND THE MINIMALLY INVASIVE SPINE SURGEON

A host of medical-related occupations tend to use radiation-emitting equipment on a daily basis. Amongst these are included, radiology technicians, interventional cardiologists, radiologists, pain physicians, urologists, orthopedic surgeons, and spine (orthopedic and neuro) surgeons. All of us are exposed to so much radiation, and yet, very few of us tend to wear sufficient protective gear, or monitor our radiation dosage.

Vertebroplasty

Radiologists, orthopedic surgeons, spine specialists as well as pain physicians are nowadays performing vertebroplasties. In view of the multitude of physicians involved in the care of the osteoporotic vertebral compression fracture, knowledge

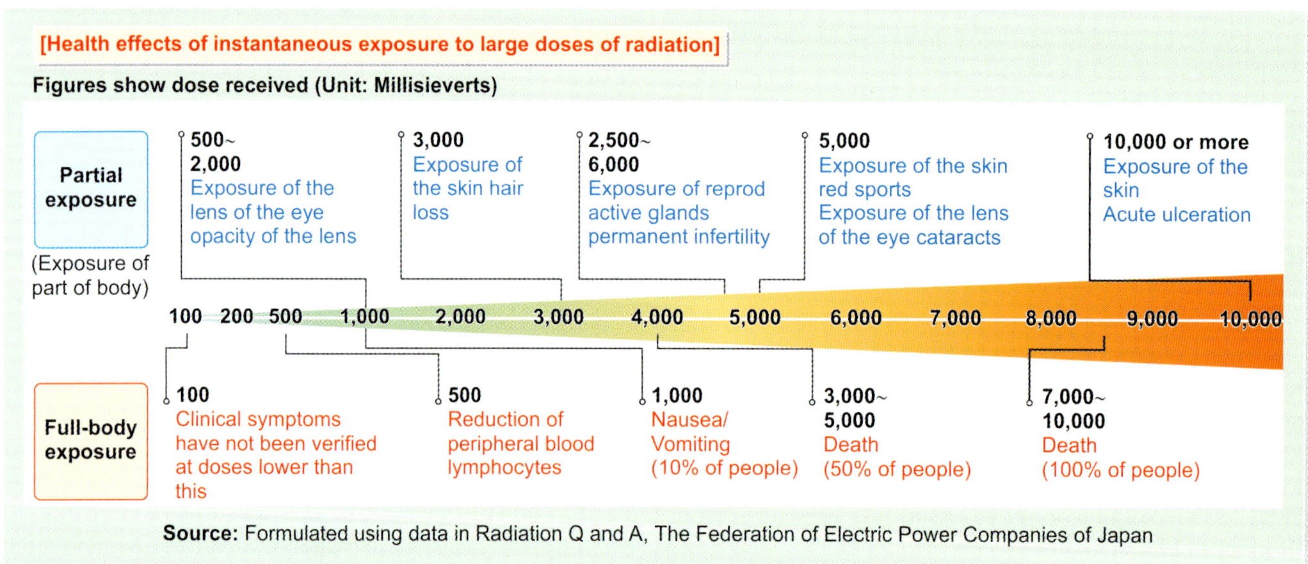

Figure 1: Health effects of acute exposure to large dosage of radiation

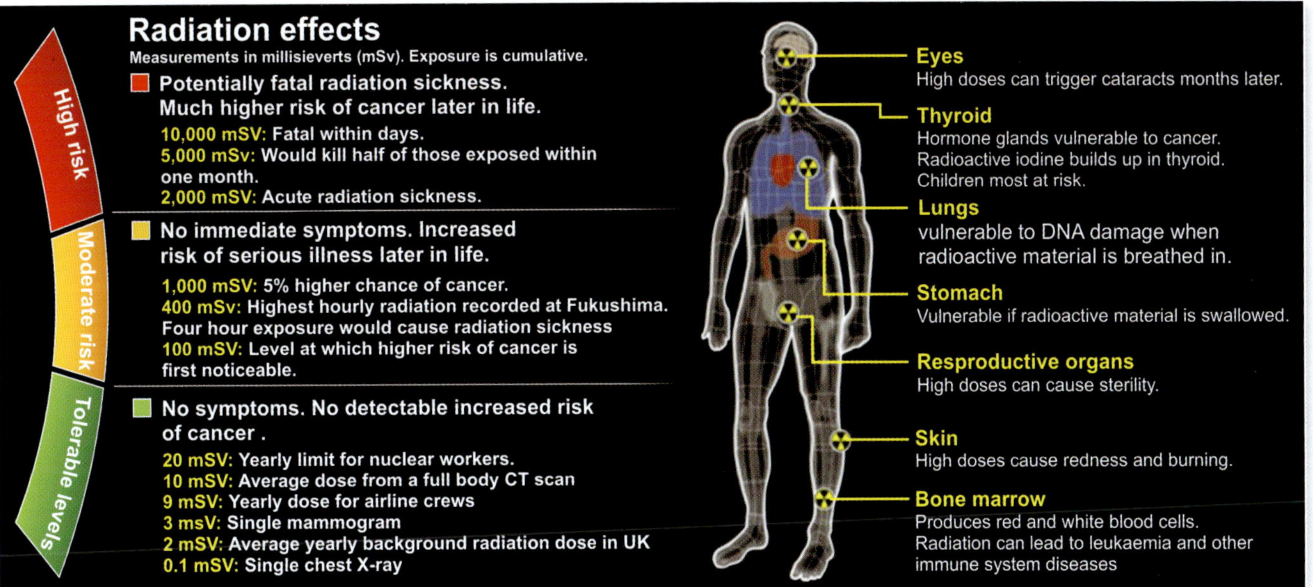

Figure 2: Radiation effects when exposure is cumulative

Source: Google web images

regarding the hazards of radiation needs to be disseminated amongst all these medical fraternities.

A study conducted by the Orthopedic department at the University of Bern, on two spine surgeons, has showed that there is a very small risk of developing a fatal cancer of the thyroid (0.0025%), and a small to medium risk of developing cancer (0.025%) with vertebroplasty. They quoted similar findings for developing radiation-induced cataract, and skin related cancers. They, however, did recommend appropriate surgical technique as well as using shielding devices as percutaneous vertebroplasty exposed the surgeon to a significant amount of radiation.[5]

On the other hand, personal dosimeters of all medical personnel working around radiation emitting equipment were assessed at a University Hospital, and the only physician whose personal dosimeter exceeded the legal limit of 1 mSv/month, was that of the physician performing percutaneous vertebroplasty. Also, this was assessed with the radiologist standing approximately 50 cm from the irradiated areas wearing lead protection gloves. They moved the X-ray tube on the side opposite to the operator, and using lead gloves reduced radiation exposure to the hand by 30–40%.[6]

A similar finding was quoted by Synowitz et al. where they evaluated radiation exposure to glove-protected and unprotected left hands of two surgeons. They showed that lead gloves lead to reduction of radiation from 1.81 mSv to 0.49 mSv (75%) if the hand was protected.[7]

Tappero et al. compared the patient and operator exposure using either fluoroscopy alone or with CT during percutaneous vertebroplasty, and demonstrated significant reduction in radiation exposure using combined CT and fluoroscopic guidance for PVP. Mean operator dose was noted as 0.8 mSv for the combined procedures compared to 5.8 mSv for only fluoroscopic guided procedures. Similarly, patient dosages were also less with the combined (6 mSv) as compared to the fluoroscopic (8 mSv) PVP procedures.[8]

Kyphoplasty

Kyphoplasty necessitates inflation of the balloon, and usually, a slightly greater amount of cement, as compared to vertebroplasty. This leads to marginally increased fluoroscopy times with kyphoplasty, in comparision with verterbroplasty **(Figures 3A to E)**.

Perisinakis et al. conducted an experimental study using a humanoid phantom and concluded that skin injuries were unlikely to occur if the source to skin distance was 35 cm or more, although such injuries may occur if total fluoroscopy time was more than the mean of 10.1 +/- 2.2 min for kyphoplasty at single level.[9] A study conducted by the orthopaedic department at a level one trauma center was able to demonstrate that unprotected individuals working at twenty four inches or less receive significant radiation, whereas those at thirty six inches or greater, received extremely low radiation.[10]

Boszczyk et al. studied 60 consecutive kyphoplasty procedures and demonstrated significantly reduced fluoroscopy times, 2.2 min in the lateral plane and 1.6 min in the anteroposterior plane, using biplanar fluoroscopy. They also recommended using large C- arms and to use the radiation exposure judiciously.[11]

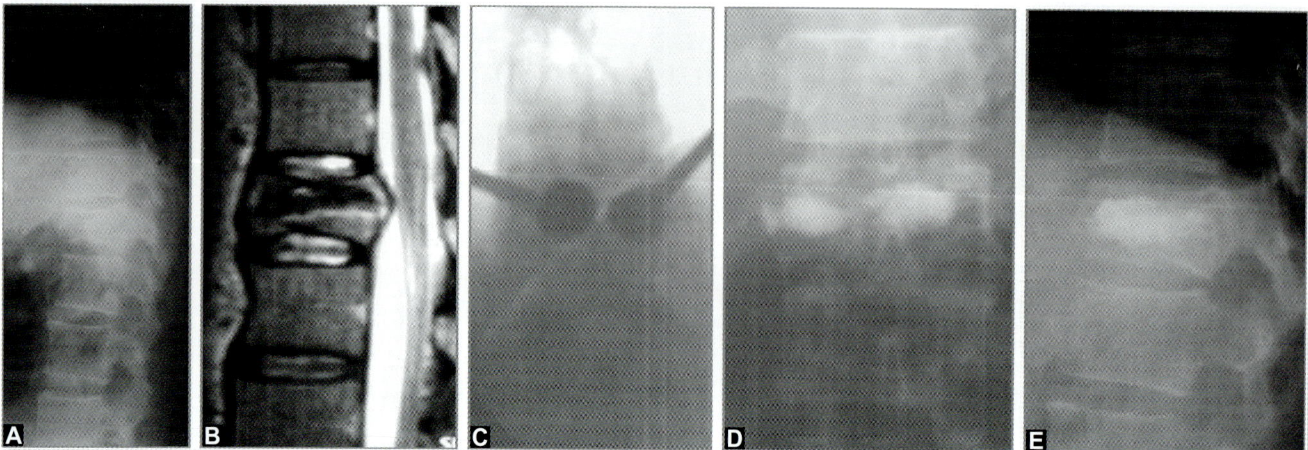

Figures 3A to E: Kyphoplasty: (A) Osteoporotic vertebral fracture at D12; (B) MRI showing minimal retropulsion on bone without significant spinal cord compression; (C) Kyphoplasty balloons at time of inflation with radioopaque dye; (D and E) Postoperative AP and lateral X-rays

Lieberman et al. evaluated the radiation dosages received by the surgeon and patient, using dosimeters outside and underneath lead aprons and thyroid collars. They found that the exposure for single level cases was 5.7 minutes as compared to two (3.9 min) or three level (2.9 min) cases. They concluded that without eye or hand protection, the total radiation exposure dose to these areas would exceed occupational exposure limit after 300 cases per year. They recommended that surgeons should wear lead lined glasses and keep their hands out of the radiation beam while doing kyphoplasty.[12]

Minimally Invasive Microdiskectomy

Lumbar microdiskectomy has gone minimal invasive with most surgeons performing the traditional surgery through a tiny incision, be it through the posterolateral or the transforaminal route. However, all these minimal invasive systems require precise location of incision, thus necessitating significant fluoroscopic guidance.

Mariscalco et al. conducted a study to compare the radiation exposure to the surgeon during 10 traditional open microdiskectomy versus 10 minimally invasive lumbar microdiskectomy. Exposure to the thyroid, eye, chest and hand were noted, and a 10-20-fold increase in radiation was noted in all areas exposed with the minimally invasive procedures. Detailed exposures according to region are tabulated in **Table 1**. They also demonstrated that surgeons standing in a sub-sterile room adjacent to the operating room were exposed to 0.2 mR radiation per case.[13]

Ahn et al. prospectively evaluated radiation exposure to surgeons' neck, chest, arm and both hands during percutaneous endoscopic lumbar diskectomy (PELD). Mean fluoroscopic time was noted as 2.5 minutes. Lead collar and apron reduced the radiation dose by 96.9% and 94.2%, respectively, and on that basis, they calculated, that a surgeon performing PELD can do 5379 cases per year using a lead apron, but only 291 cases, if he does not use it. They also showed that the maximum limit for occupational radiation exposure to hand was reached at 683 cases per year (500 mSv).[14]

Table 1

Detailed radiation exposures with open and minimally invasive lumbar microdiskectomy

Organs	*Open microdisk*	*MIS microdisk*	*Increase*
Thyroid/ eye	0.16 ± 0.22 mR	1.72 ± 1.52 mR	10 times
Chest	0.21 ± 0.23 mR	3.08 ± 2.93mR	15 times
Hand	0.20 ± 0.14 mR	4.45 ± 3.75 mR	20 times

Minimally Invasive Transforaminal Lumbar Interbody Fusion (TLIF)

Performing minimally invasive TLIF requires insertion of pedicle screws under fluoroscopic guidance. Highly accurate needle positioning and direction of trajectory is required, prompting surgeons to shoot at higher radiation dosages; and also to perform the same repeatedly depending upon the number of levels to be fused in the construct. This leads to significant radiation dosing to the surgeon as well as his team **(Figures 4A to F)**.

Bindal et al. measured the radiation absorbed by the surgeon and patient during placement of pedicle screws during MI-TLIF. Mean fluoroscopy time was noted as 1.69 minutes per case (0.82 – 3.73 min.) with the surgeon's hand receiving 76 mRem, protected waist receiving 27 mRem and the unprotected thyroid receiving 32mRem. They

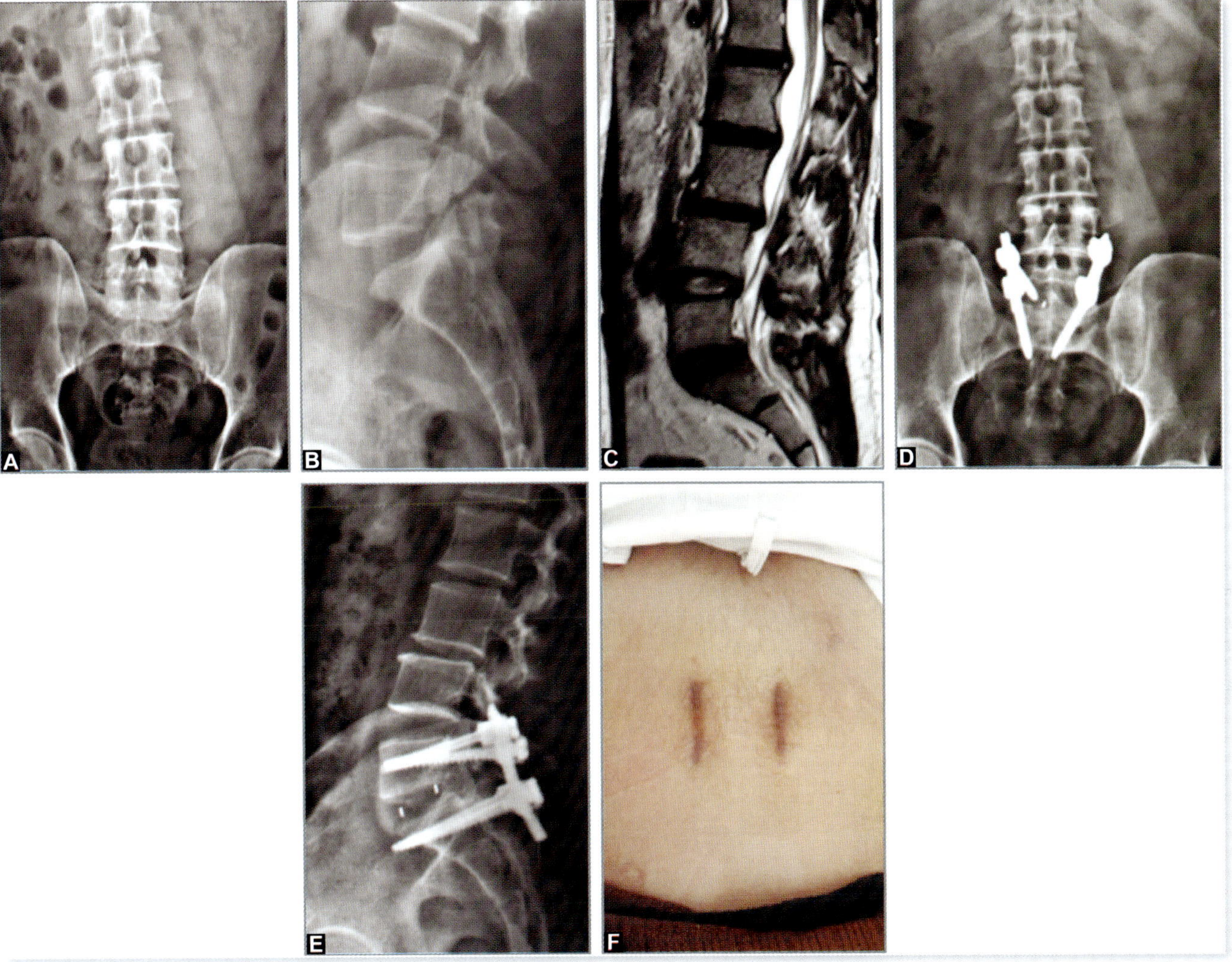

Figures 4A to F: Minimally invasive transforaminal lumbar interbody fusion: (A and B) AP and lateral X-rays of patient with L5–S1 spondylolysis with spondylolisthesis; (C) MRI of same patient with degenerated lumbosacral disk and Grade I listhesis; (D and E) Postoperative images following minimally invasive transforaminal lumbar interbody fixation and fusion; (F) Postoperative scar

recommended monitoring surgeon exposuers, as annual dose limits could easily be exceeded at centers performing large number of these fluoroscopically guided procedures.[15]

Clark et al. used a combination of low-dose pulsed fluoroscopy and digital spot imaging techniques to reduce the fluoroscopy time and radiation dose in their series of 50 patients. Mean fluoroscopic time was noted to be 18.72 seconds (7–29 seconds), and the mean radiation dose was noted to be 0.247 mGy/sq mt. They did not require any revision surgery in any of these patients, suggesting accurate placement of their pedicle screw placements.[16]

The radiation exposure to surgeons' chest as well as the operation theatre personnels' genitals was significantly increased during MIS-TLIF's in obese indiviudals (BMI >25).[17] No significant differences were found in surgical time, EBL and fluoroscopic exposure time, however, higher scatter radiation caused by higher radiation outputs and larger body surface areas might increase the surgeons' radiation doses in overweight patients.

TIPS AND SUGGESTIONS TO REDUCE FLUOROSCOPIC RADIATION EXPOSURE

Many authors have detailed their experiences, and methods to reduce the fluoroscopic radiation exposure to the surgeon as well as the assistants. Some of the noteworthy suggestions are as follows:

1. Keep the X-ray tube on the opposite side of the table, to reduce direct exposure to the scattered radiation, preferably below the operating table.[6,14]

2. The surgeon should maintain at least 60 cm distance from the direct beam of the IITV.[10]
3. The surgeon should use the "hands off" technique. If not possible, hold the needle or wire with a long handle instrument.[14]
4. The assistant, technician and anesthetist all should be more than 3 feet away from the source of radiation.[10]
5. All personnel should be wearing lead aprons, thyroid protection lead collars, and the operator should preferably have lead gloves and lead glasses.[6,7]
6. All personnel exposed to fluoroscopic radiation on a regular basis must be allocated a pair of radiation dosimeter badges, which would then be checked on an annual basis.[14]
7. Use low-dose pulsed fluoroscopy, combined with spot images, rather than "live" fluoroscopy, preferably in the automatic mode.[14-16]
8. The technician should collimate and center all images, as that reduces the scatter generated while taking images.[18]
9. Monitor your fluoroscopy usage, and next time, try to "better your score," thus effectively reducing the overall minutes of fluoroscopic radiation required per case.
10. Avoid performing a huge number of radiation dependent procedures.[12]
11. Using alternative techniques, such as navigation or robot-based techniques, would allow the surgeon to undertake a greater number of radiation-dependent procedures, although at a higher cost.[19,20]

Adherence to most or all of the above suggestions would significantly reduce the radiation exposure to the minimally invasive spine surgeon as well as his team. Knowledge of the potential hazards from ionizing radiation should be percolated through to all personnel involved in the minimally invasive spine surgeries and due precautions be taken to ensure reduction of their exposure.

REFERENCES

1. Jonathan D Cherry, et al. Galactic cosmic radiation leads to cognitive impairment and increased aβ plaque accumulation in a Mouse Model of Alzheimer's Disease. PLoS One. 2012; e53275.
2. USNRC – US Nuclear Regulatory Commission website– www.nrc.gov
3. Smith-Bindman R, Lipson J, Marcus R et al. Radiation dose associated with common computed tomography examinations and the associated lifetime attributable risk of cancer. Arch Int Med. 2009;169(22):2078-86.
4. Brenner DJ, Elliston CD, Hall EJ, Berdon WE. Estimated risks of radiation-induced fatal cancer from pediatric CT. Am J Roentg. 2001;176(2):289-96.
5. Harstall R, Heini PF, Mini RL, Orler R. Radiation exposure to the surgeon during fluoroscopically assisted percutaneous vertebroplasty: a prospective study. Spine. 2005;30(16): 1893-8.
6. Von Wrangel A, Cederblad A, Rodriguex-Catarino M. Fluoroscopically guided percuatenous vertebroplasty: assessment of radiation doses and implementation of procedural routines to reduce operator exposure. Acta Radiol. 2009;50(5)490-6.
7. Synowitz M, Kiwit J. Surgeon's radiation exposure during percutaneous vertebroplasty. J Neurosurg Spine 2006;4(2): 106-9.
8. Tappero C, Barbero S, Constantino S et al. Patient and operator exposure during percutaneous vertebroplasty. Radiol Med. 2009;114(4):595-607.
9. Perisinakis K, Damilakis J, Theocharopoulos N et al. patient exposure and associated radiation risks from fluoroscopically guided vertebroplasty or kyphoplasty. Radiology. 2004; 232(3):701-7.
10. Mehlman CT, DiPasquale TG. Radiation exposure to the orthopaedic surgical team during fluoroscopy: "how far away is far enough?". J Ortho Trauma. 1997;11(6):392-8.
11. Boszczyk BM, Bierschneider M, Panzer S et al. Fluoroscopic radiation exposure of the kyphoplasty patient. Eur Spine J. 2006;15(3):347-55.
12. Mroz TE, Yamashita T, Davros W, Lieberman IH. Radiation exposure to the surgeon and the patient during kyphoplasty. J Spinal Disord Tech. 2008;21(2):96-100.
13. Mariscalco Mw, Yamashita T, Lieberman IH et al. Radiation exposure to the surgeon during open lumbar microdiskectomy and minimally invasive microdiskectomy: a prospective controlled trial. Spine. 2011;36(3):255-60.
14. Ahn Y, Kim CH, Lee JH et al. Radiation Exposure to the Surgeon During Percutaneous Endoscopic Lumbar Diskectomy. Spine. 2013;38(7):617-25.
15. Bindal RK, Glaze S, Ghosh S et al. Surgeon and patient radiation exposure in minimally invasive transforaminal lumbar interbody fusion. J of Neurosurg Spine. 2008;9(6):570-3.
16. Clark JC, Jamer G, Marciano FF et al.Minimally invasive transforaminal lumbar interbody fusions and fluoroscopy: a low dose protocol to minimize ionizing radiation. Neurosurg Focus. 2013;35(2):E8.
17. Funao H, Ishii K, Momoshima S et al. Surgeons' exposure to radiation in single and multi-level minimally invasive transforaminal lumbar interbody fusion; A prospective study. PLOS One. 2014;9(4)e95233.
18. Srinivasan D, Than KD, Wang AC et al. Radiation safety and spine surgery: systematic review of exposure limits and methods to minimize radiation exposure. World Neurosurg. 2014 Dec; 82(6):1337-43.
19. Kim CW, Lee YP, Taylor W, et al. Use of navigation-assisted fluoroscopy to decrease radiation exposure during minimally invasive spine surgery. Spine J. 2008;8(4):584-90.
20. A Jay Khanna. 11 Tips to Help Decrease Radiation Exposure During Spine Surgery and Other Procedures. Becker's Spine Review, World wide web – www.beckerspine.com.

Diagnostic and Therapeutic Applications of Percutaneous Transpedicular Approaches to the Spine

Mihir R Bapat, Susmit Naskar, Amandeep Gujral

ABSTRACT

Pedicle serves as a gateway to the vertebral body and is used in a plethora of diagnostic and therapeutic procedures. Having a sound knowledge of surgical anatomy is paramount as the needle serves as an extension of the surgeon's hand. With an advent of percutaneous techniques, soft tissue trauma can be greatly minimized. A surgeon has to depend on tactile and visual orientation during surgery. This chapter aims to provide guidelines for the same.

INTRODUCTION

Since the advent of pedicle screw, researchers in insertion techniques have proposed numerous innovations.[1-6] While these addressed problems pertaining to screws, complications relating to tissue trauma and devascularization surfaced.[7-9] Introduction of percutaneous pedicle screws emerged from preexisting knowledge of percutaneous cannulation of pedicles for like biopsy and vertebroplasty.

The first biopsy was attempted in 1935 by Robertson and ball,[10] the first vertebroplasty in 1987 at France by Galibert for treatment of painful cervical vertebral hemangioma[11] and the first reported percutaneous pedicle screw was by Magrel et al. in 1982.[12]

Percutaneous screws have minimized tissue dissection and devascularization of muscles. Limited bleeding and approach related morbidity in the elderly/obese and significantly improved infection rates are the advantages of percutaneous screws.

Technological advances in magnification, retractor systems, instrumentation and neuromonitoring established array of procedures termed as 'minimal access spine surgery'.

APPLICATIONS

Percutaneous transpedicular corridor can be utilized for:

1. Approach to lesions of vertebral body.
   A. Biopsy: Trucut needle inserted into vertebral body under radiological guidance allows optimal tissue sampling often proving advantageous over fine needle aspiration cytology.
   B. Pain control and stabilization: In painful fractures (osteoporotic or neoplastic), percutaneous vertebroplasty or kyphoplasty allows rapid alleviation of pain and restoration of function. This is particularly beneficial in elderly patients with medical co-morbidities in whom prolong bed rest causes rapid wasting.
2. Three column spinal fixation. Percutaneous pedicle screw minimize tissue trauma (PLIF/TLIF), minimize morbidity (polytrauma/elderly/metastasis) and help manipulate the spine (scoliosis/spondylolisthesis).

TECHNIQUE

Safe cannulation of pedicles requires:

1. Sizing the pedicle
2. Getting oriented to radiological pedicle and facet contours
3. Insertion technique
4. Tips of safe manipulation
5. Errors and bail out.

Sizing the Pedicle

The preoperative assessment for pedicle screws involves planning the trajectory in sagittal and coronal plane. A standing AP and lateral radiograph reveals the direction of each pedicle under physiological load. The rotation of the spinous process (pedicle) is unmasked. Lateral deviation from the plumb line should also be noted. This is vital to allow smooth maneuvering of the rod through more than 3 screws.

CT scan is useful to measure the mediolateral width of pedicles and to optimize screw size. The sagittal width is more than mediolateral width and the later assume importance in screw placement.[13-16] The pedicle morphometry varies in patients and also at different levels in the same patient.[17]

Bone mineral densitometry (BMD) is invaluable in osteoporotic spine to gauze the pull out strength and to plan augmentation techniques to improve fixation.[18-21]

MRI along with CT helps delineate disease process that affects the pedicle and or vertebral body morphology (lytic lesion as a result of neoplasm or infection).[22,23]

Pedicle Contours and Orientation

A pedicle insertion has three parts: pilot hole, pedicle and vertebral body. All three can be mapped prior to insertion of the screw.

On the AP projection, the mouth of the pedicle has an 'owl eye' appearance at the superolateral edge of the vertebral body with the spinous process in the center. This is uniform in the lower dorsal spine below D7 through to L5. The craniocaudal dimension is longer than mediolateral width. Above D7 the pedicle eye is difficult to visualize. At S1 the medial border is sharp but the lateral border may be ill defined.

Posteriorly, the facet joint overlaps the mouth. The lateral edge of the facet overlaps the lateral edge of the pedicle mouth. This fact should be considered while planning the entry to avoid facet violation.

Rotation of the vertebral body distorts the owl eye in the concavity of the curve. To see both pedicles end on, the table should be tilted to neutralize the rotation in the AP projection.

caudal tilt of the C-arm overlap the near and distal cortical lines of the end plate and allow visualization of the pedicle 'owl eye' in AP projection.

In the lateral projection too, tilting the C-arm cranio-caudally allows the near and far pedicle contours to overlap. This allows a sharp delineation of the superior and inferior border.

Insertion Technique (Tips and Errors)

The patient is positioned prone either on bolsters or on Jackson's frame. The aim is to keep abdomen free to recreate lordosis and minimize intra-abdominal pressure. The hips can be flexed or extended to control pelvic tilt.

The pedicle is an elongated cylinder that begins postero-laterally and joins the body anteromedially.

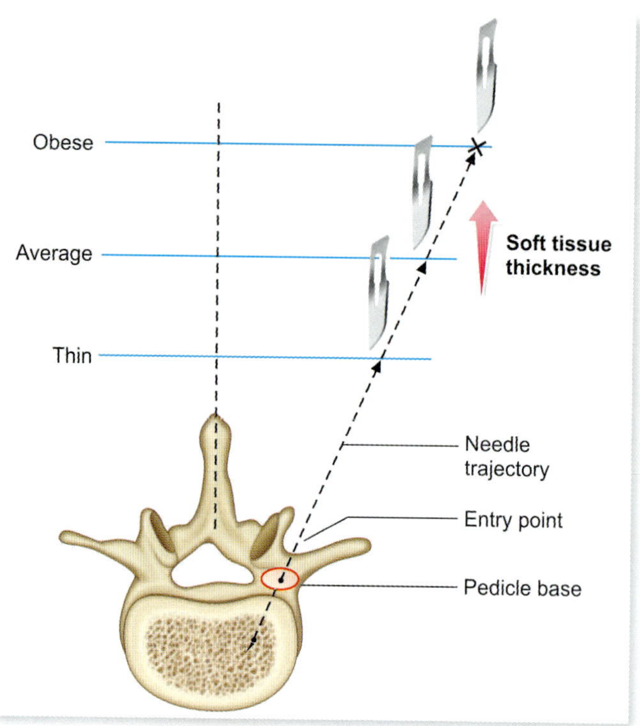

Figure 1: Site of skin incision depending upon soft tissue depth

The entry point on the skin starts 2–3 cm lateral to the lateral edge of the pedicle to allow entry into the pedicle cylinder **(Figure 1)**. The size of the incision allows the pedicle screw holder to enter smoothly without causing trauma to skin edges. The fascial incision is longer than the skin incision and finger dissection splits the muscle. The palpating finger can feel the rounded facet in most cases **(Figure 2)**. In a biopsy, the skin incision is a 5 mm stab to allow needle penetration.

The Jamshedji needle (11gauge) is inserted and docked 2–3 mm outside the lateral edge of the pedicle to avoid facet violation **(Figure 3)**. The entry is usually in the middle of the lateral edge. However, it can be shifted a little above or below to optimize the angulations in the sagittal plane (lateral C-arm image).

The cortical opening can be made manually or by tapping with a hammer. In an optimally positioned C-arm, needle is advanced toward the medial pedicle margin and stopped just short of it **(Figure 4)**.

A lateral C-arm Image is taken. Ideally, the tip of the needle should cross the junction of the pedicle and body ensuring intact medial wall **(Figure 5)**. If the needle is seen in the pedicle cylinder, the medial inclination should be reduced. Likewise if the needle extends deeper in the body, then trocar should be withdrawn and the base palpated with a guide wire. If a lateral cutout is appreciated, the needle can be repositioned with a medial trajectory. It is safer to accept a little lateral trajectory. Intraoperative neuromonitoring helps monitor nerve root irritation due to errant screw.

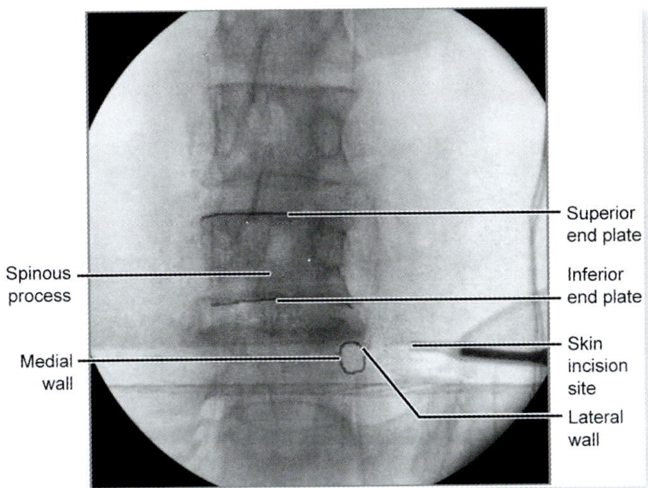

Figure 2: Anatomical landmarks of percutaneous transpedicular approach

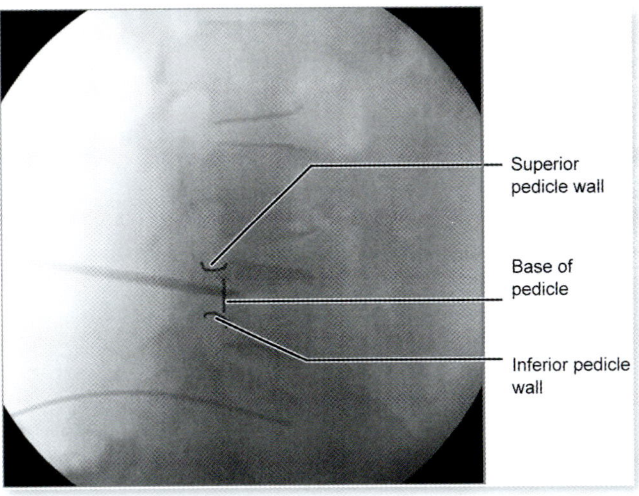

Figure 5: Lateral projection shows J needle has already crossed the pedicle base confirming proper trajectory

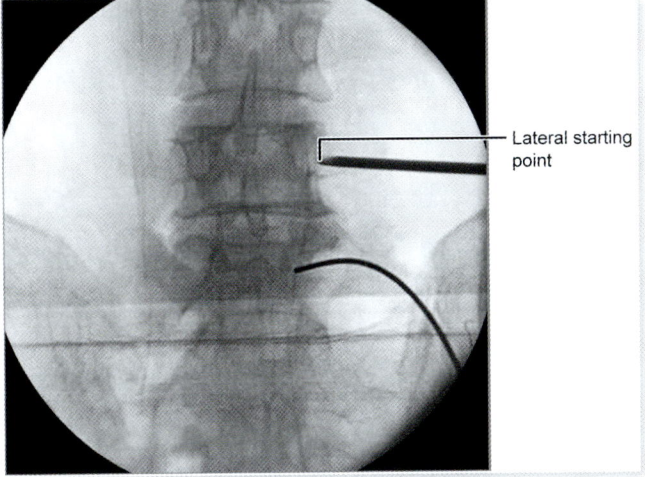

Figure 3: Pedicle entry point should start just lateral to lateral pedicle wall

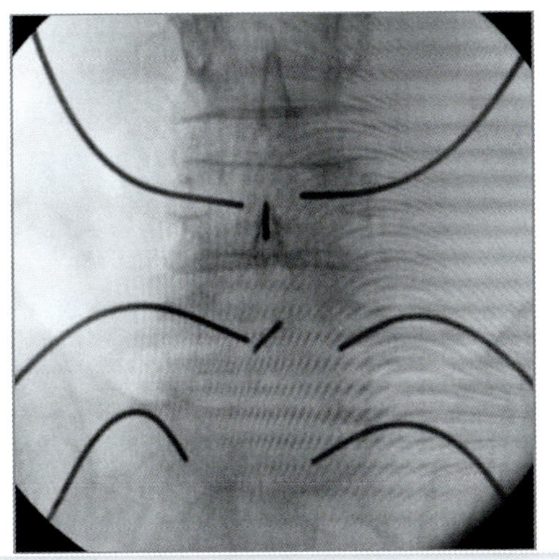

Figure 6: Final guidewire positions in AP view

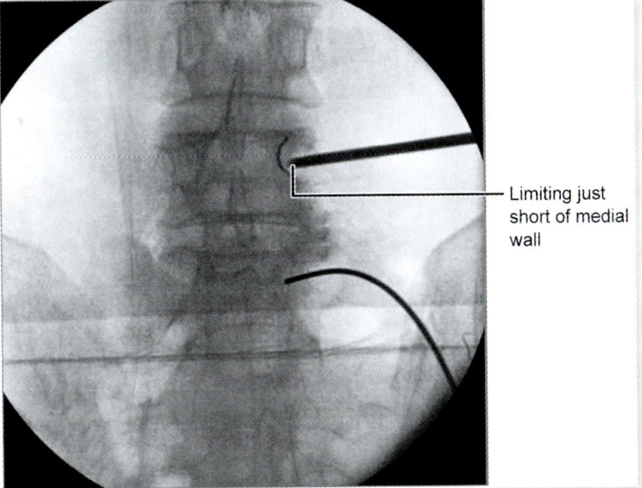

Figure 4: AP projection showing needle should stop just short of medial wall

The needle is then advance into the anterior third of the vertebral (up to 80%) body. Second cortex purchase is sought only in the sacrum or discreetly in osteoporotic vertebrae being cautious about anterior vasculature. In the AP projection the needle should be seen at or on the ipsilateral side of the spinous process. If the needle crosses the midline, medial cortex violation, long screw and vertebral rotation should be evaluated **(Figures 6 to 8)**.

Once the position of the needle is optimal, the steps pertaining to individual procedure are followed:

1. **Biopsy:** before advancing the needle in to the vertebral body, the trocar is removed. The hollow needle when introduced further retrieves a tissues sample for histopathology. The needle direction can be altered to get multiple samples.
2. **Vertebroplasty/kyphoplasty:** The cement can be injected into the vertebral body under fluoroscopy with constant vigilance for leakage. Leakage can be

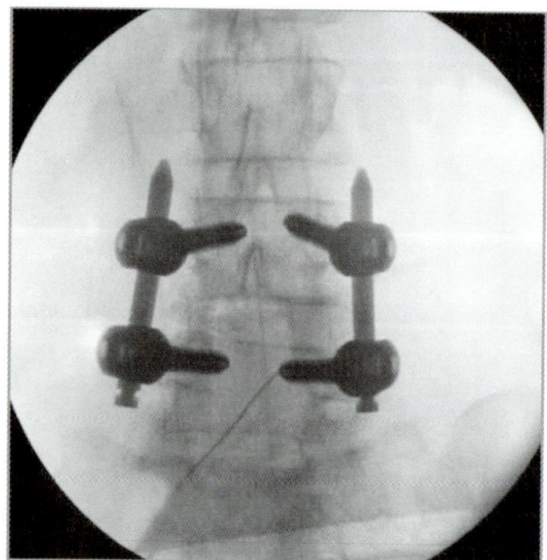

Figure 7: AP image

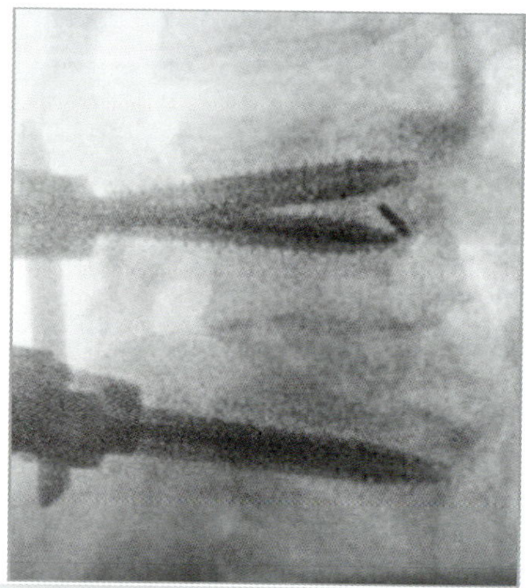

Figure 9: Improper direction of screw can cause bending of guide wire even breakage

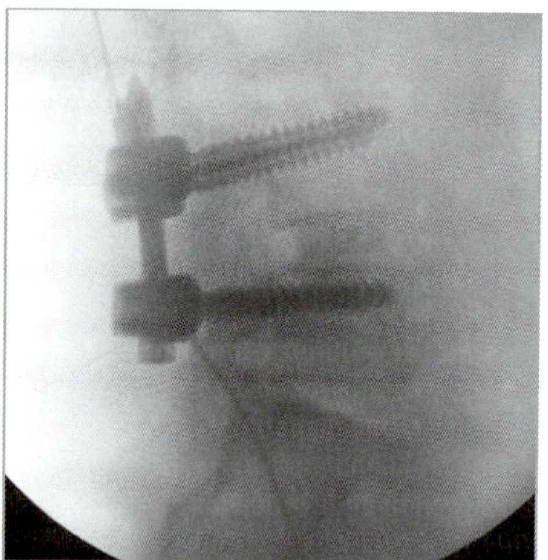

Figure 8: Lateral image

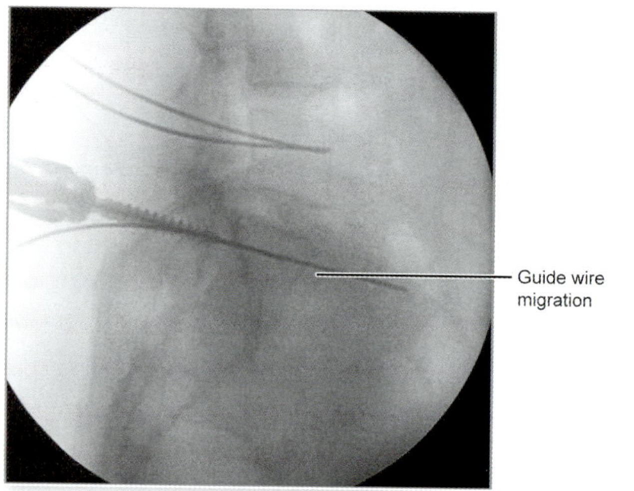

Figure 10: In osteoporotic spine anterior cortex can be broken with forceful guidewire penetration and may injure anterior vital structures

intravenous, intradiscal, perivertebral soft tissue, and the most dreaded epidural.

3. **Screw insertion:** The trocar is removed and a guidewire is inserted. The needle is withdrawn holding the wire in place. Cannulated tap and screw placement instruments are used to insert optimal size screw minimizing soft tissue trauma. It is imperative to take frequent X-rays to ensure that the screw follows the wire path without bending it. Once the screw crosses the pedicle into the body the wire should be withdrawn with a gentle outward tapping.

Slight change in the screw direction can be achieved by bending the wire. Excessive bending can result in wire getting stuck or breaking **(Figure 9)**. Wire migration through the anterior cortex into anterior viscera can be avoided by holding the tip of the wire during insertion **(Figure 10)**.

Thoracic Percutaneous Pedicle Screw Placement

Percutaneous cannulation in the thoracic spine is challenging due to small pedicle size (lowest in T4–T6-average 3.6–3.9 mm),[24-28] narrow canal[29] and prismatic shape of the body requiring a steep trajectory.[30]

Due to overlapping ribs and shoulder joint at proximal thoracic spine, visualization of lateral fluoroscopic image is suboptimal.[31]

These limitations can be minimized by the use of intra operative navigation, robotics and CT scan which render a three-dimensional image for ideal screw placement.

In our center we practice PT vertebroplasty and biopsy where indicated but we do not have experience of PTS fixation in upper thoracic spine.

Through numerous literatures[32-34] shows successful proximal thoracic percutaneous screw fixation, the high rates of screw cutout-related complications should be weighed in terms of risk-benefit ratio.

Minimizing Radiation

Role of protective garments, such as thyroid and eye shields, body jackets and radiation attenuation gloves is paramount in limiting radiation exposure to OR team. An expert C-arm technician and proper anatomical orientation aids in limiting the number of shoots. We routinely practice single shot C-arm images instead of video fluoroscopy at following critical steps:

- AP skin incision (2–3 shoots)
- Needle docking at 3/9'o clock (right and leftside) position on lateral pedicle edge (2–3 shoots)
- Advance up to medial pedicle edge (2–3 shoots)
- Advance up to body and exchange with guidewire (nil)
- Tapping of screw path (nil)
- Screw advancement up to pedicle hold at 20–30 mm (1 shoot)
- Screw advancement till it docks on facet (2 shoots)

In our practice average shoot for a single pedicle screw insertion is approximately 10–12.

Over the period as the surgical team gains experience judicious use of tactile feeling and C-arm minimizes radiation exposure.

Electrophysiological Monitoring

Lile spinal navigation, electrophysiological monitoring is another tool in a spinal surgeon's ambit to reduce complication rates in percutaneous procedures. SSEP have been used widely, but SSEP has several limitations in relation to monitoring for nerve root injury with pedicle screw placement.[35] In SSEP monitoring, the findings are not nerve root specific due to crossover of multiple roots in any given peripheral nerve; thus, the nerve roots that are not compromised can hide the response of the involved root. Moreover, SSEPs does not necessarily reflect changes in motor function, which have greater clinical significance.[36] The EMG monitoring/MEP of specific muscle groups monitors individual nerve roots and provide real-time feedback of nerve root injury.

RECENT ADVANCES AND FUTURE DIRECTIONS

A few advanced centers in the world are using O arm, spinal navigation and robotics which are a step ahead from fluoroscopy-aided procedures.[37,38] These technological advances provide a surgeon a three-dimensional vision which further minimizes surgical complications[39-41] but significantly increases surgical cost.

REFERENCES

1. Mark B Kabins, James N Weinstein. The history of vertebral screw and pedicle screw fixation. Iowa Orthop J. 1991;11:127-36.
2. Aebi M, Etter C, Kehl T, Thalgott J. Stabilization of the lower thoracic and lumbar spine with the internal spinal skeletal fixation system: Indications, techniques, and first results of treatment. Spine. 1987;12:544-51.
3. Harrington PR, Dickson JH. Spinal instrumentation in the treatment of severe progressive spondylolisthesis. Clin Orthop. Rel. Res. 1976;117:157-63.
4. Henstorf JE, Gaines RW, Steffee AD. Transpedicular fixation of spinal disorders with Steffee plates. Surg R Ortho. 1987; 3:35-43.
5. Jacobs RR, Montesano PX, Jackson RP. Enhancement of lumbar spine fusion by use of translaminar facet joint screws. Spine. 1989;14:12-15.
6. Karlstr6m G, Olerud S, Sjstrm L. Transpedicular segmental fixation: Description of a new procedure. Orthopaedics. 1988; 11:689-700.
7. Cole CD, McCall TD, Schmidt MH, Dailey AT. Comparison of low back fusion techniques: transforaminal lumbar interbody fusion (TLIF) or posterior lumbar interbody fusion (PLIF) approaches. Curr Rev Musculoskeletal Med. 2009;2(2): 118-26.
8. Hey HWD, Hee HT. Lumbar degenerative spinal deformity: Surgical options of PLIF, TLIF and MI-TLIF. Ind J Ortho. 2010;44(2):159-62.
9. Fan S, Hu Z, Zhao F, Zhao X, Huang Y, Fang X. Multifidus muscle changes and clinical effects of one-level posterior lumbar interbody fusion: minimally invasive procedure versus conventional open approach. Euro Spine J. 2010;19(2):316-24.
10. Robertson RC, Ball RP. Destructive spine lesions: diagnosis by needle biopsy. J Bone Joint Surg. 1935;57:749-58.
11. Galibert P, Deramond H, Rosat P, et al. Preliminary note on the treatment of vertebral angioma by percutaneous acrylic vertebroplasty. Neurochirurgie. 1987;33:166-8.
12. Magerl FP. Stabilisation of the lower thoracic and lumbar spine with external skeletal fixation. Clin Orthop Relat Res. 1984;189:125-41.
13. Berry JL, Moran JM, Berg WS, Steffee AD. A morphometric study of human lumbar and selected thoracic vertebrae. Spine. 1987;12:362-7.
14. Krag MH, Weaver DL, Beynnon BD, et al. Morphometry of the thoracic and lumbar spine related to transpedicular screw placement for surgical spinal fixation. Spine. 1988;13:27-32.
15. McLain RF, Ferrara L, Kabins M. Pedicle morphometry in the upper thoracic spine: limits to safe screw placement in older patients. Spine. 2002;27:2467-2471.
16. Datir, Sandeep P, Mitra Sajal RM. Morphometric study of the thoracic vertebral pedicle in an indian population. Spine. 2004; 29(11):1174-81.

17. Yu CC, Yuh RT, Bajwa NS, Toy JO, Ahn UM, Ahn NU. Lower thoracic pedicle morphometry: male, taller, and heavier specimens have bigger pedicles. Spine (Phila Pa 1976). 2015;40(6):E323-31.
18. McLain RF, Fry MF, Moseley TA, et al. Lumbar pedicle screw salvage: Pullout testing of three different pedicle screw designs. J Spinal Disord. 1995;8:62-8.
19. Wittenberg RH, Lee KS, Shea M, et al. Effect of screw diameter, insertion technique, and bone cement augmentation of pedicular screw fixation strength. Clin Orthop Relat Res. 1993;296:278-87.
20. Becker S, Chavanne A, Spitaler R, et al. Assessment of different screw augmentation techniques and screw designs in osteoporotic spines. European Spine Journal. 2008;17(11):1462-9.
21. Coe JD, Warden KE, Herzig MA, McAfee PC. Influence of bone mineral density on the fixation of thoracolumbar implants. A comparative study of transpedicular screws, laminar hooks, and spinous process wires. Spine 1990;15(9):902–907.
22. Rodallec MH, Feydy A, Larousserie F, Anract P, Campagna R, Babinet A, et al. Diagnostic imaging of solitary tumors of the spine: what to do and say. Radiographics. 2008; 28(4):1019-41.
23. Greenspan A. Radiologic evaluation of tumors and tumor-like lesions. In: Orthopedic imaging: a practical approach. 4th ed. Philadelphia, Pa: Lippincott Williams and Wilkins. 2004; pp 529-70.
24. Zindrick MR, Wiltse LL, Doornik A, Widell EH, Knight GW, Patwardhan AG, et al. Analysis of the morphometric characteristics of the thoracic and lumbar pedicles. Spine (Phila Pa 1976). 1987;12:160-6.
25. Panjabi MM, Takata K, Goel V, Federico D, Oxland T, Duranceau J, Krag M. Thoracic human vertebrae. Quantitative three-dimensional anatomy. Spine (Phila Pa 1976). 1991;16:888-901.
26. Rao G, Brodke DS, Rondina M, Dailey AT. Comparison of computerized tomography and direct visualization in thoracic pedicle screw placement. J Neurosurg. 2002;97:223-6
27. Kim YJ, Lenke LG, Bridwell KH, Cho YS, Riew KD. Free hand pedicle screw placement in the thoracic spine: is it safe? Spine (Phila Pa 1976). 2004;29:333-42.
28. Carbone JJ, Tortolani PJ, Quartararo LG. Fluoroscopically assisted pedicle screw fixation for thoracic and thoracolumbar injuries: technique and short-term complications. Spine (Phila Pa 1976). 2003;28:91-7.
29. John L. Sherman, Patrie Y. Nassaux,Charles M. Citrin. Measurements of the Normal Cervical Spinal Cord on MR Imaging. AJNR. 1990;11:369-72.
30. Mitra SR, Datir SP, Jadhav SO. Morphometric study of the lumbar pedicle in the Indian population as related to pedicular screw fixation. Spine (Phila Pa 1976). 2002;27(5):453-9.
31. Carolyn A. Hardin, Shahid M. Nimjee, Isaac O. Karikari, Abhishek Agrawal, Richard G. Fessler,1 and Robert E. Isaacs. Percutaneous pedicle screw placement in the thoracic spine: A cadaveric study. Asian J Neurosurg. 2013;8(3):153-6.
32. Park DH, Thomas AO, St Clair S. "Percutaneous lumbar and thoracic pedicle screws, a trauma experience," Journal of Spinal Disorders and techniques. 2014;27(3):154-61.
33. Hardin CA, Nimjee SM, Karikari IO, Agrawal A, Fessler RG, Isaacs RE. Percutaneous pedicle screw placement in the thoracic spine: A cadaveric study. Asian J Neurosurg. 2013;8(3):153-6.
34. Bledsoe JM, Fenton D, Fogelson JL, Nottmeier EW. Accuracy of upper thoracic pedicle screw placement using three-dimensional image guidance. Spine J. 2009;9(10):817-21.
35. Owen JH, Kstuik JP, Gornet M, et al. The use of mechanically elicited electromyograms to protect nerve roots during surgery for spinal degeneration. Spine. 1994;19(15):1704-10.
36. Epstein NE, Danto J, Nardi D. Evaluation of intraoperative somatosensory evoked potential monitoring during 100 cervical operations. Spine. 1993;18(6):737-47.
37. Martirosyan NL, Kalb S, Cavalcanti DD, Lochhead RA, Uschold TD, Loh A, Theodore N. Comparative analysis of isocentric 3-dimensional C-arm fluoroscopy and biplanar fluoroscopy for anterior screw fixation in odontoid fractures. J Spinal Disord Tech. 2013 Jun;26(4):189-93.
38. 38 Kerry G, Ruedinger C, Steiner H-H. Intraoperative three-dimensional fluoroscopy after transpedicular positioning of Kirschner-wire versus conventional intraoperative biplanar fluoroscopic control: A retrospective study of 345 patients and 1880 pedicle screws. Craniovertebral Junction & Spine. 2014;5(3):125-30.
39. Yang BP, Wahl MM, Idler CS. Percutaneous lumbar pedicle screw placement aided by computer-assisted fluoroscopy-based navigation: perioperative results of a prospective, comparative, multicenter study. Spine (Phila Pa 1976). 2012;37(24): 2055-60.
40. Bourgeois AC, Faulkner AR, Bradley YC, Pasciak A, Barlow PB, Gash JR, Reid WS Jr. Improved Accuracy of Minimally Invasive Transpedicular Screw Placement in the Lumbar Spine with Three-dimensional Stereotactic Image Guidance: A Comparative Meta-analysis. J Spinal Disord Tech. 2014. [Epub ahead of print]
41. Mason A, Paulsen R, Babuska JM, Rajpal S, Burneikiene S, Nelson EL, Villavicencio AT. The accuracy of pedicle screw placement using intraoperative image guidance systems. J Neurosurg Spine. 2014;20(2):196-203.

2

SECTION

MIS in Cervical Spine

Section Outline

8

CHAPTER

Anterior Cervical Diskectomy without Fusion

CE Deopujari, Shumayou Dutta

ABSTRACT

The surgical technique for anterior cervical disckectomy has gradually evolved over time. Since the advent of interbody cages and plates, there is much doubt regarding the role of the traditional anterior cervical disckectomy without graft and/or added instrumentation. In this chapter, we focus on the technique of cervical disckectomy and weigh the clinical benefits of cervical instrumentation over the cost implications and complications associated with its use. Interestingly, our understanding of surgical strategy has also evolved from a 'one shoe fits all' approach before, to appreciating that the surgery offered should be tailor-made, considering the patient's clinical history and radiological findings. Bearing this concept in mind, the authors describe the technique and outcomes of anterior cervical diskectomy (ACD) in symptomatic, single level herniated cervical disks without any instability. Shorter hospital stay, lesser operative time and lower complication rates without any significant negative influence on overall cervical sagittal balance, favors its continued role in modern day surgery. Instrumented fusion procedures also have their own value after diskectomy and should be used whenever indicated, depending on the local biomechanics of the patient's spine and the number of levels operated.

EVOLUTION AND INDICATIONS

Commonly accepted indications for anterior cervical diskectomy (ACD) include myelopathy and persistent radiculopathy of diskal origin which is unresponsive to nonsurgical measures.[1,2] The most common surgical techniques are diskectomy with or without fusion of the two adjacent intervertebral bodies. Robinson and Smith[3-5] introduced the anterior cervical decompression technique, and achieved fusion by inserting a bone graft harvested from the iliac crest of the patient. Hankinson and Wilson[6] improved the procedure with the use of an operating microscope. They performed the surgery without leaving a graft behind and interestingly, the results of both types of surgery were entirely comparable.[7,8] With time, several modifications of these surgical techniques have appeared. Performing anterior cervical diskectomy has proven to be successful in relieving arm pain and has been considered equivalent to anterior cervical diskectomy and fusion (ACDF) in terms of clinical outcomes in a single level involvement.[9] In Europe ACD alone is still being used as a surgical procedure. In our institution, the prerequisite for performing an ACD is normal lordosis not associated with any obvious instability or subluxations preferably in a single level involvement.

APPLIED ANATOMY AND TECHNIQUE

Technique

Preoperative Planning

In revision surgery, it is appropriate to get a preoperative otolaryngology consult to evaluate vocal cord paralysis.[10] If a vocal cord paralysis exists, the approach should be made on the ipsilateral side to avoid a potential bilateral paralysis. An approach on the right side at C5-6 may put the recurrent laryngeal nerve at more risk, while a low approach on the left side may put the thoracic duct at risk.

Preoperative Imaging

The preoperative radiographs are examined to identify unique anatomic features. Knowledge of the ventral osteophytes are particularly helpful to the surgeon and reassures that the proper level has been reached. To confirm the proper levels during the approach intraoperative radiography should be used. The vertebrae are labeled by level. Anatomically "short" necks where the lower cervical levels are at or below the level of the clavicle may alert the surgeon to potential difficulty accessing these lower levels during a standard approach.

Intraoperative Procedures

Prophylactic antibiotics (usually ceftriaxone 1 g) are given half hour before incision to minimize the risk of infection. The patient is placed supine on the operating table. The neck should be stabilized (preferably with a hard collar) while moving the patient. A folded sheet is placed in the interscapular area. Folded sheets are placed under the shoulders and the foam doughnut under the head are adjusted to obtain ideal neck extension. It is rare that any support other than the doughnut is needed under the head. In patients with a short neck, the shoulders are strapped down to enable intraoperative radiographic visualization. The inferior towel is usually at the sternal notch, the superior towel is around the chin, the ipsilateral towel is as low as possible, the contralateral towel is severalcentimeters lateral to midline to accommodate a midline-crossing incision. The carotid tubercle, thyroid cartilage, and cricoid cartilage can be palpated as landmarks. An incision is marked in a neck crease if possible, crossing midline as needed. Larger transverse incisions with less retraction (skin stretching) tend to heal better than a smaller incision with stretched skin edges. Vertical incisions are avoided as they leave unappealing scars **(Figure 1)**.

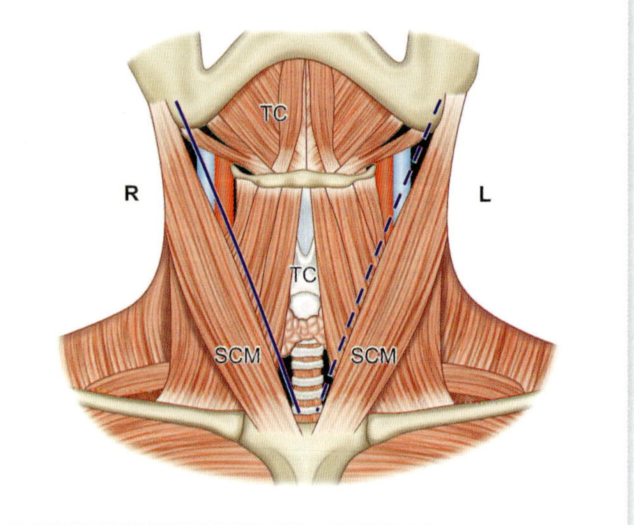

Figure 1: Incision – horizontal for 1 and 2 levels and vertical for 3 or more. SCM, sternocleidomastoid muscle; TC, thyroid cartilage

The incision should be located in the inferior third of the levels to be decompressed because it is easier to mobilize skin in a cephalad rather than a caudal direction and the disk spaces angle cephalad. Understanding local anatomy may help guide incision level **(Figure 2)**. Depending on the surgeons requirement, the skin may or may not be injected with 0.25% marcaine with epinephrine as early as possible, since the epinephrine takes time to work (ideally 10 minutes). Cut strips of adhesive barrier drape (Ioban) are used to seal the edges after the incision is marked. A scalpel is used to incise the epidermis and dermis. Leaving an intact corner of dermis at the ends of the wound protects against stretching, thereby allowing for a more cosmetically pleasing closure. Using the cut function on the electrocautery will minimize charred tissue, but small veins will often need the coagulate function. The platysma is cut transversely in line with the incision. The platysma is undermined cranially and caudally with spreading scissors, blunt finger dissection, and cautery. The interval between the sternocleidomastoid and medial strap muscles is identified. The external jugular vein may be mobilized preferably to the lateral side. Preserving the sternocleidomastoid fascia by starting the dissection closer to the strap muscles will minimize bleeding. Spreading scissors, blunt finger dissection, and cautery are used to dissect through the interval between the alar fascia (carotid sheath) and the visceral fascia (trachea and esophagus) **(Figure 3)**.

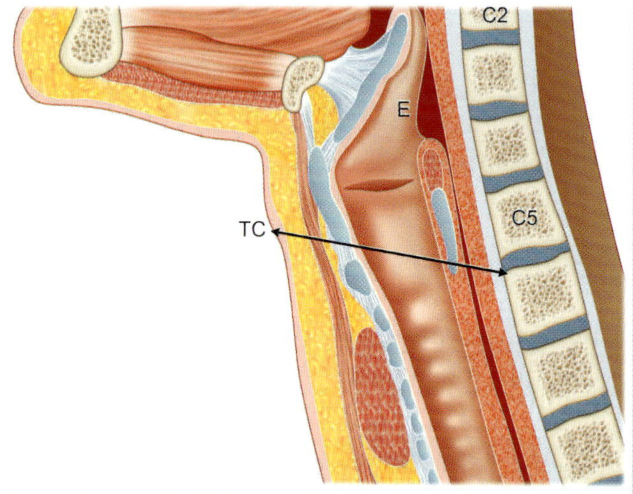

Figure 2: Relationship of the C5–6 disk space to the thyroid cartilage, which serves as a surface making

The carotid pulse can be palpated and kept lateral. In the interval, the ventral cervical spine and longus colli muscles can be palpated. Blunt finger dissection can widen the defect longitudinally, although there may be less bleeding with the spreading scissors technique. Crossing nerves that should be preserved include the glossopharyngeal and hypoglossal nerves at the very top of the approach and the superior laryngeal nerve above the superior thyroid artery. The recurrent laryngeal nerve may be at the bottom of the approach, especially on the right side. It is acceptable to take the inferior, middle, and superior thyroid vessels, if necessary.

Larger crossing vessels may need to be tied. A wall bleeder can be very difficult to stop, if it represents a side-opened vessel; in this case, a bipolar technique will often slow bleeding enough to allow packing with a hemostatic agent and cottonoid patty.

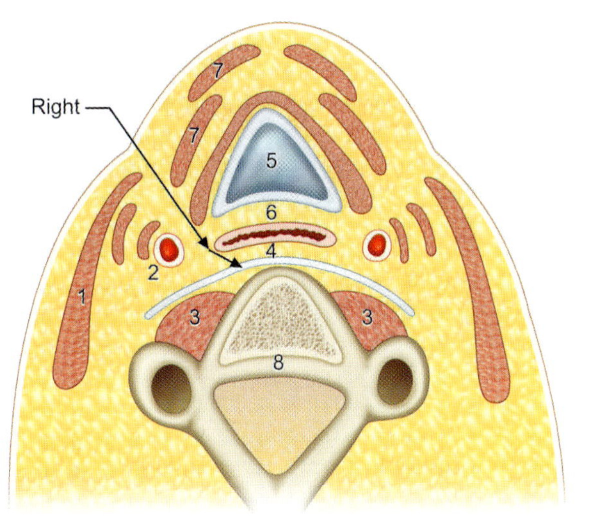

Figure 3: Diagrammatic representation of the structures and the plane of dissection through the neck. 1. sternocleidomestoid muscle; 2. carotid sheath; 3. longus colli; 4. prevertebral facia; 5. trachea; 6. oesophagus; 7. medial strap muscles; 8. vertebral body

A hand-held retractor is placed medially to pull the trachea and esophagus over the midline to see the ventral aspect of the cervical spine. The omohyoid muscle crosses the field around C6 and can be divided with lower-level dissections with no adverse effects. The muscle can be elevated and then divided with electrocautery.

The carotid tubercle, usually at C6, and ventral osteophytes can be palpated to estimate levels. The prevertebral fascia is cleared off the disks (hills) and vertebral bodies (valleys) using scissors and forceps with a nick-and-spread technique. The hand-held retractor is then replaced under this layer. A bent 12 mm, 14 mm, or 16 mm spine needle (based on preoperative radiographic measurement) is placed in the disk space of choice and the level is confirmed radiologically.

The carotid tubercle and/or ventral osteophytes can be used to predict the level. Dissection can continue while the film is being processed. The microscope is then brought into the field. The "valley" of the ventrolateral aspect of the vertebral body above and below the suspected disk is cauterized to get the segmental arteries and perforating branches. The longus colli is elevated off the vertebral body.

Bleeding bone on the front side of the vertebral body under the elevated longus can be coagulated with bone wax used as needed. If bleeding starts from the undersurface of the longus or out laterally, a hemostatic agent and a large cottonoid patty can be used. The self-retaining retractors are placed underneath the elevated layer of the longus colli. The hand-held retractor is used to move the esophagus so that the self-retaining retractor blade can be safely placed under the longus.

An assistant's hand on the medial self-retaining retractor handle can stabilize downward and keep it correctly positioned. The vertebral body just cranial and caudal to the disk space is prepared for insertion of the Caspar retraction posts. Caspar pins (usually 14 mm or 16 mm) based on preoperative and localizing radiographs) are inserted by hand. Careful insertion is important, if the patient is very myelopathic or stenotic. The Caspar pins can be inserted slightly diverging to allow for lordosis. Excellent visualization of the bodies before placing the posts will help to avoid errors at this step. Centering with reference to the spine is more reliable than centering with reference to the patient's chin and sternal notch. The cranial angulation of the disk space should be parallel to the path of the Caspar pin in the sagittalplane. It can be helpful to identify the disk space with a #15 blade if the surgeon is unsure of the location or angle.The posts must diverge or be parallel when inserted to lordose the spine and prevent the cephalad post from entering the end plate, given the upward sloping nature of the end plate. If the Caspar pins are not placed divergently, the threads of the cephalad post may be encountered while burring out the end plate. A #15 blade is used to cut the width of the ventral annulus (the cutting portion of a #15 blade is 11 mm exactly). Multiple passes are made through the disk, going no deeper than the cutting portion of the blade while turning the blade vertically at the lateral edges of the disk space. A pituitary rongeur is used to remove initial disk fragments. The Caspar retraction can be increased once the ventral anulus has been excised. A curette (Codman Microsect 4B) can be held like a dagger or a pencil while scraping the disk thoroughly. A side-to-side motion is safe as far lateral as the uncovertebral joint allows. The path of the curette should be smile-shaped during the initial passes, not just horizontal. Resting the hand on the patient with all manoeuvres will give stabilization and control. A pituitary rongeur is again used to remove numerous pieces of disk. A smaller curette (Codman Microsect 2B) can be used to get into foramen by first using a twisting or scooping motion to get the cartilage out of the uncovertebral joint and then using an upward pulling motion to get the uncovertebral process to break and come out of the foramen ventrally. The microscope should be tilted to angle into the intervertebral space optimally. Suction in the nondominant hand should rest on the patient for control and stability while in the disk space. The PLL may need to be removed only if the surgeon is going after an extruded disk. Inadequate foraminal decompression may lead to residual radicular symptoms.

Postoperative Management

For single-level anterior cervical diskectomy and fusion, an appropriately sized soft collar is placed before extubation, and the patient is instructed to wear it as needed for comfort. Patients can remove it for eating and cleaning (approximately 1 hour a day) but otherwise to wear it for 6 weeks. Patients are observed overnight in the hospital with a continuous pulse oximeter to watch for airway compromise from postoperative hematoma/seroma.

COMPLICATIONS OF ANTERIOR CERVICAL DISKECTOMY

Complications following anterior cervical diskectomy are infrequent but can be life threatening.[11] In addition to neurologic deterioration, dural injury, and inadequate decompression with persistent or recurrent symptoms, injuries to vital structures in the neck including the esophagus and the vertebral artery have been reported. These must be promptly recognized and properly treated to minimize patient morbidity.

Soft tissue swelling associated with prolonged retraction, hematoma, seroma, and implant/graft dislodgment can all contribute to airway compromise. Dysphagia and dysphonia occur following ventral cervical approaches and have traditionally been underreported in the literature. Most of these will resolve with time but in recalcitrant cases should be referred for otolaryngology evaluation.Vertebral artery injuries require direct repair, stenting, and/or ligation. Immediate bleeding should be controlled by direct pressure. Avoid injecting hemostatic agents directly into the cerebral vascular system. If available, obtain an emergent consultation with a vascular surgeon or interventionalist who can perform an angiogram to assess collateral circulation and potentially stent or occlude the lesion.

Esophageal injuries may not be detected with intraoperativedye. If any suspicion of esophageal injury exists, it is prudent to keep the patient nil per os (NPO) and obtain consultation from a thoracic or head and neck surgeon.

Airway compromise is an emergency with which all personnel caring for postoperative ventral cervical spine surgery patients should be familiar. Voice changes to a high-pitched squeak, difficulty in swallowing, and dyspnea are all causes for alarm. Immediate evaluation and treatment are mandatory. A tracheostomy may be considered. Emergent consultation with an anesthesiologist and/or otolaryngologist should be obtained.

Persistent postoperative neck and interscapular pain have also been reported after an ACD procedure. Sagittal profiles of the cervical spine have been hypothesized to influence loads on spinal tissue and influence outcome after spinal surgery.[12] It is believed that ACDF maintains sagittal alignment superiorly to ACD surgery, which should result in a better outcome after surgery and thus on the long-term in less disability for the patients. However, it is interesting to note that it has been published that single-level ACD procedures may lead to a local kyphosis, but this does not influence the regional sagittal alignment and does not lead to a deterioration of results over time. **(Figures 4 to 6)**.[13]

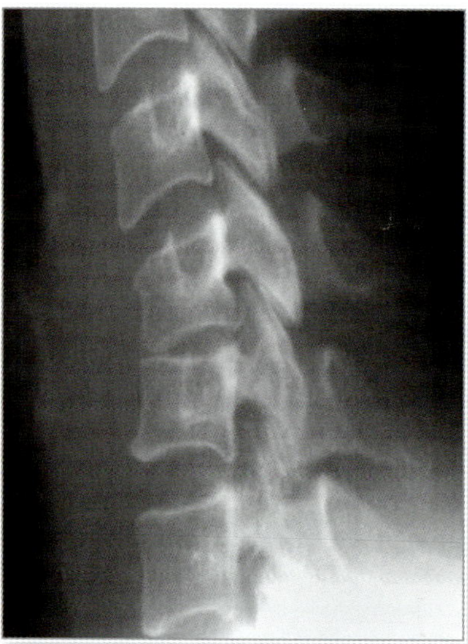

Figure 4: Anterior cervical diskectomy: Immediatly postoperative radiograph

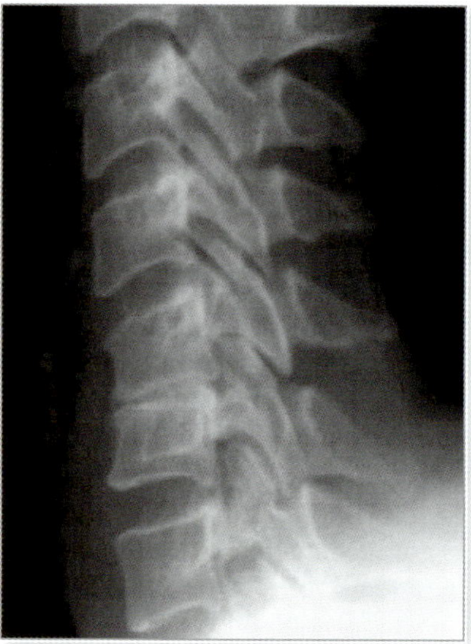

Figure 5: Postoperative photograph of ACD

Anterior Cervical Diskectomy Vs Anterior Cervical Diskectomy with Fusion

A few studies have compared ACD techniques and they all do not show any superiority of anterior cervical diskectomy with fusion (ACDF) compared to ACD without fusion.[14-17] Avoidance of the use of implants reduces the cost of surgery. More importantly, these studies revealed that ACD alone resulted in a shorter surgical procedure, hospital stay and

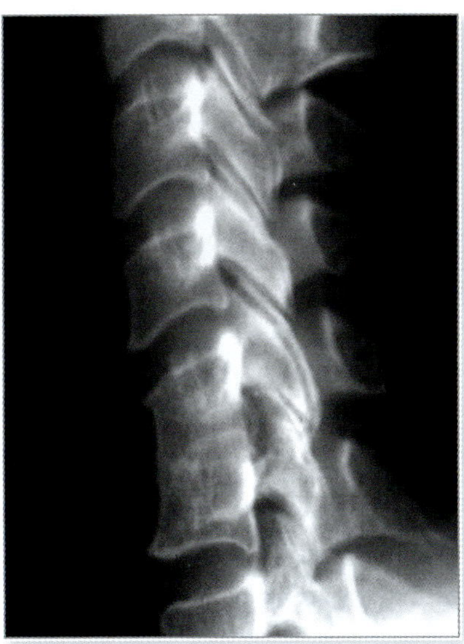

Figure 6: Anterior cervical diskectomy: One year postoperative photograph

sick leave[18,19] A frequently reported complication of ACDF is autologous grafting from the iliac crest causing post-operative pain at the donor site, which has been reported to result in up to 22% additional morbidity.[20]

AUTHOR'S EXPERIENCE

In over 15 years of experience the author has done over 350 cases of anterior cervical diskectomy with/with-out fusion following the pre-requisites and indications mentioned above. In a retrospective comparative study conducted in Bombay Hospital[21] for a period of 6 years, the author reports the outcomes of ACD, ACDF and ACDFI (anterior cervical diskectomy and fusion with instrumentation).

Results obtained were as tabulated in **Table 1.**

COMPLICATIONS

In the ACD group 3 patients had local complications (1 each of hoarseness of voice, postoperative weakness, opposite side radicular pain) and 2 had systemic (1 inferior wall MI, 1 right frozen shoulder). In the ACDF group 1 patient had graft site pain, and in the ACDFI, there was one patient who had implant failure in the form of the top screws backing out.

Nurick grading was used to chart neurological recovery and no statistically significant difference was found in the recovery pattern of either group.

SUMMARY

Like all other surgeries, anterior cervical diskectomy too has evolved over time. Instead of trying to decipher which surgical procedure is the best, the new age outlook would be to understand that not any one procedure is the best but all the procedures have their specific indications wherein they provide the best clinical outcomes. Surgery should be tailor-made, taking into account patients clinical history and radiological findings. Having understood this concept, in its most simplistic viewing, the authors feel that ACD has its place in symptomatic, single level herniated cervical disks without any instability. Apart from shorter hospital stay, lesser operative time and lesser complication rates, a substantial advantage of ACD over its counterparts is the absence of graft related complications and the reduced financial burden imposed on the patient and the healthcare industry when animplant is not added.Instrumented fusion procedures have their own value and could be used as required after assessing the biomechanics of the spine in individual patients.In this era of value based spine care, as specialists we have the onus of responsibility on us to provide affordable, high quality health care, tailored for each patient's specific needs and lifestyle.

Table 1

Parameter	*ACD*	*ACDF*	*ACDFI*
Number of patients	56	12	12
Mean Age (years)	45.4	48.4	53.7
Myelopathy **(Figures 7A to D)**	26.7%	16%	0%
Radiculopathy	42.8%	33.3%	83.3%
Myeloradiculopathy	30.3%	50%	16.6%
Mean postoperative hospital stay	5.1	5.4	6.3
Mean time for improvement to start (days)	6.76	7.75	16
Patient satisfaction	E(13),G(35),F(5),P(3)	E(2),G(8),F(2),P(0)	E(0),G(8),F(3),P(1)

E, excellent; G, good; F, fair; P, poor; ACD, anterior cervical diskectomy; ACDF, anterior cervical diskectomy with fusion; ACDFI, anterior cervical diskectomy and fusion with instrumentation

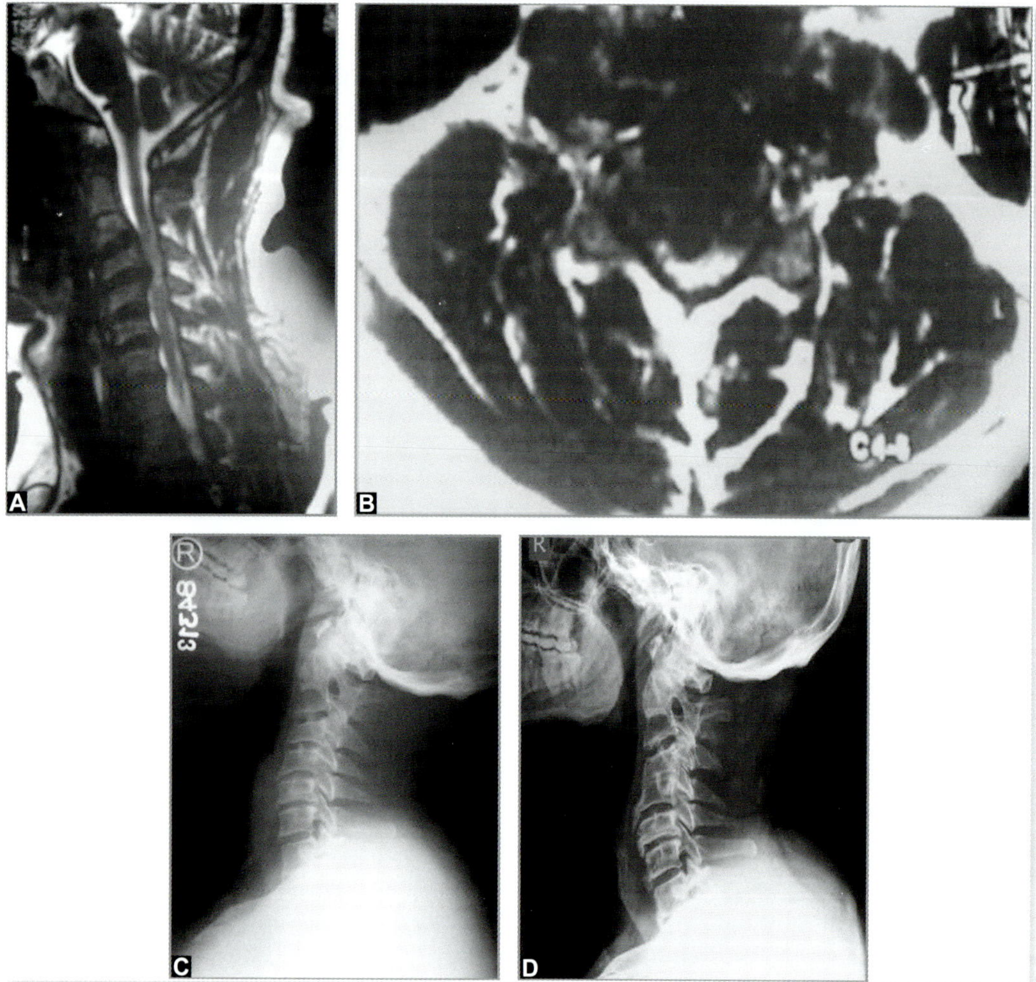

Figures 7A to D: C4,5 ACD done for a C4,5 disk prolapse causing myelopathy. (A to C) Preoperative images; (D) C4 at 1 year follow-up

REFERENCE

1. Rhee JM, Yoon T, Riew KD: Cervical radiculopathy. J Am Acad Orthop Surg. 2007;15:486-94.
2. Riew KD, Buchowski JM, Sasso R, et al: Cervical disk arthroplasty compared with arthrodesis for the treatment of myelopathy. J Bone Joint Surg [Am]. 2008;90(11):2354-64.
3. Robinson RA, Smith GW. Anterolateral cervical disk removal and interbody fusion for cervical disk syndrome. Bull John Hopkins Hosp. 1955;96(Suppl):223-4.
4. Robinson RA. Anterior and posterior cervical spine fusion.Clin Orthop. 1964;35:34-62.
5. Smith GW, Robinson RA. The treatment of certain cervical-spine disorders by anterior removal of the intervertebral disk and interbody fusion. J Bone Joint Surg. 1958;40:607-24.
6. Hankinson HI, Wilson CB. Use of the operating microscope in anterior cervical diskectomy without fusion. J Neurosurg. 1975;43:452-6.
7. Abd-Alrahman N, Dokmak AS, Abou-Madawi A. Anterior cervical diskectomy versus anterior cervical fusion, clinical and radiological outcome study. ActaNeurochir. 1999;141(10):1089-92. doi: 10.1007/s007010050487. Dowd GC, Wirth FP.
8. Anterior cervical diskectomy: is fusion necessary? J Neurosurg. 1999;90(1):8-12.
9. Jacobs WCH, Anderson PG, Van Limbeek J, Willems PC, Pavlov P. Single or double-level anterior interbody fusion techniques for cervical degenerative disk disease. 2004; Cochrane Database Sys Rev 4:CD 004958.
10. Paniello RC, Martin-Bredahl KJ, Henkener LJ, Riew KD. Preoperative laryngeal nerve screening for revision anterior cervical spine procedures. Ann Oto Rhino Laryngol. 2008; 117(8):594-7.
11. Complications of anterior cervical diskectomy without fusion in 450 consecutive patients. Eur Spine J. 2007;16(9): 1411-6. Published online 2007 Jan 30. doi: 10.1007/s00586-007-0309-y PMCID: PMC2200758.

12. Colloca CJ, Harrison DD, Harrison DE, Janik TJ. Influence of spine morphology on intervertebral disk loads and stresses in asymptomatic adults:implications for the ideal spine. Spine J. 2005;5(3):297-309. doi: 10.1016/j.spinee.2004.10.050.
13. Johnson JP, Lauryssen C, Cambron HO, Pashman R, Regan JJ, Anand N, Bray R. Sagittal alignment and the Bryan cervical artificial disk.Neurosurg Focus. 2004;17(6):E14.
14. la Torre M, Martinez-Quinones JV, Isla A, Arguello C, Bendala A, Casado J, Blazquez MG. Anterior cervical diskectomy with and without bone grafting. Multicentric comparative study. J Bone Joint Surg Br.1995;77B(Suppl 1):24.
15. Dowd GC, Wirth FP. Anterior cervical diskectomy: is fusion necessary?JNeurosurg. 1999;90(1):8–12.
16. Martins AN. Anterior cervical diskectomy with and without interbody bone graft. J Neurosurg. 1976;44:290-5. doi: 10.3171/jns.1976.44.3.0290. [PubMed] [Cross Ref].
17. McConnel JR, Freeman BJ, Debnath UK, Grevitt MP, Prince HG, Webb JK. A prospective randomized comparison of coralline hydroxyapatite with autograft in cervical interbody fusion. Spine. 2003;28(4):317-23. doi: 10.1097/00007632-200302150-00002.
18. Dowd GC, Wirth FP. Anterior cervical diskectomy: is fusion necessary?JNeurosurg. 1999;90(1):8-12.
19. Rosenorn J, Hansen EB, Rosenorn MA. Anterior cervical diskectomy with or without fusion: a prospective study. J Neurosurg. 1983;59(2):252-5. [PubMed].
20. McConnel JR, Freeman BJ, Debnath UK, Grevitt MP, Prince HG, Webb JK. A prospective randomized comparison of coralline hydroxyapatite with autograft in cervical interbody fusion. Spine. 2003;28(4):317-23. doi: 10.1097/00007632-200302150-00002. [PubMed]
21. Rajiv Kumar, CE Deopujari, Rajan Shah, Ashish Kumar. A study of anterior cervical diskectomy with or without fusion. Bombay Hospital Journal. 2010;52:30-41.

9

CHAPTER

Tubular Retractors in Cervical Spine

G Balamurali, T Ganesh Keshav

ABSTRACT

The tubular retractors have revolutionized the approach to the pathologies of the cervical spine. It provides satisfactory visualization of the determined structures and also has advantages of causing lesser tissue trauma and earlier mobilization, specially in obese individuals. This chapter will deal with the indications of using these retractors, techniques and complications of the procedure.

INTRODUCTION

Tubular retractors have revolutionized the way we approach pathologies to the spine in the last few decades. Posterior approaches to cervical spine was initially popular for disk prolapse and cervical decompression[1] until the advent of anterior approaches in the early 1950s.[2,3] Anterior approach to the spine was able to deal with total disk removal, vertebral body resection, correction of Kyphosis and attain good fusion rates. The approach-related morbidity was significantly less in experienced hands, and postoperative pain was minimal. Traditional open posterior approached needed a moderately large incision to achieve good visualization during the deep dissection though very tough musculature. To visualize the lateral mass completely for instrumentation requires significant muscle retraction. This causes severe muscle spasm, postoperative pain and sometimes wasting of muscles. The advent of tubular retractors using minimally invasive techniques minimizes these complications, and hence, some of these procedures have regained popularity to approach certain pathologies, especially laterally placed disk prolapse. It offers direct anatomical visualization of the operative field and minimizes tissue trauma. By this approach, unilateral herniated cervical disk, cervical stenosis and intradural pathologies can be approached. These benefits of reducing the approach related incisional morbidities are clearly documented. Attention to the technique and orientation, understanding of the anatomy and proper selection of patients will minimize complications and improve outcomes.

TUBULAR RETRACTOR SYSTEMS

A tubular retractor is a surgical instrument which the surgeon can employ to hold back underlying organs and tissues, so that the area of interest or operating field under the incision could be accessed. The visibility can be improved with a powerful light source from an endoscope, microscope or LED lights that fix to the retractor.

Advancements in the design of tubular retractors have drastically improved and expanded the reach of MISS. Retractors can be broadly classified in **Table 1**.

The flexible arm and easy change of tube direction help cover multiple spinal segments from a single incision. Understanding the detailed anatomy, including the tubular anatomy and having good surgical orientations are key essentials to the tubular- retractor system based surgeries.

Table 1

Classification of tubular retractor

Holding mechanism	*X-ray imaging*
Hand held	Lucent (PEEK, carbon)
Self-retaining	Semi-lucent (titanium and aluminum)
Table fixed (e.g. tubular retractors)	Opaque (stainless steel)

TYPES OF TUBULAR RETRACTORS

Nonexpandable Tubular Retractors

These are retractors of a fixed length and diameter and are usually used for a single spinal level surgery (e.g. single level fusion, microdecompression, etc.). The retractors are oval or circular which allow it to be placed in deep surgical site **(Figure 1)**. An arm extends from the retractor to get attached on the operating table **(Figure 2)**. The oval design has maximal craniocaudal exposure helping better instrumentation and minimizing mediolateral soft-tissue pressures. A well-positioned retractor gives the surgeon a good operating window and prevents soft-tissue intrusion into the surgical field. Limitations of the nonexpandable retractor are the restriction of the amount of angulation and the fixed long narrow working window which needs specialized instruments and surgical expertise with a longer learning curve.

Expandable Tubular Retractors

The deeper part of the retractor can be widened in these retractors. Used for multiple adjacent level surgery. This has a similar arm attachment to the operating table. The addition of an expandable mechanism at the distal end of the tube enlarges the deepest part of the retractor usually from 2.5 to 8 cm depending upon the manufacturer **(Figure 3)**. This enlarged surgical window allows the simultaneous visualization of adjacent level pedicles for screws/rod placement during single level fusion surgery. Limitations include the static narrow proximal view facilitates the need for specialized instrumentation and hence limits the angulation potential in spite of a wider deep window. Also the expandable retractor needs a significant amount of soft-tissue dissection for the enlarged deeper window.

Expandable Blade Retractors

These blades could be used independently to expand in a craniocaudal or in a mediolateral direction to expand the view accordingly **(Figures 4 and 5)**. These independently expandable retractor blades give a larger exposure of the surgical field and thus allows better visualization of the anatomy which is familiar to the surgeon. With this we can also perform instrumentation, insert interbody cages safely and significantly reduces the learning curve. These can also be used for intradural tumor surgery where a wider exposure is necessary. Some frames allow intermittent release of tension, thereby reducing the soft-tissue pressures during longer surgeries. Limitations include the soft-tissue damages owing to larger exposures and operating window resulting in significant postoperative pain. Occasionally, soft tissue enters between the blades on maximum extension and needs removal. Also, some complicated blade assemblies extend the intraoperative time.

ADVANTAGES AND DISADVANTAGE OF TUBULAR RETRACTORS

Advantages

The advantages of tubular retractor system are (i) it offers direct visualization of the operative field, (ii) minimizes soft tissue damage and (iii) provides anatomical familiarity

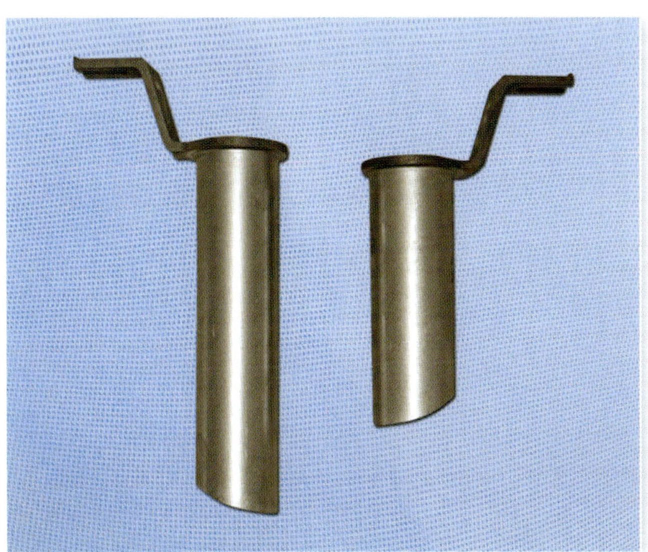

Figure 1: Nonexpandable tubular retractor

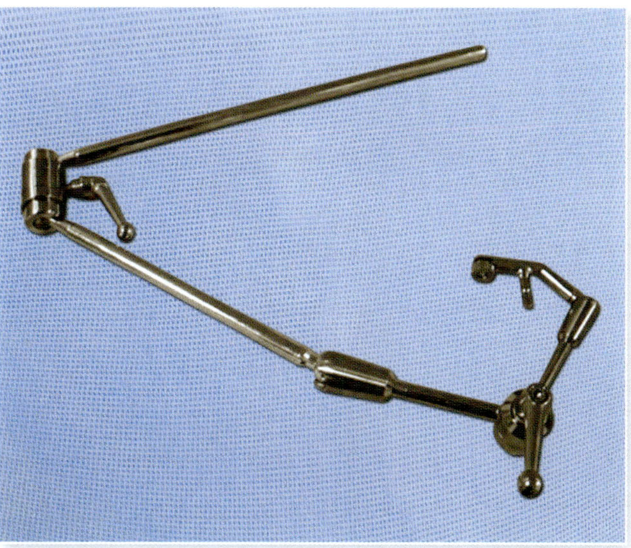

Figure 2: Attachment arm from the tubular retractor to the operating table

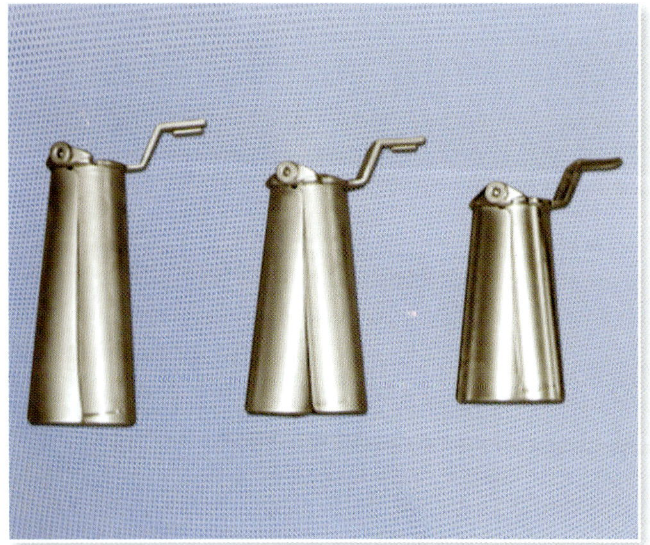

Figure 3: Expandable tubular retractor

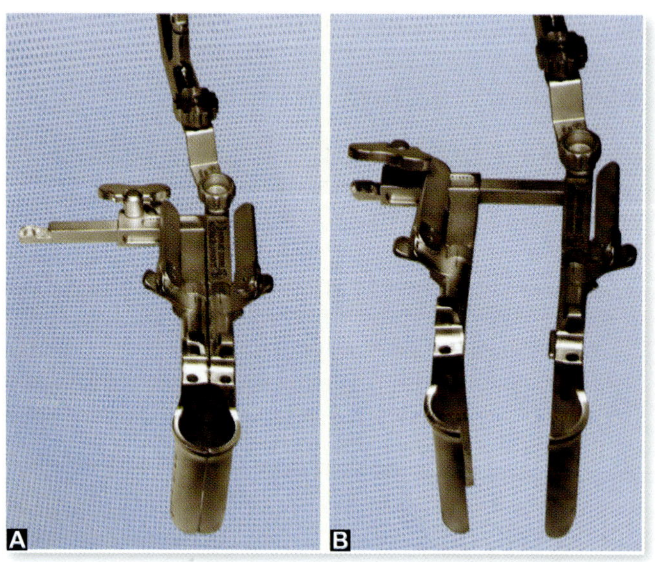

Figure 4: Expandable blade retractors. (A) Blades closed in the cranio caudal direction; (B) Blades open in the cranio caudal direction

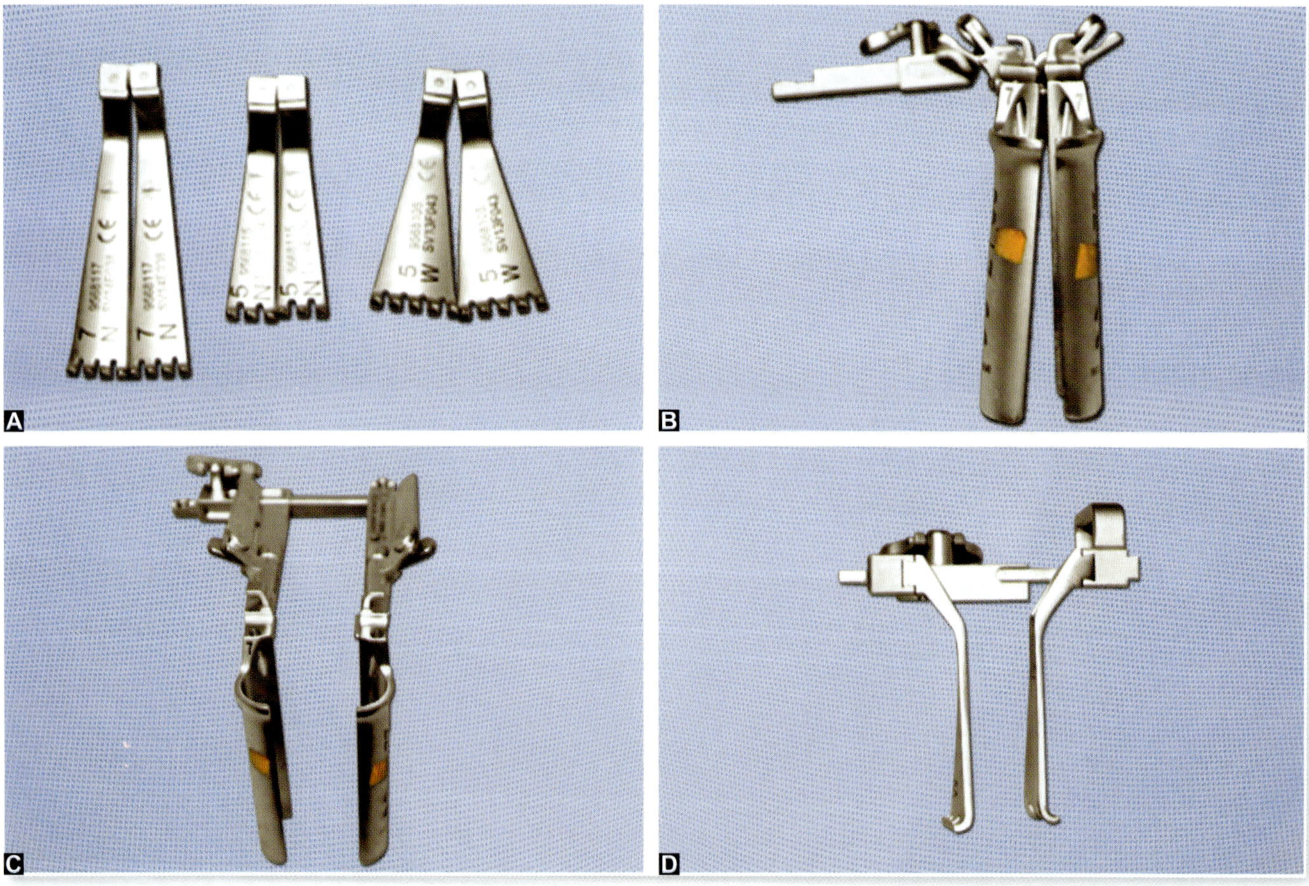

Figures 5A to D: Attachments for expandable blade retractor. (A) Different sizes of narrow and wide blades; (B) Retractor blades closed; (C) Retractor blade open in cranio caudal direction; (D) Retractor blade open in mediolateral direction

to surgeons. The retractors provide access to deeper areas especially in very obese patients where open surgery even for a single level diskectomy involves a large incision with significant retraction for visualization. The flexible arm allows angulation of the retractors in the craniocaudal and mediolateral direction facilitating multilevel surgery with single incision. With the tubular retractor, contralateral spinal decompression can be achieved from ipsilateral approach. With the advancements in the tubular retractor systems, a variety of spinal pathologies, including herniated disks, spinal stenosis, synovial cysts and intradural pathogenesis can now be treated. The advantages are summarized below.

Advantages of Tubular Retractor System

1. Good visualization of operative field with illumination
2. Minimizes soft-tissue damage
3. Anatomical familiarity
4. Deep visualization through small incision (obese patients, thoracic region)
5. Angulation for multiple levels
6. Expandable up to 2–3 levels
7. 2D and 3D visualization possible
8. Contralateral surgery with ipsilateral approach.

Disadvantages

Some of the disadvantages of the retractor systems are: They can be very complex to assemble and involve multiple tedious connections and adjustments. This can be very time consuming and frustrating when they do not assemble well. It is always best to connect them before the procedure to make sure that there are no missing components. The retractor systems are not universally designed for pediatric use and in very thin patients. A certain amount of muscle mass is needed to hold the retractors in place and sometimes even the smallest blade will be too large and cumbersome. This however happens less often. Tubular retractor systems require special bayonetted long instruments and buss extensions to work in a narrow corridor. The use of microscope and endoscopes demands a longer learning curve. Despite very meticulous use of dilators, sometimes soft tissue can enter into the tubular retractor system, especially when the expandable blade retractors are open, and if there is an uneven docking surface, there is a need to remove soft tissue. Controlling bleeding, suturing the dura and accessing the contralateral side can all be challenging. A good familiarity with open procedures is needed before embarking on access through tubes to manage such situations and familiarize with the operative anatomy. Accurate localization of the level of pathology is necessary to avoid wrong placement of tubes which will defeat the purpose of minimal access.

Disadvantage of Tubular Retractor System

1. Complex assembly of some retractor systems
2. Requires special bayonetted instruments, including burr handles
3. Difficult to use in very thin and pediatric patients
4. Difficult to control bleeding and repair dura sometimes
5. Soft-tissue interference after the retractors are placed.

APPLIED ANATOMY OF POSTERIOR CERVICAL SPINE

It is important to know the muscular and bony anatomy of the posterior cervical spine and the distance from the midline for skin incision to reach the desired pathology and the angulation that is required to tackle the problem. The two common procedures performed in the posterior cervical spine using tubes are a posterior cervical foraminotomy and posterior cervical decompression either for canal stenosis or to reach an intradural pathology. The other rarer indications are to insert lateral mass screws and deal with pathology in the CV junction.

The nuchal ligament is a fibroelastic septum that extends from the external occipital protuberance on the skull to the spinous process of C7 vertebra **(Figure 6)**. It gives septa to the spinous processes of each cervical vertebra and longitudinally divides the cervical paravertebral muscles. This is an avascular plane which is used for open procedures, but in minimally invasive procedures this access is not used.

On incising the skin and underlying subcutaneous tissues, cervical fascia is exposed. Sharp incision on the fascia allows for easier passage of sequential dilators with minimal force taking excess care when the patient in on-

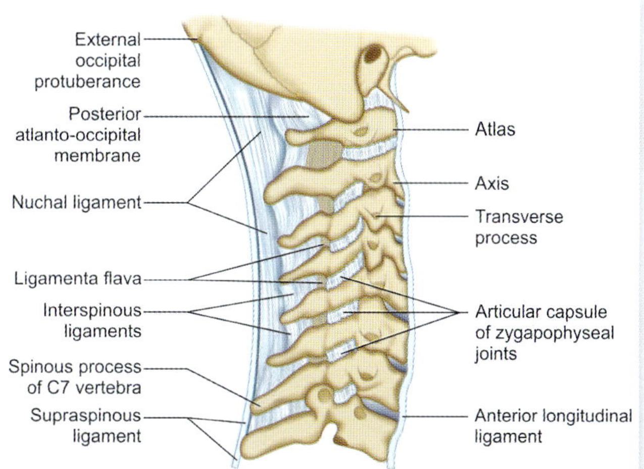

Figure 6: Midline nuchal line which gives a significant strength to the bony neck structures and attachment to neck muscles (right lateral view)

head pins. Then the posterior cervical muscles are seen in three layers, (a) superficial layer consisting of the trapezius muscle which originates from all the spinous processes of the cervical vertebrae **(Figure 7)**, (b) intermediate layer consists of splenius capitis that inserts occipital bone after originating from the ligament niche and the spinous processes of C7 vertebra and first three thoracic vertebrae **(Figure 8)** and (c) deep layer has three further layers which from superficial to deepest are semispinalis capitis inserting onto the occipital bone, semispinalis cervices and the multifidus muscles **(Figure 9)**. The exposed fibers run in an oblique or longitudinal fashion and hence the dilating tubes can be inserted with minimal tissue trauma by muscle splitting and stretching. The tubular system is set in the desired position, the electro-cautery with a long tip is used to remove the remaining muscles and soft tissue overlying the cervical facet and lateral mass. It is recommended to start using the diathermy laterally where the bone is well felt and work medially. Most often the ligamentum flavum is thinned or absent near the lateral edge of the interlaminar space, posing a risk of entering into the spinal cord.

Once the bone is visualized, it is important to appreciate the anatomy. For a posterior cervical foraminotomy, the inferior articular process of the superior lamina, facet joint and the medial edge of the lateral-mass facet junction is exposed underneath the tube **(Figure 10)**. If a decompression is planned the laminae and medial part of the lateral mass alone is only needed to be exposed. Up to three levels can be exposed with the expandable blade retractors. The retractors are angulated in the mediolateral or the craniocaudal direction for visibility.

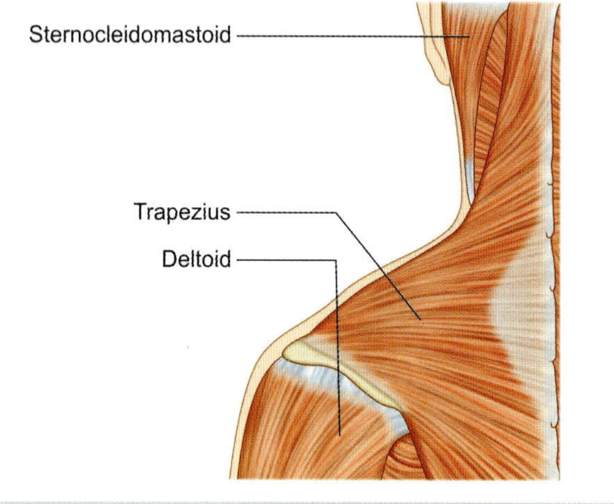

Figure 7: Superficial layers of the neck muscle showing attachment of the trapezius muscle

Indication

The tubular retractors system was commercial available for the first time in 1997 by Medtronic SofamorDanek, Memphis, TN, USA.[4] This was used in the lumbar spine for diskectomy procedures and then the system has been made available much wider. In the cervical spine the system has been, used for the following indications:

1. Posterior cervical foraminotomy
2. Posterior cervical decompression
3. Posterior cervical lateral mass instrumentation
4. Posterior C1–C2 stabilization
5. Posterior approaches to intradural tumors
6. Anterior cervical foraminotomy
7. Anterior cervical diskectomy.

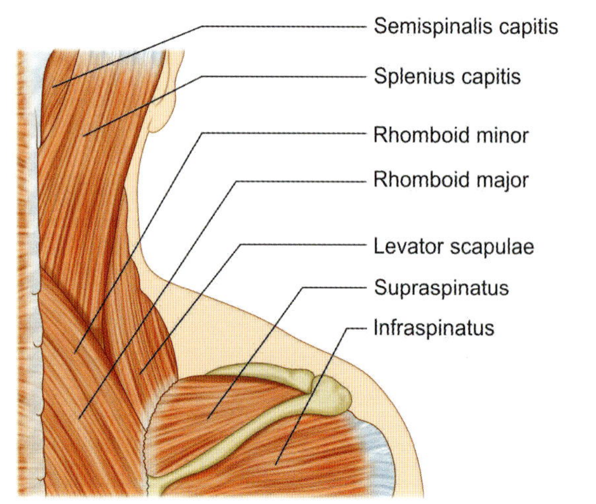

Figure 8: Intermediate layer of neck muscles

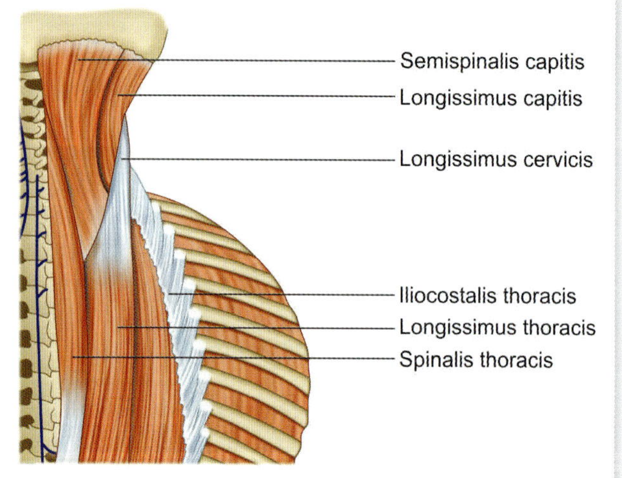

Figure 9: Deep layer of the neck muscle

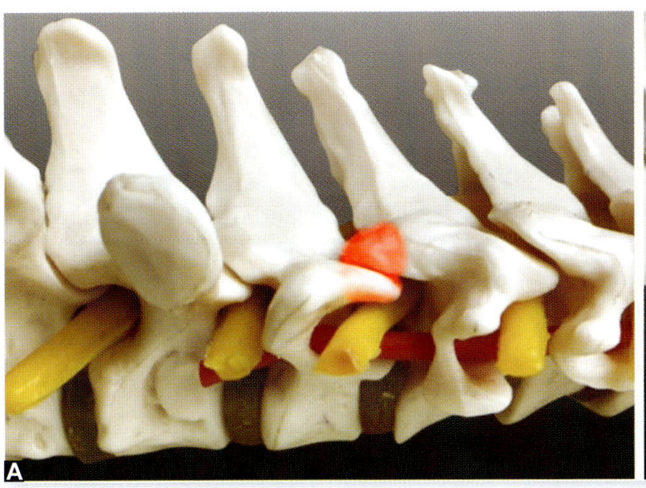

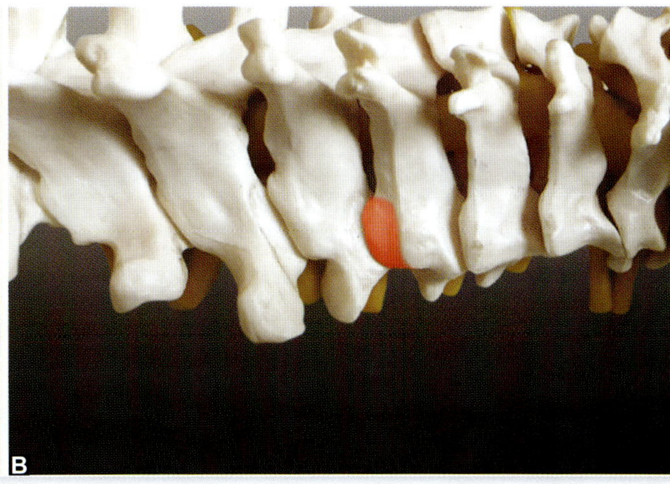

Figures 10A and B: Posterior cervical spine. (A) Lateral and (B) Posterior view, of bone required to be removed for posterior cervical foraminotomy

Contraindication

The tubular retractors must be used with caution in the cervical spine especially during the learning phase. One should learn to use with confidence in the lumbar spine before being able to use in the cervical spine though the principles are similar. Some of the contraindications for use of tubular retractors for the spine are as follows:

Posterior Approach

1. Revision posterior cervical surgery
2. Bilateral same level posterior cervical foraminotomy
3. Posterior cervical foraminotomy for centrally placed disk
4. Gross or segmental kyphosis.

Anterior Approach

1. Revision anterior surgery
2. Deformity surgery
3. Adjacent segment diskectomy and fusion
4. Following radical neck dissection or radiotherapy.

Instruments Required

1. Intraoperative fluoroscopy
2. Microscope
3. Sequential dilators
4. Tubular retractors with mounted retractor arm
5. Microscopic instruments:
   a. Bayonetted high speed burr
   b. Long Kerrison punches
   c. Pituitary roungers
   d. Bayonet curettes
   e. Bayonet suction
   f. Microinstruments.

Preoperative Work-up

1. Detailed history (including symptoms duration)
2. Physical examination corresponding to imaging findings.
3. Laboratory investigations—routine bloods, group and save.
4. Dynamic X-rays of cervical spine to assess instability (need for fusion).
5. MRI scan to look for soft or hard disk (para-sagittal T1-weighted filming is useful in determining the severity of foraminal stenosis).
6. CT scan is helpful to assess the extent of bony osteophyte compression or calcified disk (axial views).
7. Neurophysiological study in cases with multilevel root compression is present to ascertain the symptomatic level.

Patient Positioning and Theater set-up

After endotracheal intubation, the patient can be positioned for a minimally invasive posterior cervical spine surgery either in a semisitting procedure or a modified prone procedure **(Figure 11)**. The patients neck should be above the heart to reduce venous pressure and bleeding from the epidural plexus around the nerve roots. A Mayfield clamp is used to fix the head and a 30-degree reverse Trendelenburg position is used with a neck flexed mildly in order to bring the cervical spine parallel to the floor. In a semisitting position **(Figure 12)** has the advantages of lowering the bleeding and hence reduced blood loss,[5] improved visualization and better access to cervicothoracic junction thereby resulting in reduced operating time.

During a semisitting position, a precordial Doppler can be used to detect air embolism. Due to the limited incision size and reduced operative time, the risk of air embolism is slim, and therefore, a central line or precordial Doppler are not usually needed for a posterior cervical foraminotomy. Continuous intraoperative somatosensory evoked-potential monitoring (SEEP) and motor-evoked potentials (MEP) could be utilized to assess the spinal cord function, especially during posterior cervical decompression for myelopathy or intradural pathology. An electromyography (EMG) to watch out for impending motor root damage is not routinely indicated. Urinary catheter is used for procedures lasting longer than 90 minutes. We use a single dose of cefuroxime 1.5 g as a stat dose, and it is repeated if procedure lasts longer than 4 hours.

The surgeon will stand on the same side as pathology for foraminotomy procedures and for cervical decompression right-handed surgeon will stand on the left side of patient unless the symptoms are more the contralateral side. The C-arm is placed on the head end of the patient throughout the procedure and microscope is brought in from the opposite side **(Figure 13)**. The assistant stands opposite to the surgeon and the theatre scrub sister stand by the side of the surgeon with the television and C-arm monitor placed on the opposite side. Anesthetic personnel and equipments are usually placed at the foot end of the table.

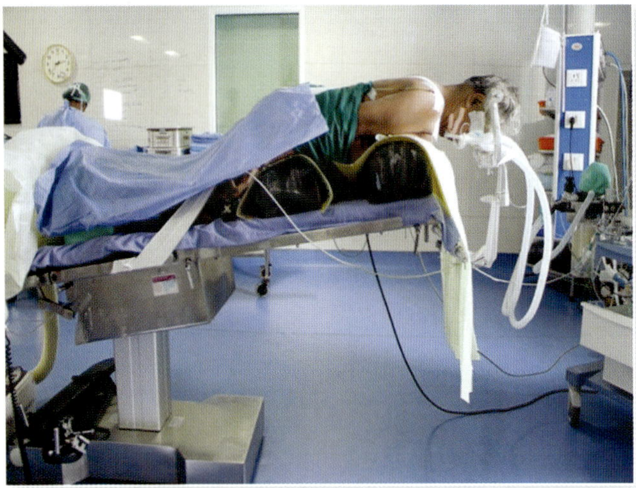

Figure 11: Modified prone reverse Trendelenburg position for posterior cervical spine surgery

TECHNIQUES

Posterior Cervical Foraminotomy

Indication

1. Single or multilevel paracentral or foraminal herniated soft disk.
2. Single or multilevel osteophyte or ligamentous foraminal stenosis.
3. Persistent foramina stenosis with radicular symptoms after anterior cervical diskectomy or cervical disk replacement.
4. Contraindications to anterior approach: infection, tracheostomy or anterior cervical radiationtherapy, radical neck surgery or disk herniation at C7/T1 level.

Contraindication

1. Central disk herniation or osteophytes
2. Myelopathy from central canal stenosis
3. Ossified posterior longitudinal ligament
4. Segmental kyphosis of spine
5. Cervical segment instability

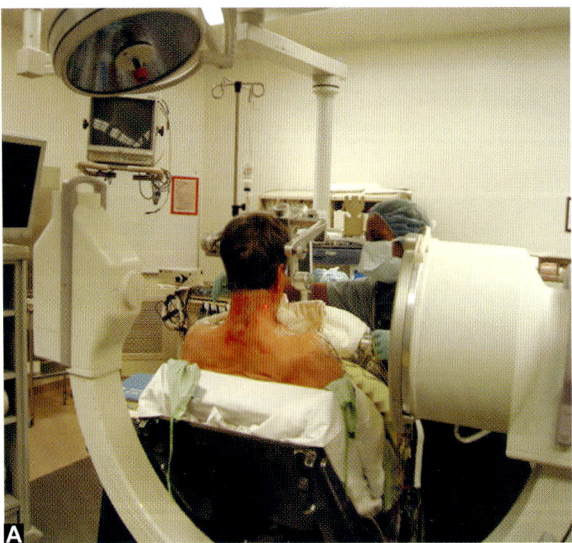

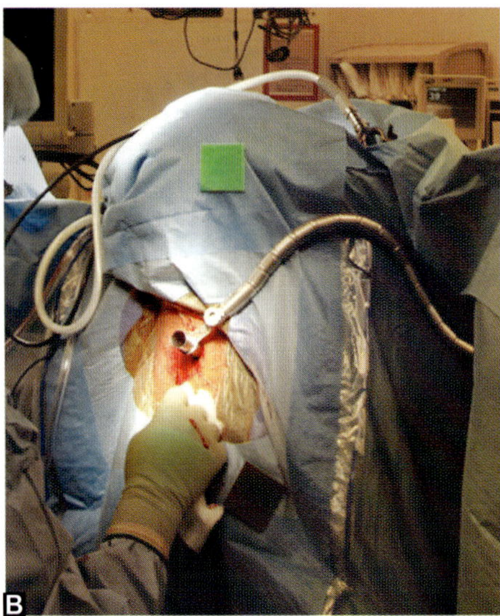

Figure 12: Sitting position of patient. (A) With C-arm positioned in the side; (B) Nonexpandable retractor in position

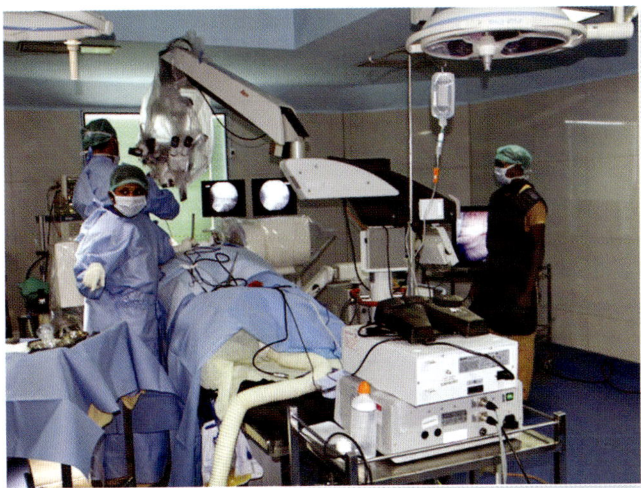

Figure 13: Operation theater set-up with the surgeon and scrub nurse on the side of pathology, microscope on the opposite side, C-arm and anesthetic machine at the head end, C-arm and TV machine on the opposite side

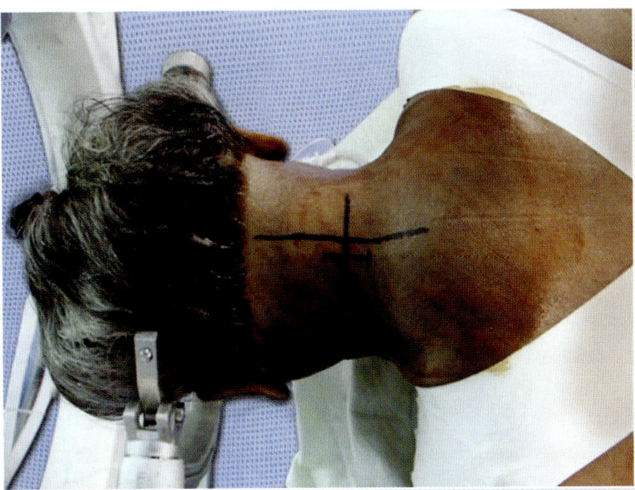

Figure 14: Skin incision 1.5 cm lateral to midline for posterior cervical foraminotomy

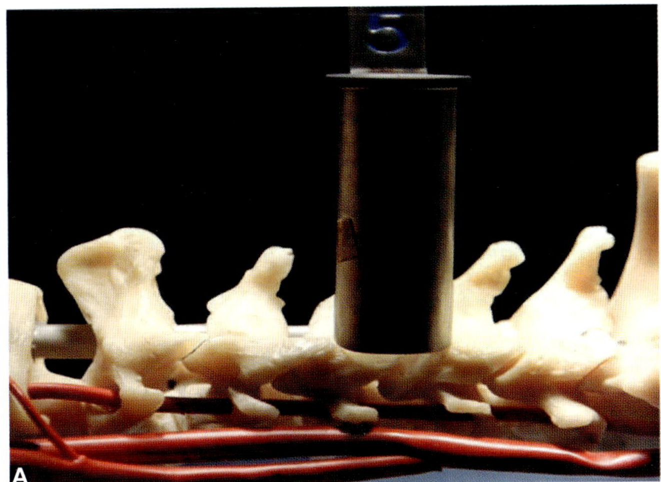

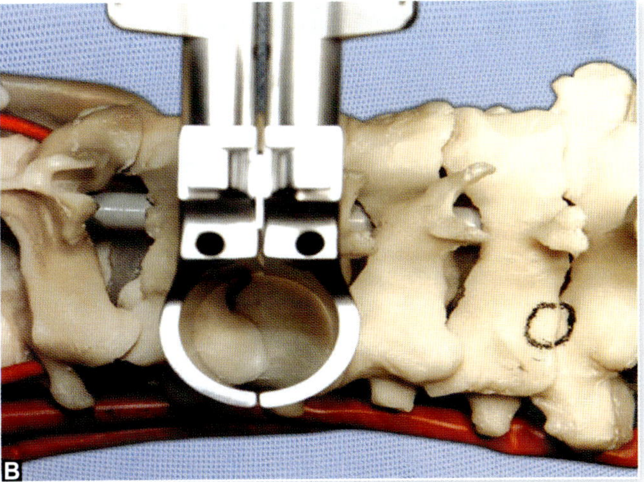

Figure 15: Model of the spine. (A) Position of the nonexpandable tubular retractor in the lateral view; (B) Surgical view showing the facet joints in the center of the tube

Procedure

Using fluoroscopy, the level of interest is marked with the needle on the lateral view. Then a 1.5 cm skin incision is made 1.5 cm lateral to the midline on the side of the pathology **(Figure 14)**. A sharp fasciotomy is done and the little finger in used to dilate the muscle gently. A K-wire is then passed to the appropriate facet joint and confirmed with fluoroscopy. Serial dilators are passed over the K-wire to dilate the muscles. After the final dilator a 14 mm or 16 mm on-expandable tubular retractor is inserted and fixed onto the operating table mounted retractor arm. A lateral fluoroscopy is used to confirm the level and direction and soft tissue over the facet is cauterized using a diathermy. The bone is exposed from lateral to medial and facet joint identified. Using a high-speed burr, the medial third of the inferior articular process of the superior vertebra is removed until the superior articular process of the inferior vertebra is seen and is thinned down **(Figure 15)**. The amount of facet joint resection must not exceed 50% in order to preserve the spinal stability **(Figure 10)**. After the bone is thinned, the ligamentum flavum and bone are separated using a 2 mm Kerrison roungers. The venous plexus is usually exposed and control of bleeding should be carefully done with hemostats and bipolar at low energy with irrigation. After the foraminotomy is complete the nerve root is mobilized gently and soft disk or osteophyte is removed. A curette can be used to widen the foramen of any osteophytes. After this is completed, a fine hook or probe, is used to check the foramen laterally. The wound is then irrigated and the tubular retractor system is removed following which multilayer wound closure of the fascia, subcutaneous tissue and skin.

Complication and Avoidance

Complications is usually due to approach and placement of the tubular retractors, foraminotomy using burr, nerve root manipulation and diskectomy, venous bleeding,[5] durotomy[6] and late complications of neck pain, segmental kyphosis and instability. In this chapter we will discuss how to avoid the complications related to placement of the tubular retractor:

1. The skin incision should be at least 1.5 cm lateral to the midline to avoid entering medially.
2. Incise the fascia with knife or monopolar diathermy to avoid undue pressure on the neck during serial dilatation.
3. Do not use the sharp end of the K wire to avoid entering the spinal canal medially or vertebral venous plexus laterally. K wire and serial dilators must be passed under fluoroscopy guidance in all cases. The guide wire must be in contact with bone before using the dilators.
4. Dock the tubular retractors on the facet joint directly and check the position and angulation on the fluoroscope before attaching the retractor mount.
5. Start diathermy coagulation to remove and expose the soft tissue from lateral to medial to avoid entering the spinal canal at the medial lamina–lateral mass junction.

Posterior Cervical Decompression

Indication

1. Cervical spondylotic myelopathy
2. Ossified ligamentum flavum
3. Ossified posterior longitudinal ligament (OPLL)
4. Access to intradural extramedullay tumors.

Contraindication

1. Revision cervical surgery for post-laminectomy kyphosis
2. Prolonged surgery with risk of anesthesia
3. Severe cervical stenosis with neurological defects (relative).
4. Trauma with central cord syndrome and cord edema.

Procedure

After careful intubation avoiding neck extension, neuromonitoring can be used in selective cases where there is severe myelopathy clinically or radiologically. After the patient is positioned in Mayfield clamps a 1-inch skin incision is performed about 1.5 - 2 cm lateral to the spinous process between C4–5 for a multilevel decompression (C3–C6) under C arm guidance.

Background

The aim of this work is to present a novel decompression technique that approaches cervical spine posteriorly, but through minimal invasive method using tubular retractor avoiding detachment of posterior musculature.

Methods

Six patients underwent minimally invasive posterior cervical decompression using the tubular retractor system and surgical microscope. Minimally invasive access to the posterior cervical spine was performed with exposure through a paramedian muscle-splitting approach. With the assistance of a specialized tubular retraction system and deep soft tissue expansion mechanism, multilevel posterior cervical decompression could be accomplished. This approach also allows safe docking of the retractor system on the lateral mass, thus avoiding the cervical spinal canal during exposure. A standard operating microscope was used with ×10 magnification and 400 mm focal length. The hospital charts, magnetic resonance imaging studies, and follow-up records of all the patients were reviewed. Outcome was assessed by neurological status and visual analog scale (VAS) for neck and arm pain.

Results

There was no significant complication related to operation. The follow-up time was 4–12 months (mean, 9 months). Muscle weakness improved in all patients; sensory deficits resolved in four patients and improved in two patients. Analysis of the mean VAS for radicular pain and VAS for neck pain showed significant improvement.

CONCLUSION

The preliminary experiences with good clinical outcome seem to promise that this minimally invasive technique is a valid alternative option for the treatment of cervical spondylotic myelopathy.

After subcutaneous dissection, fascia is incised sharply for the entire length of the skin incision. Gentle finger dissection is done to palpate the lamina and facet joint. Serial dilators are used to spread through the muscle fibers to place the tubular retractor under C-arm guidance. We prefer to use an expandable blade retractor (Quadrant Medtronic) which expands up to 3 levels. The retractors are positioned safely on the laminae and angulated in a 10–15 degrees depending in the depth of the neck musculature. The operating microscope is introduced and the soft tissue is removed using electrocautery and pituitary roungers. Careful ipsilateral hemilaminectomy is performed to expose the underlying ligament with high-speed drill. After unilateral hemilaminectomy, the working tube is angled more medial to the base of the spinous process and patient tilted away from the surgeon to undercut the base of the spinous process with the high-speed drill **(Figures 16A and B)**. After adequate thinning of the bone Kerrison's

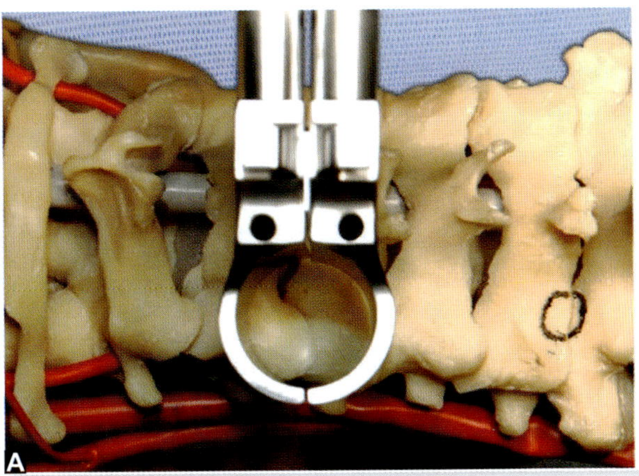

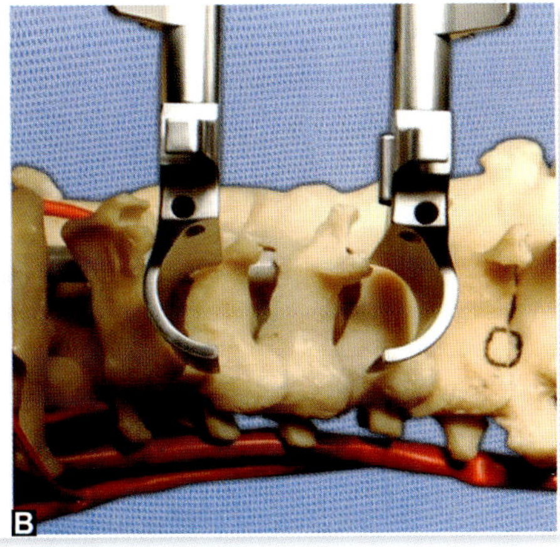

Figures 16A and B: Model of the spine showing. (A) Position of expandable blade retractor in the closed position; (B) In the open angulated position for posterior cervical decompression

rongeurs are used to removal of the lamina. The ligament is left intact at this point to protect the spinal cord. The lamina of the contralateral side is undercut up to the medial aspect of the contralateral facet. After adequate bone removal has been accomplished, the ligamentum flavum is carefully removed using upward Kerrison upcuts. The canal is hence widened without damaging the interspinous ligament. The central canal decompression can be combined with focal foraminal decompression for radiculopathy. The decompression is continued cranially and caudally to the extent of the decompression by angulating the tubes. Hemostasis is controlled and the tubular retractors are removed. Closure is done in layers from fascia, subcutaneous tissue and skin.

Complications Avoidance

Through the tubular retractor up to 4 levels of cervical laminectomy can be performed comfortably through the same incision without disturbing the midline. However, a postoperative neck pain and kyphosis should still be kept in mind. In addition, cerebrospinal fluid (CSF) leakage, wound problems, postoperative kyphosis, and instability are not uncommon. Some of the complications related to the tubular retractor are as follows:

1. Place the skin incision 1.5 - 2 cm lateral compared to the postcervical foraminotomy as we need to angle the retractors to see the contralateral side.
2. Tubular retractors need to be tilted half way through the surgery to operate on the contralateral side. During this process soft tissue can enter the field and bleeding can be a problem. Hence, proper planning is needed this maneuver must be done meticulously.
3. When operating at a depth in some patients the high speed burr should be used carefully and resting on the tubes should be avoided.
4. Placing the medial blade can be a problem when the spinous process is bifid and large; hence, the spinous process must be shaved, if needed.

Discussion

Posterior cervical foraminotomy using a microscope or endoscope can be performed safely,with results comparable to the open posterior approach using tubular retractors. It avoids the approach-related morbidity encountered in open posterior approaches to the posterior paraspinal muscles. The advantages of the using tubular retractors have been discussed,but the potential for recurrent disk herniations, the added time for surgery and the requisite learning curve for the techniques must be taken into consideration when suboptimal set up is available. Though a laminotomy or laminoplasty are straightforward options they can result in persistent neck and shoulder pain,[7] postoperative kyphosis and spinal instability due to trauma to the extensor cervical muscles. These serious complications can be avoided by using tubular retractors and miscrosurgical techniques to achieve the same through minimal access. The indication for surgery should be carefully considered. Posterior cervical foraminotomy is the most common indication for the use of cervical tubular retractors in the cervical spine; however, laminectomy is being increasingly performed both for myelopathy and intradural accesses. The safety and feasibility of this has been well proven in several studies.[8] Multilevel decompression is possible with this minimal invasive approach.[9] Those pathologies that need reconstruction of the kyphosis or anterior disk pathology, should be done through an anterior approach. Dynamic X rays must be done to exclude instability.

REFERENCES

1. Vincenzo Denaro, Alberto Di Martino. Cervical Spine Surgery: An Historical Perspective. Clin Orthop Relat Res. 2011; 469(3): 639-48.
2. Smith, George W, and Robinson, Robert A. The treatment of certain cervical-spine disorders by anterior removal of the intervertebral disc and interbody fusion, J. Bone and Joint Surgery. 1958; 40A:607-24.
3. Cloward, Ralph B. The anterior approach for removal of ruptured cervical disks. J Neurosurgery. 1958;15:602-17.
4. Young Baeg Kim, Seung Jae Hyun. Clinical Applications of the Tubular Retractor on Spinal Disorders. J Korean Neurosurg Soc. 2007;42:245-50.
5. Fessler RG, Khoo LT. Minimally invasive cervical microendoscopic foraminotomy: an initial clinical experience. Neurosurgery. 2002;51(5 Suppl):S37-45.
6. Adamson TE. Microendoscopic posterior cervical laminoforaminotomy for unilateral radiculopathy: results of a new technique in 100 cases. J Neurosurg. 2001;95(1 Suppl): 51-7.
7. Hosono N, Yonenobu K, Ono K. Neck and shoulder pain after laminoplasty. A noticeable complication. Spine. 1996;21:1969-73.
8. Wang MY, Green BA, Coscarella E, Baskaya MK, Levi AD, Guest JD. Minimally invasive cervical expansilelaminoplasty: An initial cadaveric study. Neurosurgery. 2003;52:370-3
9. Hur JW, Kim JS, Shin MH, et al. Minimally invasive posterior cervical decompression using tubular retractor: The technical note and early clinical outcome. Surg Neurol Int. 2014;15;5:34.

10

CHAPTER

Cervical Laminoforaminotomy

Satish Rudrappa

ABSTRACT

The technique of cervical laminoforaminotomy has been devised to remove bone or portion of prolapsed disk to get relief from arm pain. The procedure is performed using principles of minimally invasive techniques and provides adequate working window to treat the pathology. It can be microendoscopic, endoscopic assisted or with tubular retractors. It is also very effective and cheaper alternative to anterior diskectomy but clinical trials are needed to assess benefits and compare between these procedures.

INTRODUCTION AND HISTORY

Cervical radiculopathy is a condition that produces radiating pain, paresthesia, motor weakness and/or diminished reflex associated with impingement of one or more cervical nerve roots.[1] Reported incidence of cervical radiculopathy in US population is 1.79/1000 persons.[2] Approximate incidence in India is unknown, though it is very commonly encountered in clinical practice.

Cervical radiculopathy due to compression of nerve root by lateral disk herniation was first described by Semmes and Murphy in 1943[3] and soon after by Spurling and Scoville in 1944,[4] Elliot et al. in 1945[5], etc. Mechanism of pain generation by friction or forceful traction of the involved nerve root was later described by Frykholm in 1951.[6]

Most patients with cervical radiculopathy can be managed conservatively. Non-surgical options have been shown to have up to 92% success rate in long term.[7] Surgical treatment may be required in case of intractable pain, myelopathy or any other neurological deficits.

Posterior approach for treatment of myelopathy due to cervical spondylosis was first described by Northfield in 1955.[8] Later with the introduction of anterior cervical approach and fusion in 1958,[9] as it can decompress spinal cord and root for almost all the pathology and relative ease of performance, use of posterior approach for disk pathology became less and less. For almost last five decades, posterior foraminotomy was rarely used and they relied mainly on open keyhole approach performed through a midline incision.

Williams reintroduced cervical foraminotomy using microscope in 1983, as an alternative procedure for intractable radiculopathy. In 2001, Adamson published his results of 100 cases of endoscopic-assisted microscopic foraminotomy for unilateral radiculopathy.[10] Fully endoscopic technique was later published by Ruetten in 2007 in 87 patients with results equivalent to other conventional procedure.[11] Since then multiple reports of similar procedures have been published describing its advantages, disadvantages and complications. With recent advancement in minimally invasive techniques, there is again a resurgence of interest in posterior minimally invasive approach for laterally herniated disk.

In this chapter, we will be discussing about the indications, advantages, disadvantages, complications, technique and outcome of posterior cervical foraminotomy.

INDICATIONS

1. Cervical radiculopathy[12] due to:
   i. Posterolateral soft disk herniation
   ii. Osteophytes originating from the facet joint
2. Isolated lateral foraminal bony stenosis
3. Persistent radiculopathy despite anterior cervical diskectomy and fusion (ACDF)
4. Cervico-thoracic disk herniation and radiculopathy[13]
5. Cervical calcified ligamentum flavum.[14]

CONTRAINDICATIONS

Contraindications for posterior laminoforaminotomy[15] are:
1. Myelopathy—clinical/radiological
2. Diffuse degenerative disk prolapse
3. Significant instability
4. Kyphotic deformity at involved level
5. Local skin infection
6. Lack of congruity between clinical and instrumental findings.

ADVANTAGES

Advantages of posterior foraminotomy are as follows[12, 16-17]
1. Involved nerve root can be visualized directly
2. Avoid damage to the vital structures located anterior to cervical spine
3. Avoid structural and biomechanical damage to the remaining vertebral disk.
4. Obviated need of fusion.
5. Reduces adjacent segment disease as complete disk is not removed.
6. There is no/less chance of instability and limited surgical morbidity.

DISADVANTAGE

Major disadvantage of the procedure is significant neck pain and spasm due to damage to semispinalis and multifidus, acting as dynamic stabilizers of lamina and facet joints.

ANESTHESIA AND POSITIONING

Usually general anesthesia is used. Patient is positioned either prone or sitting. Sitting position reduces blood loss with clear surgical field. But has high risk of air embolism and relative hypotension. Hence prone is usually preferred. Head is fixed by pin fixation with neck in neutral or slight flexion so as to get a minimum two finger breadth between chin and sternum. Chin is slightly retropositioned to obtain martial posture of neck. Superior thoracic and iliac crest foam rolls are used. Bed is adjusted in Trendelenburg position. Shoulders were pulled down with an adhesive tape. Then C-arm is used to localize the level of pathology. Compressive stockings were applied to lower limb.[15]

SURGICAL TECHNIQUES

Open Laminoforaminotomy

In open foraminotomy (OF), skin incision can be a vertical 3 cm midline incision at the level of the pathology[18] or a 2 cm longitudinal incision, 1 cm off the midline.[19] In the former, avascular plane along ligamentum nuchae is used whereas later approach is through the semispinalis cervicis and multifidus to expose lateral part of the lamina, medial part of facet joint and their junction. After exposure a self-retaining retractor applied and further procedure continued using microscope. Care should be taken while dissecting and not to violate the facet capsule.

Conventionally, lateral portion of two adjacent lamina and medial part of facet were removed to expose foraminal course of nerve, its axilla and shoulder.[20] Later a semicircular laminotomy involving inferior aspect of cephalad lamina is used for pure lateral soft disk herniation, as disk space is located above the leading edge of caudal lamina.[21] For more cephalad or caudal extrusion of disk, more extensive laminotomy or complete hemi laminectomy may be required.[12] Bony decompression and skeletonisation of proximal part of root is then done using 2 mm burr and ronguer.[18] Recently, a modified cervical laminoforaminotomy is described where the inferior limit is inferior border of superior facet, superior limit is superior border of superior facet, lateral limit will be a vertical line joining the junction of lamina and facet to the lateral end of superior limit.[22] The extent of facet resection required during laminoforaminotomy is typically 25% and rarely exceeds 50%.[23-24] Inclined undercutting of facet provide 60–70% sparing of facet with adequate exposure of foraminal root.[19]

Epidural venous plexus with ooze can be controlled by topical hemostatics or coagulation using bipolar cautery, beginning medially and extending laterally along the nerve root sleeve. Then divided sharply to expose the thecal sac and exiting nerve root.

After foraminotomy, nerve root is seen laying on inferior pedicle, which is retracted rostrally, because herniated fragment is frequently located inferior to the root. Most of the neurological deficits develop due to retraction on dural sac and nerve root and there are intradural variant of cervical nerve fibers connecting adjacent segmental roots.[25] To prevent retraction on nerve root and its complications, pedidulotomy is advised by many. In pediculotomy, supero-medial border of inferior pedicle is drilled.[12,15,26] After pediculotomy and gentle root retraction, extruded part of disk is removed without piercing the annulus.[15] Wound closed in layers following adequate hemostasis **(Figures 1 and 2)**.

Minimally invasive Laminoforaminotomy

It can be a microendoscopic, purely endoscopic or tubular retractor assisted foraminotomy **(Figure 3)**. Adamson initially described endoscopic assisted microscopic foraminotomy for unilateral radiculopathy.[10] Later, a fully endoscopic technique was reported by Ruetten in 87 patients with 2 years follow-

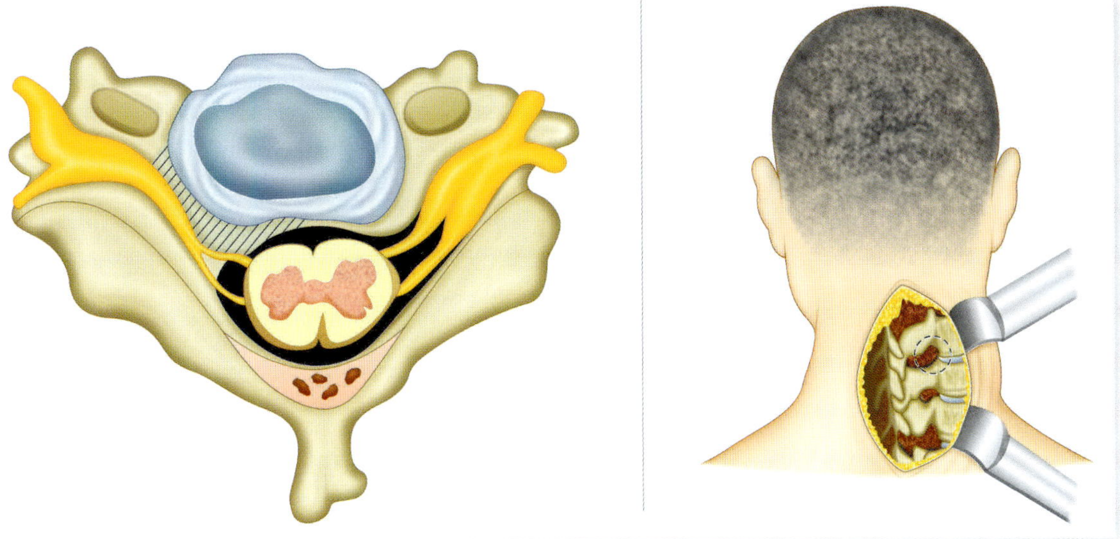

Figure 1: Open laminoforaminotomy.

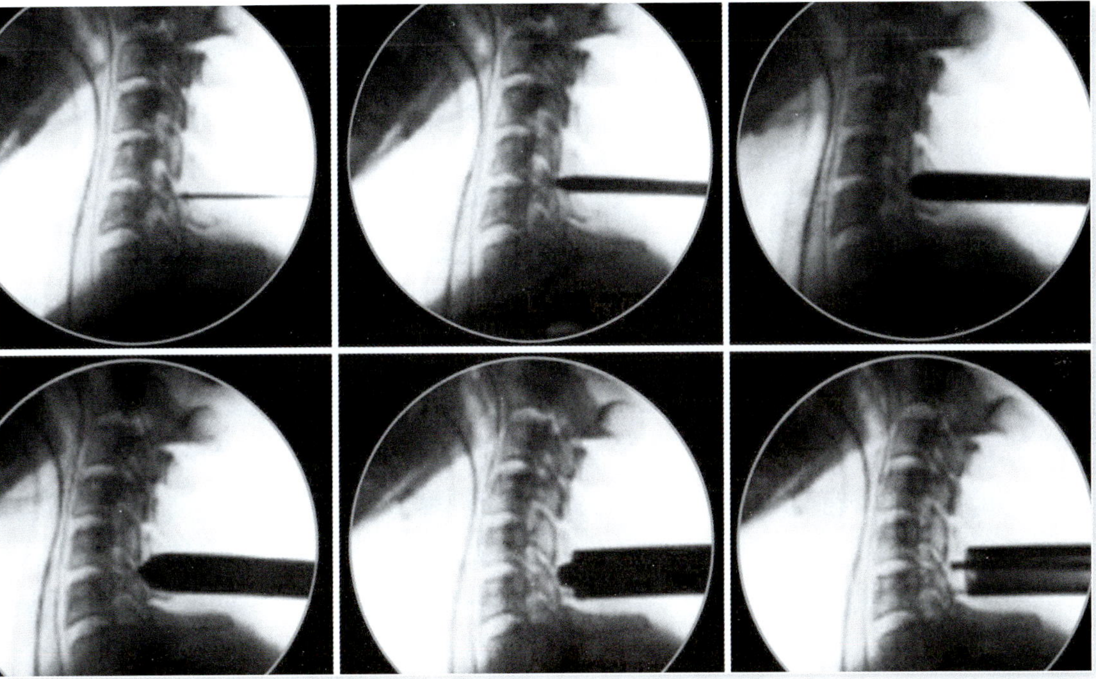

Figure 2: Localization and sequential dilation

up. Results were comparable to conventional procedures without any serious surgical complications.[11] Foleys et al. later described tubular retractor assisted endoscopic diskectomy for lumbar disk.[27] Following these, similar procedure was introduced for cervical laimnoforaminotomy.

Usually a smaller paramedian vertical or curvilinear incision is used at the level of pathology. In endoscopic procedure, a hand held rigid 0° endoscope is used for navigating. In tubular assisted foraminotomy (TAF), a 5 mm off midline puncture is made. A K-wire is passed through the muscle under continuous fluoroscopic guidance. K- wire is docked on the bone at the inferomedial edge of the rostral lateral mass at the target level. Skin incision extended around the K-wire. Cervical fascia and muscle cut sharply using monopolar cautery and serial tubular dialators (METRx System, Medtronic Sofamor Danek, and Memphis, USA) are placed around the K-wire. After dialation is complete, a final working channel (16 mm or 18 mm) is placed over

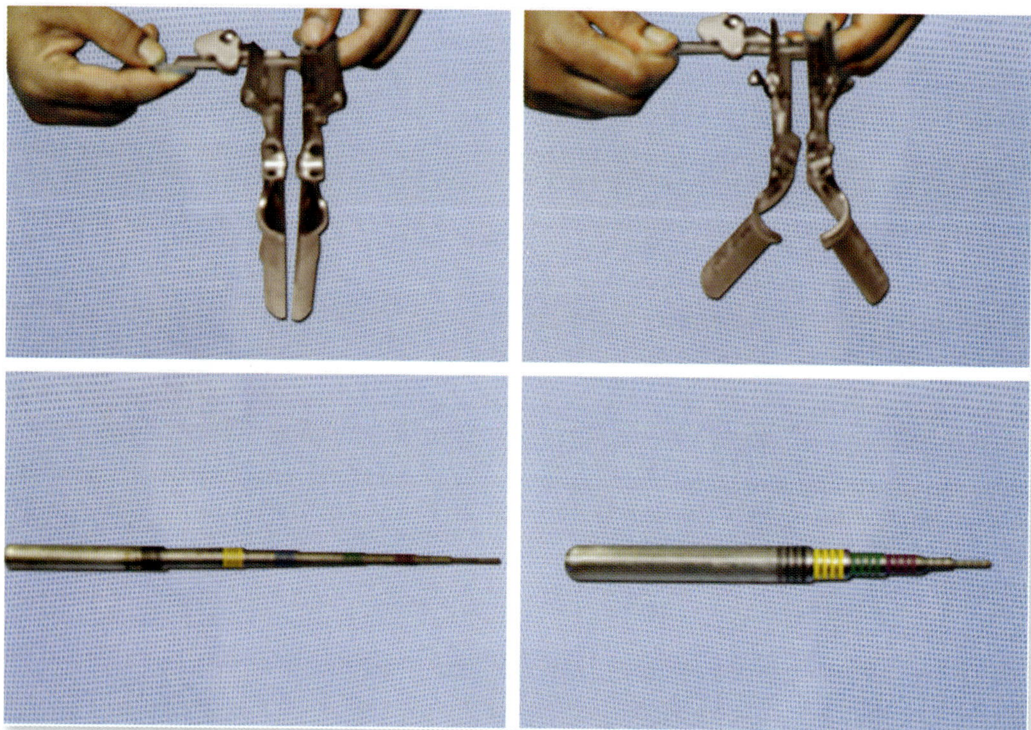

Figure 3: Tubular retractor system

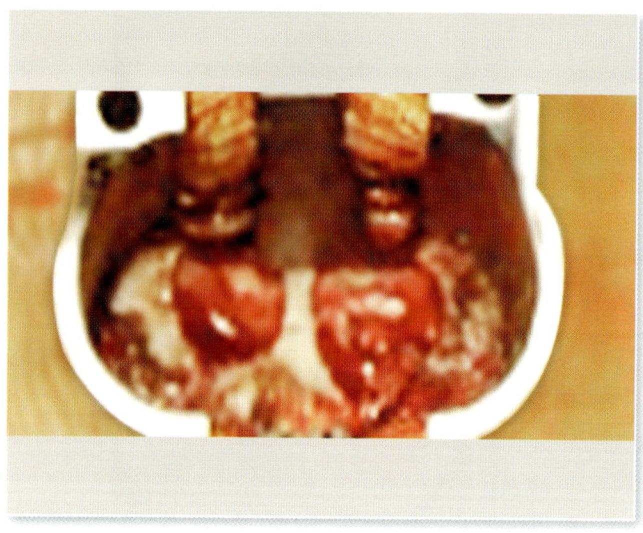

Figure 4: Tandem keyhole foraminotomy

the dialators and fixed over the lamina-facet junction with a table mounted flexible retractor arm and then dialators removed. Additional skin incision may be required at this point to prevent skin necrosis. Further procedure is same as in open foraminotomy using microscope.[18]

TAF is an easy and safe procedure.[28] For lateral disk prolapse involving adjacent segment, tandem keyhole foraminotomy is done where the incision will be between the two adjacent facet joints **(Figure 4)**.[1] Multisegmental laminoforminotomy for multilevel disk is also equally effective and a safer alternative **(Table 1)**.[29]

Table 1

Comparison between percutaneous and open cervical foraminotomy[17,30-31]

Percutaneous	*Open*
Smaller incision	Larger incision
Reduced blood loss	More blood loss
Reduced post-operative pain	More pain and need of analgesia
Longer surgeon learning curve	Shorter learning curve

Postoperatively patient can be mobilized on the same day. It is advised to wear a soft cervical collar for 2–4 weeks.

COMPLICATIONS

Posterior laminoforaminotomy is relatively safe. Though few complications specific to this approach are described in literature[10,12,19,24,32] **(Table 2)**.

1. **CSF fistula:** Durotomy with CSF leak is the most common complication.
2. **Increased epidural bleed:** Venous bleed from the epidural venous plexus is very common. Excessive blood loss from epidural plexus is very common in obese patients in prone position. Relative hypotension with cord and brain ischemia is reported in few patients, especially with sitting position.[12]
3. **Vertebral artery injury:** A very rare complication encountered while drilling the lateral part of facet.

Table 2

Complications and its avoidance

Complications	Avoidance	Treatment
1. CSF fistula	Careful drilling Use blunt dissector or hook	Direct repair if possible Fat and glue application Lumbar drain if needed
2. Cord and Root injury	Avoid traction on nerve root	Physiotherapy
3. Epidural bleeding	Use blunt bipolar tip at low current with continuous irrigation	Apply surgical and pressure
4. Vertebral artery injury	Avoid drilling lateral part of facet	Use 1mm ronguer if required

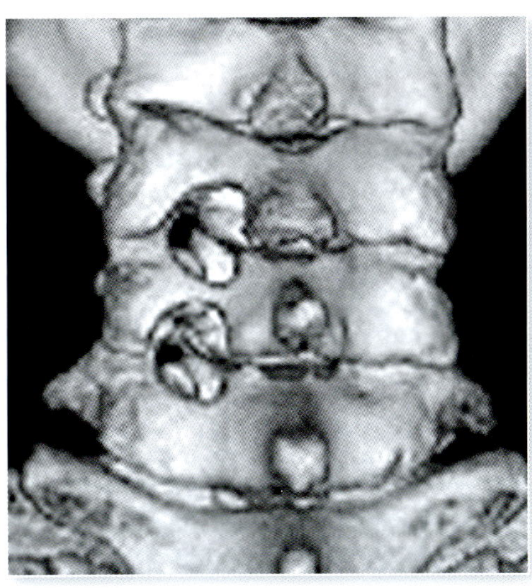

Figure 5: Postoperative 3D CT

4. **Cord and root injury:** Both can be due to inadvertent traction on the exiting nerve root while doing diskectomy. Motor nerve palsy is reported in 2.8% cases. In that 22% patients had C5 motor palsy.[32] C5 root usually covers the entire disk space and therefore needs more excessive retraction than any other nerve root.[26] This can be reduced significantly by performing pediculotomy as described earlier.
5. **Recurrence.**

OUTCOME

Posterior cervical foraminotomy for a single level lateral/foraminal soft disk protrusion causing radiculopathy are comparable with anterior microdiskectomy and probably less invasive due to fewer complications.[33] Complications range from 0–9%.[34] Pain relieved in 82–97% of patients.[18,35] Motion preservation was achieved in 93–96%.[36] Recurrence rate is very low. Recurrence at same level of diskectomy is ~3.3% and at adjacent level it is 4.4%.[19] When overall cost of posterior foraminotomy was compared to ACDF, cost of anterior diskectomy and fusion was 89% more than posterior surgery, as there is no need for fusion or instrumentation in later **(Figure 5)**.

CONCLUSION

Posterior laminoforaminotomy is an effective, safer and cheaper alternative to the anterior diskectomy, especially in lateral soft disk prolapse with radiculopathy. Though it is difficult to recommend one procedure over the other. More structured and thorough trials to be designed to clarify the risks and benefits associated with each of these procedures.[37]

REFERENCES

1. Terai H, Suzuki A, Toyoda H, Yasuda H, Kaneda K, Katsutani H, et al. Tandem keyhole foraminotomy in the treatment of cervical radiculopathy: retrospective review of 35 cases. J Orthop Surg Res. 2014;9:38.
2. Schoenfeld AJ, George AA, Bader JO, Caram PM, Jr. Incidence and epidemiology of cervical radiculopathy in the United States military: 2000 to 2009. J Spinal Disord Tech. 2012;25(1):17-22.
3. Semmes R E MF. Syndrome of unilateral rupture of sixth cervical intervertebral disk. JAMA. 1943(121):1209-14.
4. Spurling R SW. Lateral rupture of cervical intervertebral disk, a common cause of shoulder pain. surg gyne obs. 1944(78):350-8.
5. FA Elliott MK. Brachial pain from herniation of cervical intervertebral disk. The Lancet. 1945;245(6332):4-8.
6. Frykholm R. The mechanism of cervical radicular lesions resulting from friction or forceful traction. Acta Chir Scand. 1951;102(2):93-8.
7. Murphy DR, Hurwitz EL, Gregory A, Clary R. A nonsurgical approach to the management of patients with cervical radiculopathy: a prospective observational cohort study. J Manipulative Physiol Ther. 2006;29(4):279-87.
8. W NND. Diagnosis and treatment of myelopathy due to cervical spondylosis. Br Med J. 1955;2(4954):1474-7.
9. SMITH GW RR. The treatment of certain cervical-spine disorders by anterior removal of the intervertebral disk and interbody fusion. J Bone Joint Surg Am. 1958;40-A(3):607-24.
10. Adamson TE. Microendoscopic posterior cervical laminoforaminotomy for unilateral radiculopathy: results of a new technique in 100 cases. J Neurosurg. 2001;95(1 Suppl): 51-7.
11. Ruetten S, Komp M, Merk H, Godolias G. A new full-endoscopic technique for cervical posterior foraminotomy in the treatment of lateral disk herniations using 6.9-mm endoscopes:

prospective 2-year results of 87 patients. Minim Invasive Neurosurg. 2007;50(4):219-26.
12. Caglar YS, Bozkurt M, Kahilogullari G, Tuna H, Bakir A, Torun F, et al. Keyhole approach for posterior cervical diskectomy: experience on 84 patients. Minim Invasive Neurosurg. 2007; 50(1):7-11.
13. Harrop JS, Silva MT, Sharan AD, Dante SJ, Simeone FA. Cervicothoracic radiculopathy treated using posterior cervical foraminotomy/diskectomy. J Neurosurg. 2003;98(2 Suppl):131-6.
14. Takayama S, Kuribayashi K, Miyamoto Y, Nakasu Y, Handa J. [Ossification and calcification of the cervical ligamentum flavum--case reports]. No To Shinkei. 1993;45(9):859-63.
15. Franzini A, Messina G, Ferroli P, Broggi G. Minimally invasive disk preserving surgery in cervical radiculopathies: the posterior microscopic and endoscopic approach. Acta Neurochir Suppl. 2011;108:197-201.
16. Barakat M, Hussein Y. Anatomical study of the cervical nerve roots for posterior foraminotomy: cadaveric study. Eur Spine J. 2012;21(7):1383-8.
17. Fessler RG, Khoo LT. Minimally invasive cervical microendoscopic foraminotomy: an initial clinical experience. Neurosurgery. 2002;51(5 Suppl):S37-45.
18. Kim KT, Kim YB. Comparison between open procedure and tubular retractor assisted procedure for cervical radiculopathy: results of a randomized controlled study. J Korean Med Sci. 2009;24(4):649-53.
19. Kwon YJ. Long-term clinical and radiologic outcomes of minimally invasive posterior cervical foraminotomy. J Korean Neurosurg Soc. 2014;56(3):224-9.
20. Wael Fouad EE. An anatomical study of different neurosurgical approaches of the cervical spinal cord. Alexandria Journal Of Medicine. 2011;47(1):43-51.
21. Ebraheim NA, Xu R, Bhatti RA, Yeasting RA. The projection of the cervical disk and uncinate process on the posterior aspect of the cervical spine. Surg Neurol. 1999;51(4):363-7.
22. Figueiredo EG, Castillo De la Cruz M, Theodore N, Deshmukh P, Preul MC. Modified cervical laminoforaminotomy based on anatomic landmarks reduces need for bony removal. Minim Invasive Neurosurg. 2006;49(1):37-42.
23. Raynor RB, Pugh J, Shapiro I. Cervical facetectomy and its effect on spine strength. J Neurosurg. 1985;63(2):278-82.
24. Zdeblick TA, Zou D, Warden KE, McCabe R, Kunz D, Vanderby R. Cervical stability after foraminotomy. A biomechanical in vitro analysis. J Bone Joint Surg Am. 1992;74(1):22-7.
25. Perneczky A, Sunder-Plassmann M. Intradural variant of cervical nerve root fibres. Potential cause of misinterpreting the segmental location of cervical disk prolpases from clinical evidence. Acta Neurochir (Wien). 1980;52(1-2):79-83.
26. Webb KM, Kaptain G, Sheehan J, Jane JA, Sr. Pediculotomy as an adjunct to posterior cervical hemilaminectomy, foraminotomy, and diskectomy. Neurosurg Focus. 2002;12(1):E10.
27. Perez-Cruet MJ, Foley KT, Isaacs RE, Rice-Wyllie L, Wellington R, Smith MM, et al. Microendoscopic lumbar diskectomy: technical note. Neurosurgery. 2002;51(5 Suppl):S129-36.
28. Uehara M, Takahashi J, Kuraishi S, Shimizu M, Ikegami S, Futatsugi T, et al. Mini Open Foraminotomy for Cervical Radiculopathy: A Comparison of Large Tubular and TrimLine Retractors. Asian Spine J. 2015;9(4):548-52.
29. Habib HEAAM. Management of cervical polyradiculopathy through multisegmental laminoforaminotomies. Alexandria Journal Of Medicine. 2014;50:359-64.
30. Winder MJ, Thomas KC. Minimally invasive versus open approach for cervical laminoforaminotomy. Can J Neurol Sci. 2011;38(2):262-7.
31. Branch BC, Hilton DL, Jr., Watts C. Minimally invasive tubular access for posterior cervical foraminotomy. Surg Neurol Int. 2015;6:81.
32. Choi KC, Ahn Y, Kang BU, Ahn ST, Lee SH. Motor palsy after posterior cervical foraminotomy: anatomical consideration. World Neurosurg. 2013;79(2):405 e1-4.
33. Korinth MC, Kruger A, Oertel MF, Gilsbach JM. Posterior foraminotomy or anterior diskectomy with polymethyl methacrylate interbody stabilization for cervical soft disk disease: results in 292 patients with monoradiculopathy. Spine (Phila Pa 1976). 2006;31(11):1207-14; discussion 15-6.
34. Henderson CM, Hennessy RG, Shuey HM, Jr., Shackelford EG. Posterior-lateral foraminotomy as an exclusive operative technique for cervical radiculopathy: a review of 846 consecutively operated cases. Neurosurgery. 1983;13(5):504-12.
35. Ducker TB, Zeidman SM. The posterior operative approach for cervical radiculopathy. Neurosurg Clin N Am. 1993;4(1):61-74.
36. Coric D, Adamson T. Minimally invasive cervical microendoscopic laminoforaminotomy. Neurosurg Focus. 2008;25(2):E2.
37. Clark JG, Abdullah KG, Steinmetz MP, Benzel EC, Mroz TE. Minimally Invasive versus Open Cervical Foraminotomy: A Systematic Review. Global Spine J. 2011;1(1):9-14.

11

CHAPTER

Minimally Invasive Transarticular C1–C2 Fixation (MIS-TAS)

Vishal Kundnani, Sachin Patil

ABSTRACT

Atlantoaxial instability resulting from dislocation, the nonunion of an odontoid fracture, or an odontoideum, is usually treated by fusion of C1–C2 through a posterior approach. Conventional posterior transarticular screw fixation is associated with extensive muscle dissection resulting in increased blood loss, operative time, inadvertent injury to occipitocervical junction, C2–C3 facetal injury and failure of adjunct supplemental wiring.

Minimal invasive surgery for C1–C2 transarticular screw fixation (MIS-TAS) has shown advantages of reduced morbidity, smaller incisions, immediate stability comparable fusion rate (98%) and early return to work. Utilization of minimal invasive microscopic techniques not only benefit in improved visualization due to illumination and magnification but also assist in achieving most optimal entry point and trajectory through the microscopically dissected pars and isthmus of C2. Safety, feasibility and efficacy of MIS TAS have been evaluated in past by percutaneous techniques by various authors.

This chapter highlights about the feasibility, technique, tips and tricks of minimal invasive transarticular screw (MIS-TAS) for reducible mobile atlantoaxial instability highlighting the advantages and safety of MIS–TAS over conventional open posterior approach.

INTRODUCTION

A variety of techniques for posterior C1–C2 fusion have been described, ranging from in situ fusion, wiring, clamping to those with rigid internal fixation. Until recently, wiring methods were the most popular, including the Gallie and Brooks techniques.[1,2] In these techniques, wedged or H-shaped corticocancellous structural bone grafts are keyed into the posterior elements of C1 and C2 and held in place with wires. Postoperative immobilization in halo vests or Minerva braces is usually required and breakage or loosening of wire with pseudarthrosis rates as high as 10% to 15% have been reported.[3] Also, iatrogenic neurologic injury can occur during wire placement. The Halifax clamp which compresses the two adjacent laminae has also been used for atlantoaxial fixation.[4] This device has poor rotational stability due to the differences in slopes between the arch of C1 and the lamina of C2 which can lead to clamp dislodgement and pseudarthrosis rates range from 10% to 20%. In 1979, Magerl and Seeman described the placement of transarticular screws in conjunction with traditional posterior wiring and bone grafting.[5] The technique has been described studied and validated by various authors and modifications to enhance safety have been published including modification by Sonntag et al. This construct is biomechanically superior to wiring and clamp techniques.[6-10] The rigidity of stabilization with transarticular screw has been compared both in vivo and in vitro studies (compared to wiring vs clamp vs segmental C1–C2 screw fixation) and has been found to be the strongest in flexion extension and rotational stress with almost 100 percent fusion rates. The increased rigidity of the transarticular screw constructs reduces the need of postoperative external immobilization and lowers pseudarthrosis rates associated with most conventional techniques of stabilization.[3] Currently, this technique is considered to be the standard for posterior C1–C2 fixation.[3,11,12] The screws are placed at a low angle relative to the spine starting through the skin quite opposite to T1. The technique of passing transarticular screw has been described to be a technically demanding procedure with very little margins of error in view of the surrounding neurovascular structures around a narrow bony isthmus/pars of C2 which forms the tunnel for the screw to pass through. In the original description of TAS mandatory steps to pass the TAS successfully include the posterior cervical spine exposure from C1 to T1, exposure of superior aspect of C1 arch and base of occiput for wiring of c1 arch , exposure of C2–C3 joint bilaterally for accurate entry point and excision of midline C2–C3 ligamentous structure for placement of graft and wiring construct but current practice. These surgical steps from the original description of TAS have increased the associated morbidity and incidents of spontaneous OC fusion (more in pediatric population), C2–C3 joint arthritis, increased blood loss and surgical time with unfavourable neck disability indices and neck pain indices.

Attempts to reduce morbidity of conventional TAS surgery have been made by reducing the size of incision, reducing the muscle dissection and passing TAS screw percutaneously through cannulated guide and sleeves. In the majority of cases percutaneous placement of screws is possible if exposure of entry point and trajectory of screw can be delineated limiting the exposure to only of C1 and C2. This chapter describes the Minimal invasive surgical technique of C1–C2 arthrodesis using transarticular C1–C2 screws. The advantages of minimal invasive TAS insertion for C1–C2 stabilization are redud surgical time, reduced blood loss, reduced neck pain postoperative, enhanced precision , faster recovery and return to work with higher improvement in neck disability indices with lesser inadvertent complications of OC joint or C2–C3 joint issues in long run. Surgical anatomy, indications, and preoperative assessment will be discussed. Potential pitfalls to screw placement, discuss how to avoid them, and how to deal with them if encountered are discussed in detail.

INDICATIONS

The primary indication for posterior fusion of the atlantoaxial joint is instability from traumatic or inflammatory processes **(Table 1)**. Congenital conditions, such as Down syndrome or several forms of dwartism, are also associated with atlantoaxial instability. Regardless of the etiology, atlantoaxial instability can lead to axial neck pain, radiculopathy, and myelopathy. The goals of surgery are to decompress the spinal cord, reduce the C1–C2 joint, and stabilize the segment with minimum possible morbidity of surgical steps.

Table 1

Indications for C1–C2 Arthrodesis
C1–C2 instability
Traumatic
Transverse atlantal ligament rupture
Comminuted type II dens fracture
Dens fractures in which fracture fixation is not possible
Congenital/Developmental
Downs syndrome
Odontoid hypoplasia
Os odontoideum
Occipitalization of C1 with C1–C2 instability
Inflammatory
Rheumatoid arthritis
C1–C2 osteoarthritis
Syndromic
Klippel–Feil syndrome
Ehlers–Danlos syndrome
Marfans syndrome

Traumatic C1–C2 instability occurs from rupture of the transverse atlantal ligament, fracture of the odontoid processes or, less commonly, by complex atlantal injuries. Except in young children, patients with traumatic injuries of the transverse and alar ligaments are candidates for arthrodesis. Displaced and comminuted fractures through the base of the dens (type II) heal poorly nonoperatively and may be stabilized by posterior C1–2 arthrodesis.[13] Furthermore, C1–C2 arthrodesis may be indicated in elderly otherwise active patients with type II odontoid fractures. A few authors recommend C1–C2 for unstable Jefferson fractures.[14]

Transarticular screw stabilization can also be incorporated into occipitocervical constructs if stability of the occipitocervical articulation is also compromised.

Chronic post-traumatic insufficiency may present insidiously and diagnosis may be delayed years after the index injury. Initially, the diagnosis can be missed if a patient is neurologically normal and local pain and spasm limit the amount of displacement on imaging. Careful follow-up and repeat flexion–extension radiographs after acute symptoms have helped to avoid missing these injuries.

Congenital insufficiency of C1–C2 is seen in several disorders including Down syndrome and Morquio's syndrome. The incidence of atlantoaxial instability in patients with Down syndrome may be as high as 20%.[15] The instability is because of congenital absence or laxity of the transverse ligament. Often this instability is asymptomatic, although patients may experience symptoms from pain to torticollis and even myelopathy. Patients with instability may need to be restricted from activities that put the head and neck at risk. The topic of prophylactic fusion is controversial, but traditionally fusion is recommended in those with an anterior atlantal dens interval (ADI) greater than 7 mm. Additional assessment of stability of the occipitoatlantal articulations is needed as many patients will have combined sites of instability.

A relatively common etiology of instability is hypoplasia or aplasia of the odontoid and os odontoideum. Some patients present with local mechanical irritation that causes axial pain, headaches, or torticollis, while others develop neurologic symptoms. Neurologic symptoms may be transient after an acute injury or more insidious and chronic in nature. Patients with purely mechanical symptoms usually respond to supportive measures, such as rest, immobilization, and physical therapy. They should be followed to ensure that the instability does not progress. Those with progressive neurologic symptoms, significant instability (ADI >10 mm), or significant canal stenosis (space available for the spinal cord <13 mm on axial MRI scan) should undergo posterior C1–C2 arthrodesis and decompression, if necessary.

Atlantoaxial instability is commonly encountered in rheumatoid arthritis and other inflammatory and some degenerative conditions. Traditionally, observation has been recommended in neurologically stable patients as long as the ADI is less than 9 mm. Measurement of the ADI in patients with rheumatoid arthritis can be misleading as it may not represent the true space available for the spinal cord secondary to the presence of synovial pannus. Boden recommends following the posterior atlantal dens interval (PADI) in patients with rheumatoid arthritis.[16] The PADI is the distance between the posterior margin of the dens and the anterior edge of the posterior C1 arch measured on lateral radiographs. Patients with a PADI greater than 14 mm who are neurologically stable should be observed. If the PADI is less than 14 mm, a magnetic resonance imaging (MRI) should be performed and C1–2 fusion (with decompression if necessary) is recommended if the cervicomedullary angle is less than 135º, the cord diameter in flexion is less than 6 mm, or the space available for the spinal cord is less than 13 mm.[16]

Chronic instability can develop in cases of occipitalization of the atlas or congenital fusion of C2–3 (Klippel-Feil). The increased stress on the adjacent C1–2 segment can lead to attenuation of the transverse ligament over time. Symptoms usually present themselves late because of the gradual development of laxity.

Another less common indication for atlantoaxial fusion is degenerative osteoarthrosis of the C1–2 articulations. This surgery is highly effective in patients with suboccipital neck pain with severe degeneration of the C1–2 articulations.[17]

Surgical Anatomy of C1–C2 Joint for Transarticular Screw Placement

High cervical spine is a difficult terrain and the difficulties can be minimized with a thorough knowledge of anatomy of this region . Detailed knowledge of surgical anatomy of C1-C2 junction—bony anatomy of bony terrain with anomalies and anatomical variations along with surrounding neuro-vascular structures—is imperative to safe surgery in this region. The surrounding neurovascular structures that can create surgical problems or at risk structures are: Vertebral artery laterally, Spinal cord medially, C2 ganglion and nerve root with venous plexus superiorly, C2-C3 Joint inferiorly, hypoglossal nerve and internal carotid artery anteriroly.

Transarticular screws enter the lateral mass of C2, traverse the C2 isthmus and the posterior portion of the C1–2 articulation, and are seated in the lateral mass of the atlas. Knowledge of the vertebral artery path within the axis in each patient is necessary for safe screw placement.

The C2 pedicle lies anterior to the inferior articular process of the axis and is often confused with the isthmus of the pars interarticularis. Reports in the literature indicate that placement of a transarticular screw is not anatomically possible in 10–18% of the population because of vertebral artery anomalies.[18-21] Mandel reports that when the C2 isthmus measures less than 5 mm in height or width on computed tomography (CT) scan, the placement of a 3.5 mm transarticular screw increases the risk of penetration of the vertebral artery.[18]

The vertebral artery can be divided into four parts: cervical, vertebral, suboccipital, and intracranial **(Figure 1)**. The vertebral arteries originate from the respective subclavian artery and ascend anterior to the longus coli at C7 and T1. The artery enters the spinal column at C6 and courses cranially in the transverse foramina from C6 to C3. At C2, the artery turns first laterally and then again cranially so that it occupies a far more lateral position in the C1 transverse foramen. This position relatively lengthens, or creates redundancy, of the artery which allows for large excursions of C1–2 rotation without injury or obstruction of blood flow. In C1, the vertebral arteries pass through the transverse foramen and then turn 90° medial and posterior, to lie in a groove on the superior aspect of the posterior arch of the atlas. Approximately 1.5 cm from the midline they turn cranial and anterior, perforating the atlanto-occipital membrane. They ascend first lateral to the medulla, then join anteriorly forming the basilar artery. The lateral turn at C2 gives space for the TAS to pass through safely however sometimes the lateral turn at C2 can have a large tortuosity leading to C2 entering into C1 at a higher space—HIGH RIDING VERTEBRAL ARTERY- prone to be injured by TAS—which can be detected on MRI/CAT scans preoperatively. A knowledge of HR VA is mandatory preoperatively. Analogous origin, tortuous course and dominance of VA are other anatomical variations that should be known to operating surgeons. During exposure of the laminar arches, one should take care not to injure the vertebral artery. Ebraheim has reported that the medial edge of the vertebral artery groove ranges from 8 to 18 mm from the midline on the superior surface of the C1 lamina.[22] Exposure on the superior aspect of the posterior arch of the atlas should not be carried further than 15 mm lateral to midline. In 1–2% of cases, the vertebral artery lies in a tunnel, the arcuate foramen, on the superior aspect of the posterior atlantal arch formed by a thin bony arch, the posticus ponticulous.[23]

The first cervical spinal nerve lies superiorly in the groove with the vertebral artery which is situated posterior to the lateral mass of the atlas, lateral to the spinal canal, and anterior to the atlanto-occipital membrane. The second spinal nerve lies just dorsal to the C1–2 articulation between the posterior arches. Large epidural venous sinuses are located around the C2 nerve and bleeding from these sites can be difficult to control. Use of cottonoids instead of electrocautery is recommended to minimize blood loss.

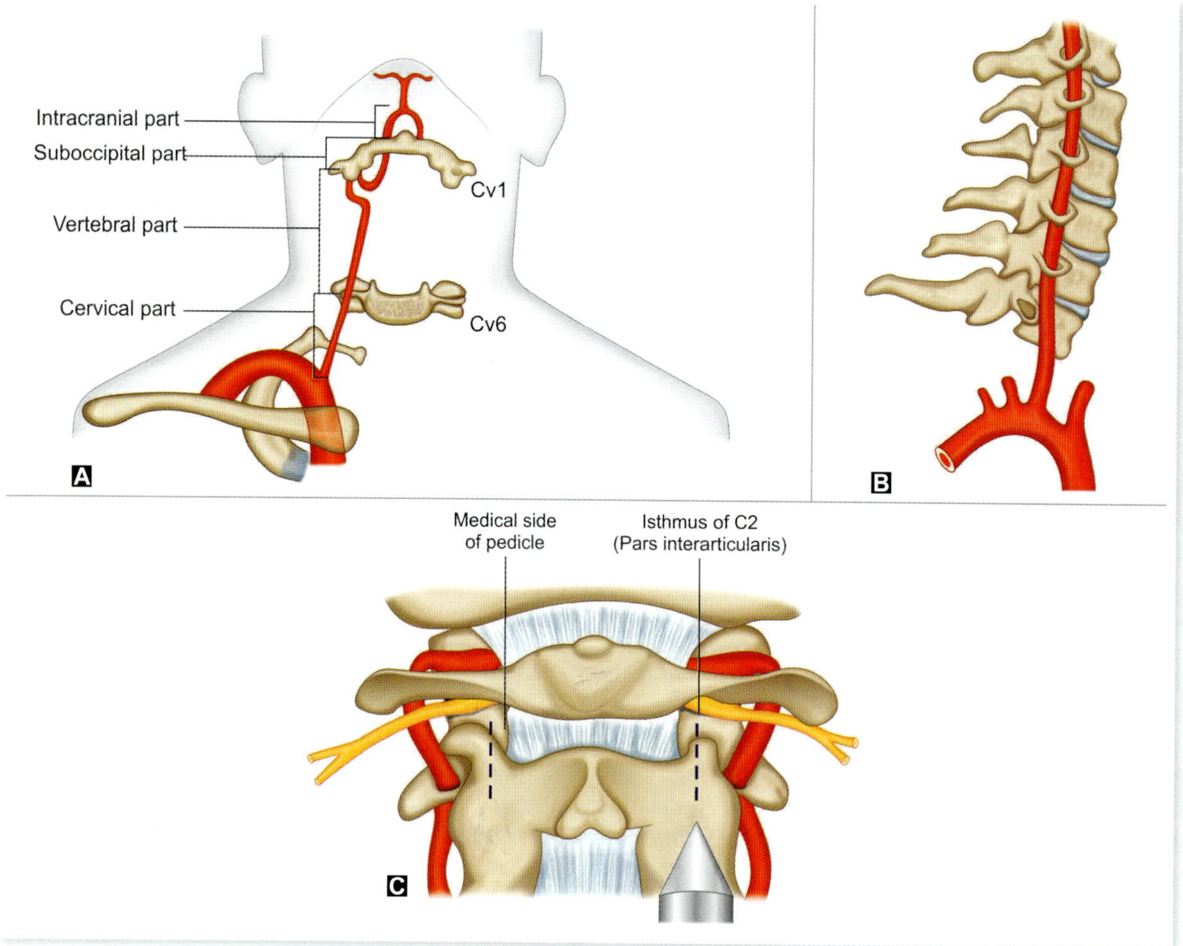

Figure 1: The vertebral artery is divided into four sections: cervical, vertebral, suboccipital, and intracranial.The artery makes two turns, first laterally and then cranial to enter the C1 foramina transversarium that is located in a more lateral position. Note the position of C2 Isthmus and relation of spinal cord medially, VA laterally, spinal nerves superiorly and C2–C3 joint capsule inferiorly

The hypoglossal nerve (CN XII) exits the skull base through the jugular foramen just anterior and lateral to the occipital condyle. It then passes anterior to the lateral part of the C1 lateral mass and C1-2 joint and can be injured if a very long screw is placed. Ebraheim reports that the optimal screw length for the transarticular technique is 38 mm; however, this number may vary depending on the individual's anatomy.[24] In order to avoid risking injury to the hypoglossal nerve, care must be taken not to past-point with the drill and the surgeon must select an appropriate length screw based on the individual patient's anatomy.

The internal carotid artery passes anterior to the lateral half of the C1 lateral on its way to the carotid foramen in the base of the skull. Currier has shown in an anatomic study that the distance between the internal carotid artery and the anterior cortex of the center of the C1 lateral mass is 2–4 mm with the head and neck in neutral rotation.[25]

PREOPERATIVE PLANNING

The close proximity of the vertebral arteries, carotid arteries, brain stem, spinal cord, and cranial nerves demand careful assessment to avoid iatrogenic injury prior to and during placement of transarticular screws. A checklist shall be prepared to keep all the mandatory preoperative steps in vigilance. To minimize the chance of inadvertent injury one shall not miss upon the contraindications of TAS **(Table 2)**

Preoperative Assessment

A thorough history and physical examination is performed. Patients may present with symptoms ranging from mechanical complaints, such as axial neck pain, neck spasm, torticollis, and headaches to myelopathy from spinal cord compression. The neurologic exam can range

Table 2

Contraindications of TAS

1. High riding VA
2. Anomalous VA making <3.5 mm bony isthmus available
3. Irreducible AAD
4. Thoracic hyperkyphosis precluding the necessary trajectory
5. Lateral Mass fracture C1–C2 precluding the hold of screw
6. Single VA –only dominant VA on side of fixation
7. Bleeding diathesis

from normal to transient quadriparesis. In cases of severe atlantoaxial instability, patients may present with brainstem symptoms, such as vertigo, syncope, respiratory distress, and stroke secondary to vertebrobasilar insufficiency from vertebral artery occlusion. Lower cranial nerve function, hypoglossal nerve, deglutition reflex and pharyngeal wall motion with gag reflex shall be checked preoperatively. Room air ABG analysis and CO_2 retention may help assess diaphragm movement apart from routine lab and fitness assessment. Body habitus is important to assess when planning a C1–C2 posterior arthrodesis. Excessive thoracic kyphosis or obesity may preclude correct screw trajectory for the C1–C2 transarticular approach.

Preoperative Imaging

Standard radiographic assessment includes an open-mouth odontoid view and lateral cervical spine radiograph centered at C2. The bony elements are assessed on these films to identify fractures, various anomalies, such as odontoid hypoplasia and os odontoideum, and severe erosive changes which may be because of various inflammatory, neoplastic, or infectious etiologies.

On the lateral view, the ADI is the distance between the posterior aspect of the anterior C1 arch and the anterior aspect of the dens. The ADI serves as a radiographic assessment of the integrity of the transverse ligament. It is normally less than 3 mm in adults and 5 mm in children, and should not change significantly from flexion to extension. Atlantal-dens intervals greater than 5 mm may be associated with spinal cord compression. The lateral radiograph may be misleading if it is taken in the supine position as the C1–2 joint may be reduced as the head falls back in extension. If the patient is alert, conscious, cooperative, and neurologically intact, lateral flexion-extension radiographs can better identify abnormal motion at C1–2. In cases of acute trauma, muscular pain and splinting may limit motion on flexion-extension films leading to a false-negative reading. Repeat flexion-extension radiographs once the acute phase spasms have resided can help avoid missing the diagnosis of C1–2 instability. All patients who are considered candidates for C1–2 transarticular screw fixation should have a CT scan with sagittal reconstruction or MRI with high-quality sagittal images to assess the course of the vertebral arteries. Although rare, there have been reports of cerebellar infarction and death following iatrogenic vertebral artery injury.[26] The size of the C2 isthmus and location of the vertebral artery can be determined on sagittal CT and MRI images. If anatomic constraints suggest that a transarticular screw cannot be safely placed, an alternate method of fixation must be performed. If a unilateral screw can be placed safely, we recommend placement of that screw combined with posterior wiring.[27]

In patients with neurologic findings, MRI evaluation should be performed to assess the spinal canal. In patients with rheumatoid arthritis, MRI also provides an assessment of the degree of synovial pannus, the space available for the cord, and the cervicomedullary angle. Signal changes within the cord representing edema or myelomalacia can give information regarding the general physiologic state of the cervical cord. Posterior sublaminar wires should not be passed in the face of canal stenosis. If reduction of the C1–2 joint will not alleviate the stenosis, decompression of the cervical cord should be accomplished by posterior C1 arch laminectomy, possibly with posterior occiput decompression and/or C2 laminotomy.

Preoperative CT scans with sagittal reconstruction or high-quality sagittal MRI images should be used to evaluate the vertebral artery and C2 isthmus to ensure that safe screw placement is possible **(Figure 2)**. If there is any question of the ability to safely place a transarticular screw on these images, screw placement should not be attempted. Satisfactory results have been achieved with unilateral screws and supplemental wire fixation.[20]

Knowledge of preoperative and intraoperative factors that needs to be kept into consideration for safe TAS and to ensure proper placement of TAS in trajectory are imperative and include checklist as mentioned in **Table 3.**

SURGICAL TECHNIQUE

Anesthesia and Positioning

General endotracheal intubation is traditionally performed, although the degree of instability and neurologic status may necessitate the rise of fiberoptic intubation. After intubation, a neurologic check is performed and then the patient is given a general anesthetic. A bite-block, gauze roll, or wine cork placed between the incisors will optimize the intraoperative visualization of the C1–2 joints on anteroposterior fluoroscopy. We recommend spinal cord monitoring with motor-evoked potentials and/or somatosensory-evoked potentials in cases of significant instability or high-grade stenosis. Mayfield tongs are placed and the patient is proned minimizing manipulation of the head and neck. The patient's chest and iliac crests are

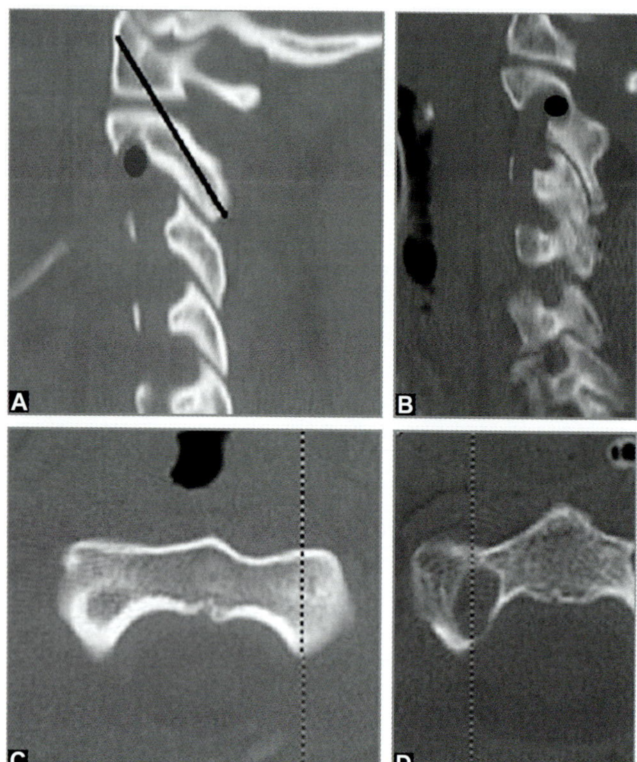

FIGURE 2: Sagittal and axial computed tomography (CT) depicting normal isthmus with screw trajectory and high riding VA precluding safe screw placement

Table 3

Safety techniques to avoid Iatrogenic injury during C1–C2 transarticular screws

Preoperative

- Prone position on Mayfeild table or Jackson table allowing C-arm imaging in AP/lateral
- Assure perfect reduction with positioning (TAS is recommended in reducible dislocations)
- Assess vertebral arteries by computed tomography and/or magnetic resonance imaging (rule out high riding VA)
- Rule out surgical contraindications

Intraoperative

- Avoid dissection on superior surface of C1 lamina greater than 1.5 mm from the midline
- Avoid screws when vertebral anomalies are present
- Use biplanar fluoroscopy
- Position screws in center of the C1 lateral mass on both anteroposterior views and lateral images
- Do not locate screws farther anterior than the posterior margin of the C1 anterior arch
- If an artery is injured, do not place a screw on the opposite side
- Avoid sublaminar wires when stenosis is present

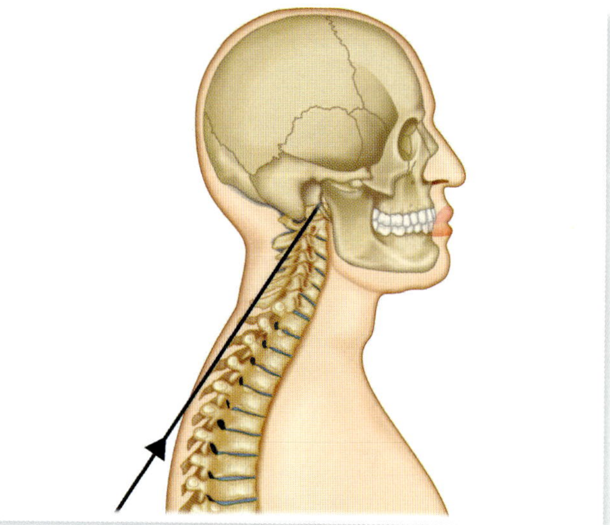

Figure 3: Positioning—Military tuck positioning with flexion at C1–C2 joint and extension at subaxial spine. Note the trajectory of percut TAS guide wire/screw entry on skin and entry on the C2 laminae

supported on gel rolls and the abdomen is allowed to fall free. The arms are positioned anatomically at the patient's side and bony prominences are padded. The C1-2 joint is reduced with gentle extension and traction of the neck while mildly rotating the chin caudally -Military tuck position **(Figure 3)**. The Mayfield is tightened and secured to the bed on a "U-frame," which allows unobstructed anteroposterior and lateral fluoroscopic views during surgery. After positioning, the reduction is confirmed by fluoroscopy. The shoulders are gently taped without excessive tension to avoid brachial plexus traction. Alternatively, the patient can be positioned prone on the Jackson table with the head held in the Mayfield device attached to the table with a special clamp. The draping is done in such a manner to keep the posterior inferior occiput to midthoracic spine exposed and covered by transparent aseptic dressing for visualization of entry point on skin for a percutaneous track of the screw at upper thoracic level

Exposure

The posterior scalp is shaved and the neck and posterior iliac crest are prepared and draped in a sterile manner. Exposure is done under microscopic guidance to ensure magnification and illuminations of the surgical wound . Minimal invasive options of TAS involve modifications in exposure so as to minimize the morbidity of exposure and yet achieve the same safe trajectory along the bony margins. Localization of C2 spinous process is done under C arm guidance and caution taken to minimize the surgical. A midline incision of 3-4 cm is made from just cephalad of C2 spinous process to the spinous process of C3. Dissection is carried sharply down to the spinous processes in the ligamentum nuchae to minimize bleeding. The posterior elements are stripped subperiosteally to the lateral margins of the C2 facet and C3 lateral mass so that the C2-3 facet joint is well visualized. The inferior aspect of posterior arch of C1 is exposed taking care not to carry the dissection further than 15 mm lateral on the posterior arch to avoid injuring the vertebral artery.

In our experience, gentle blunt dissection with a Cobb elevator on the posterior arch of C1 is effective in minimizing bleeding from the venous plexus that is found between C1 and C2 laterally. If bleeding is encountered, it is best controlled by packing with gel foam-thrombin and compression.

Due care is taken to ensure (Figure 4)

1. C2–C3 facet joint and capsule are not dissected or traumatized.
2. Keep the incision focused so as to expose the C2 spinous process.
3. Avoid exposure of superior aspect of C1 posterior arch or even Occiput.
4. Do not dissect the midline ligamentous support of C1-C2 or C2-C3 interspinous space.
5. Dissect the whole of isthmus of C2 from base of C2 inferior facet to Pars to superior surface of C2 lateral mass entering into the C1–C2 joint.
6. Carry out dissection under microscope.
7. Use cottonoids and blunt perisosteal dissectors to isolate lateral and medial margins of the isthmus isolating away the VA laterally and Spinal cord from the trajectory.
8. Decorticate the C1–C2 joint at this stage and insert graft inside the joint.

Adjunctive Wire Fixation

To increase construct rigidity and stabilize the bone graft, wire fixation is recommended using either the Brooks

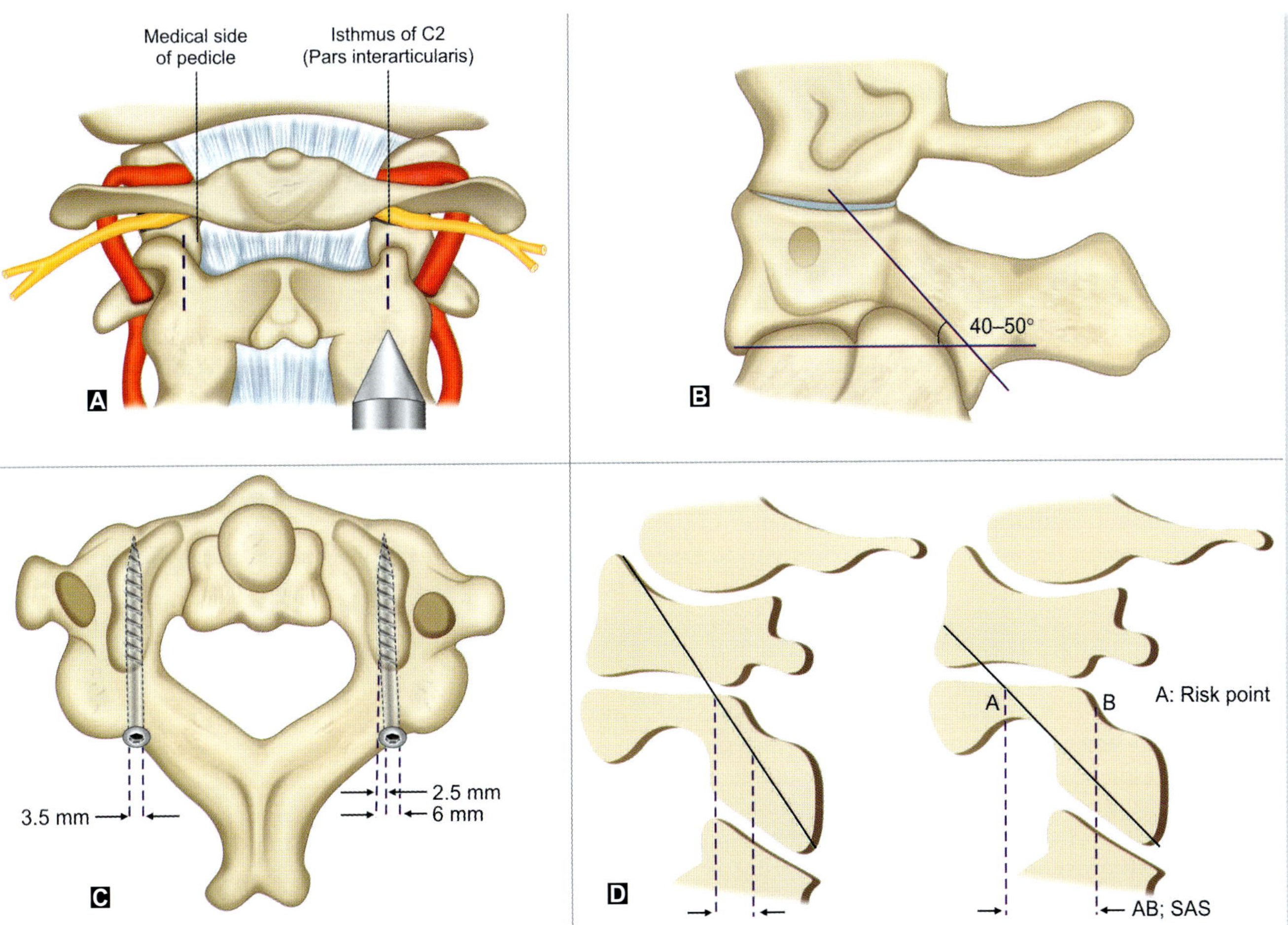

Figure 4: Exposure limited from inferior aspect of C1arch to bases of C2 spinous process and whole of isthmus isolated away from VA laterally and cord medially with cottonoids and C1–C2 joint visualized. C2–C3 joint capsule and interspinous ligament is preserved

or Gallie techniques[1,2] using titanium cables for their ease of passage, tensile strength, and image properties.[28] However, recent literature has evaluated efficacy equally efficacious with 100% fusion rate reducing the need of wiring and associated morbidity of wire related intraoperative neurological injury, wire breakage, and associated morbidity of spontaneous OC fusion reported with exposure of C1 anterior arch.

We recommend using isolated TAS without supplemental wiring with minimal invasive exposure technique under microscope guidance and in our experience fusion rates are nearing 100% in a large series of 57 patients followed up for 2 years. Wiring-related issues have not been documented in our series and no neurological worsening noted and no spontaneous OC fusion even in pediatric population.

Screw Placement

The superior and medial borders of the C2 isthmus are identified with a Penfield #4 or an angled 4-0 curette. The starting point for the transarticular screw is 3–5 mm above the C2–3 facet joint and as medial as possible without breaking through the medial aspect of the C2 pedicle. Dissecting laterally increases the likelihood of vertebral artery injury due to the oblique course that the artery takes in the axis. Using a 3 mm burr, a starting hole is made at this critical location of entry point on C2 base of lamina . We use a 2 -mm threaded guide pin to act as a drill for transarticular screws. A free guide pin is placed lateral to the neck and lateral C-arm images are used to estimate the appropriate skin entry point. A stab incision is made about 1 cm lateral to the T1 spinous process. The guide pin is inserted and advanced cranially through the paraspinous muscles until it reaches the prepared starting hole. This percutaneous method helps minimize the length of the incision. Using anteroposterior and lateral C-arm imaging, the guide pin is advanced in a sagittal plane toward the center of the C1 lateral mass on the anteroposterior view and toward the middle of the anterior C1 arch on the lateral view. The drill and subsequent screws should not extend past the dorsal margin of the anterior arch of C1. Guide pins are placed on each side to help maintain the reduction during screw placement. A free guide pin is used to measure the screw length using a subtraction technique. Hand -guided drilling over guidewire is done and drilling under c-arm guidance feeling perforation of all three cortices is ensured. Fully threaded self-tapping 3.5 mm cortical screw is placed confirming fluoroscopically that the C1–2 joint is not distracted as the screw traverses. A washer may be used if bone quality is questionable. The contralateral screw is placed in the same manner. We recommend passing a long screwdriver through the percutaneous incision first and then seating the screw on the screwdriver in the wound to avoid disengaging and losing the screw in the paraspinous muscles. Some screwdrivers lock the head of the screw to the screwdriver allowing easier percutaneous passage of the screw and screwdriver as a unit. The head of the screw should be tightened under direct vision and final anteroposterior and lateral films are obtained to confirm appropriate screws position and length **(Figure 5)**.

Guidewire, drilling and screw passage is all done through a percutaneous incision placed at T1/T2 level and passing of guide wire at entry point is always kept under visualization under microscope through the surgical site wound to prevent any slippage of guidewire or instruments. Surgical wound at C2 level is necessary not only to localize accurate entry point, monitor passage of guidewire, monitor drilling, visualize medial and lateral movement of instruments and edges of the isthmus but also to decorticate the C1–C2 joint to ensure grafting and high fusion rates which would have been impossible otherwise. Using illumination and magnification further ensure reduction of surgical wound size and also keep the primary stabilization and sound fusion intact. Further microscopic magnification also reduces the bleeding, size of sound, muscular dissection ,surgical time and postoperative healing and rehabilitation.

Bone Graft

The posterior iliac crest through a 1–2 cm incision is exposed and a 7–10 mm thick bicortical rectangular plate is harvested with an osteotome and mallet. Curettes are used to harvest separate pieces of cancellous graft. Graft is morselised and used inside the C1–C2 joint before insertion of screws and also after insertion of screws graft is laid down on laminae of C1–C2 surface **(Figure 6)**. It is Ensured that the superior surface of C1 arch and occiput are not exposed to avoid inadvertent OC fusion known to occur with this technique. Allograft from bone bank and BG substitutes can alleviate the need of BG harvesting further reducing the graft site morbidity in patients

The wounds are closed in layers with or without a drain based on the preference of the surgeon. It is important to reattach the short occipital rotator muscles to the C2 spinous process. Postoperative immobilization is in a hard cervical collar for 8–10 weeks or until there is radiographic evidence of healing.

Imaging, Microscopic and Neuromonitoring

The Procedure is carried out under strict Biplanar fluoroscopy, Microscopic illumination and magnification right from marking the level of surgery, Localization of C2 spinous process to exposure of C2 isthmus. The most dorsal and most medial aspect of Isthmus of C2 is visualized and confirmed on C arm images. Marking of entry point, localization of screw trajectory percutaneous from T1 to C2 and through C1–C2 joint into C1 lateral mass is all visualized

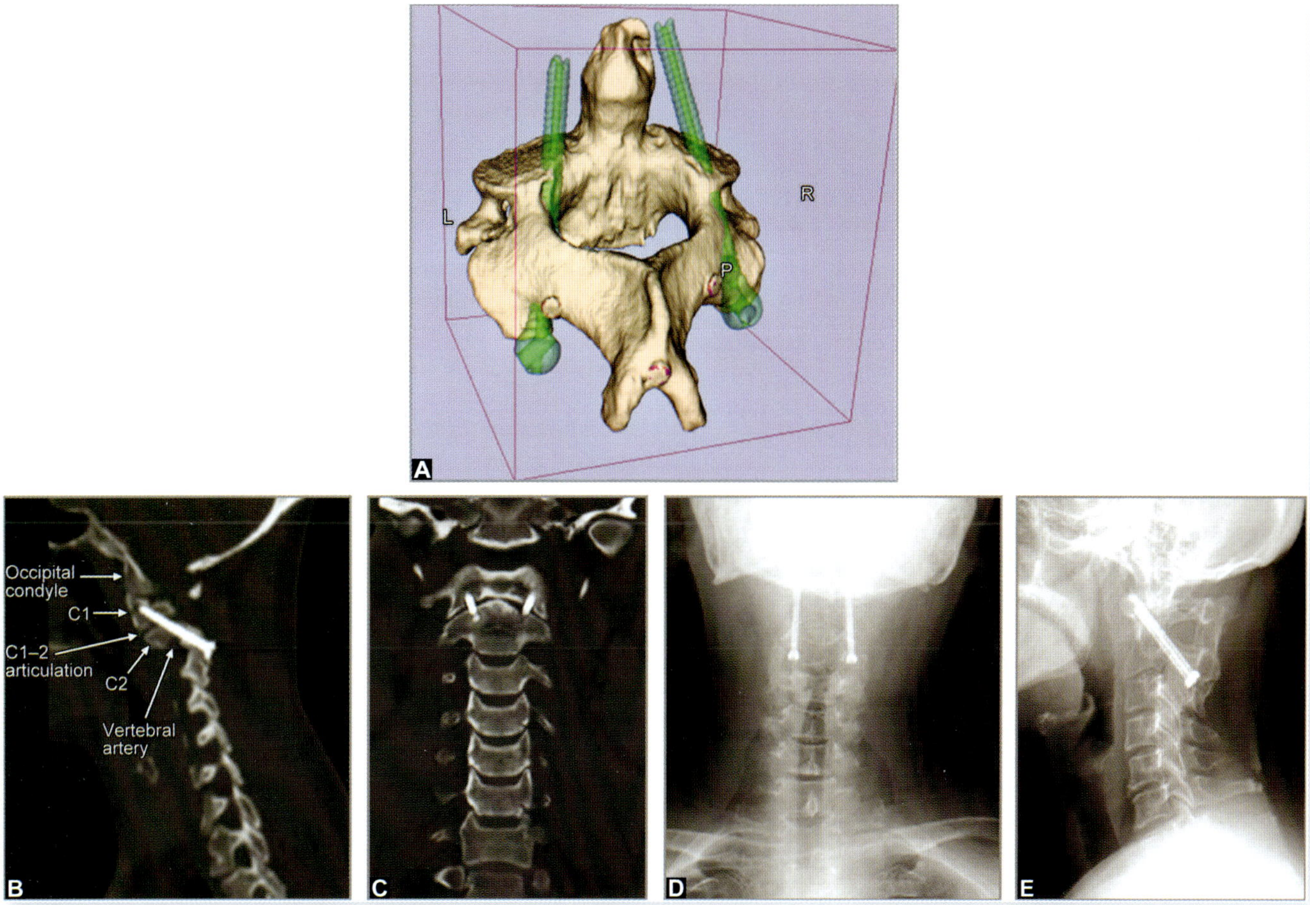

Figure 5: Placement of TAS through C2 entry point–isthmus, C2 lateral mass C1 lateral mass. Note the trajectory is 10° divulged away from midline to prevent medial perforation

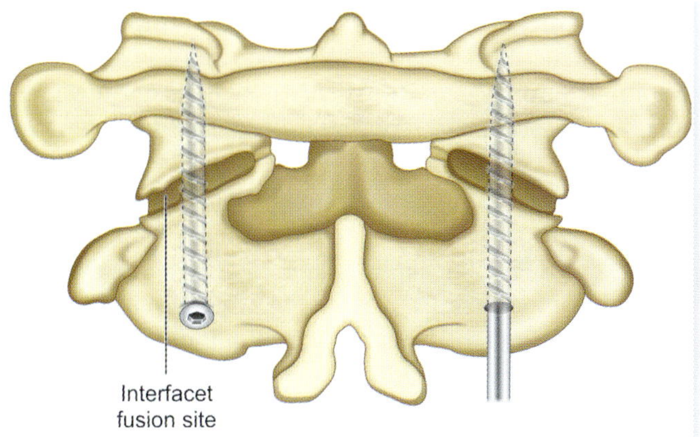

Figure 6: BG placement in the C1–C2 joint to ensure higher fusion rate of MIS TAS, it is imperative to decorticate the C1–C2 joint area for higher fusion rate

constantly under C arm IITV view, mostly lateral, AP views determine the lateral divergence of 10–15°.

Microscopic Assistance reduces the size of surgical wound to few centimeters needed to expose the C2–C3 facet and isthmus needed to guide the screw trajectory, While ensuring the minimal invasive nature of surgery with reduced surgical time, reduced surgical incision size, less blood loss , smaller recovery and rehabilitation time with faster return to work and improved NDI indices scores.

Safe placement of screw is ensured with IITV imaging intraoperative and also by Combined SSEP/NEM neuromonitoring.

POSTOPERATIVE PROTOCOL

Minimal invasive TAS placement is a safe and effective technique with reduced morbidity in management of mobile AAD. TAS placed in this manner not only provides immediate stability reducing the need of postoperative bracing, but also with added advantages of minimal invasive technique. The wound size is smaller with minimal muscle dissection and damage to paraspinal musculature, further mitigating the need of postoperative bracing.

Postoperative course involves soft cervical collar for 3–6 weeks with no additional brace support .

MIS TAS ensures faster recovery, minimal morbidity and faster return to work .

In patients with myelopathy symptoms natural course of recovery may be prolonged due to obvious reasons. However surgical morbidity with this technique is minimal and patients can often be discharged within 24–48 hours of the surgery.

Complications and Prevention

TAS is a technically challenging procedure with potential catastrophic complications **(Table 4)**. The margin of error is very narrow and can lead to problems unsalvageable at times. Prevention of these complications is possible by prompt knowledge of surgical anatomy and preoperative assessment with a meticulous surgical technique.

Placement of transarticular screws is a technically demanding procedure and even in the hands of experienced surgeons the incidence of malpositioned screws has been reported to be as high as 10%.[29] Proper screw placement requires anatomic reduction of the C1–2 during patient positioning. Failure to obtain a good reduction greatly increases the likelihood of misplacing screws and injuring adjacent neurovascular structures. Impediments to reduction such as an ossicle anterior to the odontoid or large synovial pannus can be identified on preoperative imaging.

High-quality biplanar intraoperative C-arm imaging is required to minimize screw malposition. Poor fluoroscopic visualization in either plane will increase the chance of misdirection during drilling and screw placement. Image guidance systems are an alternative.[30] In our opinion, these lack reliability because of registration difficulties and position change between C1 and C2 that occurs during surgery. Although accuracy as high as 98% has been reported, the false-negative could result in catastrophic injury.[31,32]

Careful attention should be given to the drill trajectory in both planes prior to drilling. The trajectory should be checked frequently in both planes as the drill is advanced across the joint. If the angle is too steep the tip of the screw may enter the occipitoatlantal joint, while a very flat trajectory may leave the screw inferior to the C1 lateral mass resulting in inadequate purchase. Medial deviation may leave a screw in the spinal canal, while straying laterally puts the vertebral artery at risk. Screw misdirection can be minimized by paying close attention to anatomic landmarks and radiographic images. A liberal incision of the thoracodorsal fascia aids in obtaining the appropriate trajectory by minimizing soft tissue constraints on drill positioning.

Table 4

Complications of minimally invasive TAS

Misplaced screw
VA injury
Pseudoarthrosis
Infection
Bleeding

Although rare, penetration of the vertebral artery by transarticular screw has been reported.[26] Safe screw placement may not be possible in as many as one in five patients because of anomalous vertebral artery anatomy. Wright et al. reported on a review of 2,492 transarticular screws placed in 1,318 patients and found the risk of vertebral artery injury to be 4.1% per patient.[26] The risk of neurologic injury from vertebral artery injury was 0.2% and the risk of mortality was 0.1%. Fortunately, vertebral artery injuries rarely result in neurologic injury as long as the contralateral vertebral artery is patent and the posteroinferior cerebellar artery blood flow is preserved. Demetriades[33] reports that most vertebral artery injuries can be treated by observation rather than requiring operation or embolization. The best way to avoid injury to the vertebral artery is to recognize preoperatively when the course of the artery precludes safe screw placement and perform alternative fixation.

Grob has reported unilateral hypoglossal nerve paresis from excessive length of a screw.[11] The hypoglossal nerve and internal carotid lie directly anterior to the lateral masses of C1. To avoid injuring these structures, the surgeon should be careful not to allow the drill or screw tip to pass beyond the middle of the anterior arch on the lateral C-arm projection.

OUTCOMES

Several clinical studies have shown low nonunion rates for transarticular screws despite the use of less external immobilization. Pseudarthrosis rates with posterior wiring techniques have been reported from 10% to 15%.[3] Grob et al. reported only one nonunion in a series of 161 patients undergoing C1–2 posterior fusion with transarticular screws.[11] Dickman and Sonntag reported a 2% nonunion rate for transarticular screw fixation compared with a 14% nonunion rate for posterior wiring.[3] In a separate study, Dickman reviewed the repair of 16 C1–2 nonunions with transarticular screws and reported 13 solid bony fusions, two stable fibrous unions and one failure.[3,34]

TAS without supplemental wiring has shown promising results with fusion rates of almost 100%. In initial studies 3–7% patients did not show fusion mass on normal X-rays in the posterior spinous region; however on closed analysis of AP X-rays and subsequent CT scan evaluation fusion bridges were noted anteriorly in lateral mass confirming very high fusion rates with this technique **(Figure 7)**.

Morselized grafting instead of conventional autograft blocks have shown to have similarly high rates of fusion

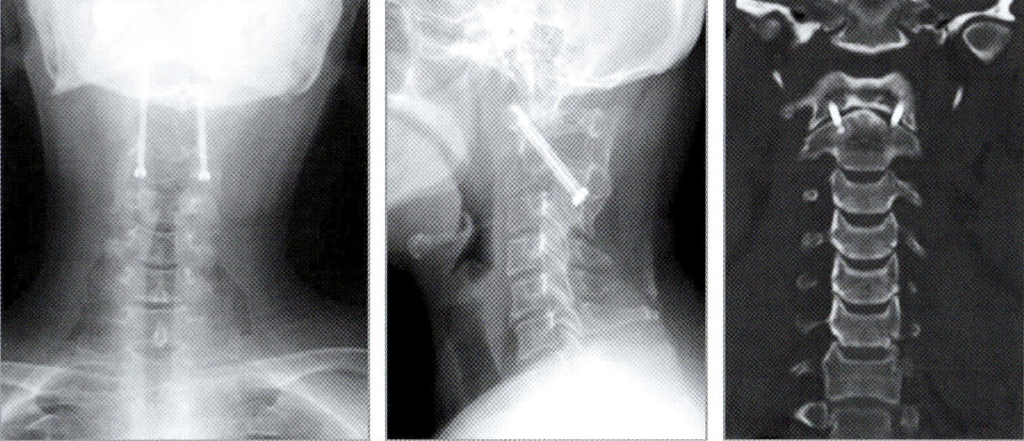

Figure 7: Fusion mass visible in posterior interspinous region, and in cases where it is not, fusion is visible in lateral masses despite poor visualization posteriorly

making autograft bone blocks un necessary as the sole criteria of fusion.

Minimal invasive techniques in exposure of C2–C3 joint have not been studied in detail but have shown promising results in initial studies. The advantages of minimal invasive exposure for TAS as described above hass obvious advantages, which cannot be neglected in coming years. The advantages of MIS in spine surgery coupled with additional safety and promising results of TAS in terms of fusion rates and immediate stability surely promise MIS-TAS as the gold standard in coming years.

CONCLUSION

Transarticular screws provide three-point fixation which is biomechanically superior to various popular posterior wiring techniques. Several clinical evaluations have proved that this biomechanical advantage correlates to improved fusion rates.[3,8,12] In addition to lowering nonunion rates, the increased stiffness of transarticular screws allows for less postoperative immobilization. Despite its many advantages, this technique is very technically demanding and should be performed by experienced surgeons. Comprehensive knowledge of the local anatomy and thorough understanding of potential pitfalls and how to avoid them will result in safe and successful placement of this screw. Minimal Invasive techniques reduce the morbidity associated with TAS access and dissection involved without compromising the benefits of this highly successful surgery . The advantages of minimal exposure and minimal invasive techniques come with an additional safety factor and involve improved disability indices and higher satisfaction rates with faster return to work . In coming years MS-TAS is going to be a successful alternative to be utilized for C1-C2 reducible dislocations and shall soon become widely practised to be termed as the gold standard of AAD management.

REFERENCES

1. Brooks AL, Jenkins EB. Atlanto-axial arthrodesis by the wedge compression method. J Bone Joint Surg Am. 1978; 60:279-84.
2. Gallie WE. Fractures and dislocations of the cervical spine. Am J Surg. 1939; 46:494-9.
3. Dickman CA, Sonntag VK. Posterior C1-C2 transarticular screw fixation for atlantoaxial arthrodesis. Neurosurgery. 1998; 43:275-80.
4. Moskovich R, Crockard HA. Atlantoaxial arthrodesis using interlaminar clamps. An improved technique. Spine. 1992; 17(3):261-7.
5. Magerl F, Seeman PS. Stable posterior fusion of the atlas and axis by transarticular screw fixation. In: Weidner PA, ed. Cervical Spine. New York: Springer-Verlag; 1987:pp 322-7.
6. Farey ID, Nadkarni S, Smith N. Modified Gallie technique versus transarticular screw fixation in C1-C2 fusion. ClinOrthop. 1999; 359:126-35.
7. Grob D, Crisco JJ III, Panjabi MM, Wang P, Dvorak J. Biomechanical evaluation of four different posterioratlantoaxial fixation techniques. Spine. 1992;17(5):480-90.
8. Hurlbert RJ, Crawford NR, Choi WG, Dickman CA. A biomechanical evaluation of occipitocervical instrumentation: screw compared with wire fixation. J Neurosurg Spine. 1999;90:84-90.
9. Naderi S, Crawford NR, Song GS, Sonntag VK, Dickman CA. Biomechanical comparison of C1-C2 posterior fixations. Cable, graft, and screw combinations. Spine. 1955;23:1946-55.
10. Henriques T, Cunningham BW, Olerud C, et al. Biomechanical comparison of five different atlantoaxial posterior fixation techniques. Spine. 2000;25:2877-83.

11. Grob D, Jeanneret B, Aebi M, Markwalder TM. Atlanto-axial fusion with transarticular screw fixation. J Bone Joint Surg Br. 1991;73:972-6.
12. Tokuhashi Y, Matsuzaki H, Shirasaki Y, Tateishi T. C1-C2 intra-articular screw fixation for atlantoaxial posterior stabilization. Spine. 2000;25:337-41.
13. Campanelli M, Kattner KA, Stroink A, Gupta K, West S. Posterior C1-C2 transarticular screw fixation in the treatment of displaced type II odontoid fractures in the geriatric population—review of seven cases. Surg Neurol. 1999;51:596-600.
14. McGuire RA Jr, Harkey HL. Primary treatment of unstable Jefferson's fractures. J Spinal Disord Tech. 1995; 8(3):233-6.
15. Ohsawa T, Izawa T, Kuroki Y, Ohnari K. Follow-up study of atlanto-axial instability in Down's syndrome without separate odontoid process. Spine. 1989;14(11):1149-53.
16. Boden SD, Dodge LD, Bohlman HH, Rechtine GR. Rheumatoid arthritis of the cervical spine. A longterm analysis with predictors of paralysis and recovery. J Bone Joint Surg Am. 1993;75(9):1282-97.
17. Ghanayem AJ, Leventhal M, Bohlman HH. Osteoarthrosis of the atlanto-axial joints. Long-term follow-up after treatment with arthrodesis. J Bone Joint Surg Am. 1996;78(9):1300-7.
18. Mandel IM, Kambach BJ, Petersilge CA, Johnstone B, Yoo JU. Morphologic considerations of C2 isthmus dimensions for the placement of transarticular screws. Spine. 2000; 25(12):1542-7.
19. Paramore CG, Dickman CA, Sonntag VK. The anatomical suitability of the C1-2 complex for transarticular screw fixation. J Neurosurg. 1996;85(2):221-4.
20. Song GS, Theodore N, Dickman CA, Sonntag VK. Unilateral posterior atlantoaxialtransarticular screw fixation. J Neurosurg. 1997;87:851-5.
21. Taitz C, Arensburg B. Vertebral artery tortuosity with concomitant erosion of the foramen of the transverse process of the axis. Possible clinical implications. Acta Anatomica. 1991; 141(2):104-8.
22. Ebraheim NA, Xu R, Ahmad M, Heck B. The quantitative anatomy of the vertebral artery groove of the atlas and its relation to the posterior atlantoaxial approach. Spine. 1998;23(3):320-3.
23. Young JP, Young PH, Ackermann MJ, Anderson PA, Riew DK. The arcuate foramen: implications for C1 lateral mass screw insertion. J Bone Joint Surg Am. 2005;87:2495-8.
24. Ebraheim NA, Misson JR, Xu R, Yeasting RA. The optimal transarticular c1-2 screw length and the location of the hypoglossal nerve. SurgNeurol. 2000;53:208-10.
25. Currier BL, Todd LT, Maus TP, Fisher DR, Yaszemski MJ. Anatomic relationship of the internal carotid artery to the C1 vertebra: a case report of cervical reconstruction for chordoma and pilot study to assess the risk of screw fixation of the atlas. Spine. 2003;28(22):E461-7.
26. Wright NM, Lauryssen C. Vertebral artery injury in C1-2 transarticular screw fixation: results of a survey of the AANS/CNS section on disorders of the spine and peripheral nerves. J Neurosurg. 1998;88:634-40.
27. Sasso R, Doherty BJ, Crawford MJ, Heggeness MH. Biomechanics of odontoid fracture fixation. Comparison of the one- and two-screw technique. Spine. 1993;18:1950-3.
28. Dickman CA, Crawford NR, Paramore CG. Biomechanical characteristics of C1-2 cable fixations. J Neurosurg.1996; 85(2):316-22.
29. Gebhard JS, Schimmer RC, Jeanneret B. Safety and accuracy of transarticular screw fixation C1-C2 using an aiming device. An anatomic study. Spine. 1998;23(20):2185-9.
30. Herz T, Franz A, Giacomuzzi SM, Bale R, Krismer M. Accuracy of spinal navigation for magerl screws. ClinOrthop. 2003; 409:124-30.
31. Kamimura M, Ebara S, Itoh H, Tateiwa Y, Kinoshita T, Takaoka K. Cervical pedicle screw insertion: assessment of safety and accuracy with computer-assisted image guidance. J Spinal Disord Tech. 2000;13(3):218-24.
32. Richter M, Amiot LP, Neller S, Kluger P, Puhl W. Computer-assisted surgery in posterior instrumentation of the cervical spine: an in-vitro feasibility study. Eur Spine J. 2000;9(suppl 1):S65-70.
33. Demetriades D, Theodorou D, Asensio J, et al. Management options in vertebral artery injuries. Br J Surg. 1996;83(1):83-6.
34. Dickman CA, Sonntag VK. Posterior C1-C2 transarticular screw fixation for atlantoaxial arthrodesis. Neurosurgery. 1998; 43:275-80.

3

SECTION

MIS in Lumbar Spine—Non-instrumented

Section Outline

12

CHAPTER

Microdiskectomy

Samir Dalvie, Pramod Saini

ABSTRACT

The lumbar microdiskectomy is one of the commonly done procedure in lumbar disk prolapse patients. This procedure has evolved over a period of time with the aim of removing the pathological cause with minimal trauma to the soft tissues and faster rehabilitation. The present chapter discusses the safer methods, trips and tricks, its complications and avoidance of performing a successful lumbar diskectomy. We have wide experience with this procedure with a satisfactory long time follow up.

INTRODUCTION

Lumbar microdiskectomy describes use of surgical microscope through interlaminar approach and a midline one inch incision to remove herniated nucleus pul posus. First lumbar diskectomy was reported by William J Mixter, a neurosurgeon along with his orthopedic colleague, Joseph Barr in 1934 at Harvard College. Their technique involved extensive removal of lamina and offending disk by transdural approach. Love, in 1939, described extradural approach for disk removal which is now commonly known as macrodiskectomy.[2] First lumbar microdiskectomy using microscope was reported in 1977 by Caspar in Germany and M. Gazi Yasargil in Switzerland separately.[3,4] Subsequently Robert Williams popularized microdiskectomy in US and later multiple studies confirmed the benefit of microsurgical techniques over open methods.[5]

Use of surgical microscope has certain technical advantages like simultaneous illumination and magnification with variable adjustment, coaxial projection of light and 3D like images. These technical advantages result in surgical benefits, such as small incision, less soft tissue trauma and blood loss, improved hemostasis due to easier identification and coagulation of epidural veins, gentle handling of neurological tissues, early mobilization and shorter hospital stay. Also, assistant has the same view of the surgical field as the surgeon; therefore it allows efficient assistance and education. But there are pitfalls to use of microscope. While using microscope surgeon loses peripheral vision. Whenever the surgical procedure moves out of microscopic field, microscope needs to be adjusted to maintain proper field of vision. Limited exposure may result in wrong level exploration or missed fragments. Technical inexperience and limited visualization of structures surrounding target area put them at risk. Therefore, microdiskectomy needs proper training and has a learning curve. Good results require meticulous planning and technique, proper positioning of the patient and correct localization of target disk level.

APPLIED ANATOMY

Anatomical structures that need to be identified to accurately localize pathology in microdiskectomy are facet, lamina, and pedicles. For better correlation between preoperative imaging and intraoperative findings, McCulloch compared a lumbar segment to three stories of a house.[6] The disk was the first storey; infrapedicle level was the second story and pedicle as the third storey. Disk herniation is most commonly limited to first storey of the same segment or the third storey of the lower segment. This three-storey concept helps surgeon accurately develop a mental picture of relationship between herniated disk and surrounding bony and neurological structures. Correlation of this three floor model with MRI and radiographs help localize the site of incision and extent of bony resection required.

Spinal canal can be divided from medial to lateral direction into zones—central, lateral recess or subarticular, foraminal and extraforaminal zone. Central zone is situated between the facet joints and occupied by dura. Lateral recess also known as Lee's entrance zone lies between lateral margin of dura and medial border of pedicle. Foraminal zone or mid zone lies below pedicle while Extraforaminal zone or exit zone lies lateral to pedicle. Microdiskectomy is indicated for all disk herniation lateral to foramen, i.e. central and parcentral. Herniations located at entrance of foramen can be removed easily by this approach, but those situated deep in foramen or are extraforaminal need alternative approaches and therefore contraindicated. Key for successful decompression is localization of pedicle and the traversing nerve root. Disk space is situated just superior to pedicle and nerve root exit spinal canal below the corresponding pedicle. Therefore, at L4–5 disk level, L4 is the exiting nerve root and L5 is the traversing nerve root.

The presenting symptoms of nerve root involvement depends on the location of disk. The central and paracentral disk will compress traversing nerve root while foraminal and extraforaminal disk compresses exiting nerve root. Therefore, a central or paracentral disk herniation at L4–L5 would compress the L5 nerve root while foraminal or an extraforaminal or far lateral disk herniation will compress L4 nerve root.

It is also important to understand relationship of interlaminar space with disk level. As we go cephalad from L5/S1 there is an increasing overlap of the superior lamina over the disk space. The disk space is interlaminar at L5/S1, partially sublaminar at L4/5 and totally sublaminar at L3/4 and higher. Therefore, higher lumbar levels require more resection of lamina to expose disk space.

INDICATION AND APPLICATION

Patient selection is critical and more important than surgical technique for achieving good outcomes. There should be a strict correlation of distribution of leg pain and imaging. Other causes of leg pain should be ruled out before proceeding with surgery.

Universally accepted indication for microdiskectomy is - failure of 6 weeks conservative treatment, severe or worsening neurodeficit and cauda equine syndrome. Delaying surgery beyond 3–4 months is associated with poor outcome because of irreversible change in nerve root.

SURGICAL TECHNIQUE: AUTHORS' PREFERENCE

Anesthesia

The procedure is performed under general anesthesia. There are reports of surgery done in local, spinal or epidural anesthesia as well. These would be in exceptional circumstances, where general anesthesia is highly contra-indicated. The patient would be uncomfortable in prone and managing airway would be challenging. Furthermore, conversion to GA would be very difficult.

Positioning

The patient needs to be positioned prone. Many positioning devices are available. The essential requirements would be avoidance of excess compression of the abdomen and chest, avoidance of pressure points, including the eyes and ease of imaging. Additional desirable elements would be positioning in a flexed position so as to open the interlaminar space. This provides access to the disk with minimal bone removal.

The most common position would be on bolsters. In this case, flexing the hips and knees would open the interlaminar space. Positioning devices, such as a Wilson's Frame would also help create a flexed lumbar spine. Knee chest and kneeling positions have also been used. These require adaptations to the operating table. Excess flexion may increase the venous pressure and also tension in muscles and nerve roots, making retraction difficult and potentially harmful. Hyperflexion of knees and hips may cause problems in elderly patients.

Initial Exposure

The surgical part is prepared for optimum asepsis. The level is marked after preparation. I insert a needle into the anticipated interspinous ligament by palpation from distal to proximal. An image intensifier is used to locate the level. The disk level is confirmed with a sagittal MRI to avoid errors. Preoperative marking is extremely hazardous, as skin markers will slip and change location after positioning, and inserting needles prior to skin preparation may introduce foreign material.

A 2.5 cm incision is made such that the interspace as well as the disk space is included. This may be placed to one side of the mid-line. Sharp dissection is carried down to the fascia. The deep fascia is sharply incised to one side of the midline leaving a small fringe for suturing. The paraspinal muscle is elevated subperiosteally till the facet. At this stage the ligamentum flavum should be visible.

Various retractor systems are available to provide access through the small incision. These have been devised by Caspar, Yassargill, McCollough etc. My personal preference is for the McCollough retractor which consists of various sizes of hooks and blades. The hook is inserted in the interspinous ligament and the blade is positioned laterally. The retractor is applied, and achieves stability by distraction between the midline and the muscles. One may use a tubular retractor system with the same technique. If there is any doubt about the level, it is wise to confirm it at this stage with another lateral image. Hemostasis is achieved at this point to prevent blood trickling into the microscopic field.

At this stage the microscope is used. The initial steps are done with a lower zoom level (2.5-4X). As the procedure advances, the zoom level may be increased.

Entry into the Canal

There are various methods to gain initial access to the neural canal. Essentially one has to safely cross the ligamentum flavum, by incising or excising it. My preferred method is entering close to the midline. At this point the dura is furthest from the ligamentum flavum, and a lateral disk is least likely to have pushed the dura dorsally. An 11 no. blade is used craniocaudally in the midline to thin the fibers of the ligamentum until the epidural fat is seen pouting from the defect. A no 1 Penfield dissector is used to push through and dissect the flavum along its fibers. The direction is towards the opposite side. Subsequently the dissector is reversed and blunt dissection is carried out to the ipsilateral side to separate the dura from the ligament. Cottonoid patties may be used to separate and protect the dura.

Alternative methods of entering the canal include disinserting the ligamentum using sharp curettes from the caudal edge of the cephalad lamina or from the lateral border of the canal.

Exposure of the Root

A no. 2 and 3 Kerrison punch is used to excise the Ligamantum flavum laterally from the midline until the lateral border of the traversing nerve root is visualized. Preferably the nerve root is freed from its origin to its exit at this stage. This is more important in cases with additional lateral recess stenosis.

Exposure of the Disk

The nerve root is carefully mobilized to expose the herniated or prolapsed disk. In most instances of posterolateral disk prolapse, the nerve root is retracted medially. In rare instances of axillary or large central prolapse, the initial access may be through the axilla of the root. However, once the tented nerve root is relaxed, further access is preferred by retracting medially.

Diskectomy

Retraction of the root usually exposes and delivers the herniated or sequestered fragment or reveals the bulge in the PLL/posterior annulus. The fragment is preferably separated using blunt dissection with a Penfield dissector so that it can be safely delivered in its entirety. In contained herniations, the annulus is probed to reveal a rent or defect, and entry into the disk space is achieved through this. A pituitary rongeur is used to remove the herniated fragments. All sequestered and herniated fragments are removed and the canal is probed to look for hidden and migrated pieces of disk. The disk space is probed for loose or easily separable pieces of disk material. I do not believe in curettage of the disk space or removal of any unseparated pieces of disk or end plate. My end point is absence of any herniated fragments, free mobility of the nerve root and absence of loose pieces of disk in the disk-space.

Epidural bleeding may be an issue and this is carefully controlled by bipolar coagulation or using cottonoid patties along with pieces of gelfoam. Irrigation of the surgical wound is performed and on confirmation of adequate diskectomy the wound is closed in layers. On releasing the retractor, muscle falls back in place. The deep fascia is sutured to the midline with strong suture. The subcutaneous tissue is closed using absorbable sutures and the skin closed using a subcuticular stitch. The skin and muscle may be infiltrated using bupivacaine for postoperative analgesia.

Postoperative Protocol

The patient is mobilized out of bed as soon as he is comfortable. In bed static lower limb and gluteal exercises are started and the patient is progressively ambulated within limits of tolerance and pain. The patient is discharged as soon as he is comfortable.

COMPLICATIONS AND THEIR AVOIDANCE

Avoidance of complications is important as they mostly end up in failed back surgery syndromes. Complications specific to microdiskectomy are wrong level, epidural bleeding, durotomy, nerve root lesion, anterior vessel and visceral injury, postoperative leg pain and residual symptoms, recurrent disk herniation and spondylodiskitis.

Incidence of wrong level exploration has been reported as 1.5% in case of very experienced surgeons and 3.3% in case of less experienced one. It occurs more commonly at L4–5 and higher levels.[7] Therefore, appropriate intraoperative radiographs need to be taken to mark correct level. Lateral X-rays should be evaluated for lumbosacral anomalies like sacralized L5 or lumbarized S1 vertebra which are responsible for last lumbar segment mismatch between MRI and X- ray. To avoid wrong level exploration counting should be done on Lateral radiographs from below upwards after identifying last formed level and this should be correlated with MRI.

Epidural hematoma resulting in postoperative deficit is one of the most feared complications of posterior spine surgery. Intraoperative bleeding occurs from two sources—arterial bleed from muscles and epidural venous plexuses. Arterial bleeders in muscle should be coagulated carefully as they can continue to bleed even after wound closure. On the other hand epidural venous bleed rarely causes cord compression as it stops after removal of disk fragment and wound closure. However, intraoperatively it obscures vision and even a small bleed appears large hemorrhage under microscope. Prevention is by proper positioning of patient with free abdomen, avoiding exploration over posterior aspect of vertebral body, retracting veins along with dura and coagulating them if they come in way. If excessive epidural bleeding occurs remove extruded disk fragment as much as possible as after fragment removal it is easier to cauterize.

Incidence of Dural tear following diskectomy ranges from 1 to 17 %.[8] Dural tears present in postoperative period with positional headache, CSF leak, wound dehiscence, and symptomatic pseudomeningocele. Pseudomeningocele can present as recurrent back and leg pain due to herniation of nerve rootlets. Dural tear most commonly occur during opening of ligamentum flavum. Once dural tear is identified, it is covered with patty and diskectomy is continued. The Author do not attempts dural closure irrespective of the size. The usual protocol is to cover the tear with fat or gelfoam and do a watertight closure of muscle and fascia with drain under gravity without suction. Patient is started on acetazolmide for reducing CSF production and put on complete bed rest for next 3–4 days. Drain is monitored for amount and nature of output. If there is a CSF leak from wound or in drain then a lumbar drain may be placed far from incision. However, if leak does not resolve spontaneously, then reoperation for closure of dura may have to be considered.

Nerve root injury has been reported in less than 1% of cases undergoing microdiskectomy.[9] Patient presents postoperatively as new or worsened neurological deficit. Causes are poor visibility, adhesions, and congenital nerve root anomalies. It is important to identify lateral border of nerve root and dural sac before entering anterior epidural space. The most vulnerable area for root injury is axilla of exiting nerve root; therefore, maneuvers for fragment removal should not be done in this area. The best measure is to stay lateral to root. Nerve root injury presents as CSF leak and herniation of rootlets. Larger defects may need suturing after reduction of rootlets while smaller ones can be covered with fat graft as any attempt to repair may result in strangulation of root.

Visceral or vessel injury occurs due to perforation of anterior annulus and ALL by instruments during grasping maneuvers in disk space. Incidence of vessel injuries is 0.045% with left iliac artery at L4–5 disk being most common (ESJ). Visceral injury incidence is 1.6–17 per 10000 cases and L5–S1 is the most common site.[10,11] Intraoperative clue to anterior annular violation is egress of fluid through the annulus and out of field. Vessel injury presents with hypotension and unexplained bleeding from annulus. If this injury is identified intraoperatively, decompression is to be stopped, wound closed and patient turned supine followed by urgent laparotomy. In spite of emergent treatment mortality rateremeined as high as 50%. Bowel injuries are uncommonly recognized intraoperatively and present in early post-operative period as persistent abdominal or flank pain, hypotension, fever, and ileus. Intra-abdominal abscesses and diskitis are seen in patients with late presentation and these cases need exploratory laparotomy. To prevent this injury surgeon has to be aware of the depth to which instruments especially pituitary roungers are inserted in the disk space and general recommendation for working depth is 25 mm.

Reported incidence of infection following diskectomy is around 0.5 %.[11] Superficial wound infection can be managed with dressings and a brief period of antibiotics. Presence of unusually marked spastic back pain in early postoperative period, even if wound is healed, should raise suspicion of Diskitis. Such patients have unusually high ESR and CRP. Plain radiographs show subchondral erosions which may be delayed by 6 weeks after onset of symptoms. MRI is the most sensitive investigation showing decreased signal intensity in adjacent bone on T1 due to edema and increased signal intensity in disk space on T2. Patients with suspected diskitis need to undergo CT guided or open biopsy to confirm diagnosis. Appropriate antibiotics, based on culture results, are continued for 6 weeks intravenously and 6 weeks orally.

Postoperative cauda equine syndrome following lumbar microdiskectomy has been reported in 0.08–1.2% of cases.[12]Urgent postoperative MRI in such cases is advised to rule out possibility of cord compression by epidural hematoma which needs emergent exploration. However most of the cases do not show any evidence of compression pointing towards vascular insult. Re-xploration in the absence of any compression may further cause neurological deterioration.

Different studies have reported Incidence of recurrent disk herniation ranging from 3 to 6%.[13] Young age, male gender, smoking, and traumatic events are associated with increased risk of recurrence. On the other hand, complete removal of disk and end plate curettage do not reduce risk of recurrence but results in accelerated segment degeneration and back pain. It is important to differentiate recurrent disk from perineural fibrosis as re-xploration in latter case may not give satisfactory results. This distinction can be made on contrast MRI. Fibrosis will enhance on MRI whereas disk will not or will show peripheral enhancement.[14,15] Repeat decompression is preferred treatment for these cases. [13,16,17]

OUTCOMES

Multiple studies have reported 80–95% excellent short and long term outcomes following lumbar microdisketomy. Findlay et al. reported 91% success rate at 6 months in 79 patients which declined slightly to 83% at 10-year follow-up. Rate of recurrence needing surgery was 6.1% in their series.[18] Moore et al. reported 88% excellent result in 100 patients followed for an average 8.6 years.[19] Williams achieved

98.8% successful result while Yasargil reported 87% overall excellent result in their series.[20,21]

Numerous authors have reported short hospital stay and earlier return to work as advantage of microdiskectomy over macrodiskectomy or open method.[22-24] But two authors, Barrios and Kahanovitz could not find any difference in long term outcomes though microsurgical method did have short term advantage.[25,26] Another prospective randomized study by katayama et al. with mean follow-up of 2 years and 8 months did not find any advantage of one method over other and concluded that both are appropriate as long as surgeon has mastery of procedure.[27]

Proponents of muscle splitting technique of tubular diskectomy suggest it to be better than subperiosteal muscle dissection of the conventional diskectomy in terms of muscle damage and outcome, but there are many reports to the contrary. Brock et al. compared tubular diskectomy to microdiskectomy and could not find any difference in post operative pain and ODI scores, but analgesic use was significantly less in tubular group.[28] Another randomized control trial evaluated extent of muscle injury between tubular and conventional diskectomy groups by using serum CPK levels and the cross-sectional area of the multifidus muscle on MRI as indicators. The trial could not find any difference between these two methods and tubular group reported more back pain during first postoperative year.[29] Similarly Muramatsu et al. showed no difference in post-operative contrast enhancement as a marker of tissue damage between tubular diskectomy and conventional microdiskectomy.[30] A recent Cochrane review evaluated available evidence about advantages of Minimal invasive diskectomy over microdiskectomy or open diskectomy.[31] This review concluded that minimally invasive diskectomy may be inferior in terms of relief of leg pain, low back pain and rehospitalization, though the difference is small but has lower incidence of surgical site infection.

REFERENCES

1. Mixter W, Barr J. Rupture of the intervertebral disk with involvement of the spinal canal. N Engl J Med. 1934;211:210-5.
2. Love JG. Removal of protruded intervertebral disk without laminectomy. Proc Staff Meet Mayo Clin. 1939;14:800-5.
3. Caspar W. A new surgical procedure for lumbar disk herniation causing less tissue damaage through a microsurgical approach. Adv Neurosurg. 1977;4:74-7.
4. Yasargil MG. Microsurgical operation of herniated lumbar disk. Adv Neurosurg 1978; 7:81
5. Williams RW. Microlumbar diskectomy: a conservative surgical approach to the virgin herniated lumbar disk. Spine. 1978; 3:175-82.
6. McCulloch J. Principles of microsurgery for lumbar disk disease. New York: Raven; 1990.
7. Kraemer R, Wild A, Haak H, Herdmann J, Krauspe R, Kraemer J. Classification and management of early complications in open lumbar microdiskectomy. Eur Spine J. 2003;12:239-46.
8. Desai A, Ball P, Bekelis K, Lurie J, Mirza SK, et al.. Outcomes after incidental durotomy during first-time lumbar diskectomy. J Neurosurg Spine. 2011;14(5): 647-53.
9. Mayer HM. The Microsurgical Interlaminar, Paramedian Approach. In; Mayer, HM ed. Minimally Invasive Spine Surgery Second Edition 283.
10. Houten J, Frempong-Boadu A, Arkovitz M. Bowel Injury as a Complication of Microdiskectomy. J Spinal Disord Tech. 2004;17:248-50.
11. Benzel EC. Spine surgery: Techniques, complication avoidance, and management. 2 nd ed. Amsterdam: Elsevier; 2005.
12. Dimopoulos V, Fountas K, Machinis T, Feltes C, Chnung I, et al.. Postoperative cauda equina syndrome in patients undergoing single-level lumbar microdiskectomy Report of two cases. Neurosurg Focus. 2005;19(2):E11.
13. Suk KS, Lee HM, Moon SH, Kim NM. Recurrent Lumbar Disk Herniation Results of Operative Management. Spine. 2001; 26:672-6.
14. Jonsson B, Stromqvist B. Clinical characteristics of recurrent sciatica after lumbar diskectomy. Spine. 1996;21:500-5.
15. Cavanagh S, Stevens J, Johnson JR. High-resolution MRI in the investigation of recurrent pain after lumbar diskectomy. J Bone Joint Surg [Br]. 1993;75:524-8.
16. Ozgen S, Naderi S, Ozgen MM, et al.. Findings and outcome of revision lumbar disk surgery. J Spinal Disord. 1999;12:287-92.
17. Cinotti G, Roysam GS, Eisenstein SM, et al.. Ipsilateral recurrent lumbar disk herniation. A prospective, controlled study. J Bone Joint Surg [Br]. 1998;80:825-32.
18. Findlay GF, Hall BI, Musa BS, Oliveira MD, Fear SC. A 10-year follow-up of the outcome of lumbar microdiskectomy. Spine. 1998;23(10):1168-71.
19. Moore AJ, Chilton JD, Uttley D. Long-term results of microlumbar diskectomy. Br J Neurosurg. 1994;8(3):319-26.
20. Williams R, Results of microsurgery. In: Williams RW, McCulloch JA, Young PH, eds. Microsurgery of lumbar spine. Rockville. Aspen;1990:211-4.
21. Abernathey CD, Yasargil MG. A 10-year follow-up of the outcome of lumbar microdiskectomy. Results of microsurgery. In: Williams RW, McCulloch JA, Young PH, eds. Microsurgery of lumbar spine. Rockville. Aspen. 1990;211-4.
22. Andrew DW, Lavyne MH. Retrospective analysis of microsurgical and standard lumbar diskectomy. Spine. 1990;15:329-35.
23. Caspar W, Campell B, Barbier DD, et al.. The Caspar microsurgical diskectomy and comparison with a conventional standard lumbar disk procedure. Neurosurgery. 1991;28:78-87.
24. Silvers HR. Microsurgical versus standard lumbar diskectomy. Neurosurgery. 1988;22:837-41.
25. Barrios C, Ahmd M, Arrotegui J, et al.. Microsurgery versus standard removal of the herniated lumbar disk. A 3-year comparison in 150 cases. Acta Orthop Scand. 1990;61:399-403.

26. Kahanovitz N, Viola K, Muculloch J. Limited surgical diskectomy and microdiskectomy: a clinical comparison. Spine. 1989;14:79-81.
27. Katayama Y, Matsuyama Y, Yoshihara H, Sakai Y, Nakamura H, et al.. Comparison of Surgical Outcomes Between Macro Diskectomy and Micro Diskectomy for Lumbar Disk Herniation: A Prospective Randomized Study With Surgery Performed by the Same Spine Surgeon. J Spinal Disord Tech. 2006;19:344-7.
28. Brock M, Kunkel P, Papavero L. Lumbar microdiskectomy: subperiosteal versus transmuscular approach and influence on the early postoperative analgesic consumption. Eur Spine J. 2008;17:518-22.
29. Arts M, Brand M, Kallen B, Nijeholt G, Peul W. Does minimally invasive lumbar disk surgery result in less muscle injury than conventional surgery? A randomized controlled trial. Eur Spine J. 2011;20:51-7.
30. Muramatsu K, Hachiya Y, Morita C. Postoperative magnetic resonance imaging of lumbar disk herniation: comparison of microendoscopic diskectomy and Love's method. Spine. 2001; 26:1599-16.
31. Cochrane Database Syst Rev. 2014;9:CD010328.

13

CHAPTER

Philosophy and Basis of PELD

Satishchandra Gore

ABSTRACT

Percutaneous procedures in the treatment of spine pathologies has been a breakthrough achievements in minimal invasive spine surgeries. The main advantages of these procedures are its small incisions, lesser tissue trauma and faster rehabilitation. Percutaneous endoscopic approach is one of its kind wherein it has wide applications with satisfactory outcomes. This chapters deals with basic aspects of percutaneous endoscopic technique, anatomy and methodology.

Understanding of back and leg pain and claudication as related to disk, facet and canal changes seen in cadaver and images have defined surgical treatment till now. Aging changes in form of disk and facet changes staged as stage of dysfunction, instability and then stabilization have been proposed in traditional degenerative cascade. Access to disk was initially transdural and then a wide laminectomy access around dural sac was promoted.

A 20 *cadaver* study based degenerative cascade by Kirkaldy Willis has led to emphasis on decompression and stabilization. The study is without clarity on neurophysiology of the changes and their timeframe. It selectively ignored nerve supply of functional spinal unit, location of dorsal root ganglion (DRG) in relation to the segment, asymmetry or so at that level, changes around DRG, and mechanism of pain, namely chemical or mechanical? Pain causation is kept in background with emphasis on anatomical variations and in turn images.

Newer understanding of degeneration as symptomatic structural failure unlike aging and symptoms as response of the nervous system to the structural failure has changed our approach to back and leg pain management. Our indications for treatment also are refined now and changed from progressive neurological deficit to much broader ones, including managing persisting pain. This refinement now includes minute structural changes in early or start of symptom generation. Symptoms are generated by response of the nervous system to the changes of degeneration at *interface* of the disk/facet structural failure and the nervous system. This interface is physiological target of treatment, and has been repeatedly ignored by over emphasis on anatomy and images of the failed structure alone. It led to many failures, e.g. in case of disk if the outline of the disk is not changed most clinicians are clueless as to what intervention is relevant? For the first time, we can now visualize this interface by awake and aware surgery under local anesthesia.[in vivo visualization] by transforaminal endoscopy.

Imaging changed from "myelography" with negative imaging of around the dural structures to CT. Advent of CT scan made us aware of cross-sectional anatomy but real change happened with MRI and its physiological correlation. But MRI still has no correlation with pain. It cannot identify painful interface.

Once MRI was available understanding of pathoanatomy changed but still neurophysiology was out of purview of the surgeons. Creating a very unusual situation where over emphasis on anatomy and pathoanatomy led to "image guided decision making" which prevails even today.

This is wrongly complemented by "untimely" and "premature" stabilizations which allegedly mimick natural end stage of degenerative cascade. Stabilization by its very nature destroys the pain generators and nerve supply. It still may not relieve the pain if all pain generators are not removed. Pain generation in common cases of radiculitis is fairly well understood. Even though in cases of stenosis it needs further refinement in understanding. Even though annular tear was noted as beginning of structural failure "nerve supply of the functional spinal unit and pain generation as concepts came in later. The importance of

DRG in foramen forming lateral wall of the safe triangle and importance of TFL ligament is not yet appreciated fully.

Microdiskectomy and further refined versions of targeting structural failure area in degeneration and changed anatomy were promoted very heavily. This highlighted better visualization of "tip of the iceberg "completely ignoring basic annular tear and inflammatory change at disk and nerve interface. It has been unnecessarily proposed as gold standard thereby stopping further change and refinements. Traditional surgery never had an inside view of the "disk" ignoring where the problem started and the mother trouble. Degenerative annular tear starts inside out. Once it reaches out it becomes symptomatic as back or leg pain depending on location and type of the tear.

The access to iceberg was gross but was refined over time. Access itself at times was promoted as treatment modality, e.g. laminectomy and "decompression" never highlighting the key target of inflammation at the say disk nerve interface. Decompression was promoted as therapeutic and refinement only came in form of use of tubes and light sources with camera and scope at site of surgery. This entirety has missed the point "where is the pain coming from and why is it persisting, how do we reach the pain generator and take care of it? [ablate, wash, irrigate, excise]. It also never highlighted interface of disk and nerve DRG and changes in this interface and how to precisely target this symptom generating structural failure. In traditional evolution *images* became supreme; ignoring minute changes enable us to distinguish chemical and mechanical causes of pain.

We need refined images of the interface where symptoms are generated. The images match the anatomy to about 87%. In refined images relevant to awake and aware approach it is noted that foraminal size increased from L1 to L5 in the ventral to dorsal and cephalad to caudal direction. Pedicle width increased from L1 to L5. Greatest width of the DRG was 6.5 mm bilaterally at L5 (range 3.2–6.5 mm). In the fourth lumbar spine, dorsal root ganglia positions were 48% IF, fifth lumbar spine 75% IF at S1 8% IF and 83% IS. Position of DRG can be ascertained by doing a epidurogram.

ANALYSIS OF DORSAL ROOT GANGLION POSITIONS

Magnetic Resonance Imaging Study of DRG Size and Location

The size and location of the lumbar and S1 DRG are as follows:

Level	Size	Location
L1	3.7 × 4.3 mm	92% in the lumbar intervertebral foramen
L2	4.6 × 5.7 mm	98% in the lumbar intervertebral foramen
L3	5.7 × 7.1 mm	100% in the lumbar intervertebral foramen
L4	6.2 × 8.4 mm	100% in the lumbar intervertebral foramen
L5	5.9 × 9.4 mm	95% in the lumbar intervertebral foramen
S1	6.2 × 11.2 mm	79% in the intraspinal region

The nerve roots occupy from 23% to 30% of the area of the intervertebral foramen. The relatively larger DRG in the lower lumbar region may be more susceptible to compression than the upper DRG, particularly with the higher propensity to disk degeneration and intervertebral narrowing in the lower lumbar region. The S1 nerve root and DRG may both be involved as a result of disk herniation or degenerative changes of the L5–S1 facet, because it is the most intraspinally located DRG of all lumbar nerve root complexes.[10]

Recently, concepts emerged about pain generation when traditional surgery was done under local anesthesia, images superseeded by "in vivo" visualization and later proposed grading of pain generating events by "Gore sign" 2014. The affect of the nerve DRG can be staged as stage of inflammation and sensitization, then added mechanical compression and may be further progressing to neuro deficit. This may not be necessarily linear in progression. But pain can be present without mechanical compression and inflammation alone can give pain. With likely proportion of the stages being 80-15-5 a new separate treatment modality in form of "pain management" emerged. It was sometimes thought as substituting surgery and other hardware based interventions. Pain can be present *only* if inflammation is present. Priming of tissue by inflammatory cytokines is must. We are not referring to symptoms of claudication or changes of stenosis becoming symptomatic. Simultaneous social changes in form of expectations from surgery and surgical morbidity, related issues about anesthesia also took center stage in debates. Old ideas about general anesthesia, morbidity, complications from surgery, access related inevitable outcomes, age and medical comorbidities related limitations and fear of surgery led to a new idea and platform "awake and aware surgery".

Refinement in answers to fundamental questions then led to stitchless surgery of the functional spinal unit under local anesthesia. Pain comes from inflammation at interface of the disk and nerve or disk change of annular tear and the anterior epidural tissue and can be reached through the foramen under local anesthesia. Ground breaking work about "pain generators and recent about pain mechanisms, effect of nucleus on nerve" made further fine tuning possible. Locationally DRG is intraforaminal at L4–5 L5-S1 thus making an access which is transforaminal almost mandatory. On clinical assessment Gore sign is proposed to identify, confirm and monitor sciatica. In early stages of inflammation and mechanosensitization, this is the *only* way to identify and monitor sciatica. It also conceptually helped us in staging sciatica and also integrating other common painful entities, namely knee pain and heel pain in "neuralgia" thread.

Once the concepts of transforaminal surgery emerged and crystallized in 2001 [Yeung and Gore] several objections emerged. These had a undercurrent of eternal conceptual rivalry between orthopedic and neuro spine surgeons. The objections were (i) indication of transforaminal interventions, treatment of back pain, (ii) uses of "fluoroscopy" and excessive radiation and (iii) "steep" learning curve. Objections were also raised about "TFE" being short on (iv) treating canal stenosis and (v) instabilities.

- Indications are inclusive of evolved thinking starting from "annular tear", staging of sciatica. The philosophy now includes treatment of symptoms at all stages and proper correlation of image, symptom, pathology and treatment modality. Rather than offering stabilization to all stages even though it may be premature, *untimely* and irreversible. The issue of facet related back pain can be tackled by facet denervation. Chronic back pain due to "non-healing ulcer" at posterior annulus can be treated by "disk fx" or by visualized treatment including cleaning and ablation and sealing of the tear.
- About radiation use of PPD, line drawing and surface marking before needle entry to understand and correctly execute access to foramen, advent of sonoanatomical understanding and use have made the radiation exposure and resulting danger least.
- Arguments about "steep learning curve" indicate that hardware zombies have till now totally ignored "chemical" aspect. It can be in form of they opposing diskography, totally neglecting clinical assessment of pain with better correlation of symptoms and pathology and always unabashedly promoting "stabilization". The learning curve then is not steep as what we really need to learn is this basic lacuna in current thinking dominated by stabilization and more stabilization ignoring refined decompression and other mechanisms over shadowed by hardware zombies.
- With refined and evolved thinking, learning objectives are now crystallized, and it really boils down to proper placement of needle and acknowledging that we do excision and also ablation, irrigation, lavage, and decompression. Stabilization may be needed in selected cases. The learning objectives are as follows:
  - Proper clinical assessment of "fundamental change of inflammation" and identifying focus of inflammation causing symptoms. Cocentrating on disk/facet and nerve DRG interface and changes there in.
  - Correlation of this understanding with images, noting images may not correlate in over 30%. Concentrating on DRG, we also acknowledge that invisible inflammation, TF Ligament, and other soft tissue variations may be "invisible" to a nontrained eye.
  - Identify anatomical and physiological target. Physiological target is almost always "inflammation".
  - *Reach* the target precisely minimizing the access related morbidity, under awake aware conditions.
  - Extend our reach even while using a rigid endoscope by articulated instruments. Instead of always trying to get the target in line of sight "extend reach by "hook" or side firing laser".
  - Confirm adequacy of surgery at the target. By realtime relief or dynamics of the local site or visualizing neural structures if need be.
  - Avoid complications in access and execution at target which is within few millimeters of the nerve or DRG. The neural tissue need not be visualized.
  - Care about further progression of changes of degeneration in time. The likely timeframe for these evolving changes is predicted so as to avoid "fusion at any cost". The wrong interpretation of data initially had led us to believe that microdiscectomy over 10 years or more stays effective is not true. The understanding of adjacent level changes even though still "unclear" is a real issue with *untimely* stabilization.
- About canal stenosis it would be prudent to understand issues like, what causes non pain symptoms in stenotic spine, how instabilities become symptomatic. Are all base symptomatic changes reversible by surgery permanently? Is it venous congestion, arterial insufficiency, dynamic physical compression? The central part of the canal can be reached by "transfacet" surgical access. Pioneered by us.[not published].
  - We had unclear concepts about stenosis that have been refined over time. This deals with causation of symptoms and even failure of surgery to relieve them.
- There are new ideas in treatment of instabilities in form of "hybrid "surgery where we combine isolation of pain generators in foramen and stabilization under local or regional "sensory" blocks. This has several key advantages. This may also be then complemented by transfacet fixation which is equally effective like transpedicular fixation. But can be done under local anesthesia and percutaneously. It can combine TFE and insertion of stand-alone cages.

Over coming all the objections about TFE thus we can say it is a easy to learn and teach methodology. It can be positioned as "safe hands" surgery for the functional spinal unit.

There are paradigm changes in basics of surgery for the symptomatic functional spinal unit in degeneration. Refined assessment is now based on Gore sign.

- Stage 1 of mechanosensitization of nerve in sciatica and back pain: treating posterior annular tear with disk fx or visualized access and sealing. Use of platelet plug is also noted.
  - Inflammation alone is treated by use of steroid or other anti-inflammatory meds at the interface.
- Stage 2 of mechanical compression in addition to inflammation tt is TFE surgery.
- Stage 3 of neural deficit needs increasing concentration on neurodeficit and presence or absence of pain noting subtle and gross changes.

There are several unanswered questions:

- How to integrate the staging and sub sets of sciatica in a comprehensive "neuralgia management"?
- How do we monitor postoperative changes in pain and lingering pain? Can it be based on monitoring inflammation?
- How do we know the recovery potential after intervention? Will all symptoms always go away? Can we predict outcome with certainty?
- How do we promote this qualitative data without images and hardware and get audience in conferences and meetings dominated by hardware?

SUMMARY

Concentrate on chemical affect, intervention under LA use of needle; as the target is precisely localized and under imaging control; stitchless access by dilatation of tissues for access; visualization of pain generator and confirming image finding; ablate, irrigate, excise, mobilize root, increase volume of the unyielding walls around DRG and root; extend reach by hook, laser, flex drill, shaver; do adequate surgery.

Added use of stabilization is advised in relevant indications using hybrid surgery combining TFE and stabilization under local regional anesthesia.

14

CHAPTER

Transforaminal Percutaneous Lumbar Endoscopic Diskectomy

Arun Bhanot

ABSTRACT

The herniated disk can be assessed through the transforaminal route. The technique of endoscopic diskectomy is based on this approach which also has advantages of causing least morbidity. The minimally invasive nature of the procedure has inherent advantages of causing lesser tissue trauma and faster rehabilitation of the patient. This chapter focuses on percutaneous approach to diskectomy, Indications and advantages of the procedure.

INDICATIONS

Indications for percutaneous transforaminal endoscopic Diskectomy are almost the same as those for a conventional open or microdiskectomy barring a few exceptions. These days, most of the paracentral, central, upmigrated and downmigrated herniations can be removed using the transforaminal approach. However, one needs to plan the trajectory and skin puncture points very precisely and specific to the individual anatomy of the herniation as well as the patient. In addition, foraminal and extraforaminal disk herniations are some of the best indications for the transforaminal diskectomy as one does not need to get inside the main disk tissue and instead focus on the herniated fragment as it lies in the direct line of access of the Transforaminal approach. Recurrent disk herniations are another good indication for this transforaminal approach as one can avoid going through the previous scar tissue and safely access the herniated fragment through a virgin terriorty of the intervertebral foramen.

However, certain highly downmigrated herniations may not be suitable for the transforaminal approach as the inferior pedicle of the foramen may impede access to the herniated fragment with conventional transforaminal instruments. With the availability of the transforaminal endoscopic burr, this limitation is also being overcome as one can drill a little bit of the superior surface of the inferior pedicle to get easy access to the highly downmigrated disk fragment. Similarly, calcified disk herniations are also not very good indications for transforaminal approach but here again, the endoscopic burr may help overcome this limitation in certain cases.

APPLIED ANATOMY

Transforaminal endoscopic diskectomy is done by a posterolateral approach accessing the herniated disk through the intervertebral foramen. This approach has the least morbidity of all the approaches to the herniated disk as it does not violate the sanctity of paraspinal musculature and protects the barrier of ligamentum flavum to the epidural space.

The key to a successful transforaminal endoscopic diskectomy is understanding of the concept of Kambin's safe triangle. As the name implies, it is a triangular working space bounded medially by the traversing nerve root, inferiorly by the superior end plate of the caudal vertebra and the hypotenuse or lateral boundary is formed by the exiting nerve root at that level (**Figure 1**). We use this safe space to access the herniated disk through the transforaminal route. The dimensions of the Kambin's triangle are different at different lumbar levels as they vary according to the width and heights of the pedicles, the take off angle of the nerve roots from the dural sleeve, etc. For a successful transforaminal endoscopy, one also needs to check for an adequate disk height and anteroposterior foraminal width that can permit the insertion of working cannula. In addition, one needs to check the location of the exiting nerve root in the intervertebral foramen to have a safe transforaminal access **(Figure 2)**. Mostly the exiting nerve root lies in the superior half of the foramen and one can safely work in the inferior half of the intervertebral foramen. However, in certain cases, the exiting nerve root lies in the inferior half of the foramen and thus falls in the direct line of working instruments **(Figure 3)**. These are not safe cases to chose for transforaminal surgery.

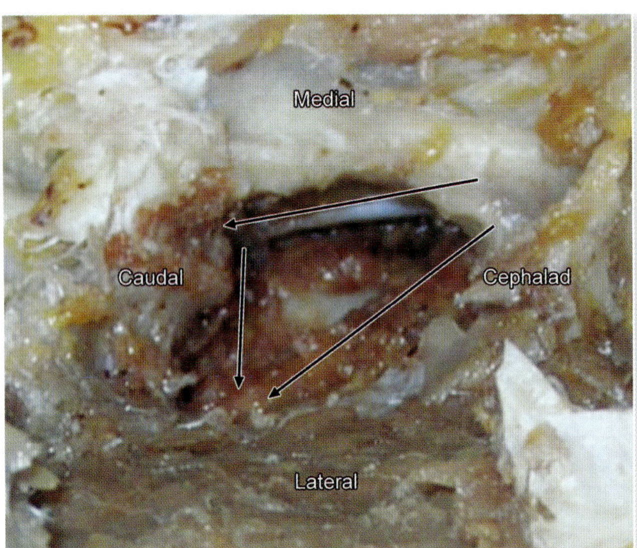

Figure 1: Kambin's triangle

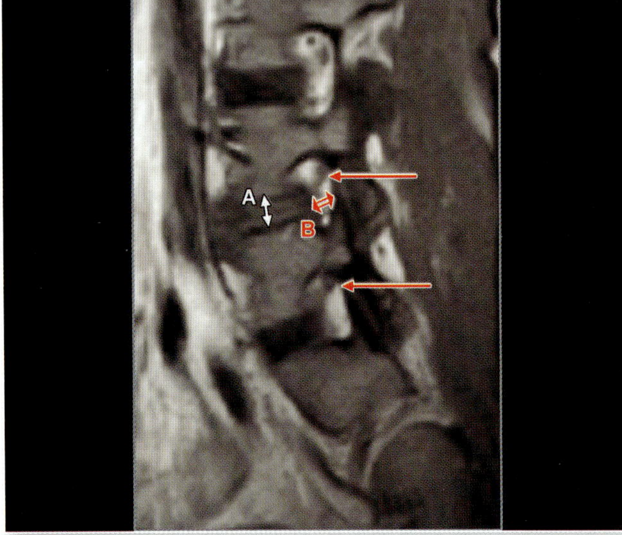

Figure 2: Sagittal MRI picture at the level of the foramen, line A measuring disk height, line B showing anteroposterior foraminal dimension, red arrrows showing location of the exiting nerve root in the superior half of the intervertebral foramen

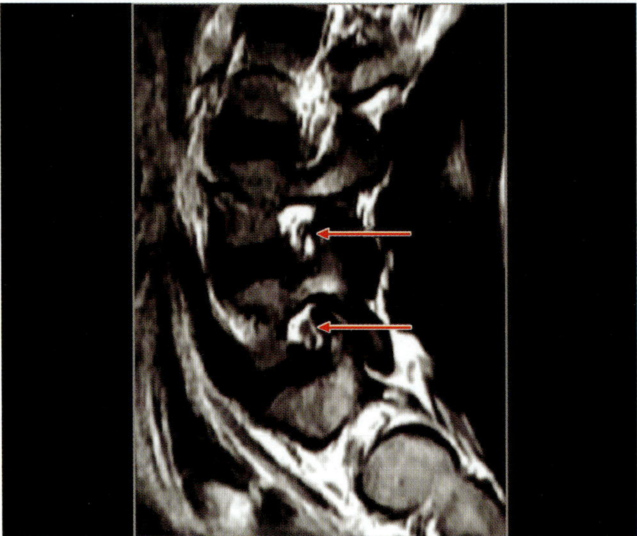

Figure 3: Inferiorly located exiting nerve roots in the intervertebral foramen (red arrows) thus rendering this patient not suitable for transforaminal endoscopy

EQUIPMENT

Transforaminal endoscopic diskectomy is usually done with a working channel endoscope. By working channel endoscope we mean that the same port is used for visualizing and use of hand instruments. The endoscope has an in built sleeve through which the working hand instruments can be introduced **(Figure 4)**. With the working channel endoscope, this surgery is done under a coaxial vision. The optics of working channel endoscope are usually between 20–30° looking upwards. This also means that you need some flexible instruments that can reach the areas that the endoscope can see but the coaxial line of work does not allow straight instruments to work adequately. One such important instrument is the flexible bipolar tip probe **(Figure 5)** that can be used for hemostasis as well as shrinking and cutting the annulus fibrosus. **Figure 6** shows the set of instruments used to create the transforaminal access starting with the 16 G needle, 1 mm guidewire, blunt obturator and various working cannulae and long endoscopic grasping forceps.

TECHNIQUE

Preoperative planning

Preoperative planning requires the surgeon to carefully read all the images (MRI, CT scan and X-rays) to correctly identify the location of the disk herniation, the adequacy of the foraminal size to permit introduction of the endoscope and anticipate any bony hindrance (e.g. high iliac crest, large

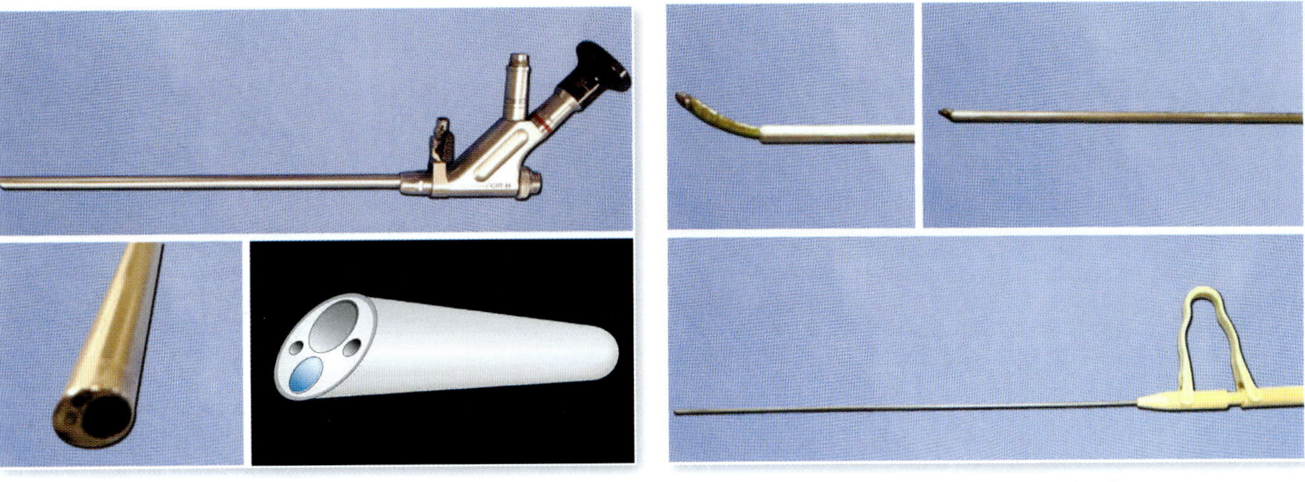

Figure 4: Working channel endoscope

Figure 5: Flexible bipolar tip

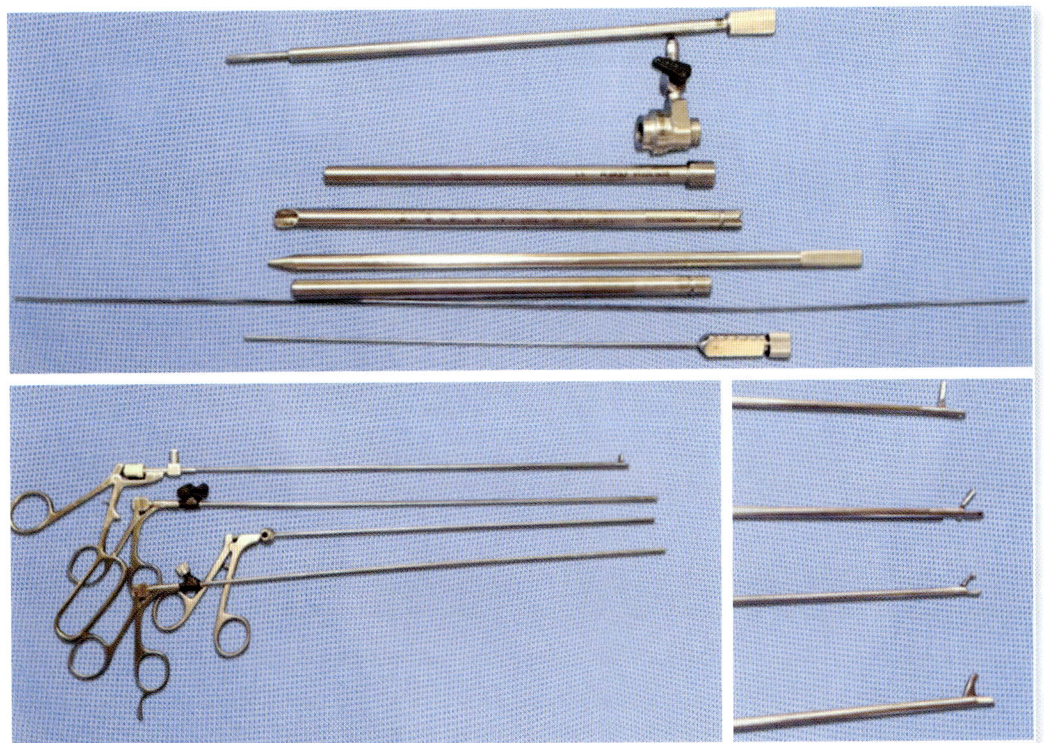

Figure 6: Instruments to create the foraminal access along with long endoscopic grasping forceps

transverse process or a hypertrophied facet joint) to the transforaminal access. The skin puncture point is calculated on special axial MRI or CT images that are taken as wide field of view (FOV) where we instruct the radiography technician to take axial images at the concerned disk level right upto the skin margin instead of the conventional axial images **(Figures 7 and 8)**.

Before doing the preoperative measurements, we need to understand the concepts of two very important points: one is the annular puncture point and the second is the skin puncture point. When we talk of the annular puncture point that means the tip of the needle when it is about to puncture the disk and how it is visualized in AP and lateral views of the intraoperaitve C-arm view. This varies according to the anatomy of the disk herniation. As a simple guide, we can take the nonmigrated herniations according to their location in the spine and how their location affects the annular puncture point in a particular situation. If the maximum volume of disk herniation is paracentral, the usual annular puncture point is taken as medial pedicle line on AP view when the needle tip is just posterior to the posterior vertebral border as seen on the lateral view on

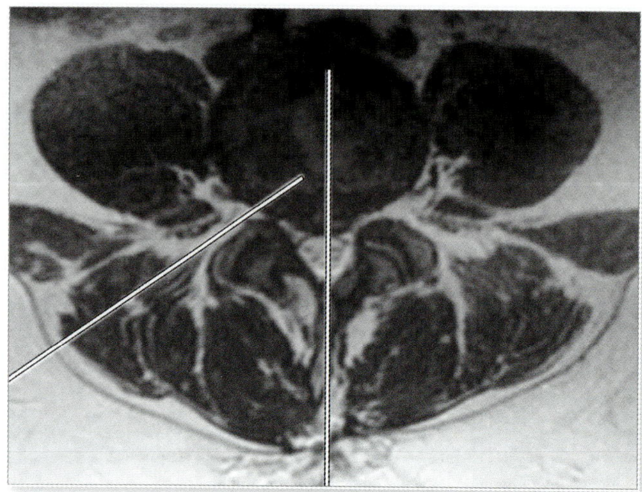

Figure 7: Inadequacy of a routine axial MRI image to measure the intended skin puncture point

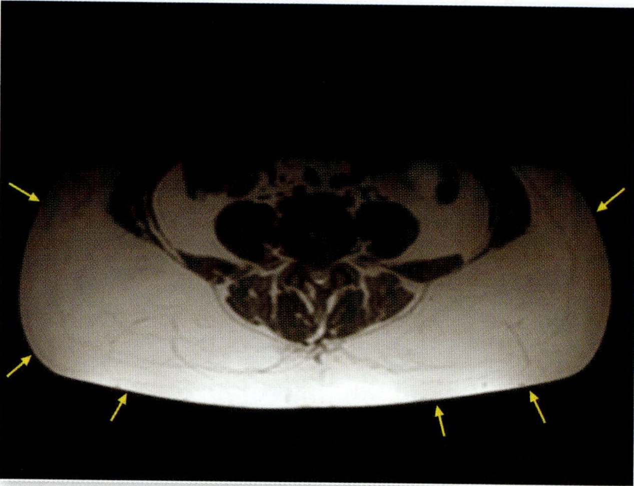

Figure 8: Special wide field of view axial image (yellow arrows) showing the margins of the skin on the axial MRI pictures

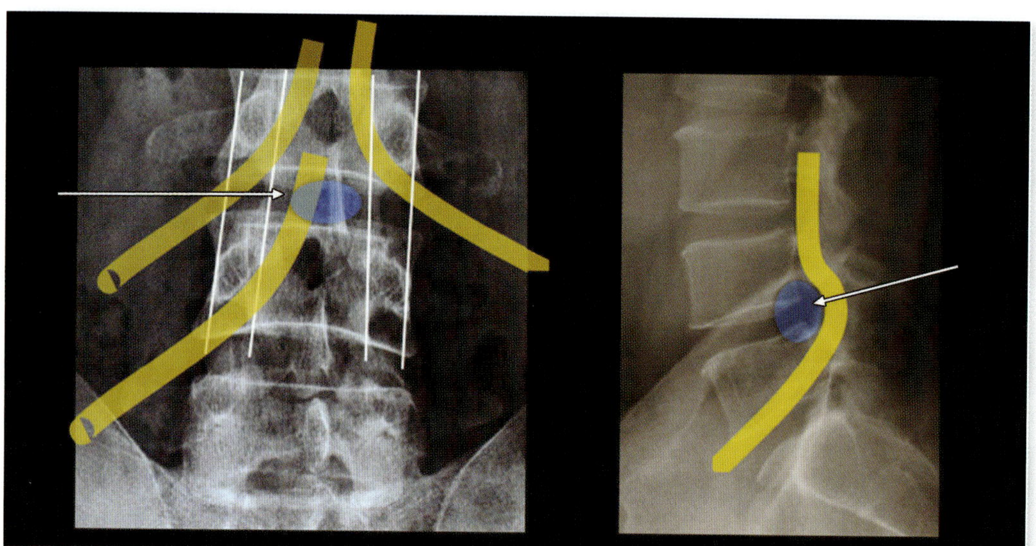

Figure 9: Intended annular puncture point for a standard paracentral disk (white arrow represents the annular puncture, blue circle is the disk herniation displacing the yellow nerve root)

C-arm view **(Figure 9)** (medial pedicle line is in reference to the inferior pedicle of the concerned disk eg. For a L4–5 disk herniation, L5 pedicle is taken as a reference for the medial pedicle border). For a central disk herniation, the annular puncture point lies just medial to the medial pedicle line **(Figure 10)**. For a foraminal disk herniation, the annular puncture point lies at the mid pedicle line **(Figure 11)** and for an extraforaminal disk herniation, the annular puncture point lies at the lateral pedicle line **(Figure 12)**.

Once the annular puncture point is decided, one can calculate the skin entry point for that particular herniation. On the axial MRI section with a wide field of view at the level of the disk, we draw a tangential line from the intended annular puncture point grazing the undersurface of the facet joint right up to the skin surface (line A, **Figure 13**). On the same axial view, we draw a line from the center of the disk bisecting the spinous process up to the posterior skin surface in the midline (line B, **Figure 13**). Then a horizontal line is drawn from line b to line a where it cuts the posterolateral skin surface of the back. This is the distance from the midline that we use to start the skin puncture with the 16 G needle.

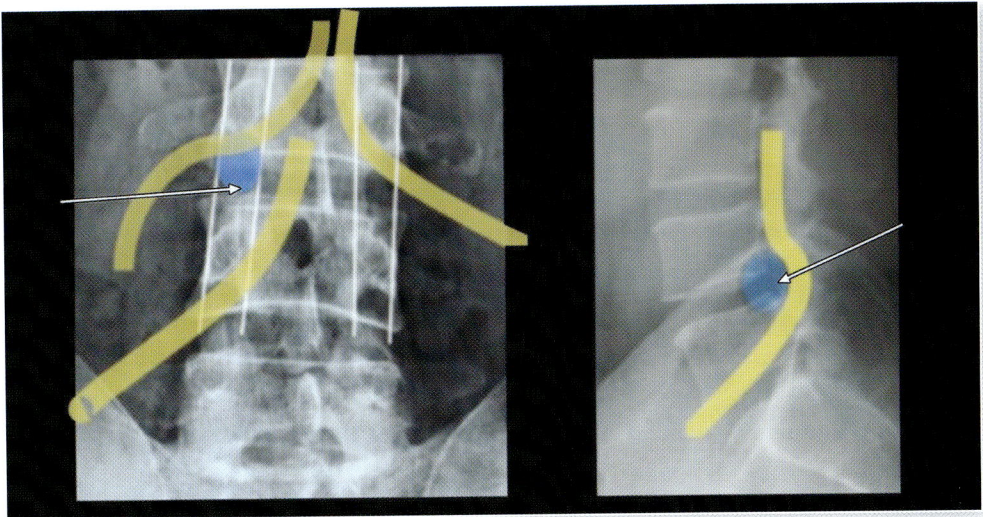

Figure 10: Annular puncture point for a central disk herniation

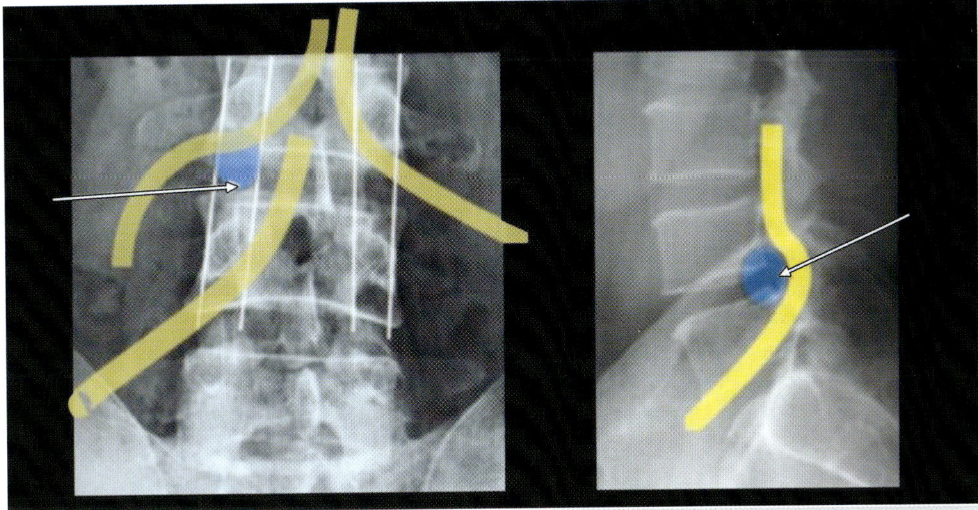

Figure 11: Annular puncture for a foraminal disk herniation

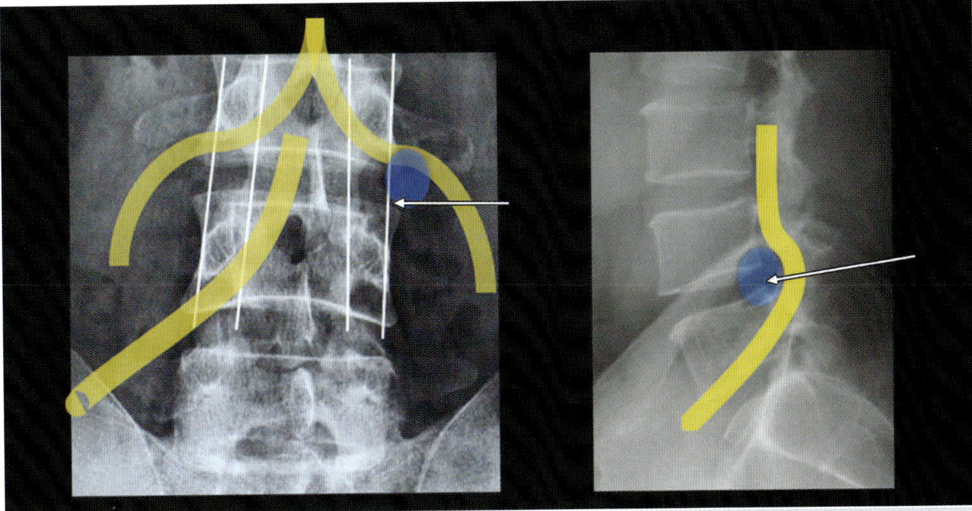

Figure 12: Annular puncture point for an extraforaminal disk herniation

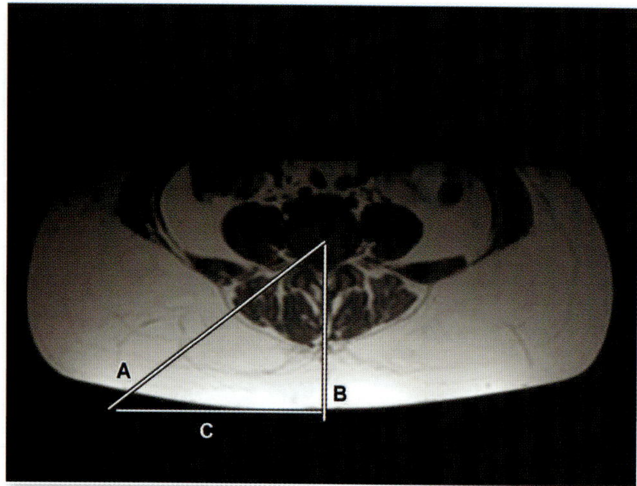

Figure 13: Showing how to measure the correct skin puncture point on MRI picture

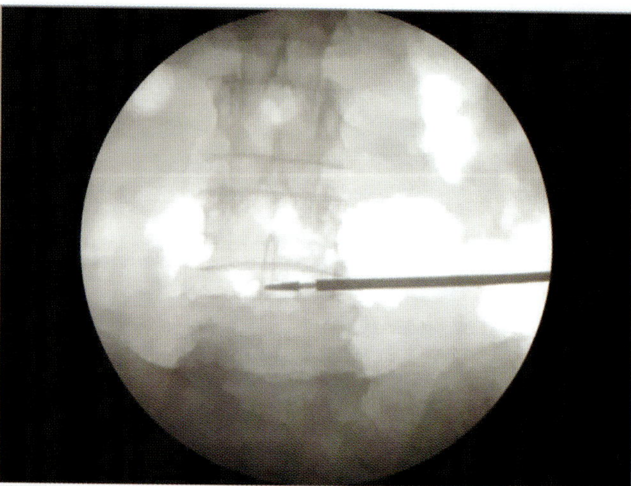

Figure 14: C-arm AP view showing parallel endplates and marking of the horizontal midline

Surgical Technique

The below-mentioned surgical technique applies for a standard paracentral disk herniation at L4–5.

I usually perform this operation under local anesthesia supplemented with intravenous sedation.

The patient is positioned prone on Jackson table or radiolucent bolsters. The image intensifier is brought in and the center and alignment of the disk is checked in true anteroposterior and lateral images **(Figures 14 and 15)**. Care is taken to visualize both the end plates of the disk as parallel. This compensates for the lumbar lordosis. Midline of the concerned disk level is marked in AP and lateral views on the skin and extended to bisect each other at the posterolateral skin surface. Skin markings are done **(Figure 16)** and the entry point from the midline is chosen as decided from preoperative measurement on MRI or CT images.

After prepping and draping the parts, 1% lidocaine is infiltrated along the surgical track starting at the correct skin puncture point right up to the facet joint. Then a 16 G long spinal needle is introduced at the skin entry point and advanced gradually towards the intervertebral foramen under frequent image intensifier guidance. The usual angle of approach is 25–30° to the flat surface of back. It is safer to first aim the needle tip to strike at the facet joint. Then withdraw it slightly, graze along the under surface of the facet and advance the needle into the foramen. At this point, the needle tip is checked in the AP and lateral views on image intensifier. The usual annular puncture point lies at the medial pedicular line, i.e. when the needle tip is seen to rest at the medial pedicular line on AP view, it should be just posterior to the posterior disk margin on the lateral view **(Figures 17 and 18)**. One can infiltrate a small amount of 0.5% lidocaine at this point to numb the annular nociceptors and make the procedure more comfortable for the patient. Now the needle is advanced

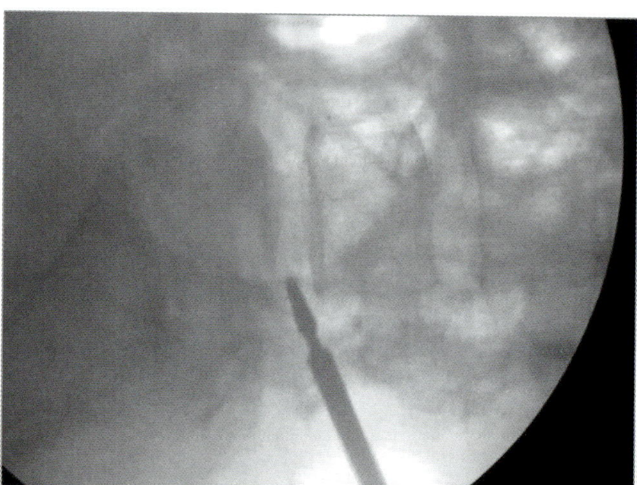

Figure 15: C-arm lateral view showing alignment of the concerned diskspace and the intended trajectory

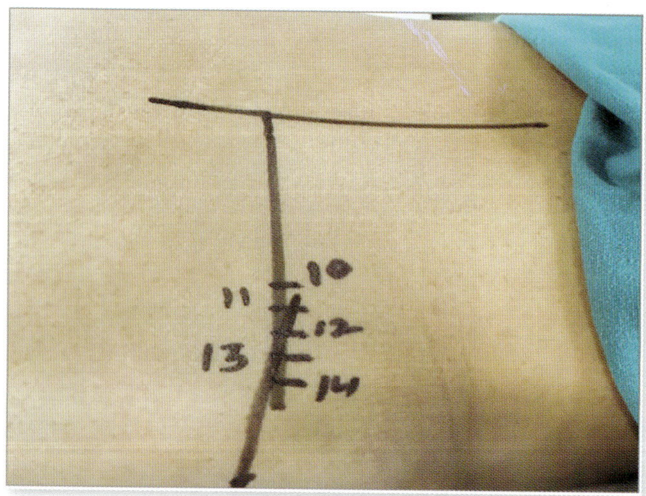

Figure 16: Skin markings

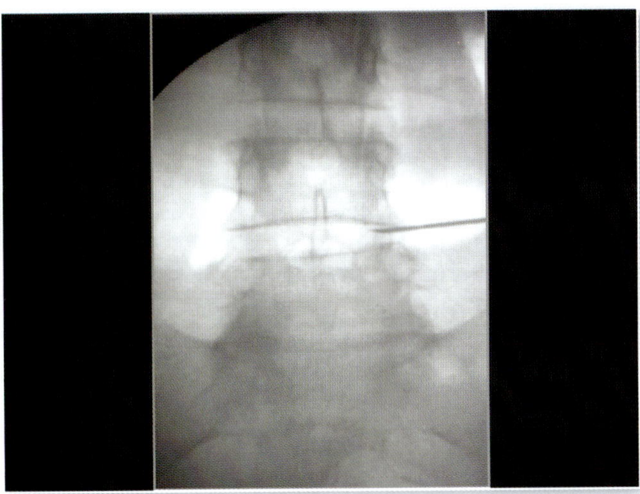

Figure 17: Needle tip at medial pedicle line in AP intraoperative C-arm view

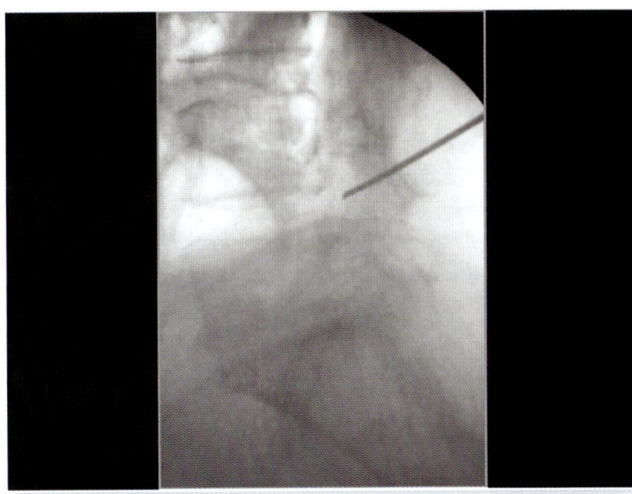

Figure 18: Needle tip just posterior to the posterior vertebral line (representing posterior margin of annulus) in the lateral C-arm view

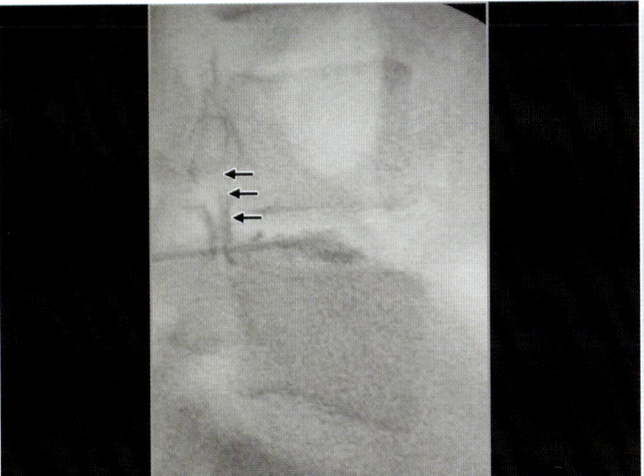

Figure 19: Intraoperative diskogram showing leakage of dye along the herniated Fragment

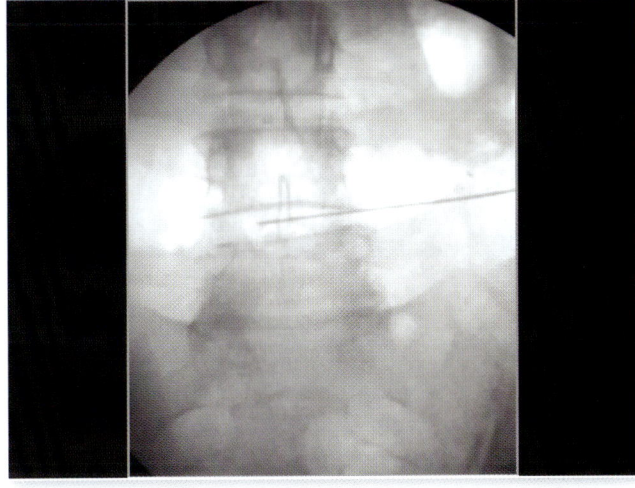

Figure 20: Insertion of 1mm guide wire through the 16 G needle

into the center of the diskspace and its position reconfirmed with image intensifier on both AP and lateral views. The stylet is removed and a diskogram is performed at this stage using a mixture of radiopaque dye (Omnipaque 300) and indigo carmine mixed in a ratio of 2:1. The dye can usually be seen leaking into the epidural space through the annular tear along the herniated fragment **(Figure 19)**. The blue colored indigo carmine helps selectively stain the nucleus pulposus blue for easy identification under endoscopic visualization. Now a 1 mm blunt guidewire is introduced through the 16 G needle and the needle is withdrawn **(Figure 20)**. A small stab incision is given over the skin and a blunt tipped obturator is threaded over the guidewire to dilate the track **(Figure 21)**. While introducing the dilator over the guidewire, it is imperative to firmly hold the guidewire and prevent it from advancing further through the diskspace and into the

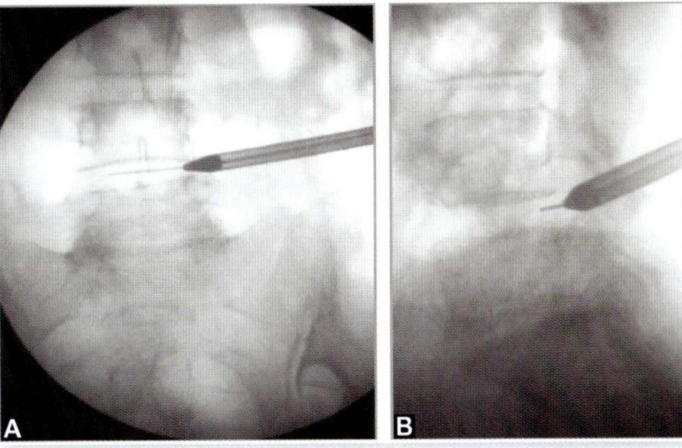

Figure 21: Insertion of blunt obturator over the guidewire being monitored constantly under (A) AP and (B) lateral C-arm views

abdominal cavity. After confirming the correct position of the obturator tip into the diskspace, the guide wire is withdrawn. An 8 mm bevelled tip working cannula is now introduced over the obturator. the working cannula is anchored on to the diskspace in such a way that half of the bevel is inside the disk and half is outside over the epidural space **(Figures 22 to 24)**. Once the working cannula is firmly anchored into the annulus, the blunt obturator is withdrawn and irrigation equipment is attached to the working cannula. I usually use a constant cold saline irrigation to flush out the debris and improve endoscopic visualization. The irrigation fluid also helps to keep the endoscopic view clear of any small bleeding points by flushing out the minor bleeding. Now a 4.1 mm, 25° working channel endoscope is introduced through the working cannula. The first look of the inside of the disk is a hyperemic vascular wooly structure because of the procedure related bleeding **(Figure 25)**. One can use the flexible tip bipolar coagulating probe (Trigger flex by Elliquence, USA) to coagulate the bleeding points. Now we orient ourselves to the coordinates. Towards 12 O'clock is the posterior disk and epidural space, 6 O'clock is anterior disk tissue, 3 and 9 O' clock are either cephalad or caudal depending upon the side to be operated. After achieving haemostasis, we search for the tear in the posterior annulus through which the nucleus pulposus has herniated and release a cuff of the annular tissue around the herniated fragment **(Figure 26)**. This can be done by using either the trigger flex probe, annular cutter or a side firing Ho:YAG laser under endoscopic visualization. Once the fragment is sufficiently mobilized it is removed by using the endoscopic grasping forceps. If the fragment is large and cannot be removed through the 4.1 mm working channel of the endoscope, one can grasp the fragment

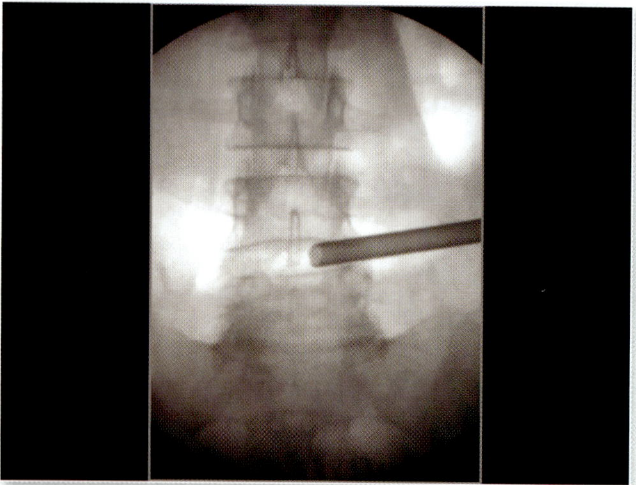

Figure 22: Final position of beveled cannula anchored at the disk in AP view

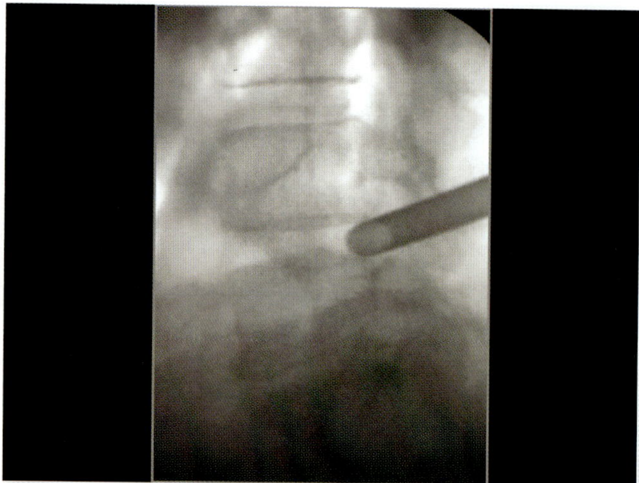

Figure 23: Showing the final position of beveled cannula anchored at the posterior annulus as seen in lateral view

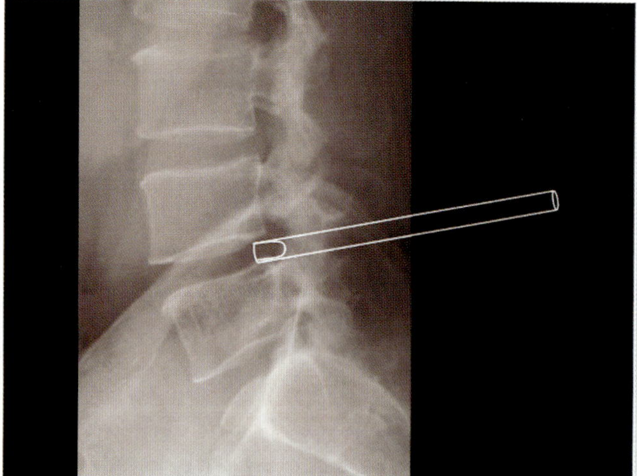

Figure 24: Animated version of the beveled cannula demonstrating "half and half" technique where a part of the cannula is anchored into the posterior annulus and a part is kept into the epidural space

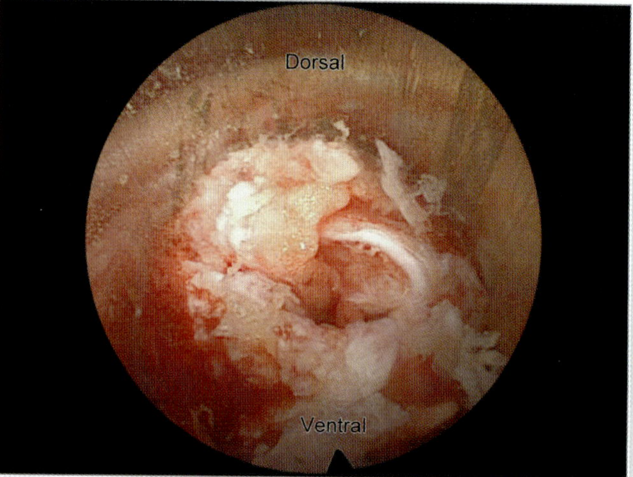

Figure 25: First view of the disk under endoscope showing hyperemic picture with bleeding points

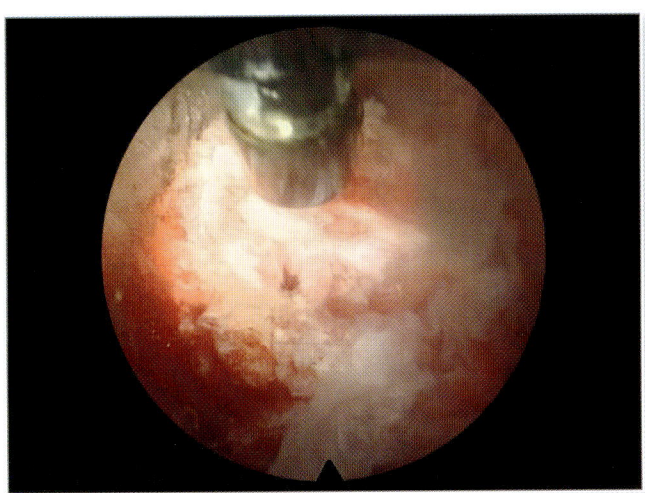

Figure 26: Use of flexible bipolar cautery for hemostasis and release of annular cuff to mobilize the herniated fragment

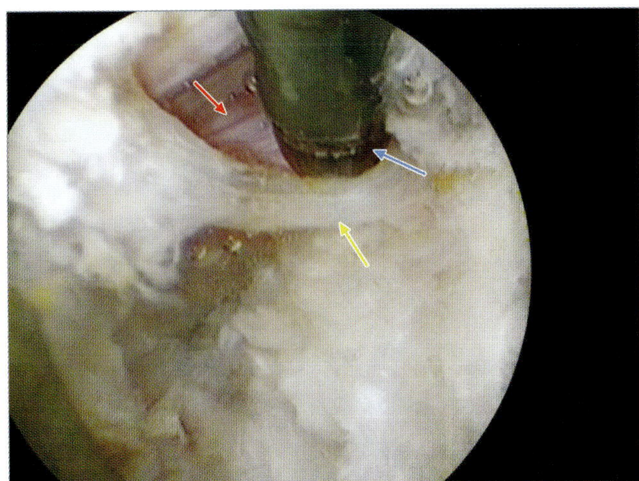

Figure 27: Decompressed traversing nerve root (red arrow) running from 1 o'clock to 10 o'clock position, blue arrow is tip of flexible bipolar probe, yellow arrow shows the posterior longitudinal ligament

and take it out along with the endoscope. After removing the fragment, one can again see a slight bleeding from the epidural veins that gets controlled with constant irrigation and bipolar coagulation. After removal of the fragment, one can see the free movement of the annular flaps or upon partial withdrawal of the working cannula, even the pulsatile thecal sac and traversing nerve root can be visualized **(Figure 27)**. This usually confirms the adequacy of the decompression and marks the end point of the surgery. One has to understand one basic difference with this approach as compared to the conventional posterior disk surgeries. In the conventional posterior surgeries, we see the thecal sac and nerve root first, retract them on the side and then visualize and remove the herniated disk fragments. Then we check for the adequacy of decompression by having a visual and tactile feel under the decompressed nerve root. However, in transforaminal Endoscopy, we are working anterior to the nerve root. So the first thing that we will see is the base of the herniation. Once the herniated disk is removed from its anterior location to the nerve root, visualization of the nerve root/thecal sac is usually the end point because that means that we have removed whatever disk fragments were lying anterior to the nerve root and the neural elements will become clearly visible only after a good decompression is achieved.

The endoscope along with working cannula is withdrawn and wound is closed with a single suture and dressed.

Postoperatively, the patient can be mobilized within a few hours after the surgery and diskharged either the same or the next day.

RISKS AND COMPLICATIONS

As the surgery is done in an awake state, the risk of neurological injury is minimal because of the active patient response. However, due to increased pressures in the intervertebral foramen due to the presence of working instruments that can cause pressure on the dorsal root ganglion, there is a possibility of dysesthesias. Postoperative hematoma formation is another possible complication. Dural tears are very unlikely but still can occur if the surgeon tries to aggressively work in the epidural space. If the irrigation pressure is increased or the surgery gets prolonged beyond an hour, there is a chance for the patient to develop neck pain and headache due to increased epidural pressure. Stray cases of seizure due to inadvertent injection of radiopaque dye into the thecal sac have also been reported. There is a risk of the guidewire or needle going through the anterior annulus and injuring the abdominal contents if one fails to monitor the advancement of these instruments under constant fluoroscopy.

TIPS AND PEARLS

Choosing a correct skin entry point, as well as annular puncture with needle tip are the key to successful transforaminal endoscopic diskectomy.

Frequent checking of the advancing instruments under image intensifier can go a long way in avoiding unnecessary complications.

Good hemostasis before attempting to remove any disk fragments is another trick to conduct a smooth endoscopic disk surgery.

For foraminal/extraforaminal disk herniations, the cannula trajectory is relatively verticle and we may not need to enter into the diskspace. Instead the round working cannula can be docked on the surface of the disk herniation and than can be gently wanded towards the herniated fragment.

RESULTS

Various series on transforaminal endoscopic diskectomy have reported a 90% and above successful outcome with this technique. Our series of first 190 patients with a minimum follow-up of 2 years have shown an excellent or good outcome in 92% of patients as judged by Oswestry Disability Index and modified Macnab criteria. 3 patients (1.5%) had a residual disk after the surgery that required conversion to open/microdiskectomy. 4 (2.1%) patients had a recurrence at the operated level (two required resurgery and the other two improved with conservative treatment) and 4 patients experienced dysesthesia that resolved within 6–12 weeks.

CASE STUDIES

Case 1: Paracentral herniation at L4–5 (Figures 28 and 29)

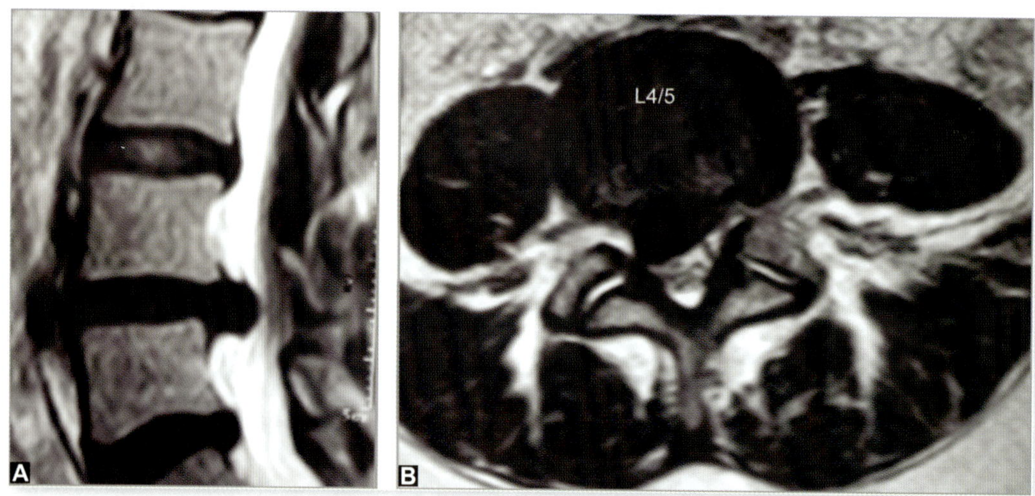

Figure 28: A large right paracentral disk herniation at L4–5

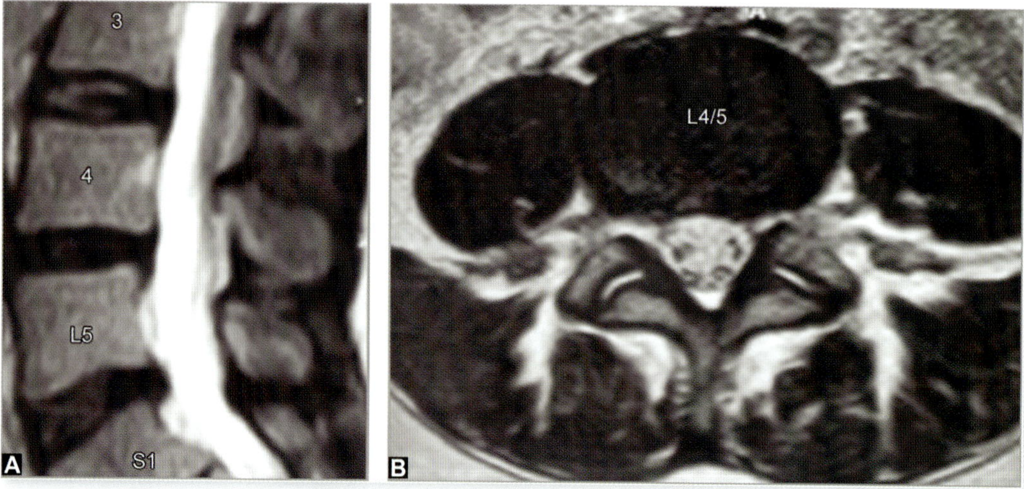

Figure 29: A 3-month follow-up MRI of the same patient as in Figure 23, complete decompression and no evidence of any scarring postsurgery

Case 2: Upmigrated and sequesterd L4–5 herniation lying besides the L4 pedicle (Figure 30)

Here the round working cannula is first docked on the surface of the disk at the level of the disk within the foramen **(Figure 31)** and then it is gently rotated and wanded superiorly towards the herniated fragment in the epidural space **(Figures 32 and 33)**.

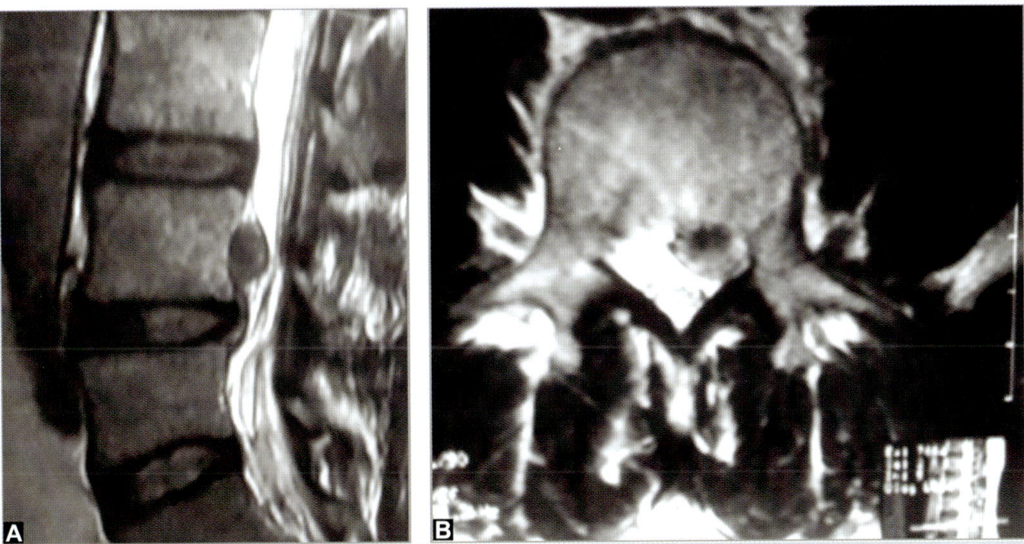

Figure 30: Sequestered and upmigrated L4–5 disk herniation and the fragment lying besides the left L4 pedicle

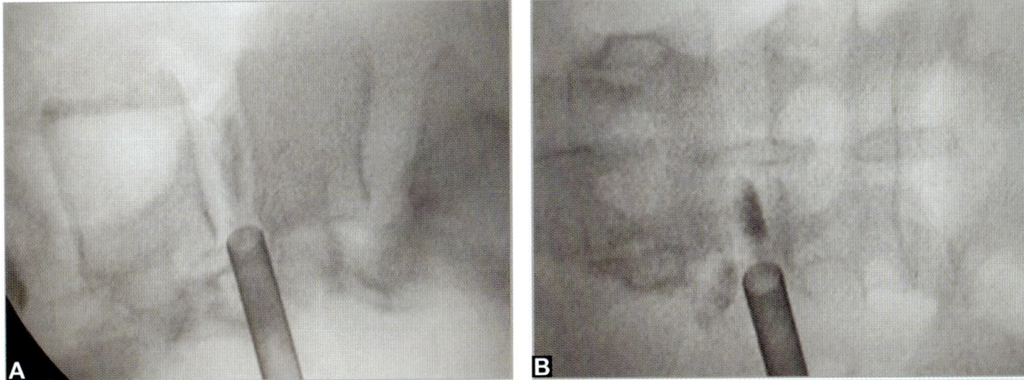

Figure 31: Intraoperative C-arm view showing the round working cannula first docked at the posterior surface of the disk within the confines of the intervertebral foramen (mid-pedicular line)

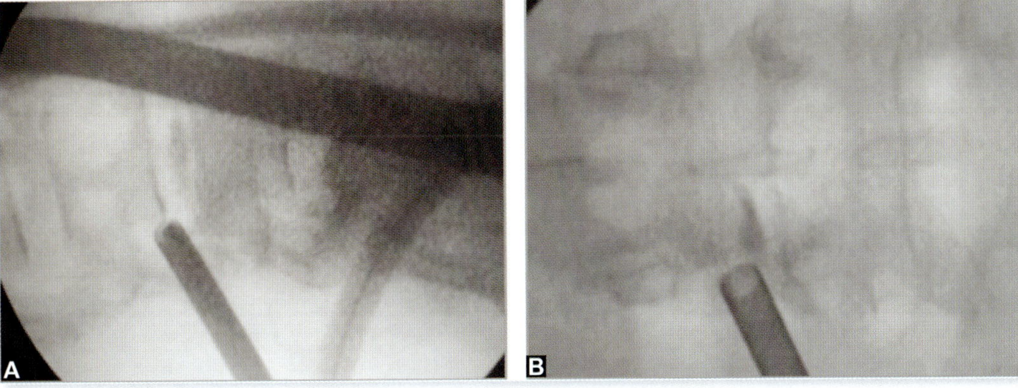

Figure 32: Round working cannula gently wanded towards the superiorly migrated disk fragment in the epidural space

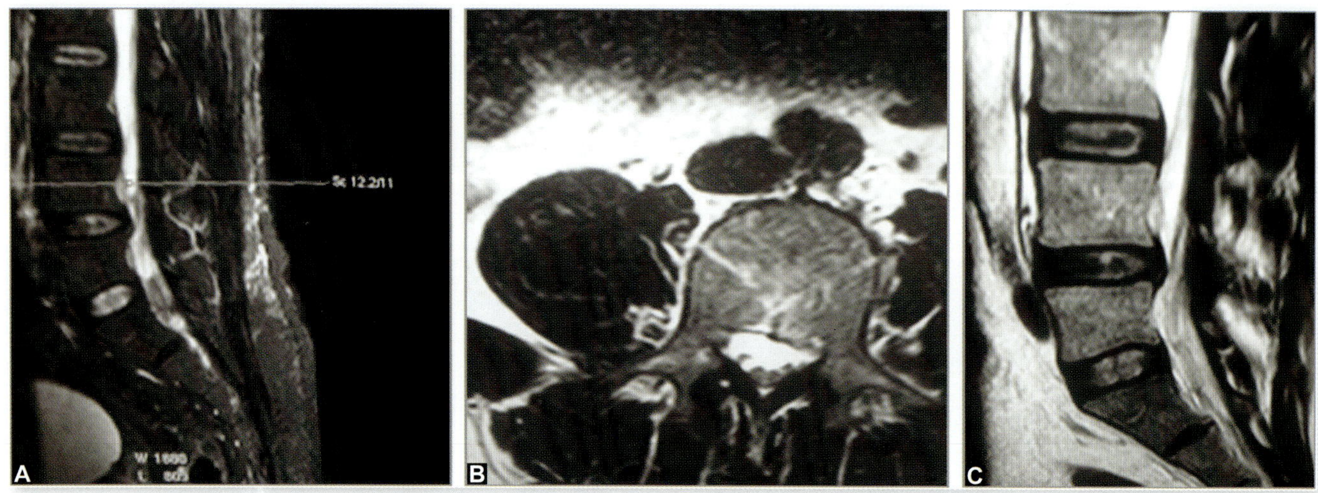

Figure 33: A next day postoperative MRI of the same patient as in Figyre 30 with complete removal of the sequestered fragement

Case 3: A downmigrated L4–5 disk herniation that reached up to the pedicle of L5 vertebra.

Such cases pose a difficulty in access due to the superior surface of pedicle hindering an adequate access to the down migrated fragment that lies medial to the pedicle. With the needle and cannula angled slightly cephalo-caudal, one can safely remove these herniations. However for severe down-migrated herniations, one may need to use alternative approach or foramen widening methods like foraminoplasty to successfully perform a transforaminal endoscopic surgery **(Figures 34 and 35)**.

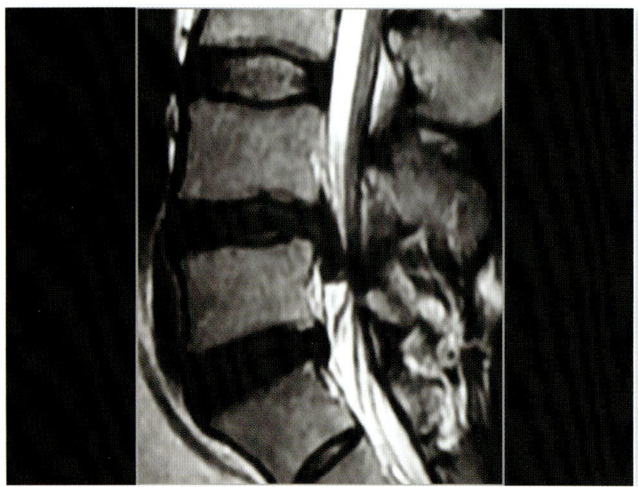

Figure 34: A downmigrated L4–5 disk herniation

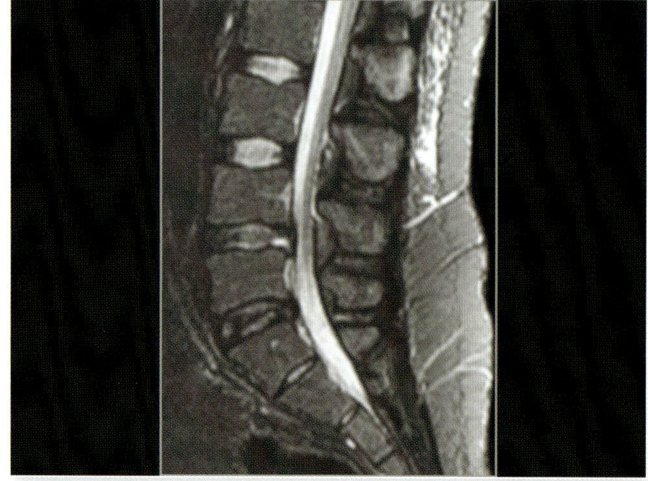

Figure 35: A postoperative MRI of the same patient with removal of the downmigrated fragment

BIBLIOGRAPHY

1. Ahn Y, Lee SH, Park WM, Lee HY, Shin SW, et al. Percutaneous endoscopic lumbar diskectomy for recurrent disk herniation: surgical technique, outcome, and prognostic factors of 43 consecutive cases. Spine. 2004;29:E326-32.
2. Bhanot A. Percutaneous Transforaminal Lumbar Endoscopic Diskectomy. In: Garg B, Malhotra R ed Mastering Orthopedic Techniques Spine Surgery, Jaypee. 2012:47-55.
3. Choi G, Lee SH, Bhanot A, Raiturker PP, Chae YS. Percutaneous endoscopic diskectomy for extraforaminal lumbar disk herniations: extraforaminal targeted fragmentectomy technique using working channel endoscope. Spine. 2007; 32:E93-9.
4. Hoogland T, van den Brekel-Dijkstra K, Schubert M, Miklitz B. Endoscopic Transforaminal Diskectomy for Recurrent, Lumbar Disk Herniation. A Prospective, Cohort Evaluation of 262 Consecutive Cases. Spine. 2008;33(9):973-8.

5. Jang JS, An SH, Lee SH. Transforaminal percutaneous endoscopic diskectomy in the treatment of foraminal and extraforaminal lumbar disk herniations. J Spinal Disord Tech. 2006;19:338-43.
6. Kambin P. NASS. Arthroscopic microdiskectomy. Spine J. 2003;3(3 Suppl):60S-4.
7. Kun Wong, Xin Hong, Bao-YI Zhou, Jun-Ping Bao, et al. Evaluation of Transforaminal Endoscopic Lumbar Diskectomy in the treatment of Lumbar Disk Herniation, International Orthopaedics. 2015;39(8):1599-1604.
8. Lee S, Kim SK, Lee SH, Kim WJ, Choi WC, Choi G, et al. Percutaneous endoscopic lumbar diskectomy for migrated disk herniation : classification of disk migration and surgical approaches. Eur Spine J. 2007;16:431-7.
9. Lee SH, Kang BU, Ahn Y, Choi G, Choi YG, Ahn KU, et al. Operative failure of percutaneous endoscopic lumbar diskectomy: a radiologic analysis of 55 Cases. Spine. 2006;31:E285-90.
10. Ruetten S, Komp M, Godolias G. An extreme lateral access for the surgery of lumbar disk herniations inside the spinal canal using the full-endoscopic uniportal transforaminal approach-technique and prospective results of 463 patients. Spine. 2005;30:2570-8.
11. Sanusi T, Davis J, Nicassio N, Malik I. Endoscopic lumbar diskectomy under local anesthesia may be an alternative to microdiskectomy: A single centre's experience using the far lateral approach, Clinical Neurology and Neurosurgery, 2015; 139:324-7.
12. Tsou PM, Yeung AT. Transforaminal endoscopic decompression for radiculopathy secondary to intracanal noncontained lumbar disk herniations: outcome and technique. The Spine Journal. 2002; 2(1):41-8.
13. Yeung AT, Tsou PM. Posterolateral endoscopic excision for lumbar disk herniation-surgical technique, outcome, and complications in 307 consecutive cases. Spine. 2002;27(7): 722-31.

15

CHAPTER

Lumbar Canal Stenosis Treated by Transforaminal Endoscopic Access

Satishchandra Gore

ABSTRACT

The endoscopic access in the treatment of lumbar canal stenosis has developed as a boon to the spine surgeons. It is the least invasive technique and helps in early mobilization and faster rehabilitation, especially in older population.This chapter deals with the technique of lumbar decompression using endoscopic access.

INDICATIONS AND CONTRAINDICATIONS FOR TRANSFORAMINAL ENDOSCOPIC INTERVENTION IN STENOSIS

The traditional candidate for surgery is a patient with severe bony or soft tissue compression of DRG or nerve root, severe leg symptoms, moderate or no neurological deficit and, except for patients with degenerative spondylolisthesis, with little or no back pain.[1] There may be a long history of low back pain but the leg symptoms lead to presentation. The symptoms are insidious, presenting in the sixth or seventh decade. The course of spinal stenosis is chronic and benign, but long-term is slow deterioration.

The patient with central canal stenosis has bilateral leg symptoms vague and often described as heaviness, soreness or weakness. The neurogenic claudication presents as numbness, weakness or discomfort in the legs; with walking or prolonged standing and is relieved by sitting or rest. The patients are able to walk further when leaning or walking uphill because spinal flexion increases the space available for the cauda equina and unfolds the ligamentum flavum. The pain-free walking distance is variable.

Patients with lateral recess stenosis present with unilateral radicular symptoms of leg pain along with numbness, paresthesia or burning that may be in a dermatomal distribution. Pain radiates from the buttock to the posterior thigh and lateral calf because most compression occurs at L4–L5. If there is a higher lumbar lesion then anterior thigh pain will be present. The symptoms may come by walking. Many times symptoms start on one side and then present on other. Cauda equina syndrome or major neurological deficits are very rare in the presence of canal stenosis.[2]

PATIENT SELECTION

Choosing a patient for intervention may be facilitated by using this questionnaire:[3] SSHQ

The 10 items on the SSHQ for diagnosis of lumbar spinal stenosis (LSS) require answers of either "yes" or "no". This contains some words patients use to describe when they have symptomatic lumbar spinal stenosis. This is given to patients with instructions "read the list, think of yourself. When you read a sentence that describes you, please circle "yes". If the sentence does not describe you, please circle "no". We always do a preoperative USG to estimate post void residual urine volume "indicative of existing neurogenic bladder", which is very helpful.

1. Numbness and/or pain in the thighs down to the calves and shins. Yes No
2. Numbness and/or pain increase in intensity after walking for a while, but are relieved by taking a rest. Yes No
3. Standing for a while brings on numbness and/or pain in the thighs down to the calves and shins. Yes No
4. Numbness and/or pain are reduced by bending forward. Yes No
5. Numbness is present in both legs. Yes No
6. Numbness is present in the soles of both feet. Yes No
7. Numbness arises around the buttocks. Yes No
8. Numbness is present, but pain is absent. Yes No

9. A burning sensation arises around the buttocks. Yes No
10. Walking nearly causes urination. Yes No

Harris and Macnab described the importance of disk degeneration in the pathogenesis of stenosis.[4] Macnab highlighted the lateral recess beneath the posterior facet joint.[5] Verbiest identified neurogenic claudication as a result of spinal canal stenosis.[6] Lumbar spinal stenosis is narrowing of the central spinal canal, lateral recess or the neural foramen. The term indicates a pathological condition causing compression of neural and vascular structures **(Figure 1)**.[7]

The lumbar spinal canal consists of a central part, two lateral parts and a posterior part corresponding to the interlaminar angle. The central spinal canal is rounded and occupied by the thecal sac. Stenosis of the central portion is almost always associated with stenosis of the lateral corners of the spinal canal reverse may not be true. The nerve-root canal is the semitubular structure through which the nerve root runs from the thecal sac to the intervertebral foramen. The proximal part of the canal, also called the sub-articular or intervertebral portion, is limited anteriorly by the intervertebral disk and posterolaterally by the superior articular process and the facet joint. The distal part of the canal corresponds to the lateral recess, i.e. the lateral corner of the vertebral foramen at the level of the pedicle. The entrance and exit of the intervertebral foramen lie at the medial and lateral borders of the pedicle. Bony hypertrophy of the inferior articular process may cause narrowing of the central portion of the spinal canal. The superior articular process contributes to the deformation of lateral portions of the nerve-root canal. Hypertrophy of the superior articular process produces narrowing of the intervertebral foramen but additional disk protrusion or any degree or region of herniation will also affect the nerves in the thecal sac and foramen.

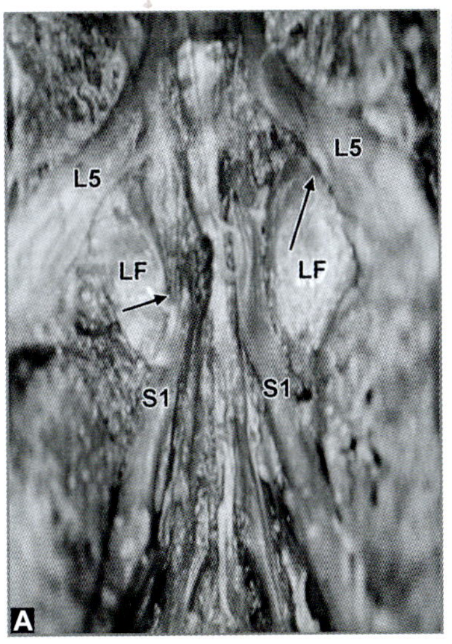

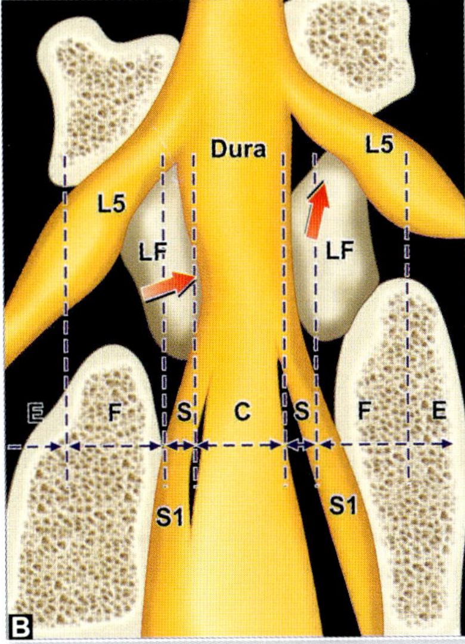

Figure 1: Coronal and sagittal view of stenotic canal for proper visualization of structures

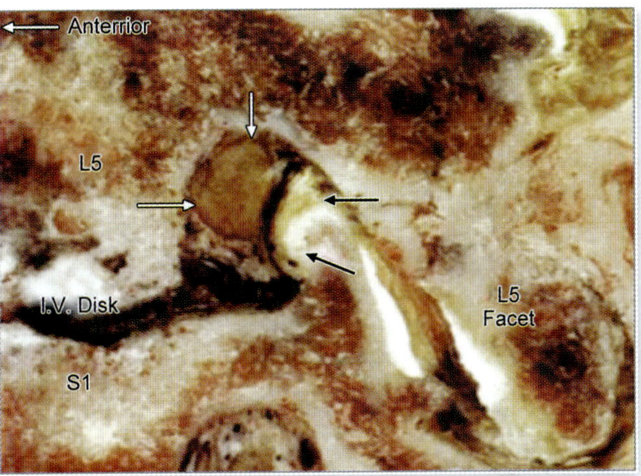

Figure 2: Shows SAP hitting nerve against pedicle or body of the vertebra

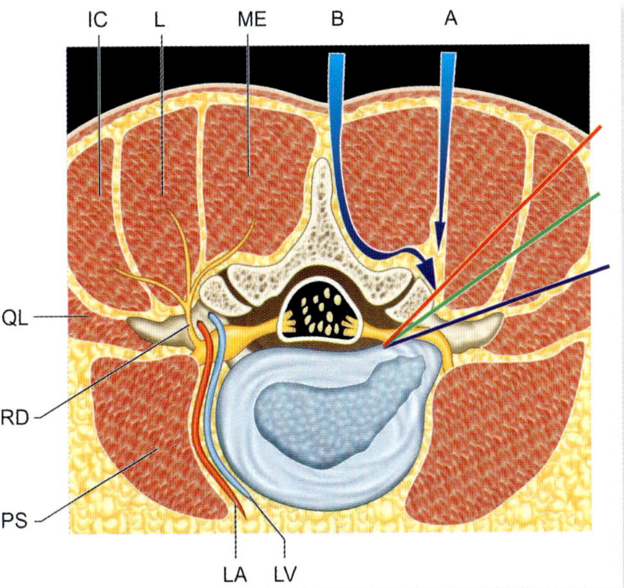

Figure 3: Changed trajectory used to access the subarticular zone or the body and under surface of the facet. Green is basic, red is for undercutting facet and blue is for flat access

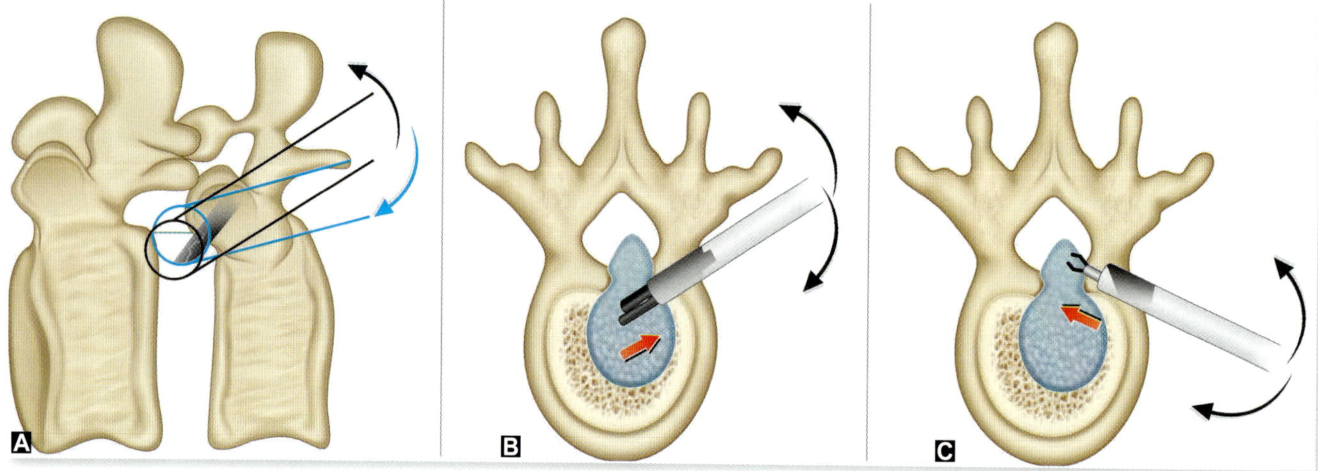

Figures 4A to C: Schematic diagrams indicate our access and maneuvers to get the decompression in stenotic canal. The newest technique is to target superior facet and walk the needle down the ventral bony facet, hugging the facet to avoid the exiting nerve and using the facet as a lever arm to perform foraminoplasty and/ or the use the facet as a fulcrum to change trajectories of endoscopic cannulas and instruments

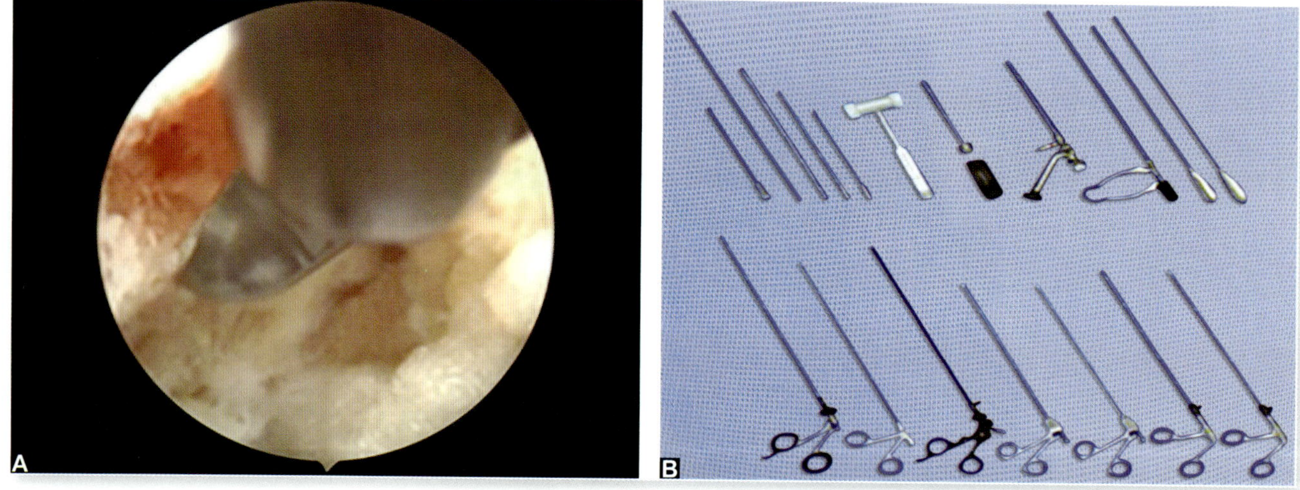

Figures 5A and B: (A) Curette working on SAP under vision, (B) Total GORE SYSTEM ® instruments set

Lee and Rauschning have described how progressive degenerative processes affect the dorsal root ganglion, the mini brain of the nerve, and how it is affected by the disk, facet, synovium of the facet, and osteophytes in the foramen.

The anatomical description of the spinal nerve root pathway, however, is not yet clinically definitive because surgeons do not see the intricacies of the microanatomy during traditional open or even microscopically guided decompression. Burton[8] divided the nerve-root canal into three portions separated by the pedicle in the cross-sectional plane, namely central, foraminal, and extraforaminal. This classification allows easy imaging diagnosis. Lee et al.[9] classified the lateral lumbar spinal canal into three zones: entrance, mild, and exit. This defined the anatomical boundaries of these zones and served as the basis for techniques of surgical decompression when clinically required.

Lumbar spinal foraminal stenosis is an important pathologic entity to recognize in patients with radicular symptoms. On MR imaging Wildermuth, et al.[10] introduced a partially quantitative classification system for grading lumbar spinal foraminal stenosis. They focused on the degree of epidural fat obliteration but did not consider direct nerve-root compression or deformity. Recently, Lee et al.[11] reported a new grading system for lumbar spinal foraminal stenosis. They considered the type of stenosis, the amount of fat obliteration, and the presence of nerve root compression. Yeung and Gore described the pathoanatomy of stenosis as seen from the foramen endoscopically. The absence of fat, vascular pulsation, scarred and fibrotic nerve roots and the axilla between the traversing and exiting nerves with hypertrophied soft tissue on its roof served as a “hidden zone” for unrecognized symptomatic stenosis **(Figure 10)**.[12]

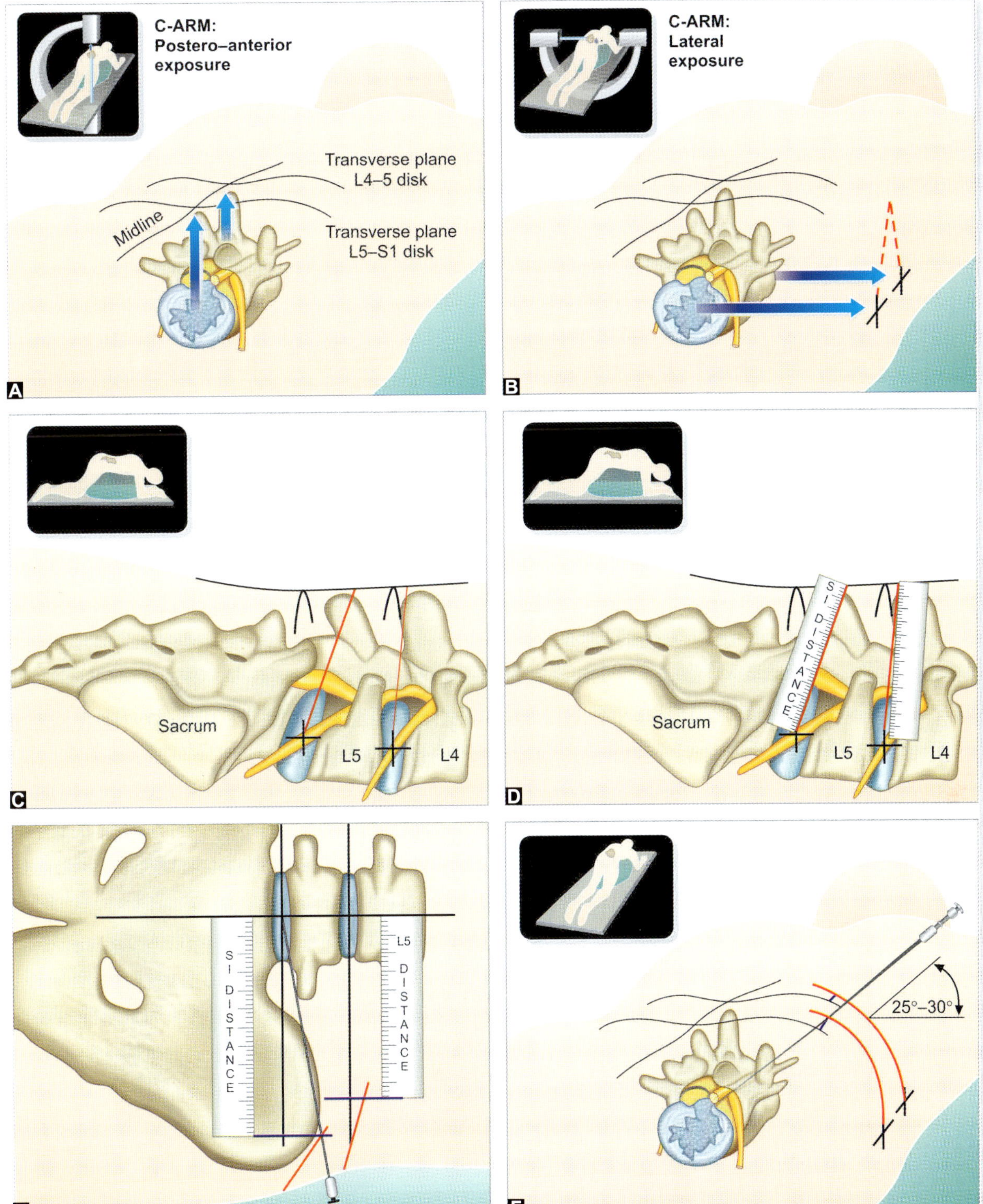

Figures 6A to F: (A) Drawing lines to detect midline and disk level as is seen; (B) Mark depth of the disk; (C) Mark disk inclination and plan for entry; (D) Measuring depth and inclination. For injections we measure up to center of disk typically it is 8 cm. Inclination is always towards the head due to lumbar lordosis; (E) Taking same distance from midline above the original disk line makes us identify point of entry of the needle; (F) Entry was initially at an angle of 25° subfacetal in the foramen thru paraspinal muscles. As techniques evolved, we started more lateral as much as 11 cm away from midline and at 20° but never at 0° because the peritoneal space and internal organs was at risk

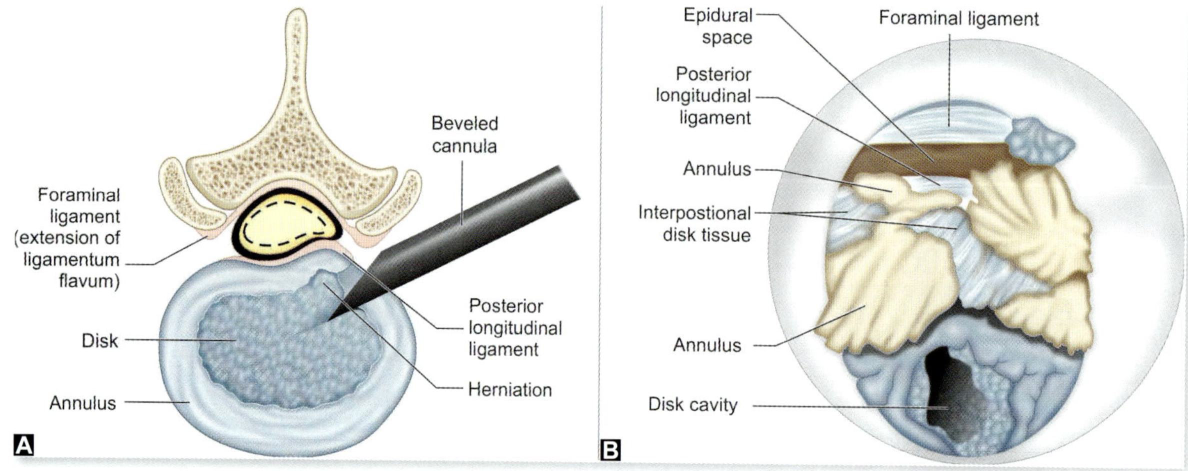

Figures 7A and B: Transforaminal endoscopic approach to the lumbar spine for diskectomy. We work more on the roof in cases of stenosis than on the floor

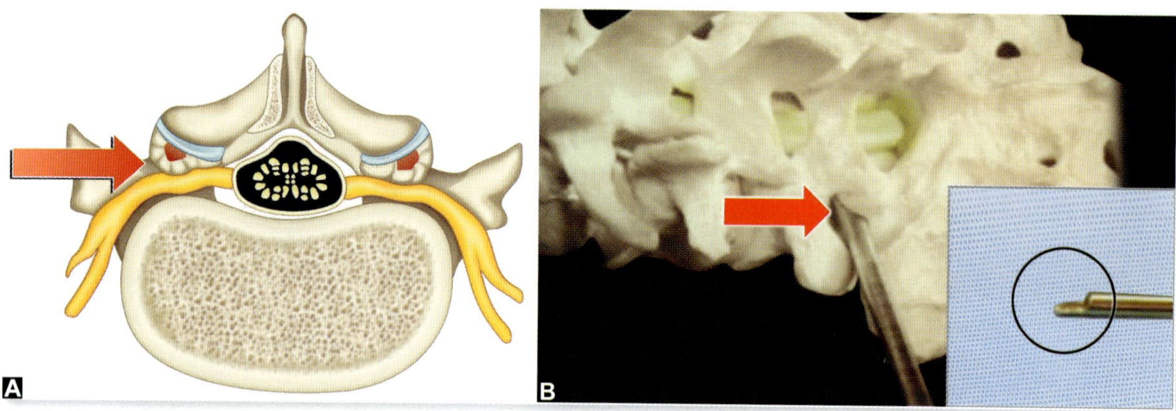

Figures 8A and B: Concept of foraminoplasty done under local anesthesia and is stitchless surgery

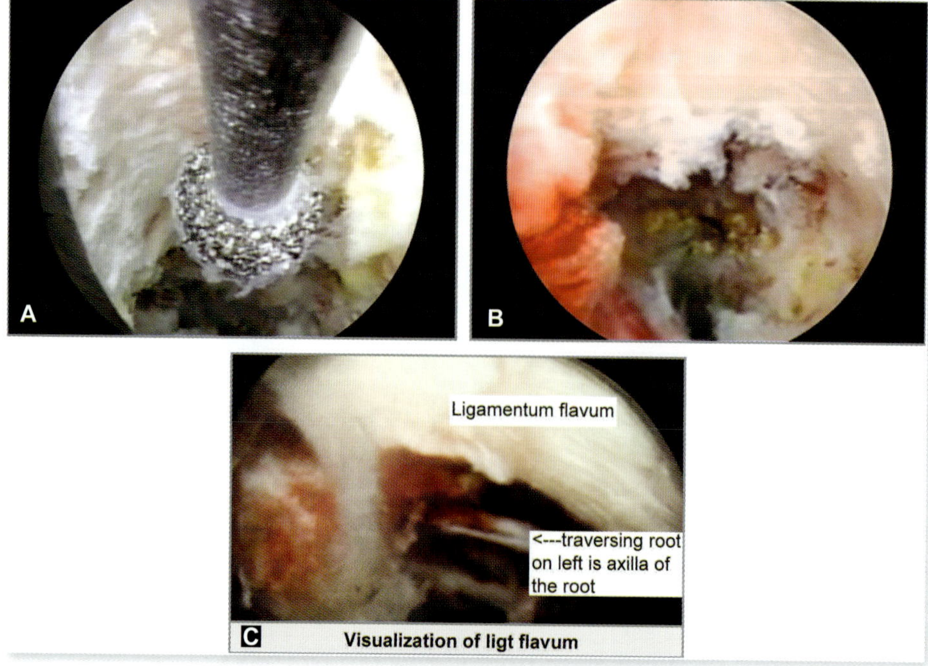

Figures 9A to C: Exposure of ligamentum flavum

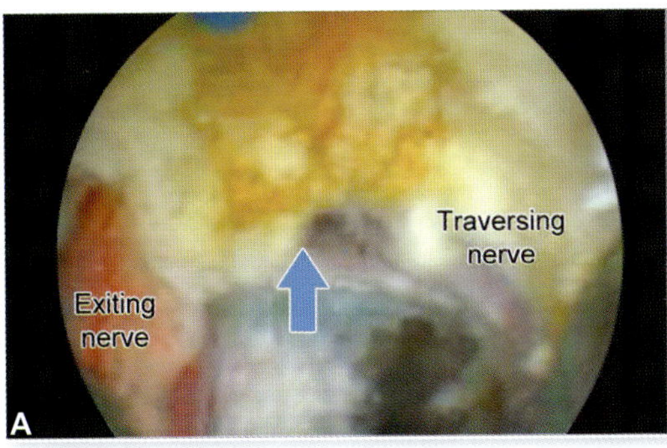

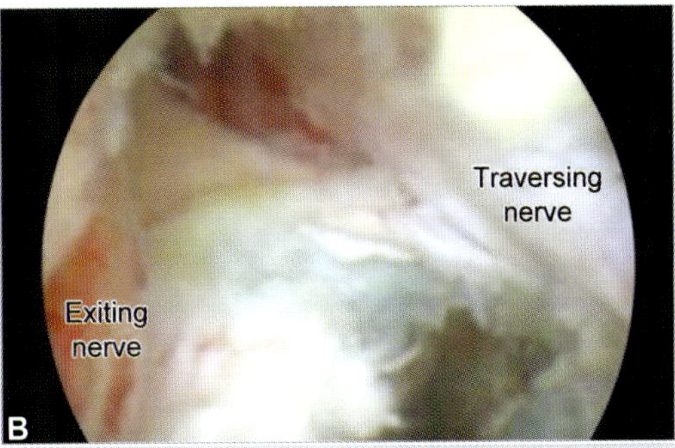

Figures 10A and B: (A) Superior foraminal ligament may tether nerve, when posible, resect; (B) Decompressed axilla confirmed

Stenosis or narrowing of the foramen can be in vertical plane due to disk degeneration and collapse. In that case we primarily look at cutting tip of the SAP. In case of narrowing in AP plane we undercut the facet. The facet at times is seen to be touching the annulus in AP plane. It is more like a curtain between foramen and contents of central canal and touches the annulus at the subarticular zone and lateral to traversing nerve. Stenosis also may be a part of residual untreated cause of pain in failed surgery **(Figures 2 to 9)**.

Stenosis usually also affects the exiting nerve. It is possible and important to avoid the exiting nerve in such a case if the stenosis is only affecting the medial and subarticular aspect of the canal and the disk protrusion, simple decompression is enough by simply making more room in the foramen. In cases, e.g. at L5–S1 with a horizontal disk trajectory and entry to disk is not below facet like normal but below isthmus and may be closer to the tip of SAP. Cutting the lateral facet will allow the excision of the medial capsule and ligamentum flavum that acts like a protective curtain between the dural sac and the foramen. This also forms the basis of "outside in" technique. Accessing the dorsal aspect of the canal is possible after cutting the facet's ventral undersurface. The enlarged portion of the foramen easily accommodates the cannula away from the DRG and nerve root.

In a hard and extreme stenosis, it is not only the size but consistency of the tissue. The annulus if too hard,collagenized or even ossified tools like simple graspers which are 3.5 mm, etc. are not very helpful and may break. Trephines, Kerrisons, burrs and specialized cutting instruments or laser are used to alter the stenotic foraminal zone.

Where we contemplate on jacking up the disk, we use fusion by OLIF and use expandable reamers in the disk. Percutaneous insertion of screws and use of cage is done under local anesthesia. In OLIF, since we are inserting the cage through foramen only a partial undercutting of facet may be adequate. There is no need for total facetectomy. This may eventually lead to stand alone intradiscal stabilization with improved intradiscal devices without traditional posterior instrumentation.

COMPLICATIONS

Exiting nerve root can be injured. To prevent it, a better image analysis may be considered. Study by Choi et al.[13] recommends measuring the distance from the exiting root to the facet [SAP] at the lower disk level according to a preoperative MRI scan. If the distance is narrow, an alternative surgical method may be considered. Shortest distance between facet and root at upper endplate level and lower endplate level is measured. If the distance is narrow alternatives may be considered **(Figure 11)**.

In endoscopic surgery through the foraminal approach, however, if a needle can be placed in the axilla between the exiting and traversing nerve and the patient receives good relief from the epidural, it is likely that a blunt obturator can be placed down the path of the needle and the exiting nerve simply gets retracted by the obturator, using the obturator to dilate the disk space enough to get a trephine or burr into the disk and foramen to enlarge the foramen in this very collapsed disk to get relief of stenotic symptoms.

POSTOPERATIVE CARE

Rehabilitation Program after Surgery

In a randomized controlled trial, the addition of a structured rehabilitation program (stabilization exercises, 30 minutes twice a week for 12 weeks) started 2 months after decompressive surgery was not found to be superior to the simple recommendation to "stay active". Best advice given to patient is to stay active once the pain subsides.[14]

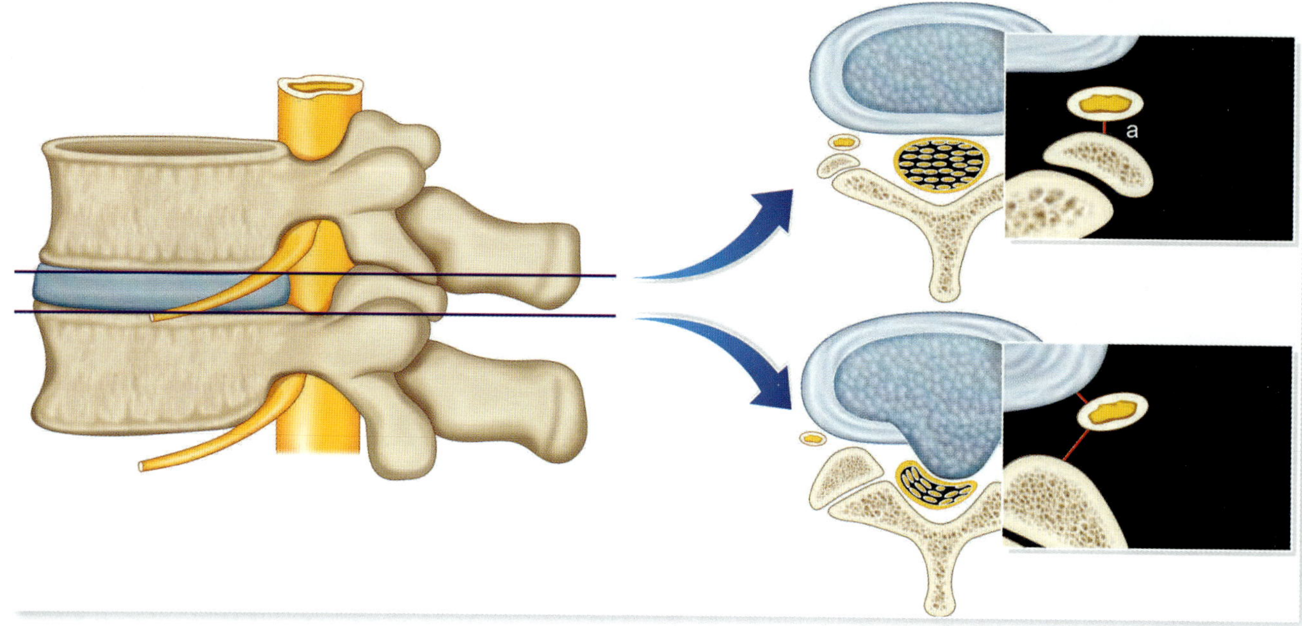

Figure 11: Transverse section highlighting distance between exiting root and facet at upper and lower endplate levels

OUTCOME

The review of the literature by Niggemeyer et al. shows that the least invasive surgical procedure can obtain the best results if the correct diagnosis is made and if the operation is carried out within the first years of the disease.[15]

The possible advantages of transforaminal endoscopic surgery are described in many articles. The procedure can be performed in an outpatient or day-surgery setting. Because of the small incision and minimal internal tissue damage, the rehabilitation period is shorter and scar tissue less. The procedure can be performed in awake patients under local anesthesia and conscious sedation, thereby avoiding the risk of general anesthesia, especially for elderly patients with comorbidities individuals. Transforaminal endoscopic surgery has a steep learning curve for some, but this translates into a long and shallow learning curve after the principles of foraminal decompression is mastered. That requires patience and experience, especially for those unfamiliar with percutaneous techniques.[15]

The literature seems to suggest that after transforaminal endoscopic surgery 69–83% of the patients experience a satisfactory outcome.[16] In our hands, the success rate is at least 85% with less than 1% permanent complication sequel. The success rate is guided by the patients' response to diagnostic and therapeutic injections performed by the surgeon and a SSHQ.

A comprehensive systematic literature review up to November 2009 to assess the effectiveness of transforaminal endoscopic surgery in patients with symptomatic lumbar stenosis was made. Two reviewers independently checked all retrieved titles and abstracts and relevant full text articles for inclusion criteria. Included articles were assessed for quality, and relevant data, including outcomes. The outcomes were extracted by two reviewers independently. No randomized controlled trials were identified in these seven observational studies. The studies were of poor methodological quality and heterogeneous regarding patient selection, indications, operation techniques, follow-up period and outcome measures. Overall, 69–83% reported the outcome as satisfactory and a complication rate of 0–8.3%. The reported reoperation rate varied from 0 to 20%. At present, there is no valid evidence from randomized controlled trials on the effectiveness of transforaminal endoscopic surgery for lumbar stenosis.[16] Randomized controlled trials comparing transforaminal endoscopic surgery with other surgical techniques are desired and needed, but in our Level 5 expert opinion and experience, the surgeon factor giving weight to surgeon experience and technical expertise, high levels results are attainable.

TIPS

1. It is possible to treat patients with severe medical comorbidities as transforaminal endoscopy can be done under local anesthesia.[17]
2. The role for shared decision making: Because patients with LSS may have potentially unrealistic expectations about the risks and benefits of surgery, it is recommended that decisions regarding surgery for LSS should be

based on a shared decision making approach. In terms of what matters most to the patient, e.g. pain relief, improved function, avoiding risk, etc. For patients with LSS, key knowledge would include the moderate benefit associated with surgery that may diminish over time, the likelihood of improvement with or without surgery, potential risk and costs.[18,19]

REFERENCES

1. Franco Postacchini Management of lumbar spinal stenosis instructional course lecture. European instructional course lectures. Vol. 2. 1995.
2. Rajgopal TS, Marshall RW. Focus on understanding and treating lumbar spinal stenosis. British Editorial Society of Bone and Joint Surgery. 2010;5-10.
3. Shin-ichi Konno, Shin-ichi Kikuchi, Yasuhisa Tanaka, Ken Yamazaki, You-ichi Shimada, Hiroshi Takei, et al. Central Open Access A diagnostic support tool for lumbar spinal stenosis: a self-administered, self-reported history questionnaire BMC Musculoskeletal Disorders. 2007; 8:102. doi:10.1186/1471-2474-8-102
4. Harris RI, Macnab I. Structural changes in the lumbar intervertebral disks; their relationship to low back pain and sciatica. J Bone Joint Surg [Br]. 1954;36-B:304-22.
5. Macnab I. Negative disk exploration: an analysis of the causes of nerve-root involvement in sixty-eight patients. J Bone Joint Surg [Am]. 1971;53-A:891-903.
6. Verbiest H. Fallacies of the present definition, nomenclature and classification of the stenoses of the vertebral canal. Spine. 1976;1:217-25.
7. Verbiest H. The significance and principles of computerized axial tomography in idiopathic developmental stenosis of the bony lumbar vertebral canal. Spine (Phila Pa 1976). 1979;4:369-78.
8. Cauthen JC (eds). Lumbar nerve entrapment: central, foraminal, and extra foraminal zones. Lumbar spine surgery: indications, techniques, failures and alternatives. Baltimore Williams and Wilkins. 1988;pp 202-7. Burton CV.
9. Lee CK, Rauschning W, Glenn W. Lateral lumbar spinal canal stenosis: classification, pathologic anatomy and surgical decompression. Spine. 1988;13:313-20.
10. Wildermuth S, Zanetti M, Duewell S, et al. Lumbar spine: quantitive and qualitative assessment of positional (upright flexion and extension) MR imaging and myelography. Radiology. 1998;207:391-8.
11. Lee S, Lee JW, Yeon JS, et al. A practical MRI grading system for lumbar foraminal stenosis. AJR Am J Roentgenol. 2010; 194:1095-8.
12. Yeung AT, Gore S. In-vivo endoscopic visualization of patho-anatomy in symptomatic degenerative conditions of the lumbar spine II: Intradiscal, Foraminal, and Central Canal Decompression. SurgTechnol Int. 2011;XXI:299-319.
13. Choi I. Jae-Ouk Ahn Seung-joon Lee, et al. Exiting root injury in transforaminal endoscopic diskectomy: preoperative image considerations for safety Eur Spine J. 2013;22:2481-7 Doi 10.1007/s00586-013-2849-7.
14. Mannion AF, Denzler R, Dvorak J, Müntener M, Grob D. A randomised controlled trial of postoperative rehabilitation after surgical decompression of the lumbar spine. European Spine J. 2007;16(8):1101-17. [PubMed: 17593405]
15. Niggemeyer O, Strauss JM, Schulitz KP. Comparison of surgical procedures for degenerative lumbar spinal stenosis: a meta-analysis of the literature from 1975 to 1995. Eur Spine J. 1997;6: 423-9.
16. Jorm Nellensteijn, Ronald Bartels, Maurits van Tulder, Raymond Ostelo, Wilco Peul, Barend van Royen. Transforaminal endoscopic surgery for lumbar stenosis: a systematic review. Eur Spine J. 2010;19:879-86. Doi 10.1007/s00586-009-1272-6.
17. Kitahama Y, Sairyo K, Dezawa A. Endoscopic transforaminal approach to decompress the lateral recess in an elderly patient with spinal canal stenosis, herniated nucleus pulposus and pulmonary comorbidities. Asian J Endosc Surg. 2013;6(2):130-3. doi: 10.1111/ases.12004.
18. Stephane Genevay, Steven J Atlas. Lumbar spinal stenosis Best Pract Res ClinRheumatol. 2010;24(2):253-65. doi:10.1016/j.berh.2009.11.001.
19. Percutaneous Endoscopic Spinal Surgery BOOK By Kai-Uwe Lewandrowski, Sang-Ho Lee, Menno Iprenburg published by JP Medical London.

16

CHAPTER

Percutaneous Endoscopic Lumbar Diskectomy in Spondylodiskitis

Pradyumna Pai Raiturkar

ABSTRACT

Sponylodiskitis involves infection of the vertebral bodies and the adjoining disk spaces. The diagnosis of spondylodiskitis is crucial. Early diagnosis and treatment play an important role in its management. The transforaminal endoscopic approach helps in diagnosis and initiation of treatment. The inherent advantages of the percutaneous endoscopic techniques are lesser tissue trauma, faster rehabilitation and lesser chances of instability. This chapter will deal with the indications, technique, tips and tricks of the technique.

INTRODUCTION

Spondylodiskitis literally means infection involving the vertebral body and the adjoining disk and it includes vertebral osteomyelitis, spondylitis and diskitis. Spondylodiskitis is relatively rare but a serious morbid condition and its incidence is increasing due to increasing susceptible population who are elderly, immunocompromised and with medical comorbidities.

Spondylodiskitis can be categorized based on the infective pathogen as pyogenic, granulomatous or fungal. Infection occurs mainly via three routes by hematogenous spread the common,[1] by direct external inoculation [post surgery or interventions including injections] or by spread from contiguous tissues. Spondylodiskitis is multifocal in 4% cases and Lumbar spine is the most common site for hematogenous route.[2]

Clinical features in spondylodiskitis are nonspecific but most distinguishing feature is pain which can be acute onset in pyogenic and more chronic course as in granulomatous and fungal infections. Pain has the red flag features which is constant progressive and with night aggravation at rest. Constitutional symptoms of fever are present in acute pyogenic infections and low-grade fever is commonly in granulomatous type. In advanced cases with significant destruction and abscess formation, there is a chance of neurological involvement with paresis and bladder bowel involvement. Deformity is also a consequence of chronic infection.

The primary goals of treating infectious spondylodiskitis are to make a prompt, accurate diagnosis, isolate the responsible organism, and prescribe effective antibiotic therapy. Nonoperative treatment is adequate for most infections and those detected early. Surgery usually is reserved for patients with failed antibiotic therapy, progressive spinal deformity or instability, epidural abscess, or neurologic deficits.[2-12]

Percutaneous endoscopic transforaminal diskectomy and drainage, a relatively new technique, is emerging because of its simplicity and apparent diagnostic accuracy from 45 to 87% according to the organism isolated as well as its therapeutic advantage.[13-18] It has been referred to as percutaneous endoscopic diskectomy and drainage PEDD or percutaneous endoscopic lavage and drainage PELD.[13,15,16,18-22]

Indications for Percutaneous Disk Decompression and lavage with biopsy:

1. Early stages of any spondylodiskitis affecting the lumbar disks or lumbosacral disk space.
2. For postoperative infective diskitis after lumbar diskectomy either open or endoscopic.
3. In elderly patients with lots of comorbid conditions with immunocompromised status, having serious medical conditions having relatively advanced infective spondylodiskitis and where a definitive open surgical method would not be feasible.

Contraindications

1. Significant neural deficit caused by large epidural abscess extending across many segments accompanying spondylodiskitis.
2. Spondylodiskitis which is advanced to cause instability.

ANATOMY OF THE TRANSFORAMINAL ENDOSCOPIC APPROACH

Percutaneous approach to the lumbar disks is through the transforaminal route popularized by Prof. Parvez Kambin,[23,25] which is gaining popularity now for all types of disk herniations **(Figure 1)**. It is through the safe triangle lying on the posterolateral aspect of the disk bound by the traversing root medially, the exiting root on the obtuse side and the superior endplate of the inferior vertebra. This approach goes through a window between the exiting root and the undersurface of the superior articular facet. A lot of cadaveric studies have found that there is sufficient place for a cannula of diameter 6–8 mm to be passed safely at most places in the lumbar spine.[26]

Rather than targeting the fragment as in case of a disk herniation for diskectomy in case of spondylodiskitis one can target the center of the disk at an angle of 45° at each level **(Figures 2 and 3)**.

In cases of higher lumbar disks one has to be careful of not violating the peritoneal space and the organs within.

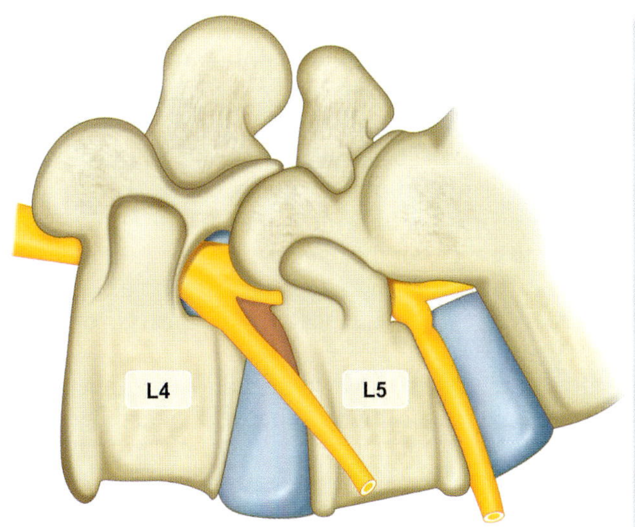

Figure 1: Kambin's safe triangle illustrated at L4–5 disk space

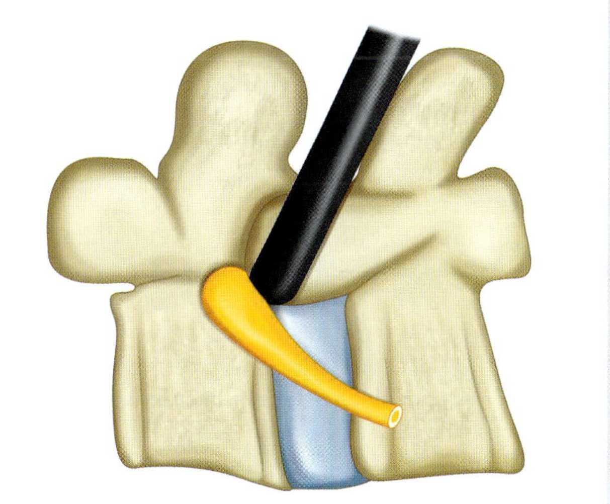

Figure 2: Transforaminal placement of access cannula

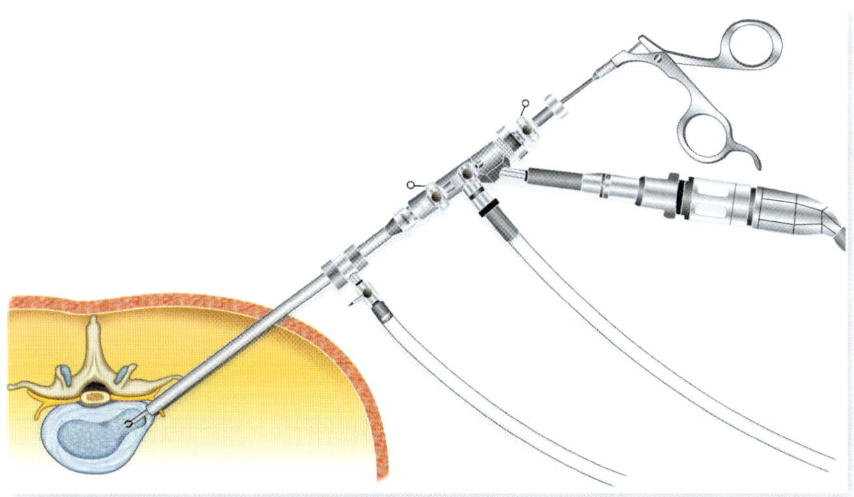

Figure 3: Schematic diagram showing the entire assembly of using the working channel endoscope for percutaneous diskectomy

PREOPERATIVE PLANNING

Most recent imaging studies including the MRI and also preferably a CT scan helps us to plan the trajectory of approach and the skin entry point from the midline to be taken. CT scan is also essential as it would give you a more fair idea of the bony destruction caused by the infective process **(Figure 4)**.

TECHNIQUE

Preferably done under local anesthesia with sedation. Local anesthetic may not act so effectively around the infected area within the disk and so patient needs to be very cooperative. If the patient is in severe pain and apprehensive then can be best done in general anesthesia but the surgeon needs to be experienced in doing percutaneous endoscopic diskectomy procedures so as to avoid complications due to wrong placement of the needle and cannula.

Prone position over horizontally placed bolsters whereby the abdomen is free. The patient is made comfortable in this position by applying cushioning wherever required.

Image intensifier positioned to have a perfect AP and lateral images of the involved level whereby the spinous processes are placed exactly in the midline in AP, and the Disk spaces are perfectly parallel with no parallax in lateral. Once a perfect position of the image intensifier is got the C-arm is fixed in that position throughout the procedure.

In cases with more advanced diskitis, the disk space is collapsed and the endplates are also not clearly visible. With bedridden patients there is also a lot of gas shadows which obscure the clarity. It is difficult to accurately position the needle and the cannula subsequently in such individuals. The quality of the image intensifier and also the technician then matters a lot **(Figure 5)**.

No antibiotic to be given preoperatively to the patient as this can affect the yields of the organisms.

Intended point of insertion is marked after drawing line along the disk space and distance from the midline as calculated on preoperative axial images **(Figure 6)**.

5–10 cc of 2% lignocaine given at this point of insertion and also along the intended trajectory of needle insertion **(Figure 7)**.

18 G needle introduced from this point toward the disk space continuously monitored by AP and lateral images so that one does not sway too vertical or horizontal **(Figures 8 and 9)**. The angle of approach varies from the disk level you are targeting. At higher lumbar levels the approach angle is steeper than at the lower lumbar levels. The exact point of disk entry for the needle is where the needle tip is located at the midpoint of the inferior pedicle on AP view and the tip is just over the posterior disk margin on lateral view **(Figure 10)**.

Giving anesthesia over the annulus surface before penetrating is usually highly effective in pain relief during diskectomy but in infective diskitis pain relief may be partial.

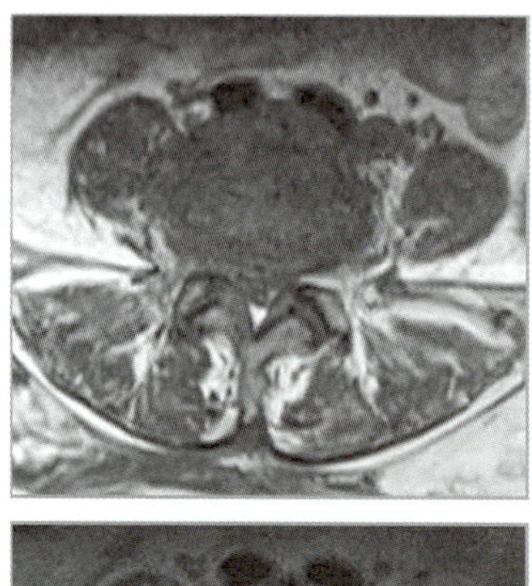
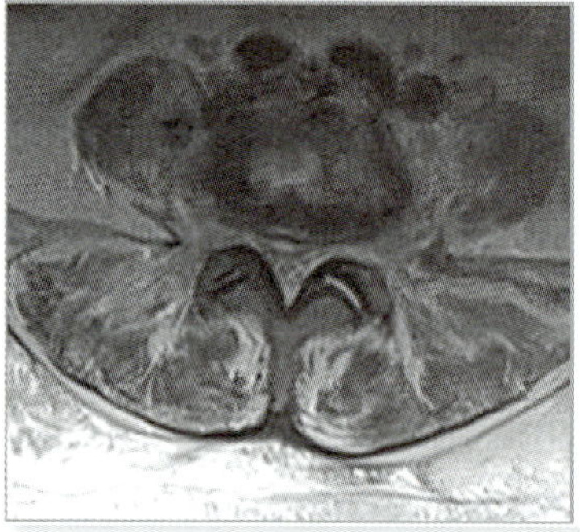
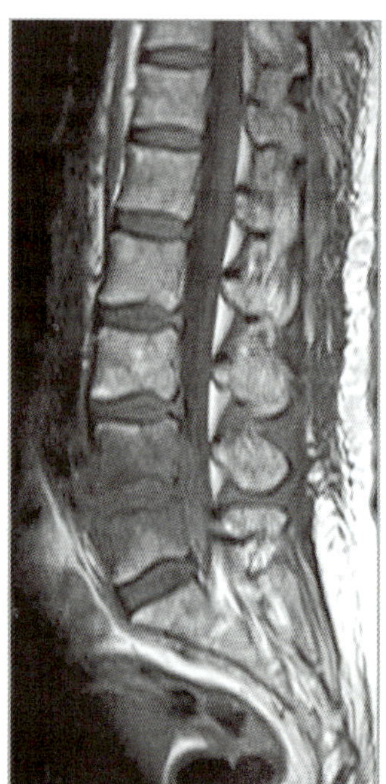
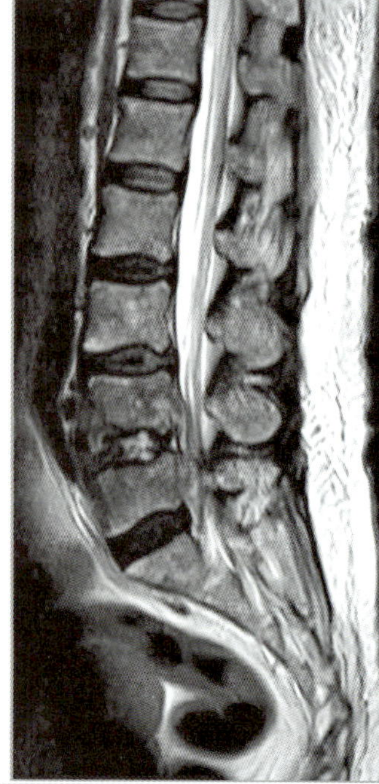

Figure 4: 62-year-old hypothyroid with chronic renal failure on twice weekly dialysis presenting with severe progressive low back pain

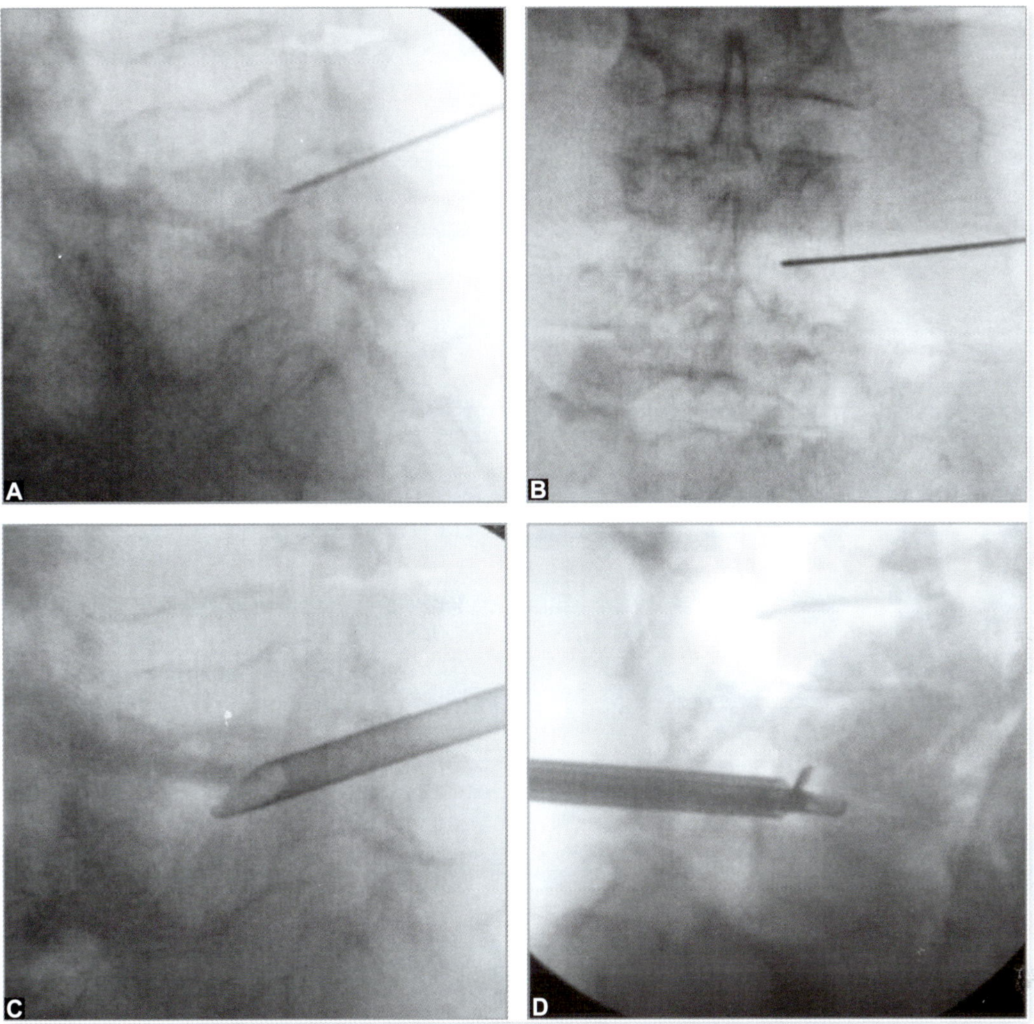

Figures 5A to D: Needle insertion is challenging with collapsed narrow disk space with significant endplate destruction

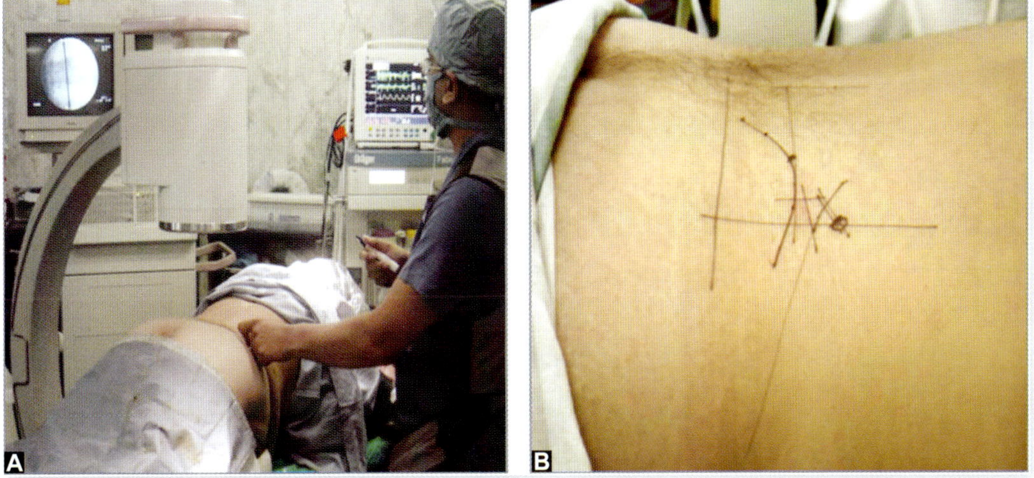

Figure 6: Entry point marked on skin under image intensifier control

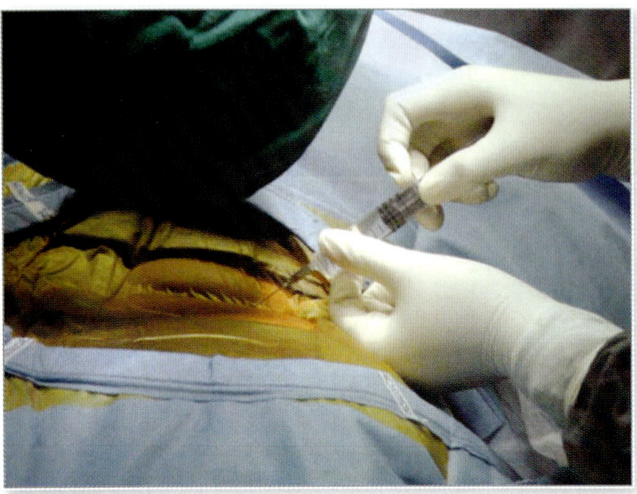

Figure 7: Local infiltration with 2% lignocaine

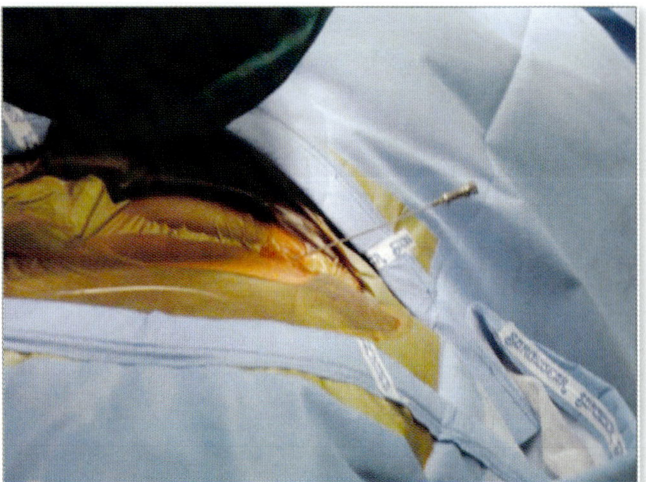

Figure 8: Entry with 18 G needle under image intensifier control

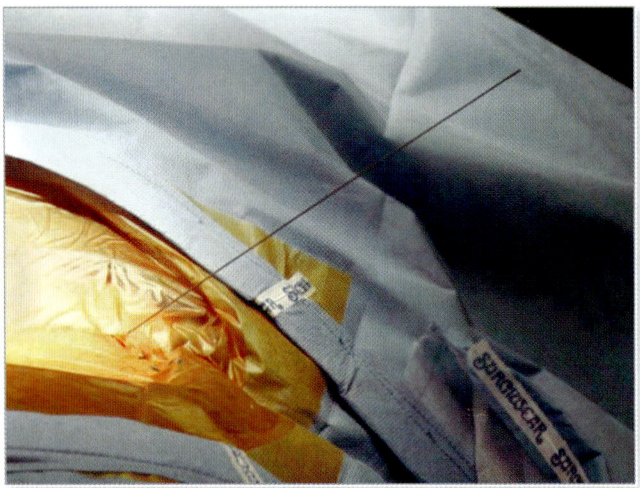

Figure 9: Guidewire introduced through the needle

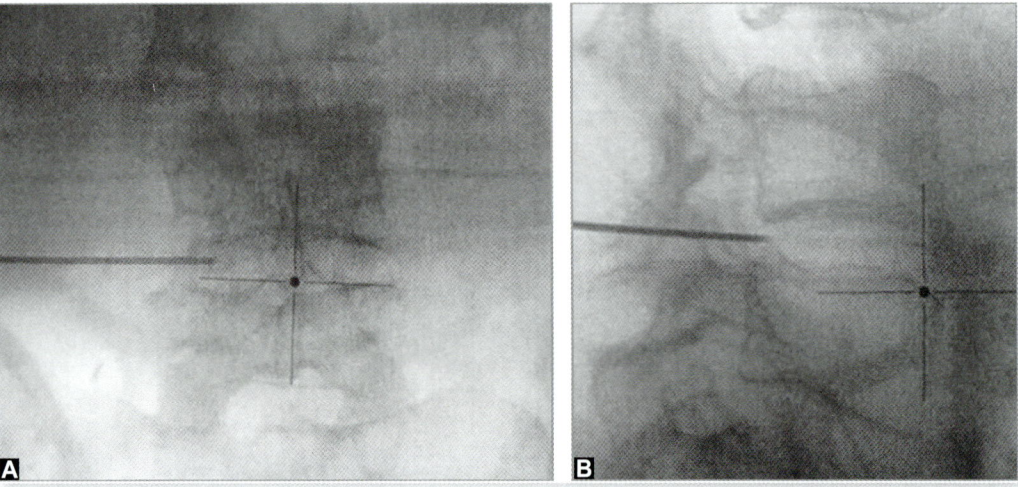

Figure 10: Perfect needle position on anteroposterior and lateral image intensifier views before entering the disk space safely through Kambin's triangle.

Once the needle is introduced in the disk space, one can aspirate for liquefied pus, if any.

A guidewire is then introduced and then after a stab incision on the skin, a dilator is slid over the guidewire gradually in the disk space. One needs to be careful that the guidewire does not migrate further while pushing the dilator inside. This is the most painful part of the procedure and one need to ask the anesthetist to top up the sedation well in advance of this step **(Figure 11)**.

A cannula is then passed over the dilator to position it intradiskally. The cannula position is in the center of the disk space **(Figure 12)**.

Through this cannula first advance a long disk forceps to have free material from disk for microbiological studies. Sufficient disk material can be obtained through this method. One must have a visual sense of how deep the disk forceps is going in the disk space each time you are using it by using an image intensifier the first time you use it.

Till this time no irrigation should be attached so as to dilute the materials to be biopsied.

Once sufficient disk material has been obtained, one can use a special disk forceps to which a normal saline irrigation can be attached so as to irrigate the disk space as you obtain more free lying infected disk tissue. Actually a manual diskectomy through such specially designed forceps is also sufficient for thorough irrigation of the disk space with 2-4 liters of normal saline. As it has been said, dilution is the solution to pollution this is very effective in controlling infection locally **(Figure 13)**.

One can then pass the working channel endoscope which has a dedicated irrigation channel and also an outflow for the liquid and remove tissue under vision **(Figure 14)**. We use the Vertebris 4.0 mm system by Richard Wolf or the 3.7mm system by Maxer endoscopy. Percutaneous debridement is performed piecemeal under vision of the endoscope using working channel disk forceps, flexible rongeurs into different

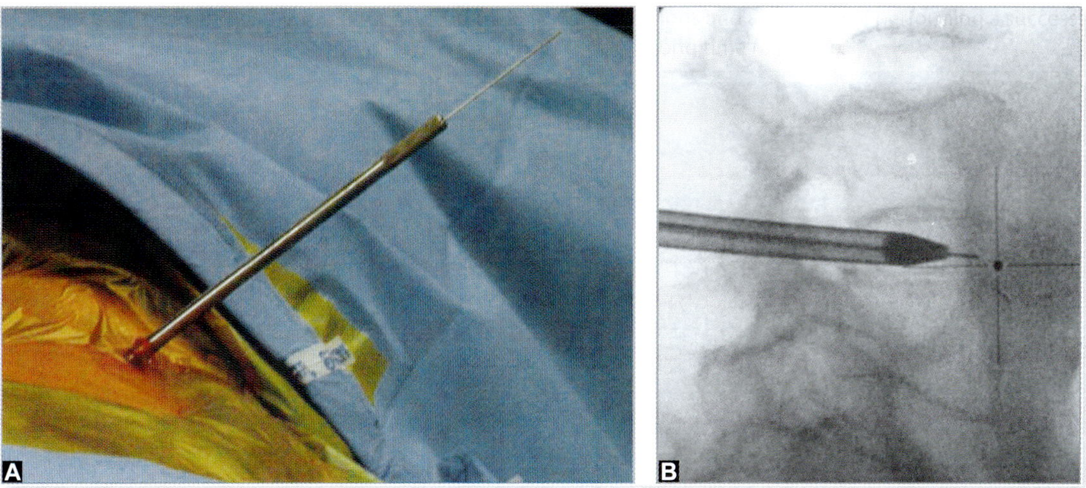

Figure 11: Dilator over the guidewire

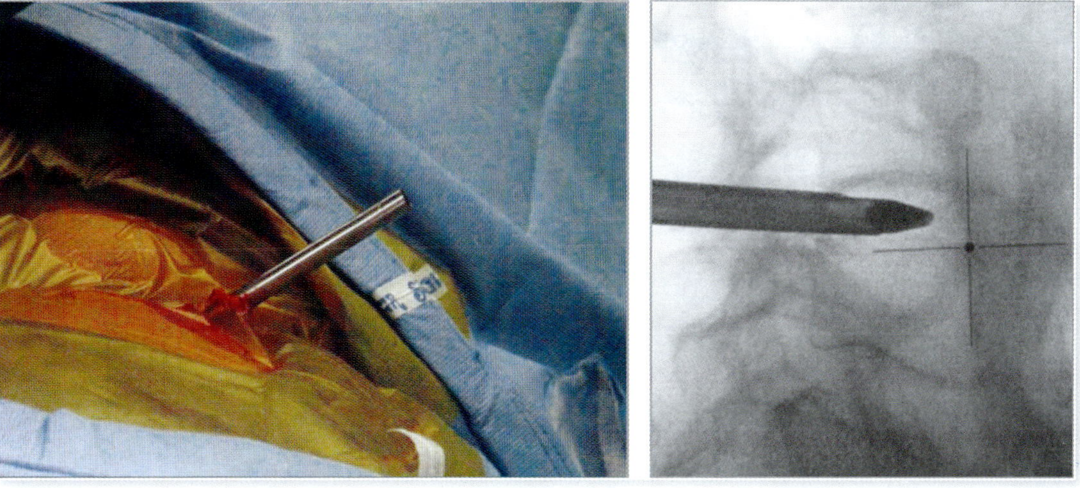

Figure 12: Cannula over the dilator introduced in the disk space

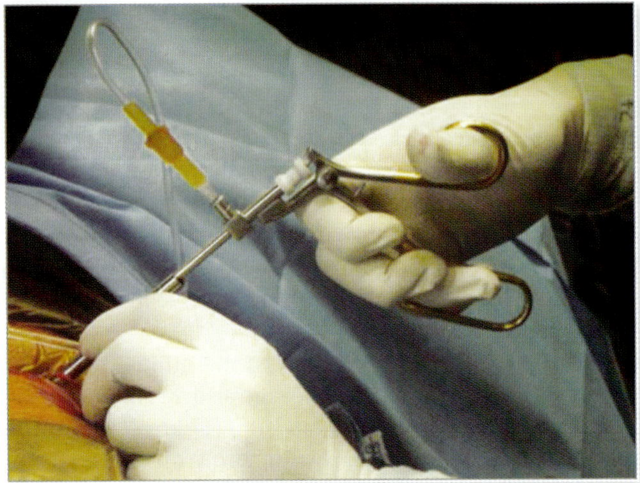

Figure 13: Disk forceps with irrigation attached

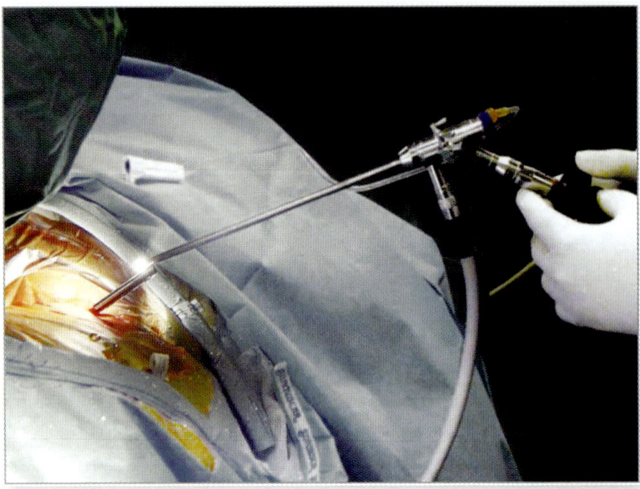

Figure 14: Working channel endoscope introduced

portions of the disk to withdraw as much infected tissue as possible. This helps to remove large free lying fragments. One can also remove large parts of loose endplates through the cannula. Bleeding from endplates is a concern for visualization but being performed under constant irrigation this problem can be tackled by increasing the pressure of irrigating fluid temporarily. Use of a hydropump may be helpful but too much pressurized fluid can also be harmful as it increases the epidural pressure with some patients immediately complaining of neck pain and headache. Bleeding from small vessels can be effectively controlled using the flexible bipolar tip [By Elliquence] attached to a 4 .1 MHz radiofrequency generator. Using this generator prevents the lateral spread of the current especially when near sensitive neural structures **(Figures 15 to 18)**.

A sufficient amount of specimen for microbiological examination is definitely obtained, but more specifically, we can get samples from different infected disk regions which thus improves the culture yield. Causative organism can be identified in about 90% of cases in which percutaneous endoscopic disk lavage is performed as compared to 47 % of cases with a CT-guided biopsy.[13]

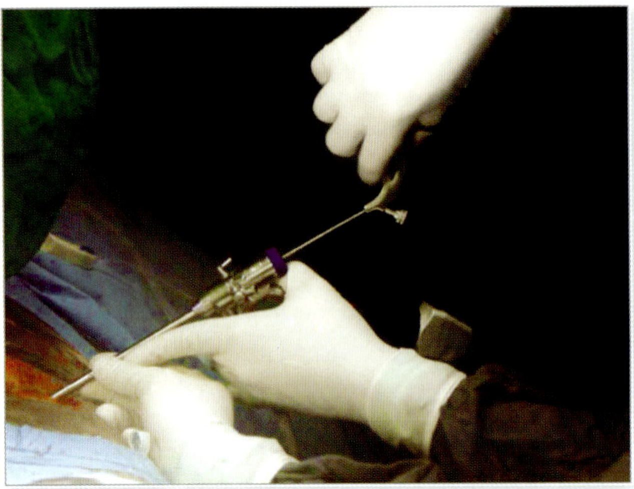

Figure 15: Furthur debridement of disk space under vision

Several authors have also tried the biportal access simultaneously whereby a similar percutaneous channel is created on the opposite side **(Figure 19)**. This aids in more aggressive debridement of the disk space. There have been others who have used irrigation from one portal and used the other portal to drain the irrigating fluid. Some even keep a continuous irrigation postoperatively with a suction attached on the other side and this is removed later.[13,15,18]

Using just normal saline is helpful but Shih-Chieh Yang et al.[16] have used a 3.5% diluted povidine iodine solution [10 lit]. According to them using povidone iodine in that concentration can help in locally acting against most pathogens including oxacillin resistant *Staphhylococcus aureus* without any resistance and so also not have any cytotoxic effects on normal cells which should not impede normal healing. Hsin-Chuan Chen et al. used normal saline solution mixed with 1 g cefazolin.[17]

Use of a drain in the postoperative phase is recommended in the acute setting of the infection. The negative pressure suction drain is left in place until the drainage is stopped or reduced to <10 mL per day for three consecutive days. One has to be extremely cautious with drain care and the duration for it is kept as it should not act as a conduit for superadded infection.

Throughout the procedure, one has to be careful that because of infection, the annulus is not very much competent and hence forceps can pass beyond the disk space easily if not controlled. If inadvertently breached can cause injury to abdominal great vessels.

The advantage of percutaneous endoscopic diskectomy and drainage is that we get sufficient material with very good yield for finding the organism causing the infective process

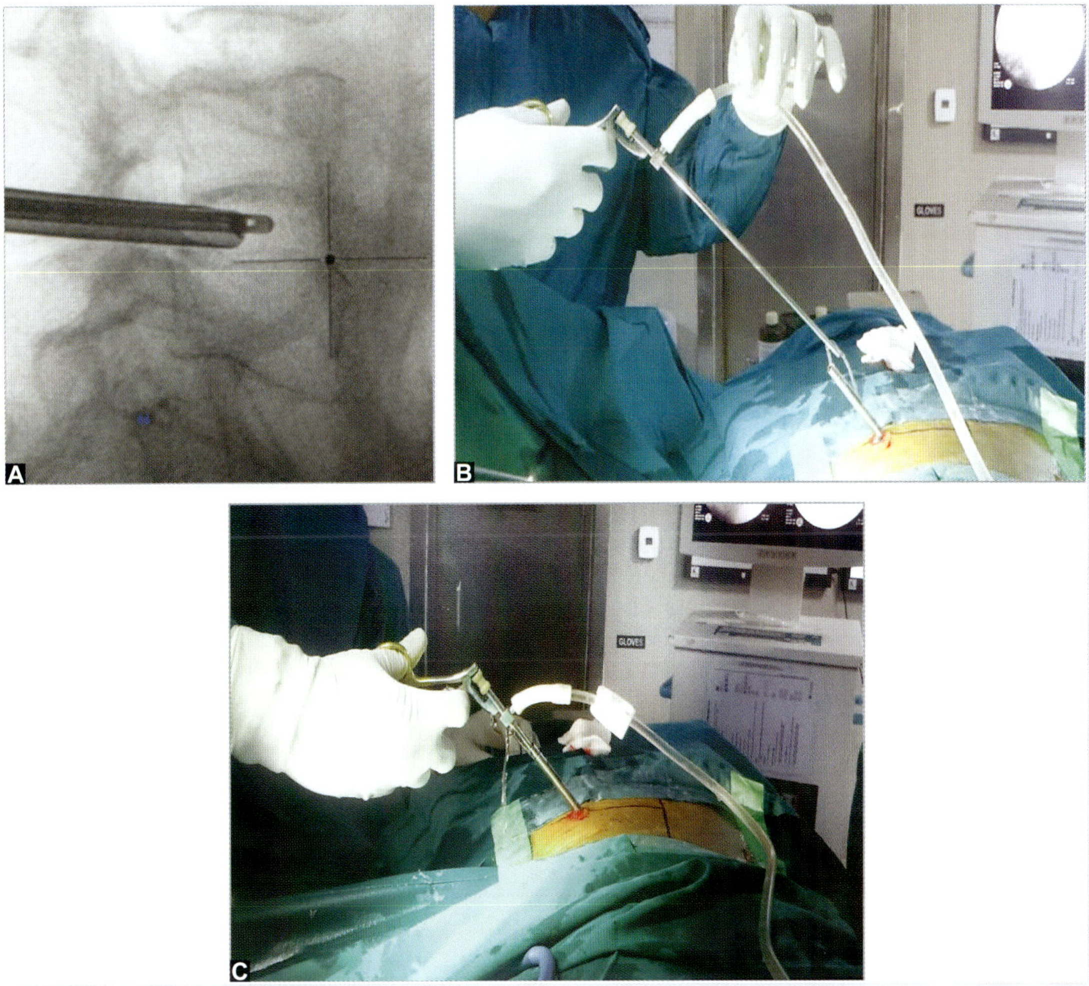

Figure 16: Use of the large special disk forceps with possibility of continuous irrigation through the forceps

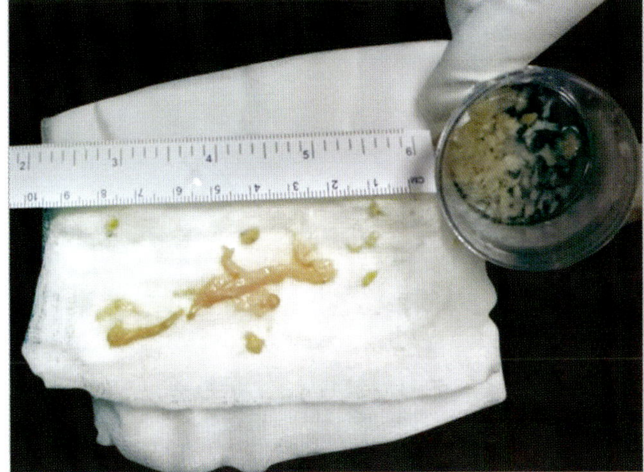

Figure 17: Slimy infected disk tissue harvested from all regions of the disk for microbiologic examination. It yielded *Staph aureus* on culture

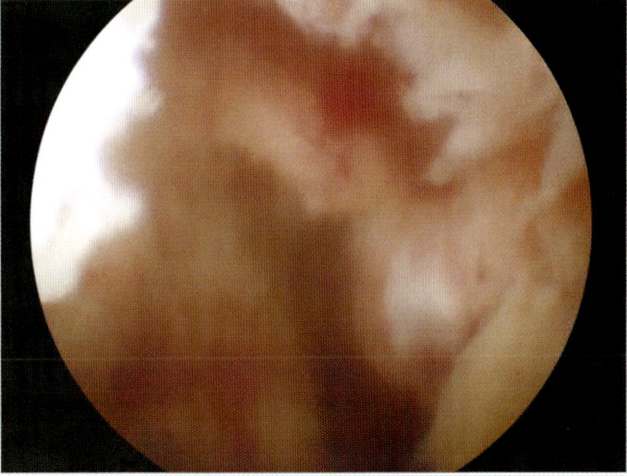

Figure 18: Endoscope image of the disk space with necrotic infected tissue. Disk space is relatively empty after debridement

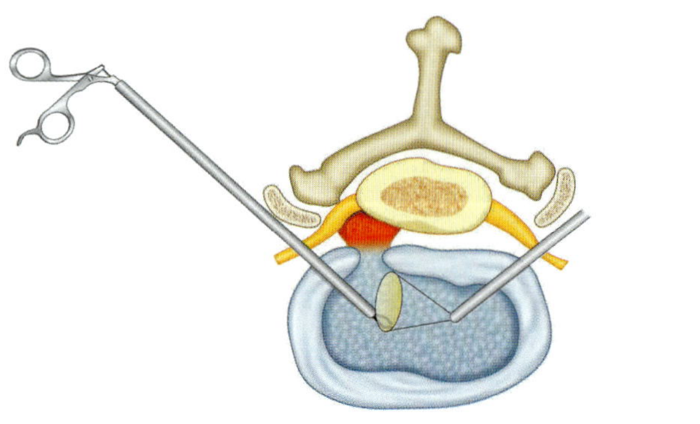

Figure 19: Schematic diagram showing the biportal technique

and also by way of antibiotic sensitivity the best antibiotic for arresting the infection. *Staphylococcus aureus* is the most common organism for pyogenic spondylodiskitis followed by *Pseudomonas aeruginosa, Streptococcus viridians,* enterococci and *Haemophilus influenza.* In addition to being diagnostic because of lavage and drainage of the infected tissue it is also of therapeutic value with significant pain relief for the patient immediately after the procedure. All authors who have used this technique are unanimous in accepting that there is dramatic immediate relief of back pain.

COMPLICATIONS

Complications can arise because of improper placement of the needle and subsequent cannula. There have been no reported major complications in literature in using it for treatment of spondylodiskitis. This is in contrast to the occurrence of complications after open spine surgery for pyogenic spondylodiskitis.[1,27,28] Throughout the procedure the blood loss is negligible and nonmeasurable. With use of endoscope and continuous visualization of structures under local anesthesia, there is no chance of neurological injury at the lumbar spine. While applying the same at the lower dorsal spine special precautions are required. Hsin-Chuan Chen et al.[17] used a CT to introduce a angiographic catheter precisely avoiding other visceral structures and then went ahead with a percutaneous diskectomy over the CT-guided catheter later in the operating room. They have used the same even at Dorsal level involvement at D89 or D11 D12.

In acute infective pyogenic diskitis, there is significant oozing through the endplates and it is necessary to put a suction drain so as to avoid any postoperative collection of blood or infective material.

Percutaneous diskectomy and lavage can be a definitive therapeutic surgery in many if followed by good adequate antibiotic therapy. But one has to counsel the patient of requirement of open anterior debridement with or without fixation in cases which progress in spite of this.

REVIEW OF LITERATURE

There have been several attempts to treat pyogenic spinal infections using minimally invasive surgical techniques.

Valls et al. reported the technique of needle biopsy for vertebral infections in 1948.[29]

With the advent of CT guided procedures the isolation of infective organism improved to about 50% and still newer techniques are devised on how to target a specific area which is detected in MRI images so as to increase the yield.[30]

In 1991, Yu, et al.,[31] reported the first two cases of spinal osteomyelitis managed with percutaneous suction aspiration; they used a nucleotome that was originally designed for percutaneous disk excision and reported good results.

Jeanneret and Magerl (1994)[32] introduced the use of per cutaneous external fixation following percutaneous suction or irrigation. The treatment consisted of percutaneous vertebral biopsy for bacteriologic diagnosis, installation of a suction/irrigation system into the intervertebral disk space, and posterior stabilization (and reduction if indicated) with an external fixator placed percutaneously. In their series of 23 patients, this was the definitive treatment for 15 patients; while in others, it was used as a stop gap arrangement.

Gebhard JS et al. (1994)[33] as well as Watters WC 3rd et al.(1994)[34] also used percutaneous diskectomy to diagnose as well as treat bacterial diskitis effectively in small number of patients and effectively rapidly reducing pain and shortening the acute clinical course.

Haaker et al.(1997)[35] reported satisfactory results of 26 patients of lumbar disk infections, treated with percutaneous lumbar diskectomy. They primarily used it as a diagnostic tool for identification of the organism but found it to be of therapeutic advantage also as only 3 of the 26 required an open interbody fusion and rest had spontaneous fusion gradually.

Hadjipavlov et al. (1998)[36-38] have used the percutaneous transpedicular approach to reach the disk for biopsy and subsequent irrigation and lavage in cases with spondylodiskitis with long-term success rate of 68%.

Hanaoka et al. [2006][39] in their study of 5 patients treated with percutaneous drainage and suction used it as a salvage procedure when antibiotic therapy had failed for 5–19 weeks. They had good pain relief in 4 of the 5 patients within 8 days in spite of doing the procedure late in the disease process. We advocate the use of percutaneous diskectomy and drainage immediately on clinical diagnosis for having a good material for diagnosing the culprit organism as well as decreasing the load thereof.

Ito et al. (2007)[19] reported their results in using posterolateral endoscopy in 15 patients with serious comorbid conditions. All had failed a conservative trial of an average of 20 weeks with a diagnosis of organism in only 6 patients. Postendoscopy a diagnosis of organism was possible in 11 of the patients. The average VAS for pain decreased from 86 preoperatively to 25 at one week post-operative. Similar decrease was observed for CRP levels.

Li J et al. (2011)[21] retrospectively reviewed the role of percutaneous diskectomy in the management of post-operative diskitis after either open or percutaneous diskectomy. In a group of 34 patients, 31 of whom were lumbar, they had a good clinical outcome both clinically with decreased CRP levels and improvement in the VAS score for pain in all the patients with none requiring open surgical intervention.

Tsai-Sheng Fu et al. (2013)[13] in their series of 14 patients managed by Percutaneous endoscopic diskectomy and drainage[PEDD] showed that all had excellent immediate pain relief, causative organism found in 12 out of 14 and 10 patients eventually getting treated completely without the need of any additional open stabilization procedure

Shih-Chieh Yang et al. (2014)[15,16] in their study operated 21 patients with percutaneous endoscopic Lavage and drainage[PELD] with advanced infectious spondylitis excluding those with instability and neurological deficits. Organism was cultured in 19 out of the 21. The overall infection control rate was impressive 86%. Value of PELD is limited in multilevel infections. It is interesting to note that in a subset with postoperative infection the infection control was 100%.

Murata Y et al. (2014)[40] compared their results after percutaneous nucleotomy with drainage with those having open anterior debridement and interbody fusion. They concluded that though more number of patients undergoing Anterior interbody fusion (97%) showed recovery, the recovery in percutaneous nucleotomy and drainage group was also an impressive 83% with much less morbidity. Thus they recommended that percutaneous nucleotomy should always be considered as the first choice before more invasive anterior approach is considered.

Li-Chen Hsu et al. (2015)[18] concluded that percutaneous endoscopic debridement with bilateral biportal approach was helpful to eradicate lumbar pyogenic spondylitis in 18 out of the 22 cases without the need of any further open procedure.

Percutaneous endoscopic lavage has also been used successfully in the management of early tubercular or fungal spondylodiskitis in very selected patients.[41,42]

With advent of percutaneous pedicle screw instrumentation, it would be a useful adjunct to provide immediate stability after percutaneous diskectomy and lavage in selected patients. There have been no clinical reports of the same other than the one by Jeannert et al.[32] who have used percutaneous spinal external fixation.

Percutaneous diskectomy with lavage and drainage is particularly suitable for patients with early-stage spinal infection or serious medical conditions. Using posterolateral spinal endoscopy enables both extensive debridement of infected sites and pressurized irrigation under clear visualization and also a higher yield of positive culture for the target organism. Yang SC, et al.[43] have demonstrated that percutaneous endoscopic diskectomy and drainage yield higher bacterial recovery rates (90%) than CT-guided spinal biopsy (47%). The best indication of this procedure should be minimal or moderate destructive changes of the vertebrae. With reduced invasiveness and immediate symptomatic relief the procedure is very patient friendly. The rate of secondary surgical intervention is also reduced after thorough debridement using percutaneous transforaminal endoscopy combined by prompt use of antimicrobial therapy. Using the transforaminal approach is more safe, suitable in treating postoperative infections after microdiskecomy as one does not have to go through previous operated and scarred tissue. Also the stability of the functional vertebral unit can be better preserved which otherwise could be compromised by more resection of the facet joint for open access.

Thus percutaneous transforaminal endoscopic diskectomy is an effective alternative for treating infectious spondylodiskitis and should be considered prior to extensive anterior surgery in selected cases.

REFERENCES

1. Carragee EJ. Pyogenic vertebral osteomyelitis. J Bone Joint Surg Am. 1997;79:874-80.
2. Goulliouris T, Aliyu SH, Brown NM. Spondylodiskitis: update on diagnosis and management. J Antimicrob Chemother. 2010;65 Suppl 3:iii11-24.
3. Khan IA, Vaccaro AR, Zlotolow DA. Management of vertebral diskitis and osteomyelitis. Orthopedics. 1999;22:758-65.
4. Schinkel C, Gottwald M, Andress HJ. Surgical treatment of spondylodiskitis. Surg Infect (Larchmt). 2003;4:387-91.
5. Frangen TM, Kalicke T, Gottwald M, et al. [Surgical management of spondylodiskitis. An analysis of 78 cases]. Unfallchirurg. 2006;109:743-53.
6. Skaf GS, Domloj NT, Fehlings MG, et al. Pyogenic spondylodiskitis: an overview. J Infect Public Health. 2010;3:5-16.
7. Di Martino A, Papapietro N, Lanotte A, et al. Spondylodiskitis: standards of current treatment. Curr Med Res Opin. 2012;28:689-99.
8. Guerado E, Cervan AM. Surgical treatment of spondylodiskitis. An update. Int Orthop. 2012;36:413-20.
9. Devkota P, Krishnakumar R, Renjith Kumar J. Surgical management of pyogenic diskitis of lumbar region. Asian Spine J. 2014;8:177-82.
10. Shetty AP, Aiyer SN, Kanna RM, et al. Pyogenic lumbar spondylodiskitis treated with transforaminal lumbar interbody fusion: safety and outcomes. Int Orthop. 2016;60(6):1163-70.
11. Tschoke SK, Fuchs H, Schmidt O, et al. Single-stage debridement and spinal fusion using PEEK cages through a posterior

approach for eradication of lumbar pyogenic spondylodiskitis: a safe treatment strategy for a detrimental condition. Patient Saf Surg. 2015;9:35.
12. Gerometta A, Bittan F, Rodriguez Olaverri JC. Postoperative spondilodiskitis. Int Orthop. 2012;36:433-8.
13. Fu TS, Chen LH, Chen WJ. Minimally invasive percutaneous endoscopic diskectomy and drainage for infectious spondylodiskitis. Biomed J. 2013;36:168-74.
14. Verdu-Lopez F, Vanaclocha-Vanaclocha V, Gozalbes-Esterelles L, et al. Minimally invasive spine surgery in spinal infections. J Neurosurg Sci. 2014;58:45-56.
15. Yang SC, Chen WJ, Chen HS, et al. Extended indications of percutaneous endoscopic lavage and drainage for the treatment of lumbar infectious spondylitis. Eur Spine J. 2014;23:846-53.
16. Yang SC, Fu TS, Chen HS, et al. Minimally invasive endoscopic treatment for lumbar infectious spondylitis: a retrospective study in a tertiary referral center. BMC Musculoskelet Disord. 2014;15:105.
17. Chen H-C, Huang T-L, Chen Y-J, et al. A Minimally Invasive Endoscopic Surgery for Infectious Spondylodiskitis of the Thoracic and Upper Lumbar Spine in Immunocompromised Patients. Biomed Res Int. 2015;2015:8.
18. Hsu LC, Tseng TM, Yang SC, et al. Bilateral Portal Percutaneous Endoscopic Debridement and Lavage for Lumbar Pyogenic Spondylitis. Orthopedics. 2015;38:e856-63.
19. Ito M, Abumi K, Kotani Y, et al. Clinical outcome of posterolateral endoscopic surgery for pyogenic spondylodiskitis: results of 15 patients with serious comorbid conditions. Spine (Phila Pa 1976). 2007;32:200-6.
20. Fu TS, Yang SC, Tsai TT, et al. Percutaneous endoscopic debridement and drainage in immunocompromised patients with complicated infectious spondylitis. Minim Invasive Ther Allied Technol. 2010;19:42-7.
21. Li J, Yan D, Duan L, et al. Percutaneous diskectomy and drainage for postoperative intervertebral diskitis. Arch Orthop Trauma Surg. 2011;131:173-8.
22. Chen HC, Huang TL, Chen YJ, et al. A Minimally Invasive Endoscopic Surgery for Infectious Spondylodiskitis of the Thoracic and Upper Lumbar Spine in Immunocompromised Patients. Biomed Res Int. 2015;2015:780451.
23. Kambin P. Arthroscopic microdiskectomy. Mt Sinai J Med. 1991;58:159-64.
24. Kambin P. Arthroscopic microdiskectomy. Arthroscopy. 1992;8:287-95.
25. Kambin P, Zhou L. History and current status of percutaneous arthroscopic disk surgery. Spine (Phila Pa 1976). 1996;21:57S-61S.
26. Mirkovic SR, Schwartz DG, Glazier KD. Anatomic considerations in lumbar posterolateral percutaneous procedures. Spine (Phila Pa 1976). 1995;20:1965-71.
27. Karadimas EJ, Bunger C, Lindblad BE, et al. Spondylodiskitis. A retrospective study of 163 patients. Acta Orthop. 2008;79:650-9.
28. Reihsaus E, Waldbaur H, Seeling W. Spinal epidural abscess: a meta-analysis of 915 patients. Neurosurg Rev. 2000;23:175-204; discussion 5.
29. Valls J, Ottolenghi CE, Schajowicz F. Aspiration biopsy in diagnosis of lesions of vertebral bodies. J Am Med Assoc. 1948;136:376-82.
30. Matsumoto T, Yamagami T, Morishita H, et al. CT-guided percutaneous drainage within intervertebral space for pyogenic spondylodiskitis with psoas abscess. Acta Radiol. 2012; 53: 76-80.
31. Yu WY, Siu C, Wing PC, et al. Percutaneous suction aspiration for osteomyelitis. Report of two cases. Spine (Phila Pa 1976). 1991;16:198-202.
32. Jeanneret B, Magerl F. Treatment of osteomyelitis of the spine using percutaneous suction/irrigation and percutaneous external spinal fixation. J Spinal Disord. 1994;7:185-205.
33. Gebhard JS, Brugman JL. Percutaneous diskectomy for the treatment of bacterial diskitis. Spine (Phila Pa 1976). 1994;19:855-7.
34. Watters WC, 3rd, Khalil MA. Percutaneous diskectomy for disk space infections. J South Orthop Assoc. 1994;3:283-9.
35. Haaker RG, Senkal M, Kielich T, et al. Percutaneous lumbar diskectomy in the treatment of lumbar diskitis. Eur Spine J. 1997;6:98-101.
36. Hadjipavlou AG, Mader JT, Necessary JT, et al. Hematogenous pyogenic spinal infections and their surgical management. Spine (Phila Pa 1976). 2000;25:1668-79.
37. Hadjipavlou AG, Katonis PK, Gaitanis IN, et al. Percutaneous transpedicular diskectomy and drainage in pyogenic spondylodiskitis. Eur Spine J. 2004;13:707-13.
38. Hadjipavlou AG, Crow WN, Borowski A, et al. Percutaneous transpedicular diskectomy and drainage in pyogenic spondylodiskitis. Am J Orthop (Belle Mead NJ). 1998;27:188-97.
39. Hanaoka N, Kawasaki Y, Sakai T, et al. Percutaneous drainage and continuous irrigation in patients with severe pyogenic spondylitis, abscess formation, and marked bone destruction. J Neurosurg Spine. 2006;4:374-9.
40. Murata Y, Kanaya K, Wada H, et al. Clinical outcome of percutaneous drainage for spondylodiskitis. J Neurol Surg A Cent Eur Neurosurg. 2014;75:7-11.
41. Ito M, Sudo H, Abumi K, et al. Minimally invasive surgical treatment for tuberculous spondylodiskitis. Minim Invasive Neurosurg. 2009;52:250-3.
42. Iwata A, Ito M, Abumi K, et al. Fungal spinal infection treated with percutaneous posterolateral endoscopic surgery. J Neurol Surg A Cent Eur Neurosurg. 2014;75:170-6.
43. Yang SC, Fu TS, Chen LH, et al. Identifying pathogens of spondylodiskitis: percutaneous endoscopy or CT-guided biopsy. Clin Orthop Relat Res. 2008;466:3086-92.

17

CHAPTER

Microlumbar Diskectomy

CE Deopujari, Shumayou Dutta

ABSTRACT

Lumbar diskectomy has witnessed an evolution in surgical technique with recent emphasis being laid on reduction of the surgical footprint via minimal invasiveness. Irrespective of the type of diskectomy offered to the patient, the principles of surgery remain the same as that described by Fager for microlumbar diskectomy. Careful patient selection, preoperative planning with due consideration given to the location of the prolapse as well as individual anatomical challenges are key to a successful outcome. In this chapter, we look at the evolution of surgical techniques for diskectomy, discuss the principles of microlumbar diskectomy, and describe the steps of performing a microlumbar diskectomy in simple (paracentral disk herniations) as well as challenging cases (lateral disk herniations). We highlight the outcomes of the various minimally invasive techniques against the gold standard of microlumbar diskectomy. Having performed over 600 microlumbar diskectomies with more than 10 years of follow-up, we also share our personal experiences.

EVOLUTION OF DISKECTOMY

Diskectomy, first reported by Mixter and Barr[1] in 1934, has changed the management of lumbar disk herniations. William J Mixter, a neurosurgeon at Harvard Medical School, and his orthopedic colleague, Joseph Barr, first elucidated the pathophysiology of the age-old curse often described as lumbago or sciatica. They reviewed and synthesized the case reports by Oppenheim, Goldthwait, Ellsberg, Bucy, Dandy, Petit-Dutallis, Schmorl, and others, added 11 cases of their own, thus providing the information substrate and the catalyst that lead to the preoperative diagnosis and the surgical cure of intractable pain. Far from minimally invasive, the lumbar diskectomy technique described by Mixter and Barr involved an extensive removal of the lamina and offending ruptured disk through an intradural approach. Their technique was used during much of the Cold War era and underwent only subtle alteration in the late 1960s. It was not until 1977 that Caspar[2] and Yasargil[3], for the first time in history, demonstrated the use of a microsurgical approach for lumbar diskectomy. The following year Williams'[4] whose referral base included Las Vegas showgirls, popularized the microdiskectomy technique in the US. He demonstrated in a series of 532 patients that surgical scars could be minimized and patients could return to work more quickly through the use of a more conservative technique of removing only the protruded portion of the offending disk to decompress the affected nerve root. Williams specified his technique to be applied when the protrusion was present at the level of the disk space and not for sequestered or migrated fragments. While Williams is often credited with the procedure, it is interesting to note that Yasargils' technique of microscopy-assisted diskectomy, with its wider indications, is more in tune with the currently performed surgical procedure. The use of the operative microscope began to gain popularity only in the late 1980s. In the 1990s, many spinal surgeons abandoned conventional diskectomy with naked-eye to pass to the routine practice of microdiskectomy. The merits of this technique are that it allows every type of disk herniation to be excised through a short approach to skin, fascia and muscles as well as a limited laminectomy. For these reasons, it has been, and still is, considered the "gold standard" of surgical treatment for lumbar disk herniation, and the method used by the vast majority of spinal surgeons.

INTRODUCTION TO MICROLUMBAR DISKECTOMY

Yasargil demonstrated that the operating microscope contributes greatly to the success of neurosurgical procedures. Stereoscopic magnification combined with intense coaxial lighting along the surgeon's line of vision increased the ability to reach fragments that were previously considered difficult to remove. Now many spine surgeons use the operating microscope during lumbar spine surgery.

Advantages of the Operating Microscope

There is sufficient evidence in literature suggesting that patients who have undergone microlumbar diskectomy (MLD) leave the hospital sooner and return to full activity sooner than do patients who have had a "standard" diskectomy.

The use of a microscope probably offers several advantages. Magnification allows the surgeon better appreciation of the anatomy. A nerve root distorted and flattened by a disk fragment anterior to it may be confused for a part of the compressed annulus and accidentally incised by a surgeon with the naked eye. The epidural veins can be recognized and preserved, to maintain venous drainage of the nerve root. Tissue planes between a nerve root and an adherent disk fragment can be more easily developed if magnification is available. If a dural tear occurs, it can be more easily repaired under magnification. A unique system of prisms in the microscope offers the surgeon stereoscopic vision, this beings its biggest advantage over 'loupes.' Currently, optical accessories for the microscope include a truly binocular viewing station for the assistant surgeon and attachments for video observation and recording of the procedure. Therefore, the assistant surgeon and the rest of the team can participate to a much greater extent than he or she can during the procedures in which the surgeons head blocks the view.

The microscope, with its stereoscopic magnification and intense coaxial lighting, allows the surgeon to work effectively in a narrow, deep operative field. Therefore, he or she can use a smaller incision and limit soft tissue trauma. The shorter incision protects the paravertebral muscles from extensive denervation, decreases blood loss, and is more cosmetic, thus increasing patient acceptance of the operative procedure. Despite all the advantages a microscope offers, the main disadvantage is the steep learning curve associated with it.

PRINCIPLES OF MICROLUMBAR DISKECTOMY

Fager[5] critically analyzed microsurgical techniques and summarized principles of MLD. First, the exposure must accomplish decompression of the neural elements before attempting to deal with the lesion itself. Following this principle will ensure no damage comes to the nerve root or dura during removal of the lesion. Second, the neural elements must be satisfactorily released longitudinally. If a nerve root or dura remains restricted cephalad or cauda to the lesion, neurologic damage may occur during excision of the lesion. If the bony removal is not extended adequately cephalad or caudad, disk fragments that may have migrated may be missed. Third, the lesion should be approached laterally, to minimise retraction of the nerve root or dura and to allow better visualization and preservation of the epidural veins. Approaching the fragment via the axilla may cause an inadvertent durotomy in a location difficult to approach for repair. These principles can be easily followed during MLD, as long as the surgeon is comfortable with the microscope and does not get distracted and frustrated handling it.

TECHNIQUE

Preoperative Evaluation and Preparation

Patients with at least 6 weeks of conservative treatment with positive nerve root tension signs, radicular pain and correlating MRI findings are offered surgical option. Also patients with worsening neurology and impending cauda equina syndrome are selected for MLD. Carefully studying the MRI for stage **(Figures 1A to D)** and location **(Figures 2A and B)** of disk heriation is crucial for localizing fragment and knowing how much disk material to be removed.

Intraoperative Medications

The disk space is avascular and, as a result, less resistant to infection. There is evidence that the risk of disk space infection may be reduced through the use of perioperative antibiotics. Half an hour before surgery IV ceftriaxone 1g is recommended. This is repeated if the blood loss exceeds 500 mL or the operative time crosses 4 hours. The dose is repeated post-surgery and a final shot is given coming morning.

OPERATIVE POSITIONING AND PATIENT PREPARATION

The preoperative placement of elastic stockings to prevent thromboembolism is recommended. A urinary catheter is usually unnecessary unless the procedure is expected to take more than 2 hours. Before the skin incision is made, the surgeon should have taken the opportunity to become familiar with the patient's particular anatomy and pathology, and the operation should have been planned. Ideally, the interpretation of the preoperative studies, how they relate to the patient, and the intraoperative plan in brief terms should be committed to the chart.

For most surgeons, the prone position on a frame works well. Obese patients are better positioned in such a manner that the abdominal panniculus hangs unimpeded, without bearing any of the patient's weight. The eyes and facial

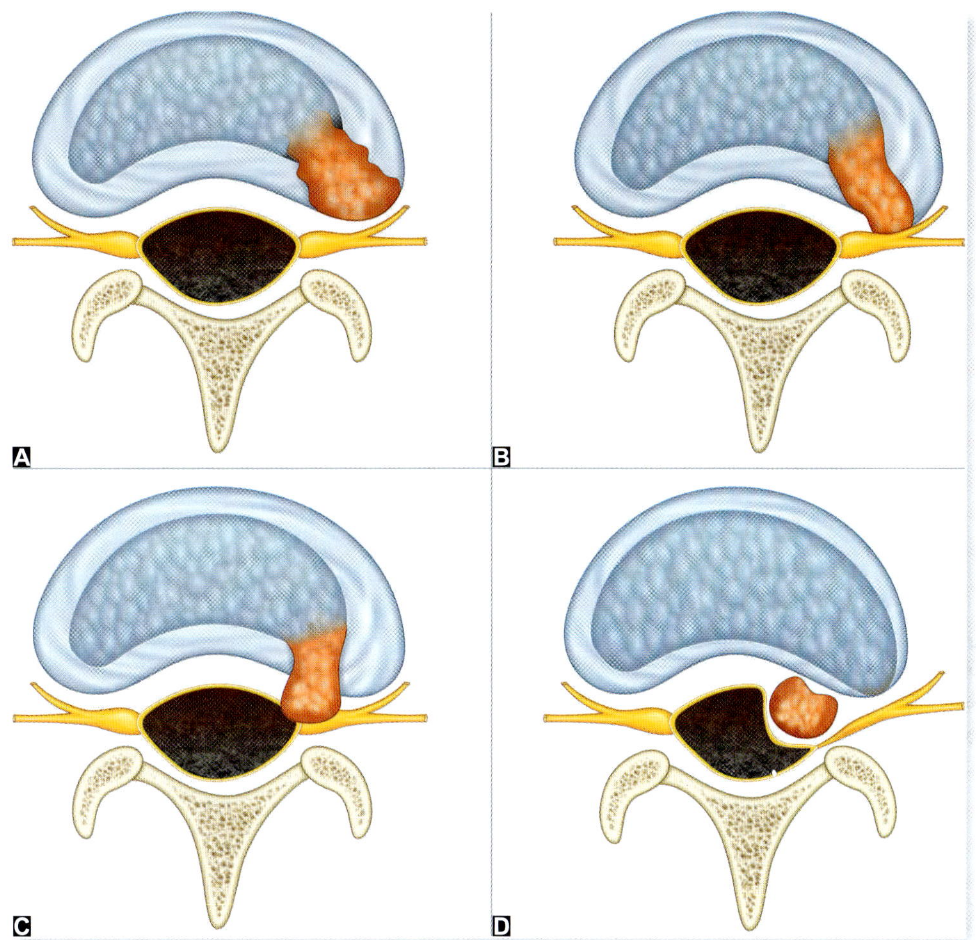

Figures 1A to D: Stage of disk herniation. (A) Degeneration; (B) Protrusion; (C) Extrusion; (D) Sequestration

prominences should be well padded and inspected after the patient is turned to the prone position because ocular pressure, or a combination of pressure and hypotension, can lead to blindness. The arms, if held abducted on arm boards, must be well padded over bony prominences and over the ulnar nerves. To prevent costoclavicular compression of the brachial plexus, care should be taken to avoid hyperabduction over 90 degrees at the shoulders and shoulder hyperextension. The radial pulse on each side should be felt. Women should bear the weight of the chest on the ventrolateral rib cage (not on the breasts, which should be moved medially). All skin that is in contact with the frame or with pads on the frame should be protected with a layer of linens; skin should not be allowed to touch the bare occlusive surface of vinyl or silicone rubber cushions.

The urinary catheter (if placed) is inspected after the patient has been turned. Male genitalia must not be subject to compression between the approximated thighs. All bony prominences of the legs must be padded; in particular, the toes must bear no weight of the foot. A diminished or absent pedal pulse may indicate femoral artery compression. The patient, when positioned, should be stable so that vigorous intraoperative manipulation will not cause movement **(Figure 3)**.

SURGICAL STEPS

The patient is scrubbed and draped for surgery. A 18G/20G needle is placed 1.5 cm lateral to the midline in the paraspinal muscles. A lateral X-ray **(Figures 4A and B)** is taken to confirm the level of the needle.

The needle location serve as a marker for planning the incision. The location of the needle is not as important as the need for the needle to be vertical. If the needle is tilted, the surgeon may plan the incision considering the tip of the needle which will not correspond with the level where it pierces the skin. In an ideal situation, for a L4/5 diskectomy, the needle will be at the L4/5 disk space. It is important to remember that the interlaminar window of interest for the L4/5 level will be slightly distal to the level of

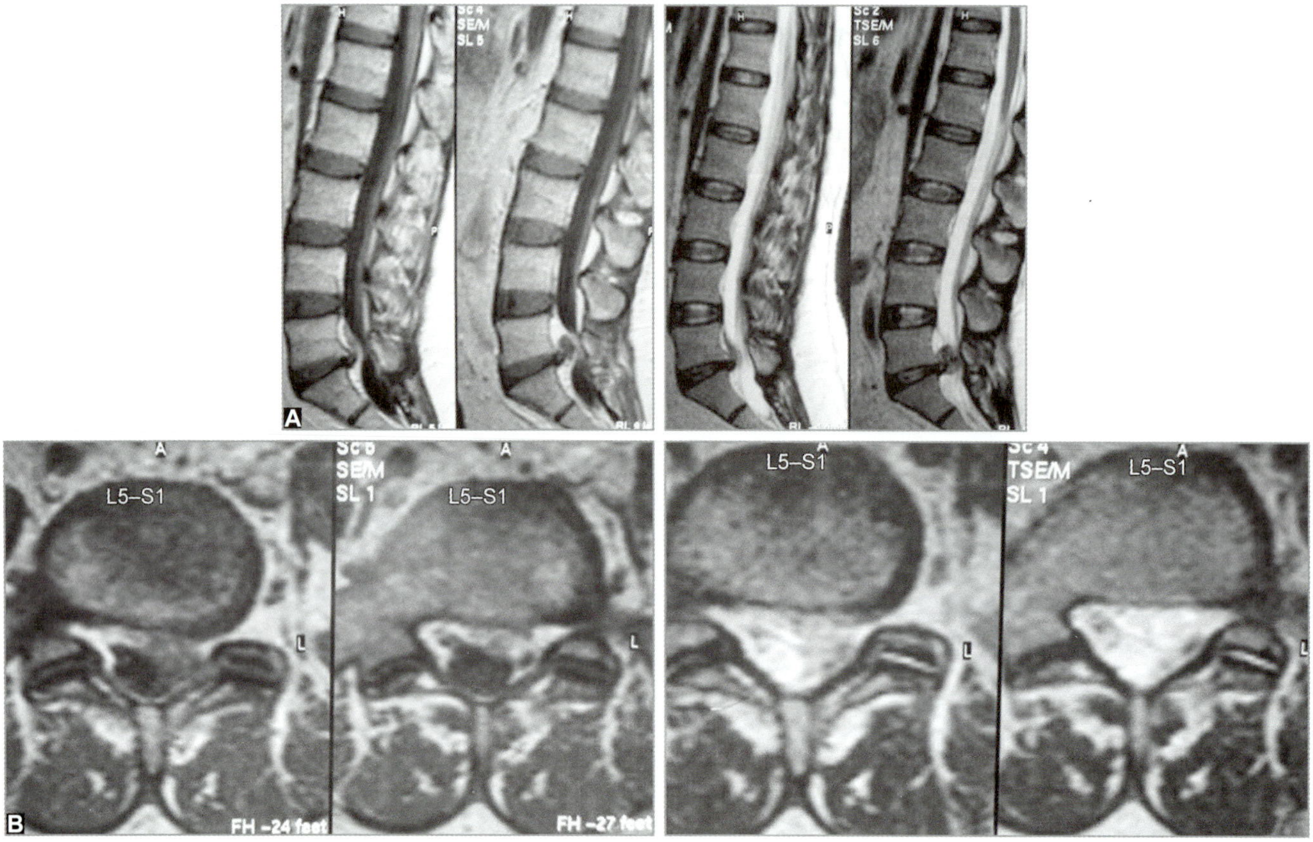

Figures 2A and B: MRI showing left paracentral disk at L5–S1

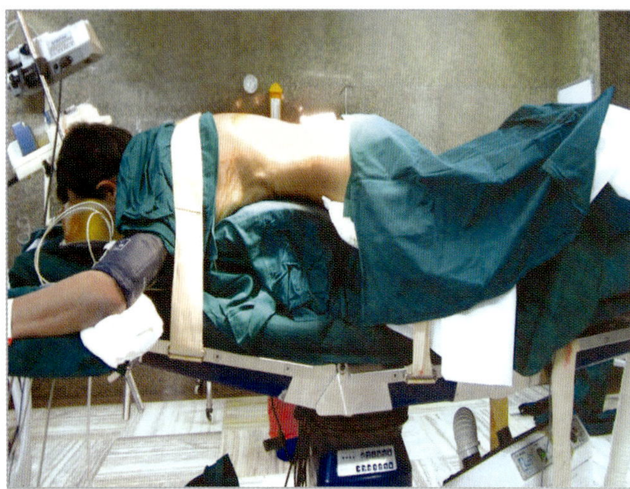

Figure 3: Patient positioned on a Wilson's frame with slight hip flexion to open the interlaminar space

the disk. In any case, obtaining an intraoperative radiograph is recommended to avoid erroneous interpretation of the level or levels exposed.

Prior to incision, the skin and subcutaneous tissue is infiltrated with 0.5% lignocaine with adrenaline, 1: 2,00,000 IU. In a MLD, a 2–3 cm incision should be sufficient for excision of the fragment. Planning for the incision should also take into consideration whether the sequestered fragment has migrated inferiorly or superiorly. After the skin has been incised, the subcutaneous tissue is divided. This can be accomplished without bleeding or trauma with blunt dissection. The lumbodorsal fascia is then exposed, and for ease of subsequent closure, it is prudent to sweep the subcutaneous fat off a short distance laterally. The fascia is then incised, just lateral to the spinous process, rather than in the midline, which allows the preservation of interspinous ligaments. Patients who have unilateral leg pain symptoms are approached from the same side or the more painful side in bilateral symptoms. The surgeon stands on the same side as the disk fragment and separates the muscles from the spinous process. Proper exposure is a crucial step in spine surgery as visualization of the lateral extent of the lamina will allow the surgeon to plan the hemilaminotomy without violating the pars interarticularis. Once exposure is complete, the self-retaining retractors are placed **(Figures 5A and B)**.

With the field prepared for bone work, the overhanging caudal lip of the rostral lamina can be partially removed, allowing for further exposure of the interlaminar ligamentum flavum. The amount of bone removal is at the surgeon's discretion and location of the herniation. The hernia and the

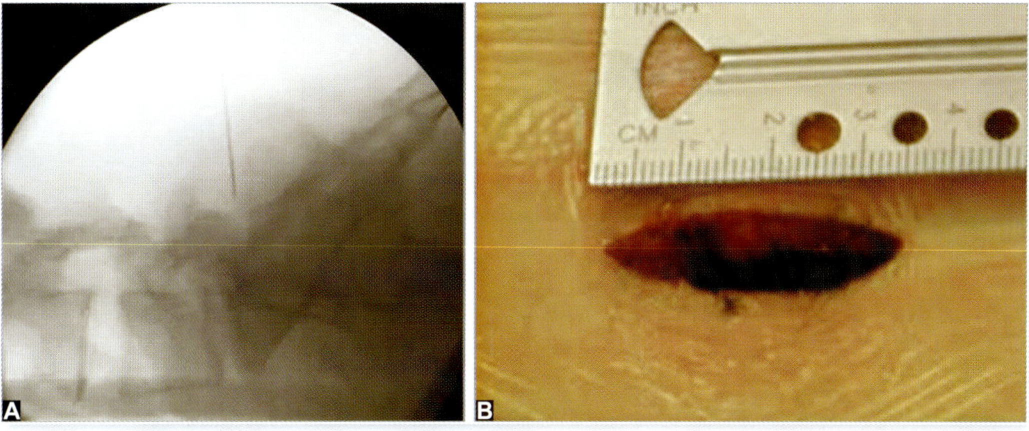

Figures 4A and B: Dateral X-ray used to localize level and 3 cm incision required for exposure

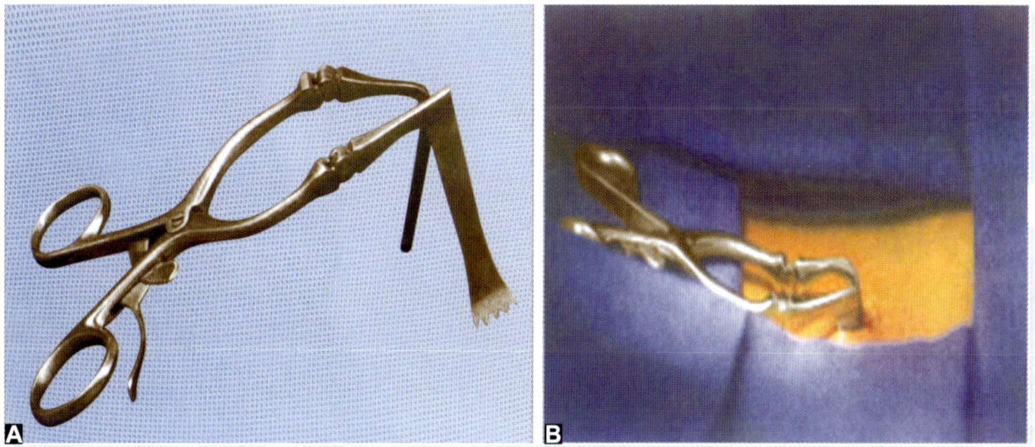

Figures 5A and B: Williams' retractor

annulus can be accessed with little or no removal of bone if one is comfortable with the amount of force necessary to retract the nerve root medially. For a lateral disk, small portion of lower border of upper lamina to get to the ligamentum flavum. A central disk can be accessed through an interlaminar approach with bilateral exposure. A paracentral disk can be reached through a standard unilateral approach. Foraminal disk will require a foraminotomy through a unilateral exposure. Extraforaminal region is accessed via drilling part of the pedicle to unroof foramen or a transforaminal approach. Excision of the flavum will enable visualization of the root and cauda equina **(Figures 6A and B)**.

A bulge in the root may be an obvious clue to the location of the disk. Other clues to a more chronic pathlogy is a decrease in the epidural fat due to chronic compression.

Large engorged epidural veins may be encounted and preserve these as much as possible. It is important to determine preoperatively on the MRI, whether the location of the disk is in the axilla or the shoulder of the nerve root. An inferiorly migrated disk is generally in the axilla of the nerve root. At times, a sequestered fragment may be impacted with the dura. Every attempt should be made to retract the root and dura medially and then releasing the disk fragment. However, an axillary impacted disk may be delivered via the axilla. In case of a shoulder disk, the nerve root once identified, can be retracted medially using a nerve root retractor. The disk is then identified.

During the course of bone removal, the underlying epidural fat is protected. The location of the foot of the punch or the edge of the curette and the location of the nerve root sleeve should be well perceived by the operating surgeon. It is worth noting that a risk of dural tear is present in every case. If a scar is present, fixing the dura mater to overlying bone, the risk of a dural tear is increased. The chance of tear is also increased in the elderly (particularly elderly women), in whom the dura mater is thin and in whom a noncompliant scar may be present, even in the absence of prior surgery.

Often, the herniated nucleus pulposus is sequestered beneath the posterior longitudinal ligament rather than being free in the spinal canal or lateral recess. A simple poke with the bipolar tips through the ligament may be all

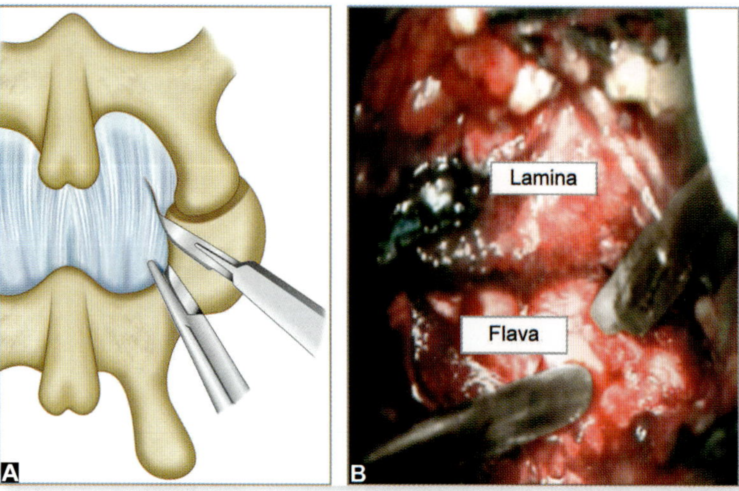

Figures 6A and B: Incision of the ligamentum flavum

that is necessary to initiate its delivery. Perhaps the most atraumatic method of removing the hernia is to grasp a small slip of the fragment with a pituitary instrument and deliver it slowly up through the ligamentous tear, serially repositioning the instrument to catch more of its bulk while doing so. The residual ligament protects the adjacent nerve root from traction.

Occasionally, the hernia represents a complete nuclear extrusion, and its attempted removal in one piece may force the nerve root medially to such an extent that injury results. It is therefore often optimal to remove it piecemeal. When the prominence has been reduced by removal of some of the herniated disk material, the nerve root is more relaxed, and more room is available for exploration with blunt angled dissecting instruments, such as a ball-ended dissector. The ventral epidural space is thoroughly palpated for any residual fragments by sweeping the dissector over the disk space. The subligamentous space is similarly palpated, as is the neural foramen rostral and lateral to the pedicle. The intervertebral disk space is then thoroughly explored and emptied of nucleus, using a combination of straight and angled pituitary rongeurs. It is often necessary to enlarge the annular tear to permit entrance of the rongeurs into the disk interspace. It is recommended that this be accomplished sharply and generously with a no. 15 or 11 blade on a long handle, fashioning a rectangular window through the annulus fibrosus. After diskectomy, the annulus, if otherwise left in the lateral recess, may prolapse or adhere to the nerve root and produce recurrent symptoms.The extent of diskectomy in contained disks has for long been a matter of debate. Nucleus material should be removed. It is neither possible nor desirable to remove all disk material. Overly aggressive curettage with removal of end-plate cartilage and excessive removal of interspace volume can result in a patulous anulus, poor mechanical support of the motion segment, and potential foraminal stenosis or instability. Removal should be limited to loose fragments that are within reach of the annular opening. Approaches range from sequestrectomy alone to aggressive curettage of the disk space, which may remain the more common procedure.

Multiple attempts are made to seek hidden disk fragments with a nerve hook till adequate nerve root decompression is performed. A pulsatile central dural sac and nerve root that is mobile is considered an adequate decompression surgery. Any epidural bleeding is controlled using a combination of bipolar cautery, bone wax and Gelfoam®.

The thoracolumbar fascia and subcutaneous tissue are closed using 2-0 Vicryl (Ethicon, Johnson and Johnson). The skin is closed using 3-0 monocryl (Johnson and Johnson Int.). A drain is often not used in MLD.

The patient is shifted to the ward and as per pain tolerance is allowed to log roll, sit and even walk. A careful physiotherapy regimen is mapped out to rehabilitate the patient to his prepathology state. Bending and lifting weights is restricted for a period of 3 weeks till soft tissues heal.

Lateral and Far Lateral Hernia

Far lateral disk hernia, with resulting compression of the nerve root in, or lateral to, the intervertebral neuroforamen, occurs in about 10% of all symptomatic annular prolapses or disks.

Extraforaminal hernia is relatively uncommon, accounting for 0.7–11.7% of all lumbar hernias. Most commonly, far lateral disk herniation occurs at L3–4, L4–5, or higher levels.

Lateral hernias occur in older patients more often than the more common dorsolateral hernias do. Lateral hernias are more likely to produce sensorimotor deficit. Radiculopathic pain may be more severe and back pain less severe than that incurred in paramedian disk hernia because of the location of the sensory root ganglion. The exposure of far lateral disks can often be more complicated than that of routine paramedian hernias. Preoperative planning is facilitated by classifying the hernia location into one of three areas and judging its accessibility accordingly. First, the lateral hernia may lie within the proximal foramen just at the medial aspect of the pedicle, and in this case can be approached through a modification of the paramedian laminotomy.

Second, it may lie in the lateral foramen and must then be approached by means of a lateral facetectomy. Third, it may lie in an extraforaminal location, in which case an extraforaminal or parasagittal approach would be necessary to avoid complete facetectomy.

A complete facetectomy may result in delayed instability and warrant an additional fusion procedure. Consequently, complete facetectomy is avoided when possible. Despite its recognition, it is still difficult to effectively treat a far lateral hernia. The most popular approach is a standard midline incision and interlaminar exposure with medial facetectomy. This approach has the advantages of greater familiarity of the surgeon with surgical anatomy, absence of bleeding, early exposure of the affected nerve root, and the ability to perform diskectomy to preclude recurrence. To gain exposure to the neuroforamen, the amount of bone that must be removed is greater than that in simple dorsolateral hernias. Tilting the table toward the operator helps greatly with visualization. Another option, building on the familiar midline exposure, is the possibility of approaching the hernia in the proximal foramen from an interlaminar approach originating from the contralateral side of the midline and proceeding across the midline and under the facet, minimizing facetectomy. Foraminotomy, with some form of partial facetectomy, is still the most popular surgical option, despite the inherent disadvantage of aggressive bone removal. Using a modification of the midline approach to address a hernia deeper within the lateral foramen, a slightly different combined interlaminar and extralaminar exposure has also been described. In the extralaminar approach, the muscle is not dissected off the spinous processes but rather incised 1 cm lateral to the midline. The facet joint is exposed, and a drill and punch are used to produce a partial lateral facetectomythrough which the rostral and caudal pedicles can be palpated. The nerve root, forced dorsally by the pathologic hernia, lies deep to the facet capsule and ligamentum flavum. It can be mobilized and retracted to address the disk hernia.

The paramedian, muscle-splitting approach has the advantage of sparing the patient the loss of bone and of providing a somewhat more oblique view of the neuroforamen. It is most useful for hernias that are within the lateral foramen or are extraforaminal. A paramedian skin and fascial incision, about 3 cm from the midline (or further lateral at lower levels), is made just over the natural plane groove between the multifidus and longissimus muscles. Descending through the paraspinous musculature between the transverse processes onto the neuroforamen from a lateral orientation, the surgeon is able to locate the lateral facet and its capsule and perhaps be able to remove only a small amount of lateral facet, if necessary.

Although the major advantage is the preservation of the pars interarticularis and the facet joint with little likelihood of instability, it has the disadvantages of surgical unfamiliarity, deeper dissection, possibly poorer visualization, difficulty enucleating the disk space, potential injury to the nerve root within the neuroforamen, This approach is exploited in tubular-assisted microdiskectomy wherein the final dilator is docked on the lamina via a paraspinal approach.

REVIEW OF LITERATURE

Advances in surgical technique and technology have seen an increase in minimally invasive (MI) techniques whereby access to the disk is gained via a tube, using a microscope or endoscope (camera) for visualization. Currently available tubular retraction systems and endoscopic systems enable simultaneous visualisation and removal of disk material via one MI working portal. MI techniques are contrasted with open microdiskectomy, which requires a larger incision and hypothetically a greater degree of muscle trauma. On the other hand, safety of the MI approach has been questioned due to the small working channel and compromised visualization. The minimal working space might make it difficult to avoid and control damage to dural and neural structures. For all the advances in surgical techniques, Steven J Kamper[6] et al. conducted a systematic review and meta-analysis in Minimally invasive surgery for lumbar disk herniation and concluded that 'there is moderate to low quality evidence of no differences in clinical outcomes between MI surgery and conventional microdiskectomy for patients with sciatica due to lumbar disk herniation. Studies comparing transforaminal MI with conventional surgery with sufficient sample size and methodological robustness are lacking.'On reviewing other techniques, such as ozone chemonucleosis, IDET and APLD, it appears that while contemplating epidural steroid injection, ozone chemonucleolysis intervention may be safe and simple, low-risk procedure that bridges between existing conservative measures and surgical diskectomy and is particularly useful in those patients without a clear-cut indication for surgical removal of the disk herniation. In studying patients undergoing ozone chemonucleolysis with a follow up of 10 years, Josip Buric et al. found that only 43.3% improved while 20% went on to require surgery.[7] A review of literature on IDET (intradiskal electrothermal therapy), a technique that involves placement of a navigable intradiskal catheter with a temperature controlled thermal resistive heating coil revealed no benefit of IDET over placebo and concluded that the evidence for efficacy of IDET remains weak and has not passed the standard of scientific proof.[8]

Chatterjee et al.[9] conducted an RCT comparing the efficacy of an automated percutaneous laser diskectomy (APLD) to the efficacy of microdiskectomy or open conventional diskectomy showed significantly worse result for patients treated with APLD (MacNab: 29% success for APLD vs. 82% success for microdiskectomy, $p < 0.001$) and concluded that the efficacy of APLD is inferior to that of microdiskectomy. Hence, it becomes clear as to why lumbar microdiskectomy is the gold standard to which all newer techniques are compared to.

Authors' Experience

In the authors' experience of over 15 years, 647 lumbar microdiskectomies have been performed with 86% excellent results and maintaining so at 10 years follow-up. 17 patients required a single **(Figures 7A to E)** revision surgery for a

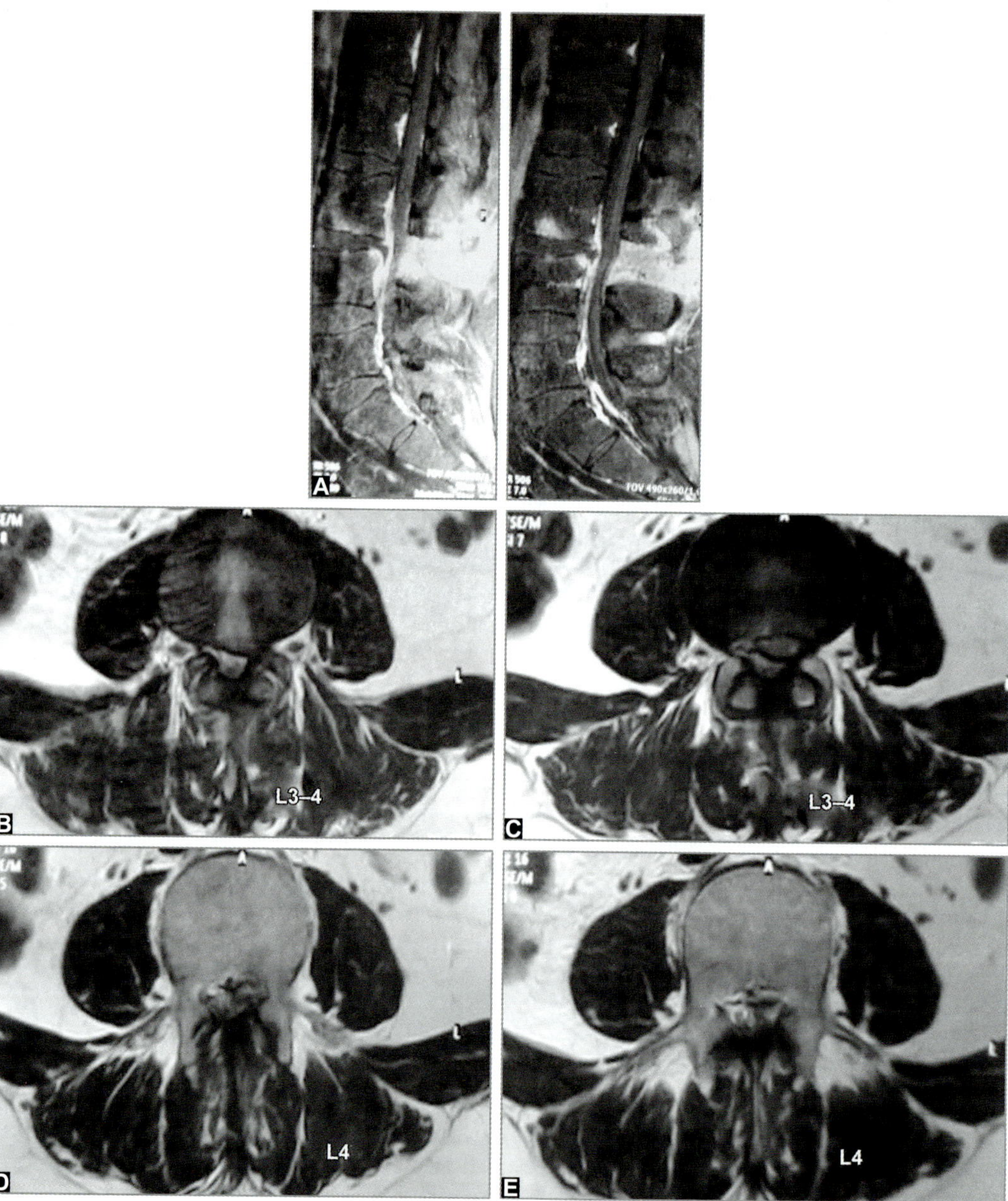

Figures 7A to E: Relapse of L3–4 after asymptomatic period

same level recurrence while 3 patients underwent revision surgery twice at the same level.

Summary

Any new adaptations of the surgical technique described above should aim to achieve either better results or at least similar results while reducing the surgical footprint. Microscopic lumbar diskectomy has further evolved into two main groups, those that use the microscope (tubular retractor assisted- interlaminar via the paraspinal approach) or the endoscope (transforaminal, interlaminar and posterolateral). While results of these adaptations are comparable to that of traditional microdiskectomy, the steep learning curve associated with them is the reason for microsurgical diskectomy remaining as the gold standard.

REFERENCES

1. Mixter WJ, Barr JS. Rupture of the intervertebral disc with involvement of the spinal canal. N Engl J Med. 1934;211:210-5.
2. Caspar W. A new surgical procedure for lumbar disc herniation causing less tissue damage through a microsurgical approach. In: Wullenweber R, Brock M, Hamer J, editors. Advances in neurosurgery. Berlin: Springer;1977. pp 74-7.
3. Yasargil MG. Microsurgical operations for herniated lumbar disc. Adv Neurosurg. 1977;4:81-2.
4. Williams RW. Microlumbar discectomy: a conservative surgical approach to the virgin herniated lumbar disc. Spine. 1978;3:175-82.
5. Fager CA. Microsurgical intervention for lumbar disc disease: a critique. 1990 Aspen p. 249.
6. Steven J Kamper, Raymond WJG Ostelo, Sidney M Rubinstein, Jorm M Nellensteijn, Wilco C Peul, Mark P Arts, et al. Minimally invasive surgery for lumbar disc herniation: a systematic review and meta-analysis. Eur Spine J. DOI 10.1007/s00586-013-3161-2. 2014;23:1021-43.
7. Josip Buric, Luca Rigobello and David Hooper. Five and Ten Year Follow-up on Intradiscal Ozone Injection for Disc Herniation. Int J Spine Surg. doi: 10.14444/1017. 2014;8:17.
8. Brian JC. Freeman. IDET: a critical appraisal of the evidence. Eur Spine J. 2006 Aug; 15(Suppl 3): 448–457.Published online. doi: 10.1007/s00586-006-0156-2. 2006; Jul 26.
9. Chatterjee S, Foy PM, Findlay GF. Report of a controlled clinical trial comparing automated percutaneous lumbar discectomy and microdiscectomy in the treatment of contained lumbar disc herniation. Spine. 1995;20(6):734-8.

18

CHAPTER

Microendoscopic Diskectomy

Aaron J Clark, Matthew T Brown, Kevin T Foley

ABSTRACT

The microendoscopic diskectomy using tubular retractor is the time-tested standard technique in lumbar prolapse and decompression surgeries. The minimal invasive nature of the procedure helps in lesser tissue trauma and faster rehabilitation. This chapter deals with the techniques, its indications and the outcomes of the procedure.

INTRODUCTION

Microendoscopic diskectomy was initially described in 1997.[1] Although percutaneous lumbar spine techniques had been previously reported, the bed-mounted tubular retractor allowed the surgeon to operate with two hands and, thus, the application of standard time-tested surgical techniques through a small incision with less muscle destruction.[2] This made possible the removal of not only contained disk herniations, but also free fragments and bony compression in the lateral recess. Subsequent modification of the tubular retractor allowed usage of the operating microscope for minimally invasive (MIS) microdiskectomy. In large part, these developments ushered in the widespread practice of outpatient lumbar spine decompression surgery. In the United States health care system, this has translated into total hospital cost savings of $5453 per procedure.[3] Importantly, similar and very favorable clinical outcomes can be expected from MIS and standard microdiskectomy.[4-6] Studies have demonstrated equivalent operative times compared to the standard open microdiskectomy, with lower blood loss and shorter hospital stays.[7-9] Furthermore, postoperative analgesia usage is significantly lower after MIS microdiskectomy. Operative times and overall rates of complications are no different for MIS microdiskectomy compared to open.[6,10] This is particularly true once surgeons have progressed along the well-documented learning curve.[11] This chapter will highlight the appropriate usage, surgical nuances, and clinical outcomes of MIS microdiskectomy.

INDICATIONS AND APPLICATIONS

The indications for MIS microdiskectomy are the same as for the standard open approach. Patients must have radicular symptoms in a distribution that correlates with imaging evidence of a herniated lumbar disk with neural compression. Patients with radicular pain of short duration should first undergo a trial of conservative management consisting of nonsteroidal anti-inflammatory medications, physical therapy, and epidural or transforaminal steroid injections. Those who fail non-operative management, those with progressive severe motor deficits, or those with symptoms of cauda equina syndrome are candidates for MIS microdiskectomy.

There are no unique contraindications for MIS microdiskectomy compared to the open approach. Patients with associated instability at the level of the disk herniation should not be treated with a decompression alone. Likewise, patients with foraminal compromise due to severe degenerative disk disease or asymmetric disk collapse due to degenerative scoliosis may require complete diskectomy with interbody grafting to increase the vertical height of the foramen. Recurrent disk herniation is not a contraindication for an MIS approach.[12] In fact, anecdotally, MIS treatment of a recurrence after a standard midline approach microdiskectomy may be slightly easier than a second midline approach as the MIS approach avoids the midline dense scar tissue from the initial operation.[13]

APPLIED ANATOMY

At the surface, the spinous processes mark the midline. Although lumbar level should always be definitively identified on fluoroscopy, the intercrest line transecting the highest points on the iliac crests usually marks the level of the L4/5 disk space **(Figures 1A and B)**. The anatomy relevant to MIS microdiskectomy relates to the superior and inferior lamina that define the interlaminar space overlying the disk herniation, the associated superior and inferior articular processes, and the pedicle **(Figures 2A and B)**.

With the patient in the prone position, the spinous process projects vertically. In the lumbar spine, the multifidus muscle arises from the mammillary processes laterally, runs superomedially to insert into the spinous process of the superior vertebral body or higher. As the bony structure begins to curve horizontally it becomes the lamina. The ligamentum flavum is located between the adjacent laminae. It inserts caudally on the anterior surface of the caudal lamina and cranially on the anterosuperior surface of the cranial lamina. This is important when bone removal from the caudal lamina is required, there is no ligamentum between the bony undersurface and the dura. The laminae are continuous with the superior and inferior articular processes by the pars interarticularis. The inferior articular process from the level above, the superior articular process from the level above, and the interposed synovial joint articulation define the facet joint which is covered by a joint capsule. In the axial plane, the angle of the facet joints becomes steeper in the upper lumbar spine compared to the lower. This becomes important when performing a medial facetectomy in the upper lumbar spine. The pedicle is located at the junction between the lamina and the pars. The nerve root exits the spinal canal below its numbered pedicle. The posterior longitudinal ligament (PLL) runs along the posterior surface of the vertebral bodies and is

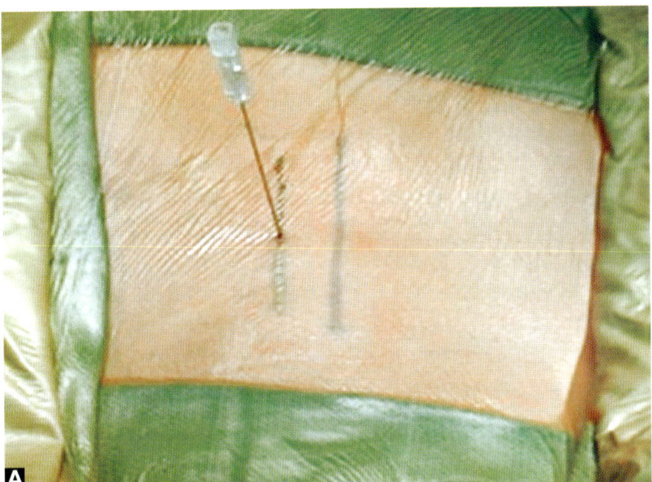

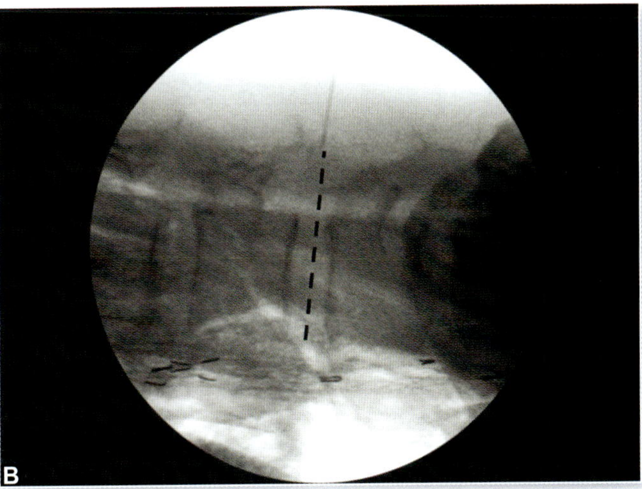

Figures 1A and B: Marking of skin incision with needle at level of disk space

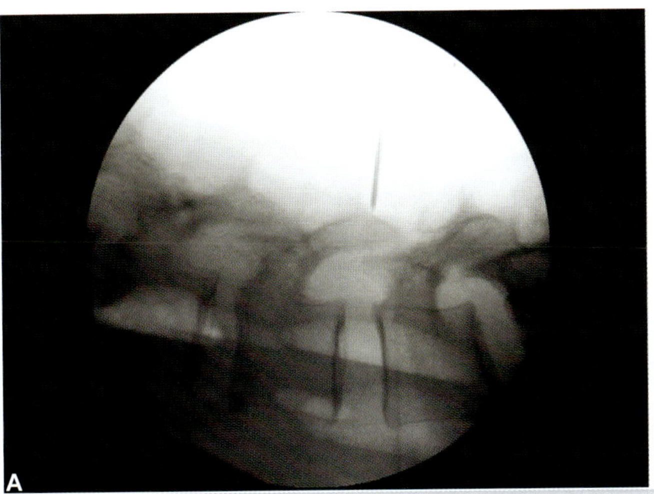

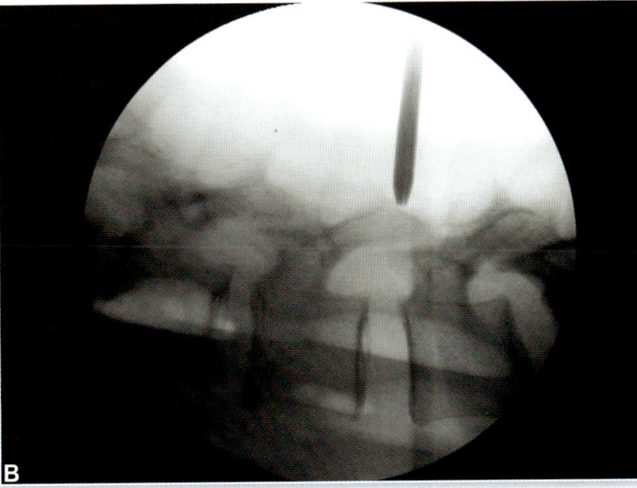

Figures 2A and B: Visualization of level with C-arm

weaker than the anterior longitudinal ligament which runs along the anterior surface. The PLL attaches to the annulus fibrosis, the fibrous rings which surrounds and contains the nucleus pulposus.

The tubular retractor is docked at the base of the spinous process on the inferior border of the superior lamina. The docking point is generally located 1.5 cm from midline.

TECHNIQUES

Preoperative planning should include magnetic resonance or CT myelographic evidence of a herniated disk at the level appropriate for the radicular symptoms obtained from a thorough history and physical examination. Lateral flexion-extension view radiographs can confirm spinal stability at the level of interest with no evidence of subluxation.

The authors prefer to perform these procedures under general anesthesia. Although the use of local or epidural anesthesia is possible, general anesthesia has the benefit of lack of patient movement during surgery and also the ability to obtain a full neurologic examination immediately on awakening. The patient is then positioned prone on the operating room table. We use the Wilson frame as it allows for suspension of the abdomen and opening of the interlaminar space. The fluoroscopy unit is then brought into position and a lateral fluoroscopic image is obtained. Care should be taken to position the patient as far as possible to the head of the bed, so that the base of the operating room table does not obstruct the fluoroscopy unit in the lower lumbar region. When draping, a wide area should be prepared as the incision has not yet been planned. The surgeon should stand on the side of the pathology with the fluoroscopy unit opposite.

The midline is marked by palpating the spinous processes. A parallel line is then drawn 15 mm ipsilateral to the side of the pathology. For morbidly obese patients and those with bulbous spinous processes, the line can be drawn a few millimeters more to the side. The incision is planned by first inserting a 22 gauge spinal needle through the skin along a trajectory that exactly bisects the disk space of interest. A 16 mm vertical incision is then made with the needle mark as the midpoint and is only carried down to the subcutaneous tissue. A sharp guidewire is then placed under fluoroscopic guidance along the same trajectory, piercing the dorsal lumbar fascia. An initial tubular dilator is passed over the guidewire. Once the dilator has passed through the fascia, the guidewire can be removed. The initial dilator is then used to palpate the lamina to ensure correct docking location. The second dilator is then passed over the initial dilator. At this point the dilators can be removed and straight Mayo scissors can be placed in the fascial defect and spread in a vertical direction to dilate the fascia and muscles. The initial dilator is then replaced followed by the second, third, and fourth **(Figures 3A and B)**. Once the trajectory is confirmed, the 16 mm tubular retractor is placed over the third dilator and docked on bone. The flexible arm is attached on the side ipsilateral to the surgeon **(Figure 4)**. Downward pressure while securing the tubular retractor prevents paraspinal muscle from entering the tube **(Figure 5)**.

The operating microscope is then brought into place. Residual soft tissue can now be removed with the pituitary rongeur **(Figure 6)**. Hemostasis is achieved with bipolar and bovie cautery. The inferior edge of the lamina is defined and the lamina is removed with the high speed drill. The lamina is removed until the superior insertion of the ligamentum flavum is visualized **(Figures 7 and 8)**. To progress superiorly, the tubular retractor can be "wanded" in which the largest dilator is reinserted into the tubular retractor, the flexible arm is loosened, and the retractor is angled superiorly while applying steady downward pressure to avoid unwanted soft tissue encroaching on the operative corridor. The ligamentum flavum is dissected free of the

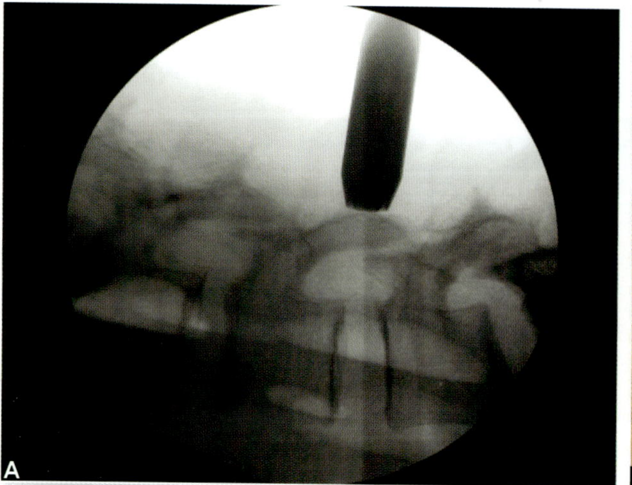

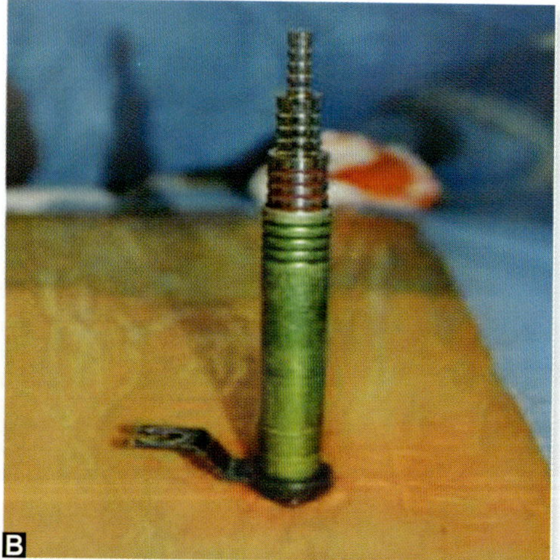

Figures 3A and B: Progressive dilatation with dilators

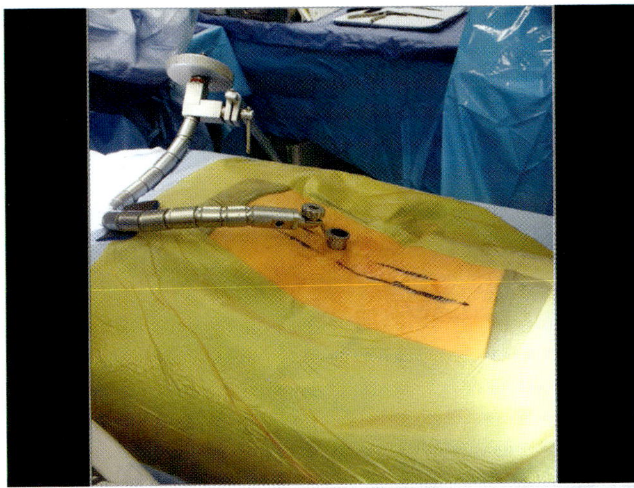

Figure 4: Banking the apparatus to the table

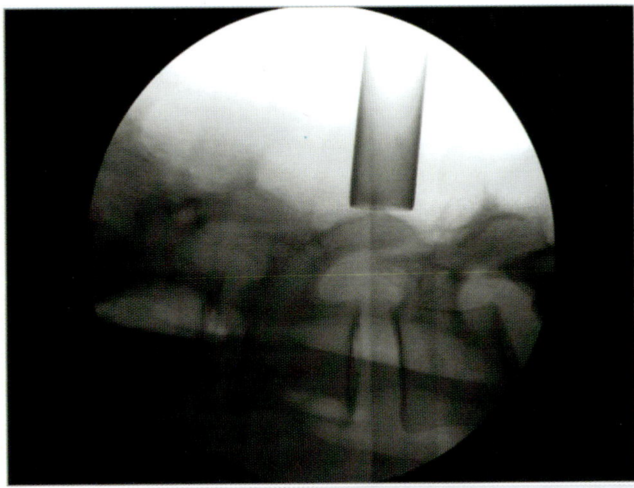

Figure 5: Final dilator on C-arm

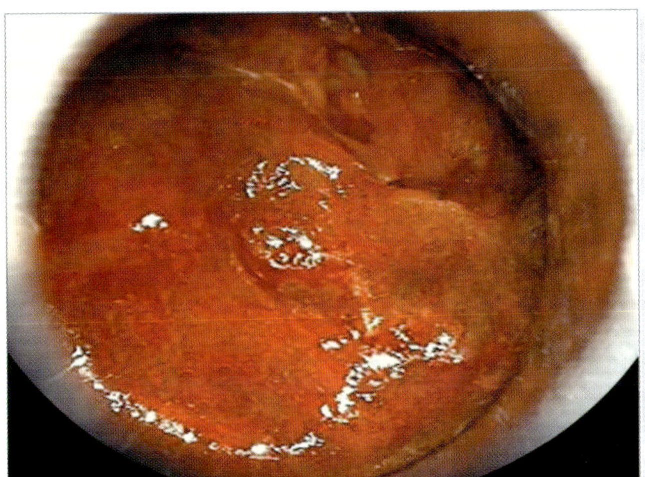

Figure 6: Paraspinal muscle dissection

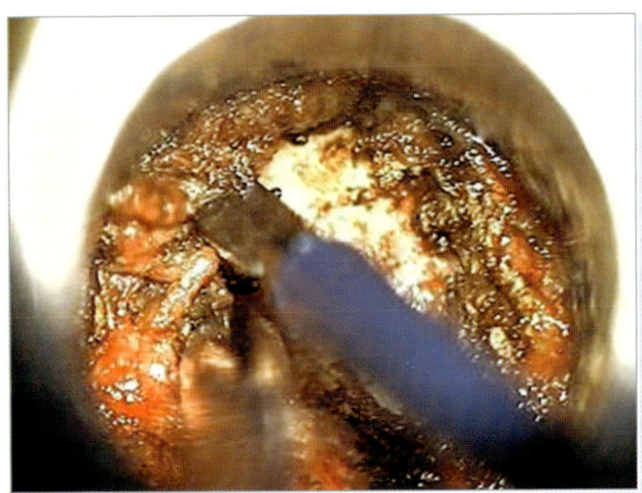

Figure 7: Lamina freed of attachments

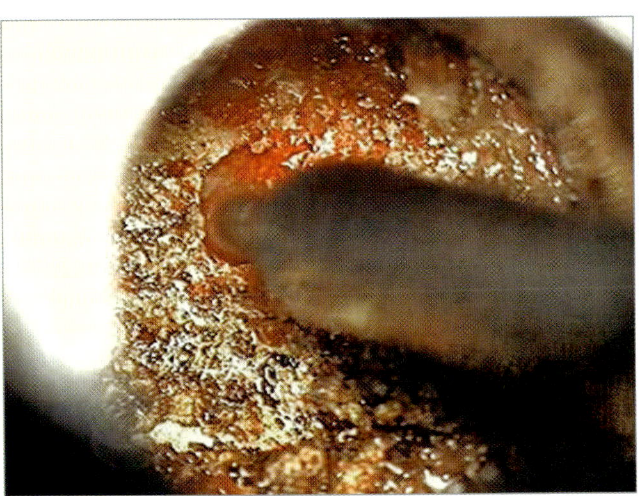

Figure 8: Laminotomy with burr

underlying dura with a modified ball dissector and is then resected with Kerrison rongeurs **(Figure 9)**. The resection should continue until the lateral edge of the traversing nerve root is visualized **(Figure 10)**. A medial facetectomy can be performed if necessary to obtain this critical visualization. When the ball dissector can easily pass along the medial border of the inferior pedicle, the dorsal decompression is complete.

The tubular retractor is then "wanded" until the trajectory is along the axis of the disk of interest. The nerve root retractor is placed to protect the traversing nerve root which is retracted medially **(Figure 11)**. Epidural veins are coagulated with bipolar cautery. Free disk fragments can be removed with the pituitary rongeur. Contained disk herniations are approached by incision the annulus fibrosis overlying the mass with a #15 bayoneted scalpel. The mass

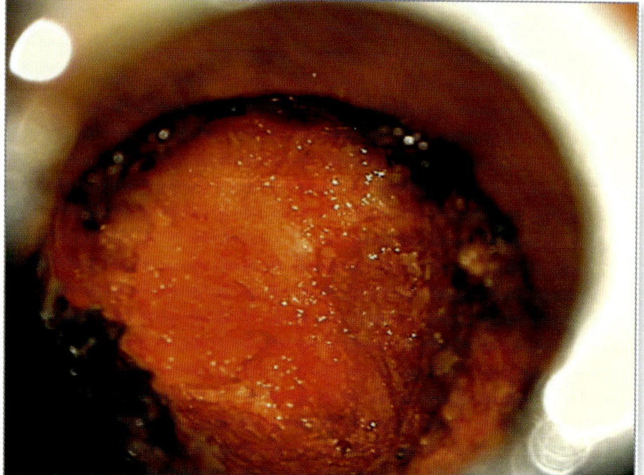

Figure 9: Visualization of flavum

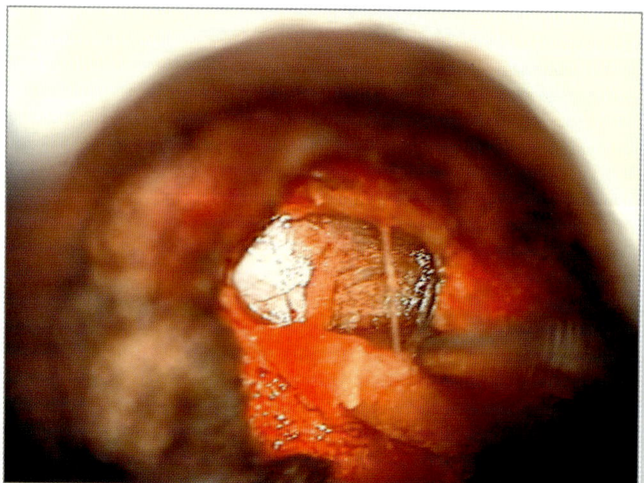

Figure 10: Flavum excision

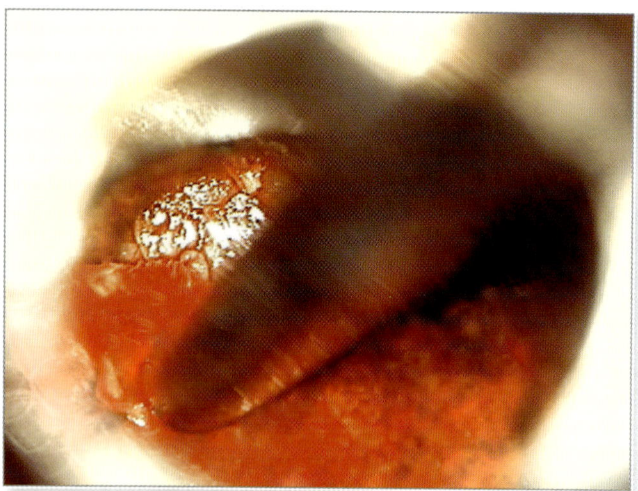

Figure 11: Visualization of root

is then decompressed with a combination of straight and angled pituitary rongeurs and curettes. The decompression is complete when a ball dissector can be freely passed beneath the traversing nerve root and thecal sac without encountering a mass and all loose fragments have been removed **(Figures 12A to C)**.

Hemostasis is obtained with gelfoam and bipolar cautery. A gelfoam sponge soaked in 40 mg Depo-Medrol can be placed on an irritated appearing nerve root. The tubular retractor is then removed while visualizing the intact muscle fibers coming together to close the potential space. A single Vicryl stitch is used to approximate the dorsal lumbar fascia. Vicryl suture is used to close the dermis in an inverted interrupted fashion. The skin is approximated with steri-strips. A waterproof dressing is applied so patients can shower.

Postoperatively, patients are mobilized immediately. They are diskharged home after a few hours of observation. Patients are prescribed 600 mg TID of oral ibuprofen for 3 weeks and low dose oral acetaminophen-oxycodone to be used on a PRN basis. They are seen in clinic in 1 week for a wound check and 6 weeks for a follow-up postsurgical visit. Most patients do not require postoperative physical therapy or rehabilitation.

COMPLICATIONS

Complication profiles are similar for MIS microdiskectomy compared to the standard open technique. Intraoperative dural tear is the most common complication. Rates range from 7–10%.[8,9,14-16] There are several technical nuances to avoid this frequent complication. First, once the tubular retractor is docked in the appropriate location, complete bony removal with the drill and rongeurs should be performed using the entire operative field within the tube. This bony decompression relieves some of the stenosis allowing for free passage of instruments adjacent to the dura. A ball dissector should be passed under the ligamentum flavum prior to flavectomy to eliminate tethering adhesions which could otherwise lead to durotomy. While removing the ligamentum flavum, the use of angled Kerrison rongeurs can avoid inadvertent entry of the dura into the jaws of the instrument. We prefer to use the 90° rongeur when progressing medially and superiorly while using the 40° instrument when removing tissue laterally and inferiorly. Lastly, using the suction to provide gentle traction on the adjacent dura when removing tissue can prevent redundant dura from billowing into the instrument. Neural injury to the traversing nerve root is a serious but rare intraoperative complication with reported rates of 0–3%.[14-16] Clear identification of the relevant anatomy is required to prevent this complication. It is particularly important to define the lateral edge of the traversing root. Free passage of the ball dissector along the inferior pedicle delineates the lateral margin of bony removal. Being able to pass the

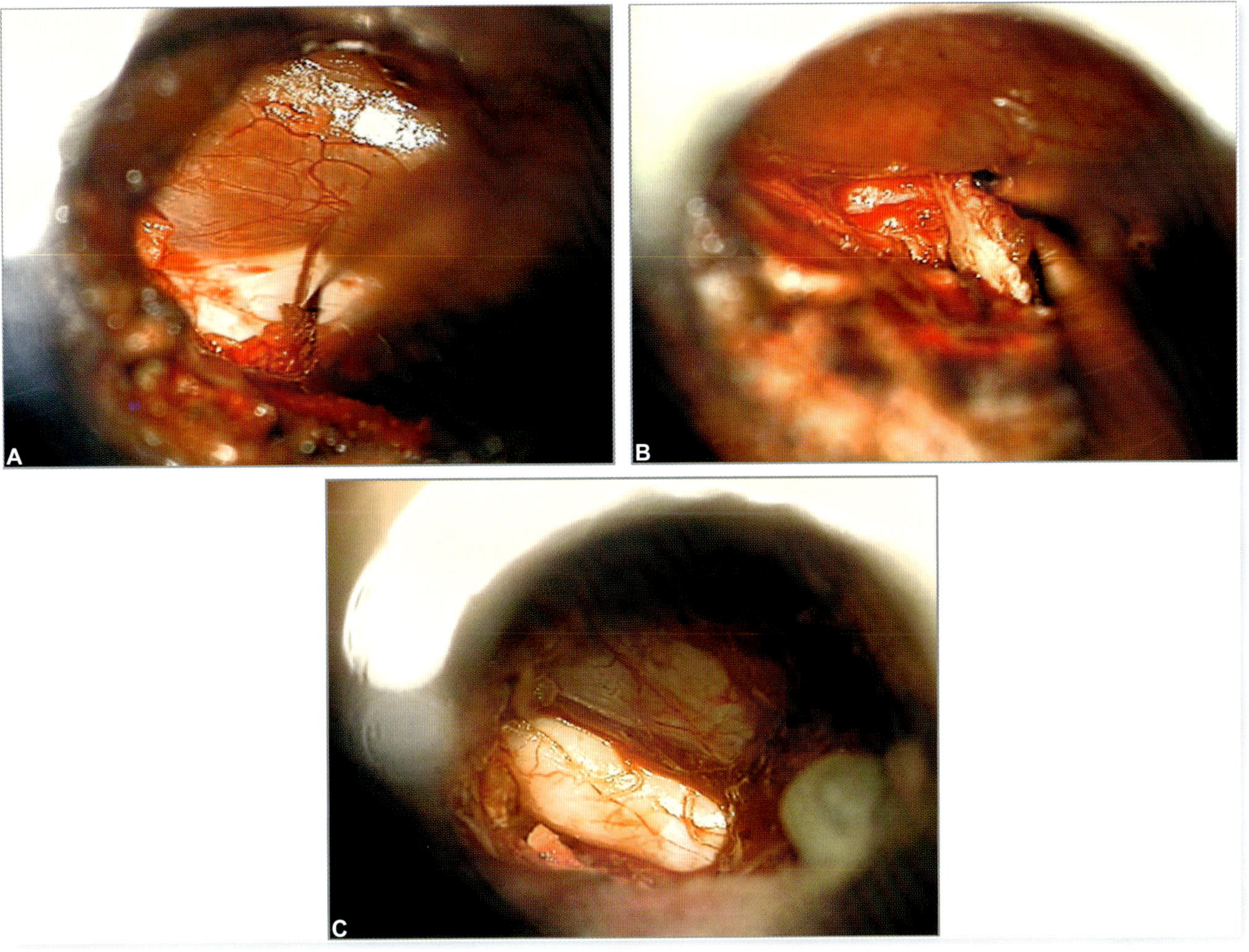

Figures 12A to C: Visualization of contralateral roots

ball dissector under the nerve root confirms that the lateral edge is being visualized. In cases of revision surgery, it is important to remove additional bone superior to the previous laminotomy to access normal dura and then follow that plane into the scarred area.

Postoperative infection after MIS microdiskectomy is extremely uncommon with a reported rate of 0.1% in a large prospectively collected database.[17] This is likely due to the smaller incision and lack of significant devascularized tissue. Most rare cases can be managed with a course of antibiotics; however, deep or persistent infections may require debridement. In our practice, we use preoperative prophylactic intravenous antibiotics and generous irrigation with antibiotic containing sterile saline at the conclusion of the operation. Postoperative painful hematoma is a rare complication with rates of 1%.[14] This can be avoided with the judicious use of gelfoam and the technique of slowly removing the tubular retractor under microscopic visualization and hemostasis with bipolar cautery. Recurrent disk herniation is a consideration after all diskectomy procedures. Published rates after MIS diskectomy range from 2 to 11%.[9,14-16] Free disk fragments are removed by fragmentectomy. Contained disk herniations are removed by annulotomy and disk exploration. All loose disk material is removed. At the conclusion of diskectomy, 10 cc of sterile saline (using a 10 cc syringe with a 8 French suction tip attached) is forcefully irrigated into the annulotomy site to loosen any residual tissue that would be at risk for re-herniation.

CONCLUSION

MIS diskectomy represents a highly efficacious surgical treatment option for patients with primary or recurrent disk herniation. In experienced hands, it is associated with favorable clinical outcomes with a low complication profile. Familiarity with the technique and relevant anatomy is required. Meticulous technique and several technical nuances can help avoid unnecessary complications.

REFERENCES

1. Foley KT, Smith MM. Microendoscopic diskectomy. Techniques in Neurosurgery. 1997;3(4):301-7.
2. Kim CW. Scientific basis of minimally invasive spine surgery: prevention of multifidus muscle injury during posterior lumbar surgery. Spine (Phila Pa 1976). 2010;35(26 Suppl):S281-6.
3. Cahill KS, Levi AD, Cummock MD, Liao W, Wang MY. A comparison of acute hospital charges after tubular versus open microdiskectomy. World Neurosurg. 2013;80(1-2):208-12.
4. Brock M, Kunkel P, Papavero L. Lumbar microdiskectomy: subperiosteal versus transmuscular approach and influence on the early postoperative analgesic consumption. Eur Spine J. 2008;17(4):518-22.
5. Righesso O, Falavigna A, Avanzi O. Comparison of open diskectomy with microendoscopic diskectomy in lumbar disk herniations: results of a randomized controlled trial. Neurosurgery. 2007;61(3):545-9; diskussion 549.
6. Ryang YM, Oertel MF, Mayfrank L, Gilsbach JM, Rohde V. Standard open microdiskectomy versus minimal access trocar microdiskectomy: results of a prospective randomized study. Neurosurgery. 2008;62(1):174-81; discussion 181-172.
7. Huang TJ, Hsu RW, Li YY, Cheng CC. Less systemic cytokine response in patients following microendoscopic versus open lumbar diskectomy. Journal of Orthopaedic Research: official publication of the Orthopaedic Research Society. 2005;23(2):406-11.
8. German JW, Adamo MA, Hoppenot RG, Blossom JH, Nagle HA. Perioperative results following lumbar diskectomy: comparison of minimally invasive diskectomy and standard microdiskectomy. Neurosurg Focus. 2008;25(2):E20.
9. Lau D, Han SJ, Lee JG, Lu DC, Chou D. Minimally invasive compared to open microdiskectomy for lumbar disk herniation. J Clin Neurosci. 2011;18(1):81-4.
10. Dasenbrock HH, Juraschek SP, Schultz LR, et al. The efficacy of minimally invasive diskectomy compared with open diskectomy: a meta-analysis of prospective randomized controlled trials. J Neurosurg Spine. 2012;16(5):452-62.
11. Sclafani JA, Kim CW. Complications associated with the initial learning curve of minimally invasive spine surgery: a systematic review. Clin Orthop Relat Res. 2014;472(6):1711-7.
12. Ahn J, Tabaraee E, Bohl DD, Aboushaala K, Singh K. Primary Versus Revision Single-Level Minimally Invasive Lumbar Diskectomy: Analysis of Clinical Outcomes and Narcotic Utilization. Spine (Phila Pa 1976). 2015.
13. Smith JS, Ogden AT, Shafizadeh S, Fessler RG. Clinical outcomes after microendoscopic diskectomy for recurrent lumbar disk herniation. J Spinal Disord Tech. 2010;23(1):30-4.
14. Arts MP, Brand R, van den Akker ME, et al. Tubular diskectomy vs conventional microdiskectomy for sciatica: a randomized controlled trial. JAMA: the Journal of the American Medical Association. 2009;302(2):149-58.
15. Lee P, Liu JC, Fessler RG. Perioperative results following open and minimally invasive single-level lumbar diskectomy. J Clin Neurosci. 2011;18(12):1667-70.
16. Teli M, Lovi A, Brayda-Bruno M, et al. Higher risk of dural tears and recurrent herniation with lumbar micro-endoscopic diskectomy. Eur Spine J. 2010;19(3):443-50.
17. Shousha M, Cirovic D, Boehm H. Infection rate after minimally invasive noninstrumented spinal surgery based on 4350 procedures. Spine (Phila Pa 1976). 2015;40(3):201-5.

19

CHAPTER

Microendoscopy for Lumbar Disk Prolapse

Amit Jhala, Dhruv Patel

ABSTRACT

Microendoscopic diskectomy is minimally invasive tubular decompression technique for lumbar diskectomy. The chapter describes the evolution and advantages of MED over other standard diskectomy. The indications, preoperative planning, technique, applications and complications are described in detail. Outcomes of the MED have been discussed. MED is safe and effective for all types of lumbar diskectomy and is considered the stepping-stone for further evolution in minimally invasive spine surgery.

INTRODUCTION

The lumbar diskectomy is one of the basic surgeries of the spine and the methods of diskectomy and lumbar decompression continue to evolve in efforts to perform a surgical decompression. A direct decompression simply requires an operative corridor to access the spinal canal and decompress the nerve root. Surgical options for lumbar diskectomy include traditional open diskectomy, which evolved to microdiskectomy later on with use of microscope giving magnification and light for better anatomical visualization. Use of microscope had advantage of smaller skin incision, less bleeding and infection and preservation of soft tissues, which reflected clinically as less postoperative pain and early return to work. In 1997, the microendoscopic diskectomy (MED) system was introduced by Foley et al. which allowed surgeons to decompress a symptomatic nerve root reliably using an endoscope.[1] This was a conceptual advance in decreasing approach related morbidity as it utilized muscle-spitting paraspinal approach with the use of tubular retractors for access. Instead of cutting or separating the Paraspinal muscles from the spinous process the tubular retractor was introduced through the muscle by sequentially dilating the paraspinal muscles and hence preserving the attachment of the paraspinal muscle to the bone. This has led to less paraspinal muscle tissue injury and muscle atrophy with clinical effect of preserving the Paraspinal muscle strength.[2-6] This procedure offers many advantages over open diskectomy and Microdiskectomy techniques like smaller skin incision, reduced tissue trauma, preservation of muscle damage due to limited retraction, early ambulation, shorter hospital stay and early return to work with proven efficacy in literature. The use of tubular retractor approach has significant advantage over microdiskectomy in subset of patients requiring lumbar diskectomy, which generally would require larger incision, which would add to morbidity especially in cases of obese patients, elderly patient with comorbidities, far lateral disk herniation and recurrent herniations. By doing tubular diskectomies it would definitely help surgeon in further evolving into this technique to decrease the learning curve for doing additional procedures through tubular approach like decompressions in lumbar canal stenosis, multilevel lumbar decompressions, lumbar interbody fusions and applying same technique in cervical and thoracic regions also. Considering the versatility of this approach in overall application of minimally invasive approach in different regions and variety of different indications in spine surgery, tubular diskectomy becomes the base of the pillar of minimally invasive spine surgery.

INDICATIONS AND APPLICATIONS

Clinical indications of doing microendoscopic lumbar diskectomy remain traditionally same. The patients should have a radicular pain, which is not relieved by adequate conservative trial for around six weeks unless the patient is suffering from major neurological deficit like cauda equina syndrome or progressive deficit in which case early intervention is required. One should be able to clinically correlate the root involved with the radiological MRI picture. It is imperative to get X-rays, including dynamic views in patients to rule out any obvious instability.

Radiologically, on MRI the classical indications are paramedian and sequestrated or extruded disk herniations. With the experience and overcoming learning curve the extended indications are central disk herniation, foraminal and extraforaminal disk herniations and recurrent disk herniations. Associated pathologies along with the disk herniations, which can be dealt with, are central and lateral canal stenosis. Technique of MED can be used after enough experience for opposite side decompressions by over-the-top technique and double herniations like L-45 and L5-S1 para median herniations on the same side with single approach.

CONTRAINDICATION

There is no absolute contraindication for MED in disk herniations as with overcoming of the learning curve almost all types of the herniations can be dealt with.

APPLIED ANATOMY

Surgical approach for microendoscopic diskectomy needs a special attention. The approach is not midline as in traditional microdiskectomy but paraspinal and working space is through the tubes and targeted to pathology as opposed to microdiskectomy. As tubular retractors spare the multifidus muscle attachments to spinous processes and gains its access through the muscle by dilating them, the anatomy on approach to bone is slightly different. This will give a focused view of the field without any peripheral view. The orientation and anatomy through the tube should be very clear. The diameter of the tube, depth of the tube, docking point on the spine and the trajectory or angle of the tube defines the orientation and tubular anatomy. The docking point for the paramedian disk herniation is at the inferior edge of the superior lamina. Sometimes, because of some muscle creep and soft tissues the peripheral view is lost and one can view only bone; hence the orientation and anatomy is lost. The tubular anatomy and orientation for diskectomy on docking is as shown in **Figure 1**.

Preoperative Planning

Preoperative evaluation should include thorough clinical examination, identifying the exact root involved giving rise to symptoms. This should be complemented by radiological identification by MRI of the root compressed by the disk herniation. Clinicoradiological correlation is extremely important as MED being targeted approach extension of approach is very difficult during the surgical procedure. The site, size and type of disk herniation and associated stenosis should be identified on MRI. The docking of the retractor depends on the type of pathology on MRI. CT scan is sparsely used but plain X-rays are useful for identifying the segmentation problems of spine to avoid wrong levels and any instability on flexion and extension views.

SURGICAL TECHNIQUE

Patient is positioned prone after general anesthesia on two transverse bolsters keeping in mind no to have excessive lumbar lordosis with hip and knee flexed and abdomen free taking care of eyes and padding for bony pressure points **(Figure 2)**. The patient should be adequately taped so that it allows for table to be tilted on either side if required during decompression.

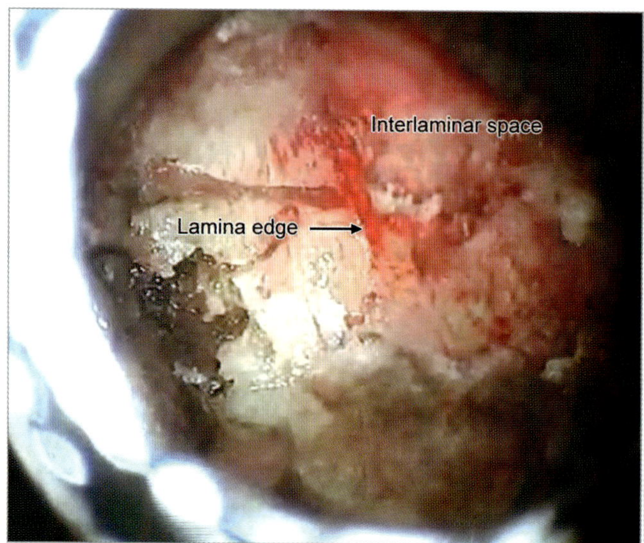

Figure 1: Anatomy as seen through tubular retractor

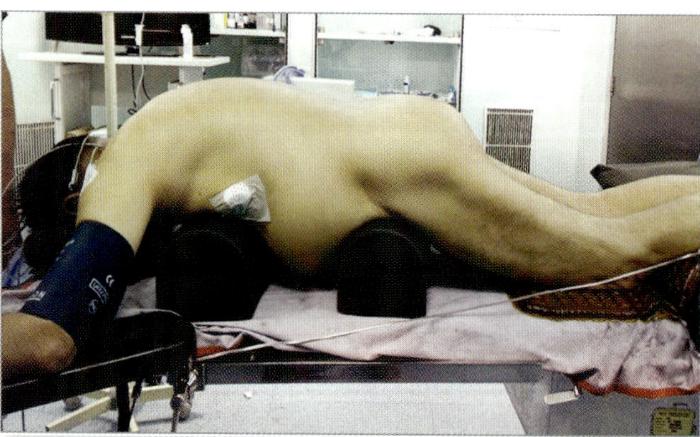

Figure 2: Position for MED

The lumbar level to be approached is confirmed by AP and lateral fluoroscopy. The operating field is prepared, painted and draped. Under fluoroscopy guidance marking is done in AP and lateral view. In AP view the docking point is marked at the inferior edge of superior lamina approximately finger breadth on the side of midline **(Figure 3)**. In lateral view, the marker should be parallel to the disk space. Vertical skin incision of approximately 18 mm is made over the marked site keeping the marking in the center of the incision. Incision length matches the desired diameter of respective tubular retractor.

After incising skin, thoracolumbar fascia is incised in the direction of skin incision. We do not use K-wire or guide-wire in our routine practice as it may accidently cause dural puncture. First, dilator is inserted and docked over the desired docking point and position confirmed under fluoroscopy. Tip of dilator is used to sweep the paraspinal muscles from the laminar edge while palpating the lamina. Care must be taken not to enter the spinal canal.

Sequential dilators are passed over the initial dilator down to the lamina **(Figure 4A)**. Dilatation should be smooth and ensure sufficient facial opening to allow the last

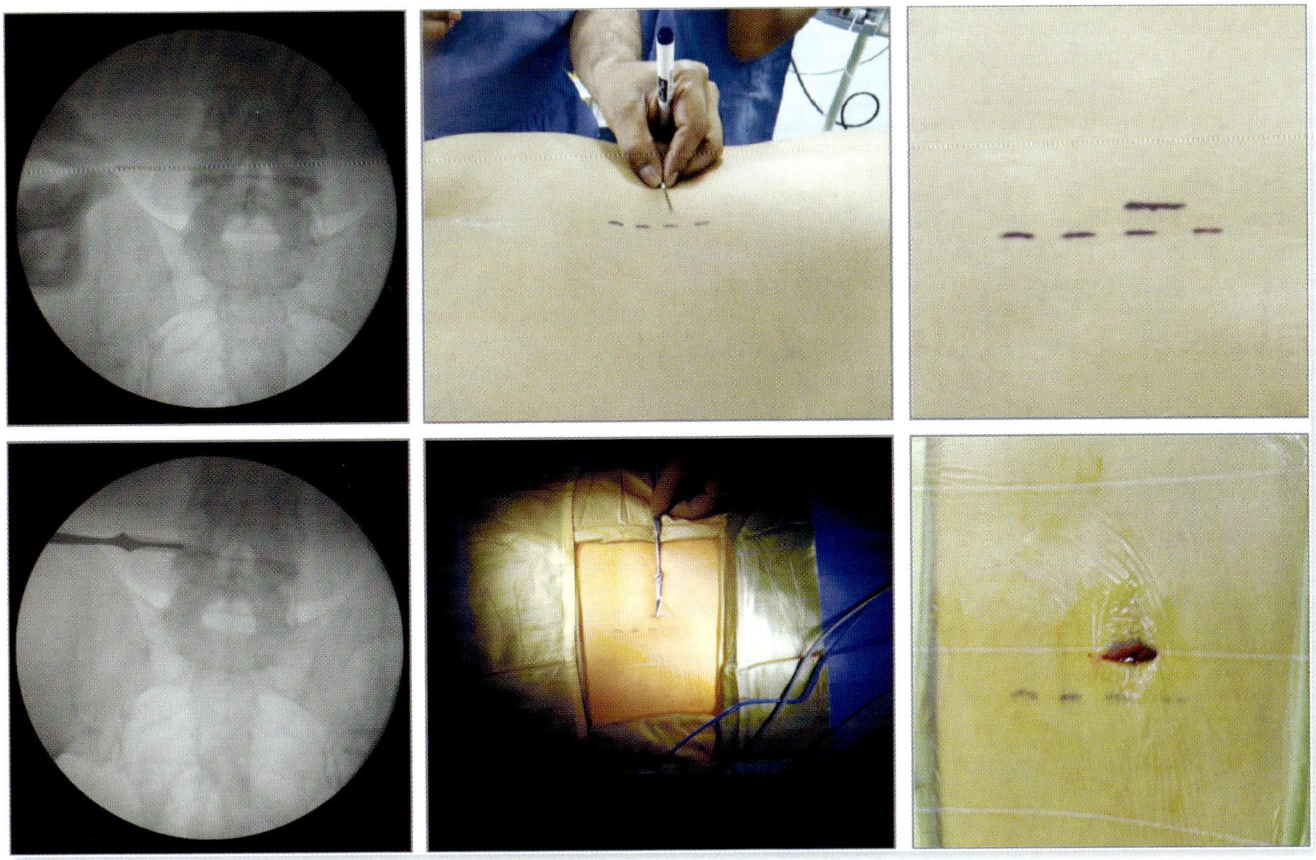

Figure 3: Docking point and marking of skin incision for diskectomy

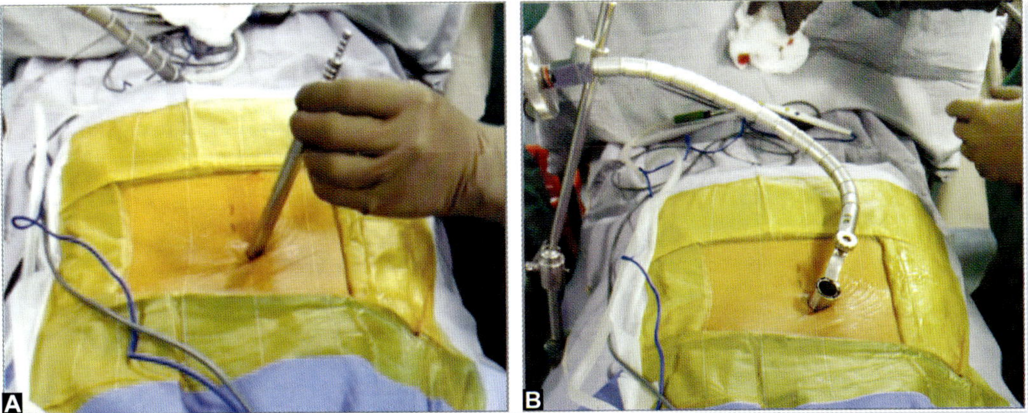

Figures 4A and B: (A) Sequential dilatation of muscles by dilators; (B) Placement of tubular retractor

dilator to glide in. Final working channel or tubular retractor is placed over the final dilator. The flexible arm, which was secured to the table, was attached to the tubular retractor to hold it firmly in place once positioned. The attachment of the flexible arm should be such that it does not come in way of the surgeon while working. The sequential dilators are then removed to establish a tubular operative corridor to the superior lamina, interlaminar space, yellow ligament and the medial portion of facet joint **(Figure 4B)**. Fluoroscopy is used to check the final positioning **(Figure 5)**.

After docking is complete either endoscope or microscope is used for further visualization to get magnification and lighting. Ensure clean view inside the tubular retractor. The soft tissue over the lamina and the interlaminar space is removed by electrocautery and inferior edge of the superior lamina is identified to start removal of the lamina for fenestration.

A hemilaminotomy is done with the help of Kerrison rongeur or high-speed burr. The lamina removal is ideally limited up to the upper margin of the ligamentum flavum to free the ligamentum flavum **(Figure 6A)**. A 90-degree Penfield is used to lift the ligamentum flavum and separating it from underlying dural sac **(Figure 6B)**. Ligament is removed piecemeal to expose the thecal sac and traversing nerve root **(Figure 6C)**. The nerve root is then retracted medially by Penfield dissector **(Figure 6D)**. Volar epidural space is then exposed and epidural veins are cauterized by bipolar. Cotton patties may be used to achieve hemostasis.

Disk space is exposed and annulotomy is performed if required with micro-knife protecting the traversing nerve root medially by retractor **(Figure 6E)**. The herniated disk is then removed by pituitary rongeur **(Figure 6F)**. After removing the disk nerve root is explored to ensure the decompression is complete **(Figure 6G)**. The wound is irrigated before closure. The flexible arm assembly is made loose and tubular retractor is removed. Retracted muscles fall back while removing tubular retractor. Any bleeding in paraspinal muscles is controlled by bipolar cautery. Fascia and subcutaneous tissue is closed with absorbable suture and skin is closed with subcuticular sutures **(Figure 6H)**.

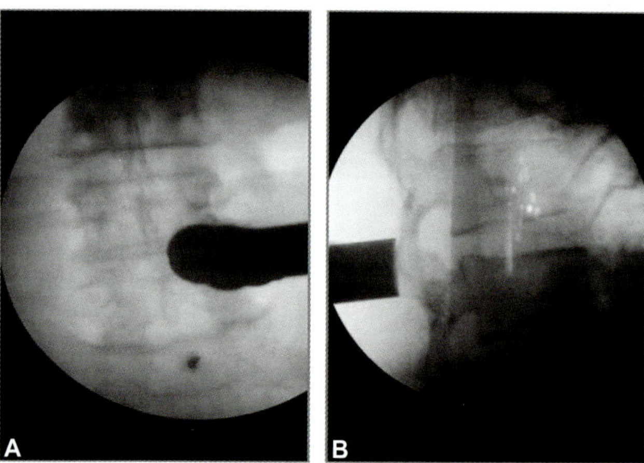

Figure 5: Fluoroscopic final position of tubular retractor

POSTOPERATIVE PROTOCOL

The patient is allowed to mobilize 6–8 hours after the operation or once the postoperative pain subsides. They are allowed to do all the activities depending on the pain. Postoperative hospitalization ranges from 1 to 2 days. Isometric back exercises are started after 2–3 weeks. Most of the patients return to work after 3 weeks of surgery.

COMPLICATIONS

The complications of MED include dural tears, root and other neurological injuries, inadvertent facet removals, residual disk or incomplete decompression, recurrent disk herniations and wrong level surgeries. The other issues, which can increase the difficulties in the procedure is during the initial learning curve. Some issues, which need to be tackled during initial learning curve, are orientation to the tubular anatomy due to highly targeted focused view, bleeding control and adequate bone removal to access the pathology to adequately mobilize the nerve roots. There are enough reports in the literature to emphasize that the complication rates are more during the initial learning curve but the rates starts to decrease, as the learning curve is overcome.

APPLICATIONS OF MED

Except for paramedian disk herniations the indications have expanded for foraminal and extraforaminal and far lateral herniations by intertransverse approach. It is also used for recurrent disk herniations.

Once the technique of MED is mastered, it can be used for other indications for decompressions. Change in docking point of the tube, different types of the tubes, angle of docking and maneuvering the tube by wanding either up or down or to the opposite side can help in dealing with wide variety of pathologies which has expanded the indications from lumbar diskectomies to central and lateral lumbar canal stenosis, facet cyst excisions, multilevel lumbar decompressions, lumbar interbody fusions, intradural tumor excisions and decompressions in thoracic and cervical regions also.

OUTCOMES OF MED

Microendoscopic diskectomy was introduced by Foley et al. in 1997 with specific advantage of decreasing the approach related muscle damage and secondary advantage of small

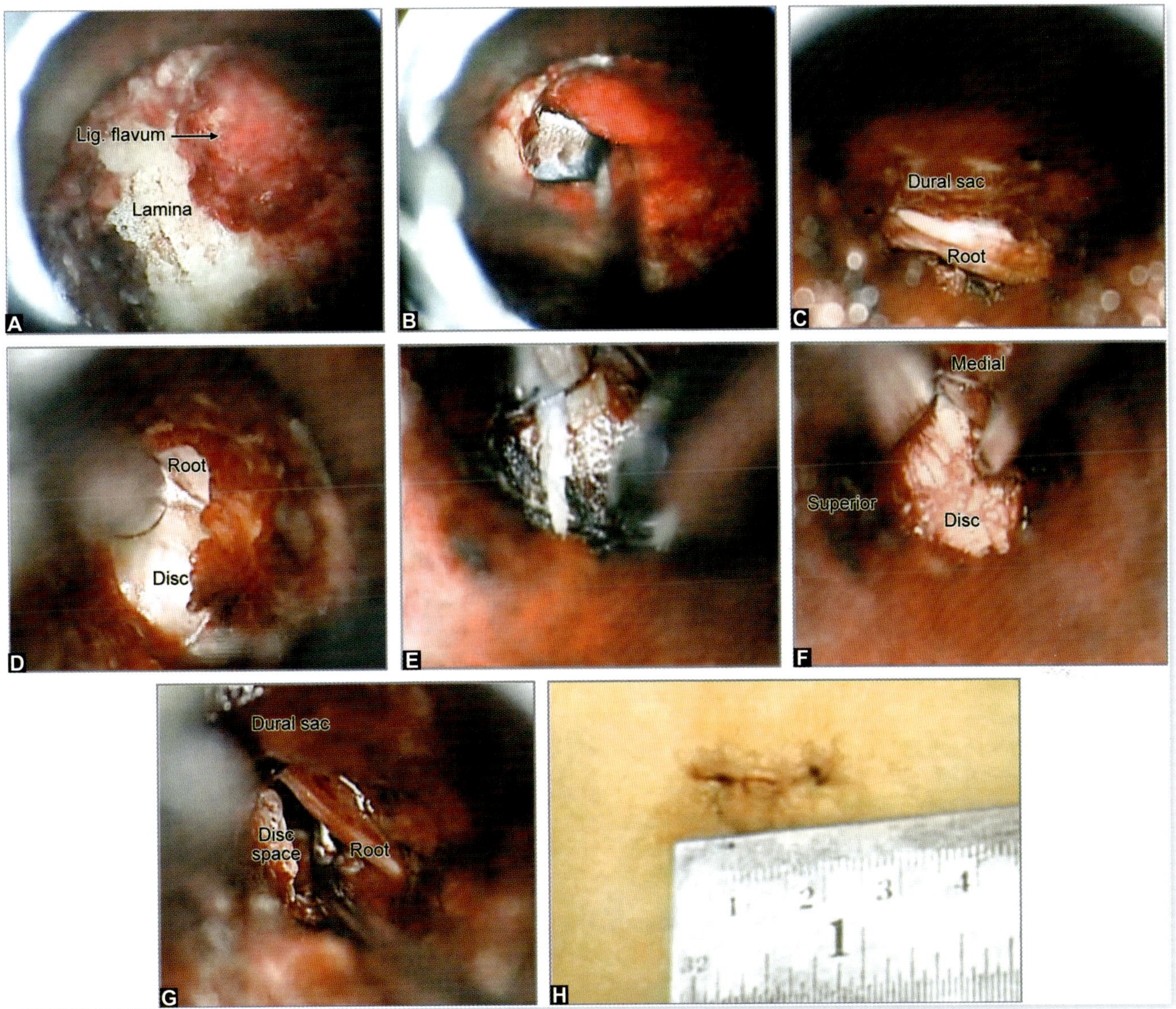

Figures 6A to G: (A) Identifying ligamentum flavum; (B) Separating ligament from under the lamina; (C) Identifying root and dural sac; (D) Retracting the root and identifying disk space; (E) Extrusion of disk material after Incision; (F) Removal of disk; (G) Probing the root after disk removal; (H) Closure and length of incision

skin incision leading to less pain, less blood loss and early return to work.[1] They reported their results in initial 150 cases with 94% excellent to good results with early return to work after 17 days. The patients had smaller skin incision and less pain.[7] After there report number of authors have reported similar results in the literature from around the world.[8-16] Since then MED was compared with the open traditional diskectomy and Microdiskectomy to assess the comparative advantage between the two techniques. MED has similar results to open diskectomy but with advantage of less invasiveness.[9,13,14,17] Not only the short-term outcomes but also even the long-term outcomes of 5 years 8 and 10 years[15] have been reported with satisfactory outcomes. The advantage of MED has been that it has less invasiveness and less iatrogenic muscle damage. The various biochemical parameters have been studied by different authors to prove that MED causes less tissue damage and is protective to the muscles.[3,4,6] There is a definite learning curve for MED. Nowitzke et al. reported on the assessment of the learning curve after MED and cutoff for overcoming the learning curve is approximately 30 cases.[18] The complication rates decreases, as the learning curve is overcome. Matsumoto et al. have studied the recurrence rate after MED which is 10.8% after mean follow up of 3.6 years which is similar to conventional diskectomy.[19] The results of redo diskectomy by MED for recurrent disk has been studied with similar results as in conventional open diskectomy.[20,21] MED technique has been applied for far lateral disk herniations with modifications in docking technique and approach. The docking is between the transverse processes as an intertransverse approach. MED has been safe and effective for far lateral disk herniations also.[22-24]

CONCLUSION

Microendoscopic diskectomy is safe and effective technique for all types of diskectomies with advantage of minimal tissue invasiveness and muscle preservation. It has the advantage of smaller incision, less pain and early return to work. It is the basic technique to move further on in the stepladder of minimally invasive spine surgery.

REFERENCES

1. Foley KT, Smith MM. Microendoscopic diskectomy. Tech Neurosurg. 1997;3:301-7.
2. Tabaraee E, Junyoung Ahn, Bohl DD, Phillips FM, Kern Singh. Quantification of multifidus atrophy and fatty infiltration following a minimally invasive Microdiskectomy. Intern J Spine Surgery. 2015;9.
3. Hara M, Takahashi H, Yokoyama Y, Wada A, Hasegawa K, Iida Y. Comparision of invasiveness of open conventional diskectomy and microendoscopic diskectomy for lumbar disk herniation: Differences in the methods of approach. Asian Journal of Endoscopic Surgery. 2015;8(1):40-7.
4. Huang TJ, Hsu RW, Li YY, Cheng CC. Less systemic cytokine response in patients following microendoscopic versus open lumbar diskectomy. J Ortho Res. 2005;23(2):406-11.
5. Kim DY, Lee SH, Chung SK, et al. Comparison of multifidus muscle atrophy and trunk extension muscle strength: percutaneous versus open pedicle screw fixation. Spine (Phila Pa 1976). 2005;30:123-9.
6. Shin DA, Kim KN, Shin HC, Yoon DH. The efficacy of microendoscopic diskectomy in reducing iatrogenic muscle injury. J Neurosurg Spine. 2008;8(1):39-43.
7. Perez-Cruet MJ, Foley KT, Isaacs RE, Rice-Wyllie L, Wellington R, et al. Microendoscopic lumbar diskectomy: technical note. Neurosurgery. 2002;51(5):S129-36.
8. Casal-Moro R, Castro-Menendez M, Hernandez-Blanco M, Bravo-Ricoy JA, Jorge-Barreiro FJ. Long-term outcome after microendoscopic diskectomy for lumbar disk herniation: a prospective clinical study with a 5-year follow-up. Neurosurgery. 2011;68(6):1568-75.
9. Garg B, Nagraja UB, Jayaswal A: Microendoscopic versus open diskectomy for lumbar disk herniation: a prospective randomised study. J Orth Surg. 2011;19(1):30-4.
10. Jhala A, Mistry M. Endoscopic lumbar diskectomy: Experience of first 100 cases. Ind J Orth. 2010;44(2):184-90.
11. Kulkarni AG, Bassi A, Dhruv A. Microendoscopic lumbar diskectomy: Technique and results of 188 cases. Ind J Orth. 2014;48(1):81-7.
12. Ranjan A, Lath R. Microendoscopic diskectomy for prolapsed lumbar intervertebral disk. Neurology India. 2006;54(2):190-4.
13. Righesso O, Falavigna A, Avanzi O. Comparison of open diskectomy with microendoscopic diskectomy in lumbar disk herniations: results of a randomized controlled trial. Neurosurgery. 2007;61(3):545-9; discussion 549.
14. Smith N, Masters J, Jensen C, Khan A, Sprowson A. Systematic review of microendoscopic diskectomy for lumbar disk herniation. Eur Spine J. 2013;22(11):2458-65.
15. Wang M, Zhou Y, Wang J, Zhang Z, Li C: A 10-year follow-up study on long term clinical outcomes of lumbar microendoscopic diskectomy. J Neurolog Surg. 2012;73(4):195-8.
16. Wu X, Zhuang S, Mao Z, Chen H: Microendoscopic diskectomy for lumbar disk herniation: surgical technique and outcome in 873 consecutive cases. Spine. 2006;31(23):2689-94.
17. Katayama Y, Matsuyama Y, Yoshihara H, Sakai Y, Nakamura H, Nakashima S, et al. Comparison of surgical outcomes between macro diskectomy and microdiskectomy for lumbar disk herniation: a prospective randomized study with surgery performed by the same spine surgeon. J Spinal Disorders & Techniques. 2006;19(5):344-7.
18. Nowitzke AM. Assessment of the learning curve for lumbar microendoscopic diskectomy. Neurosurgery. 2005;56(4):755-62, discussion 755-62.
19. Matsumoto M, Watanabe K, Hosogane N, Tsuji T, Ishii K, et al. Recurrence of lumbar disk herniation after microendoscopic diskectomy. J Neurolog Surg. 2013;74(4):222-7.
20. Isaacs RE, Podichetty V, Fessler RG: Microendoscopic diskectomy for recurrent disk herniations. Neurosurgical Focus. 2003;15(3):E11.
21. Smith JS, Ogden AT, Shafizadeh S, Fessler RG: Clinical outcomes after microendoscopic diskectomy for recurrent lumbar disk herniation. J Spinal Disorders and Techniques. 2010;23(1):30-4.
22. Foley KT, Smith MM, Rampersaud YR: Microendoscopic approach to far-lateral lumbar disk herniation. Neurosurgical Focus. 1999;7(5):e5.
23. Li SW, Yin HP, Cao ZH, Bai M, Du ZC, et al. Intertransverse approach microendoscopic diskectomy for far lateral lumbar disk herniation. Zhongguo Gushang. 2014;27(9):752-5.
24. Yoshimoto M, Iwase T, Takebayashi T, Ida K, Yamashita T: Microendoscopic diskectomy for far lateral lumbar disk herniation: less surgical invasiveness and minimum 2-year follow-up results. J Spinal Disorders and techniques. 2014;27(1):E1-7.

20

CHAPTER

Tubular Decompression Technique in Lumbar Spinal Stenosis

Arvind G Kulkarni, Ankit Patel, Sameer Ruparel, Navin Mewara

ABSTRACT

Microscopic-assisted tubular retractor system has wide indications in dealing with pathologies of different areas of spine. The minimally invasive nature of these retractors helps in lesser tissue trauma, optimum visualization of intended structures, less pain and early rehabilitation. The retractors can be used in dorsal and lumbar spine as well. This chapter deals with the technique, indications and contraindications of the tubular retractors.

INTRODUCTION:

Lumbar spinal stenosis (LSS) is the most common pathology for which spinal surgery is performed in patients over age of 65 years[1-3] Failure of conservative treatment resulting in persistent claudication pain and functional limitation is the most common indication for operative intervention in LSS.

Unless associated with instability, these patients are treated with lumbar decompression surgery alone. The techniques of treating this condition have gradually evolved extensively over the past few decades. Laminectomy is an excellent procedure and has historically been the gold standard**.** Laminectomy is associated with extensive resection of posterior spinal elements, possibly leading to postoperative iatrogenic pain and sowing the seeds of progressive segmental instability. With an aim to preserve as much bony and soft tissue integrity as possible to prevent iatrogenic instability, minimalist approaches such as laminotomy, laminoforaminotomy and bilateral microlumbar decompression technique came into vogue. The advent of tubular retractors was a revolution in the management of lumbar spinal stenosis. The ability to perform a thorough ipsilateral-contralateral decompression through a small unilateral portal with preservation of the paraspinal muscles and the stabilizing structures make it unique compared to other techniques. Tubular decompression surgeries have smaller incisions, lesser blood loss, better visualization of pathological site and faster rehabilitation without compromising the surgical outcomes. The chapter discusses the technique of tubular decompression in detail and highlights several points, which are necessary to be considered before clinical application of this procedure in day-to-day practice.

INDICATIONS AND CONTRAINDICATIONS

Indications for doing tubular decompression are not quite different from any other techniques used for lumbar spinal stenosis. Central and lateral recess stenosis can be decompressed using this technique with minimal bone removal, thus maintaining stability of the motion segment.[4-9] The technique can be used to decompress multilevel lumbar spinal stenosis using the same portal or multiple portals depending upon the anatomy. Spinal canal decompression using microendoscopic technique can also be performed for decompression and excision of synovial cysts,[10-12] and in selected cases of stenosis associated with degenerative spondylolisthesis.[13]

Absolute contraindications mainly include operating room related issues like unavailability of a working microscope, C-arm, high speed drill-burr, etc. Relative contraindications include mobile degenerative spondylolisthetic stenosis, narrow bony canal with sagittal-small facets.

ADVANTAGES

The advantages of microendoscopic decompression (MED) fall into two categories biomechanical and clinical. Since during decompression, there is no stripping of paraspinal muscles and posterior ligamentous complex and the muscular supporting structures of the spine are preserved to a large extent, MED serves to keep the biomechanics and stability of spinal motion segment intact. The amount of soft tissue trauma as compared to conventional decompression is quite less. Decompression of the central canal, bilateral lateral recesses and foramina can be achieved through one keyhole preserving the contralateral anatomy.

Minimal morbidity and pain are hallmarks of this procedure. There is minimal blood loss, almost zero infection rate,[14] reduced hospital stays and costs as compared to open destructive laminectomies. Patients can be mobilized in few hours following the surgery. It is cosmetically more appealing whilst accomplishing the same goal. The greatest beneficiaries of this procedure are patients with high BMI, who would otherwise need long incisions even for a single level surgery. It also avoids a wrong level surgery as the entry of the tubular retractor is done under image intensifier guidance.[15]

DISADVANTAGES

There is a steep learning curve to this procedure. Initially the surgical time and complications may be higher. However, with experience decompression can be safely and quickly performed. Technical challenges include working through a tube wherein there is small operative corridor and focused vision. This would make it difficult to identify proper anatomical landmarks. Working with tube would not allow much of instrument angulation during decompression and one will have to train him to work with use of parallel instruments and if angulation is required, the whole tube needs to be angulated.

Surgical Technique

Instruments for tubular decompression:

1. Tubular dilators and retractors **(Figure 1)**
2. Operating table that can tilt in all directions.
3. Specialized long bayonet instruments for use in MIS
4. Curved Kerrison ronguer
5. Long cautery tip
6. High-speed cutting burr
7. Nerve root retractor and nerve hooks and probe
8. Gel foam, bone wax, neurosurgical patties
9. Fibrin glue (TISSEL).

Preoperative workup

LSS is diagnosed after a thorough clinical history and examination. Persistence or worsening of symptoms even after a fair trial of conservative treatment is an indication for tubular decompression surgery. The surgeon should be precise about the location of the pathology as the exposure is limited. MR films should be examined to locate the level, site and side of pathology, the orientations of the facet joints and subtle signs of instability like the vacuum sign, facet fullness and presence of spondylolisthesis at the affected segments. Dynamic radiographs are done to diagnose dynamic instability. Patient with clinico-radiological correlation and no dynamic instability is a good candidate for MED.

All symptomatic levels need decompression. When operating more than one level, the author prefers a single incision at the lower lumbar levels. The natural lordosis in the lower lumbar spine makes wanding from one level to the other quiet smooth. In the upper lumbar spine, incisions can be taken on contralateral sides, or the same incision can be extended by another centimeter and decompression at both levels can be done one after the other. In the presence of sagittal facet orientation, it is important to remember to dock the tube in less of inclination to avoid inadvertent damage to the ipsilateral facet joint.

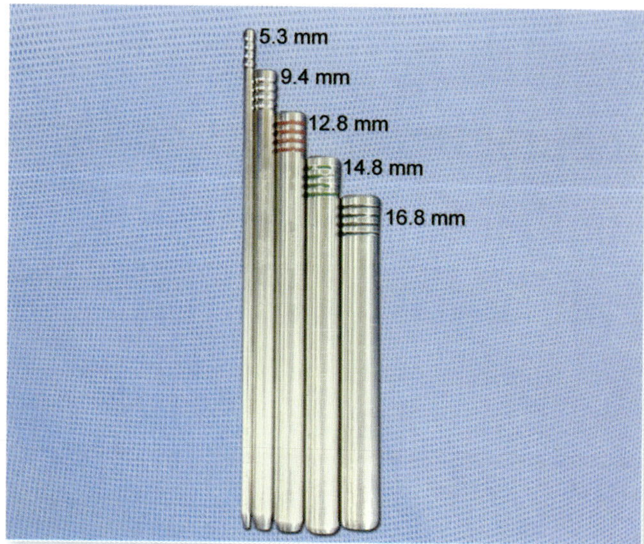

Figure 1: Different dilator sizes with color-coding

The side of port of entry is chosen on the basis of patient symptoms, facet inclination on the axial MRI and spinal alignment. In case of unilateral symptoms and no stenosis on the other side, the authors prefer to enter from the contralateral side and hence avoid encroaching into the facet joints of both sides. In patients with bilateral stenosis and symptoms, various factors need consideration, though a thorough bilateral decompression is possible from any of the sides. In general, right-sided approach is more comfortable for a right-handed surgeon. Decompression of the lateral recess and foramina is quite easier from the contralateral side as the inclination of the tube allows direct visualization of the opposite side, thus the tube can be docked contralateral to the more stenotic side. The side from which facets can be spared should be chosen. For example, the side of port insertion has to be strategic in degenerative scoliosis. There is attrition of the facet joints on the concave side making them atrophic. Hence, laminotomy on the concave side would compromise the integrity of the facet joint. The authors prefer to approach the lateral recess of the concave side from the opposite sid—the convex side. Similarly, the authors prefer to address synovial cysts from the opposite side. One advantage is that the facet joint anatomy on both sides is not compromised and the other is that one can clearly define the plane between the dural sac and the cyst from the opposite side. In situations where LCS is associated with lumbar disk herniation that needs to be addressed, it would be ideal to make the port of entry on the side of the herniated disk.

Anesthesia

The procedure is always performed under general anesthesia.

Positioning

Patient is positioned on a radiolucent table in prone position with bolsters below the chest and iliac crest, keeping the abdomen free to reduce intravenous pressure in the epidural plexus. This positioning puts the patient's lumbar spine in lordosis, thus facilitating decompression of the canal in its narrowest dimensions. A head high of 10-15 degrees is provided to avoid venous engorgement in the eyes. The foot end of the table should be flexed as the patient may slipoff as the head end of the table is raised. Pressure points should be well padded. Patient should be firmly strapped to the table to avoid slippage while turning the table. The surgeon should stand on the side that he chooses to decompress depending on the MRI findings and the leg symptoms. Lateral recess decompression is easily achieved by approaching from the opposite side as it provides a better trajectory. The table mount and flexible arm of the tubular system should be tightly secured before the incision.

Site Identification

Using lateral fluoroscopy imaging a 20 G spinal needle is inserted at the level of the involved disk space and parallel to both the end plates. The needle is inserted about 1 cm lateral to the midline and position confirmed with a lateral image on the image intensifier **(Figure 2).**

Sequential Dilator Insertion and Tube Docking (Figures 3 and 4)

About 5 cc of 0.5% bupivacaine diluted in 15 cc of saline is infiltrated for preemptive analgesia. A 2 cm incision is then centered over the needle and deepened till the fascia. Although the diameter of the tube (working portal) is 18 mm, it is better to take a slightly longer (2 cm) incision to allow for wanding of the tube and in order to prevent maceration of the skin. To avoid injury related to guide-wire, the authors has stopped using the same, and use the initial dilator to locate the inferior lamina of the superior vertebra. The initial dilator is then used to sweep off the paraspinal muscle mass and palpate the bony landmarks.

The spinous process medially and the facet joint complex laterally are felt as two mountains with the lamina as the valley in-between. Sequential dilators are then inserted while confirming the target site under fluoroscopy. The dilators have graduations marked on them to determine the depth of the tube. The marking on the final dilator at the level of skin provides the length of the tubular retractor. If the marking is between 4 and 5 then a number 5 tubular retractor should be used. 18 mm diameter tubular retractor is then docked with the flexible arm as the final working channel. The dilators should be deeply seated on the lamina to avoid "muscle creeping" into the working field. The working channel should be kept as perpendicular to the floor to maintain an easy working position for the surgeon. This can be achieved by raising the head end of the table. This is essential for decompressing the L4–5 and L5–S1 levels owing to the lumbar lordosis. Microscope is then brought into the field. As an alternative, an endoscopic camera can also be attached to the tubular retractor.

Visualization of the Anatomical Landmarks

Soft tissue is separated using a long cautery tip till the lamina can be visualized. An excellent exposure is one, wherein the inferior part of superior lamina and flavum are visualized.

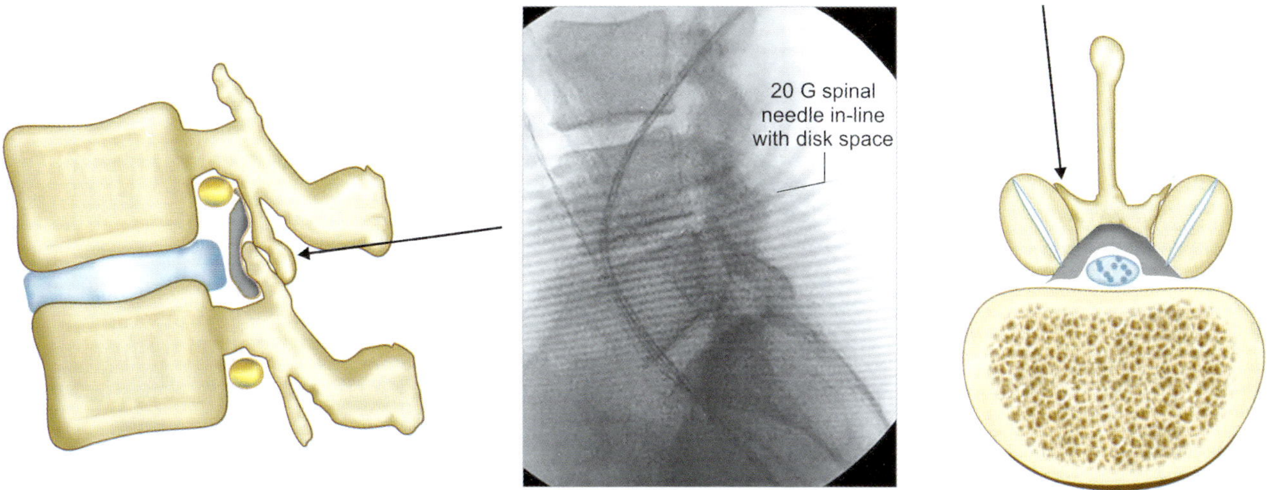

Figure 2: Level marking with 20 G spinal needle and IITV guidance. The needle is placed inline with the disk-space of interest

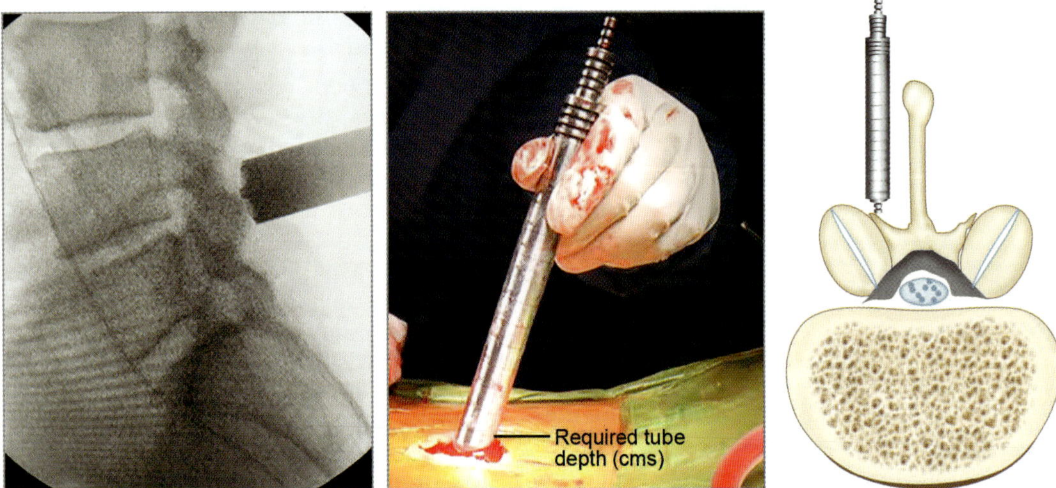

Figure 3: Serial dilatation of muscles with sequential dilators. Each successive dilator has to be rotated and kept firmly over bone to achieve adequate muscle separation

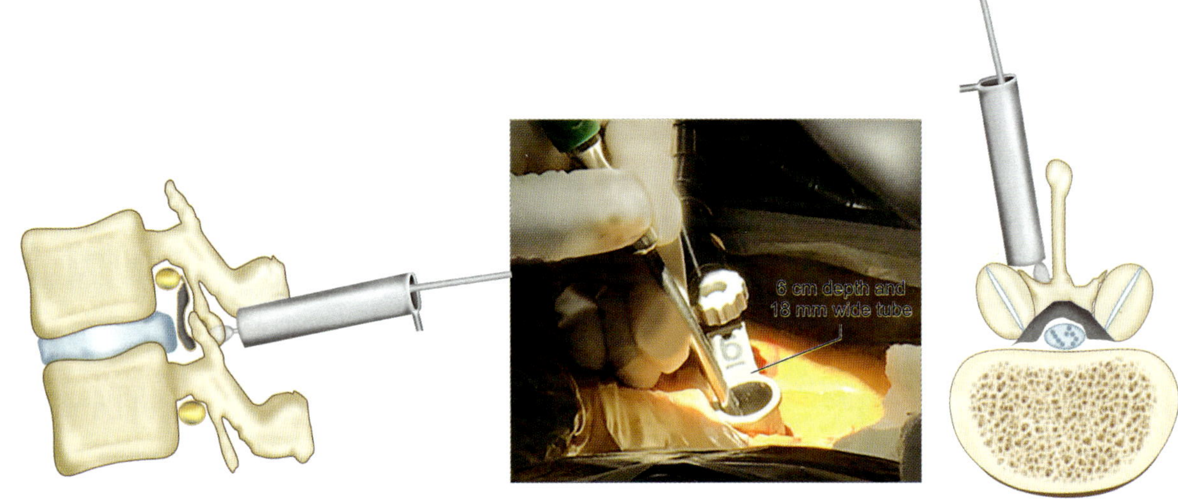

Figure 4: Appropriate length (3–9 cm) 18 mm tube docking. The reading is taken off the last dilator and tube matching the diameter of last dilator is passed over them and affixed to the flexible arm

Ipsilateral Laminotomy (Figure 5)

Lamina is then burred using a 4 mm cutting burr, till the junction of the inner cortex and ligamentum flavum is encountered. Ligamentum flavum is separated from the lamina by using a bayonet-handle angled curette. Ipsilateral laminotomy is completed using a no 2 Kerrison ronguer, leaving the flavum intact. Intact flavum protects the dural sac from injury whilst drilling the opposite side.

Going "Over the Top" (Figure 6)

In order to decompress the opposite side, the line of vision must extend underneath the spinous process and inter-spinous ligament across the midline. This is achieved by, aiming the tubular retractor medially (wanding) and tilting the table away from the operating surgeon towards the opposite side. This helps in providing a better visualization of the lateral recess of the contralateral side. The inner cortex of the contralateral lamina till the hypertrophied medial margins of the opposite facet joint are drilled with a high-speed burr, beginning at the base of the spinous process and proceeding laterally within the canal. This deroofs the canal and exposes the flavum entirely.

Contralateral Decompression (Figures 7)

The insertion of the flavum is then detached using a no 4 penfield. The intervening ligamentum flavum is then removed piecemeal thus decompressing the dural sac and

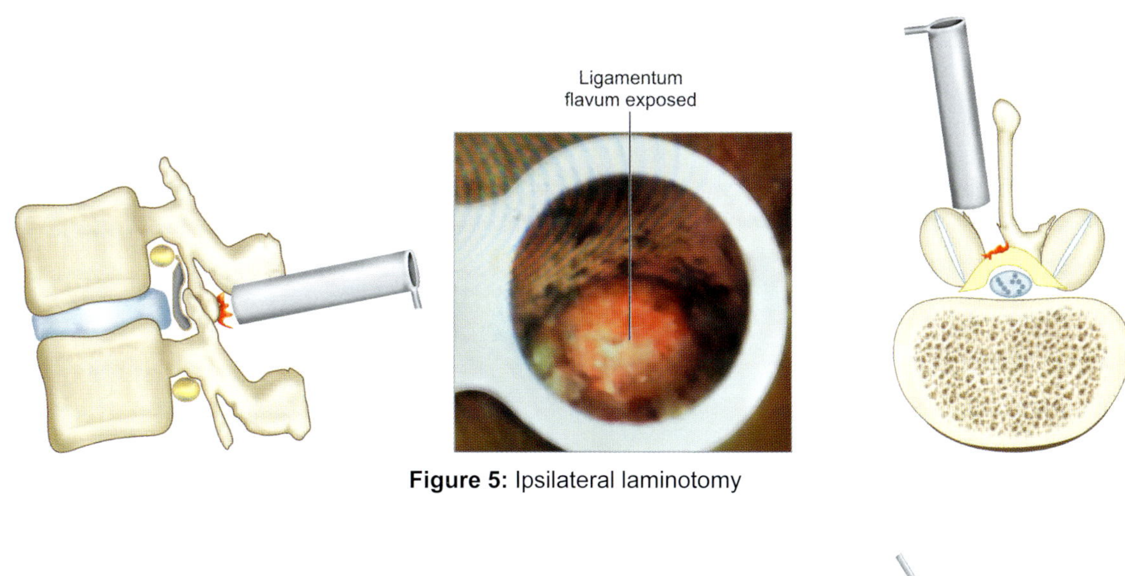

Figure 5: Ipsilateral laminotomy

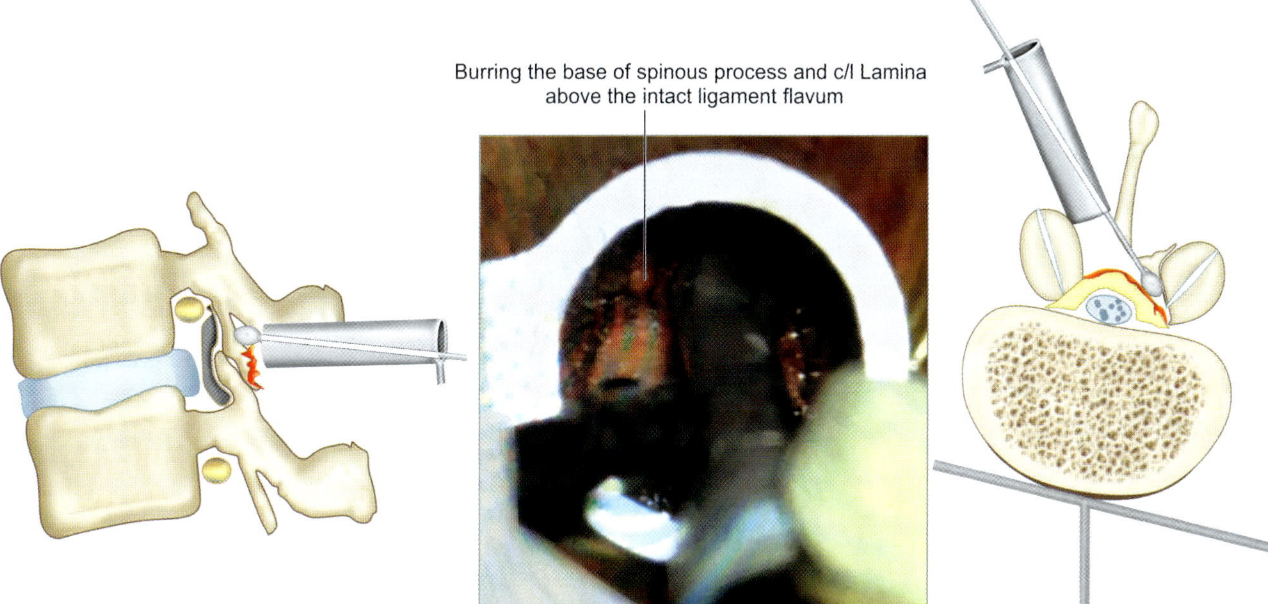

Figure 6: Over-the-top decompression

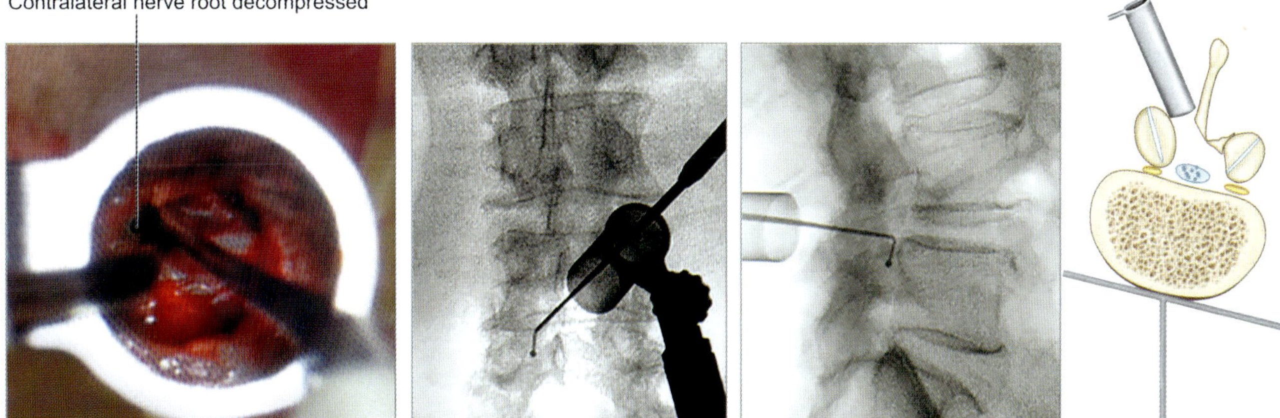

Figure 7: Contralateral nerve root decompression and ligament flavectomy

the opposite side nerve root. This successive resection is carried until the contralateral caudal pedicle is visualized. Using a curved Kerrison the lateral recess and foramen are decompressed effectively.

A dural retractor or a nerve hook is used to confirm if adequate decompression has been achieved. The nerve root is traced from its exit from the dura till it exits out of the foramen. Changing the direction of the tube superiorly and inferiorly and tilting the operating table aids in achieving this.

Ipsilateral Decompression (Figure 8)

The tube is then turned back laterally and table turned towards the surgeon and the ipsilateral side is decompressed similarly. The nerve root on this side is similarly traced.

Hemostasis and Closure

Bleeding is controlled using a combination of bipolar cautery, bone wax and gel-foam. Fascia and subcutaneous tissue are closed using 2-0 vicryl. Skin is closed using 3-0 monocryl. Steri-strips are applied to hold the skin edges together. Waterproof dressing is applied. If another level is to be decompressed the same procedure is repeated with a separate incision on the contralateral side or it is sometimes possible to decompress L4–5 and L5–S1 levels through the same incision owing to the lordosis.

TECHNICAL TIPS FOR CONTRALATERAL DECOMPRESSION (TABLE 1)

Postoperative Management

Patient is mobilized the same evening and is discharged the next day. Only one dose of intravenous antibiotics is given the same night. Injectable analgesics are given on the day of surgery and oral analgesics the next day onwards. Patient is weaned off oral analgesics by the 5th day postoperatively. Bathing is allowed immediately. Patient can go back to

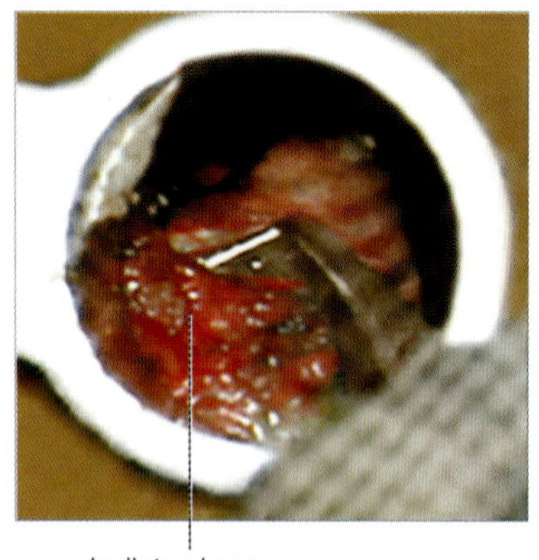

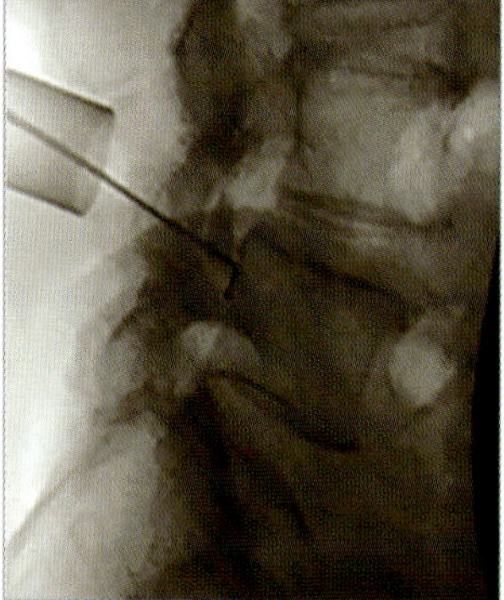
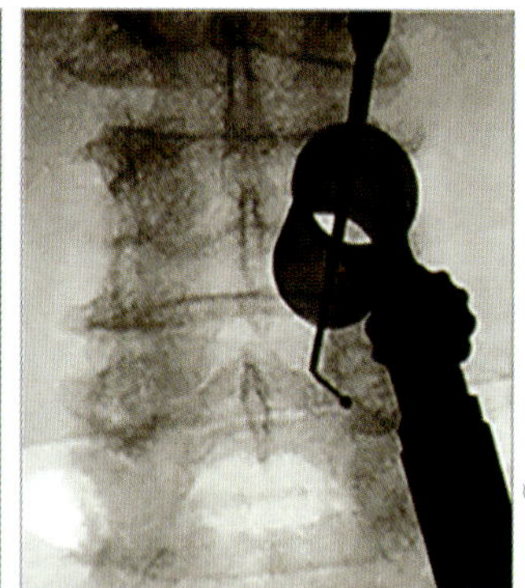
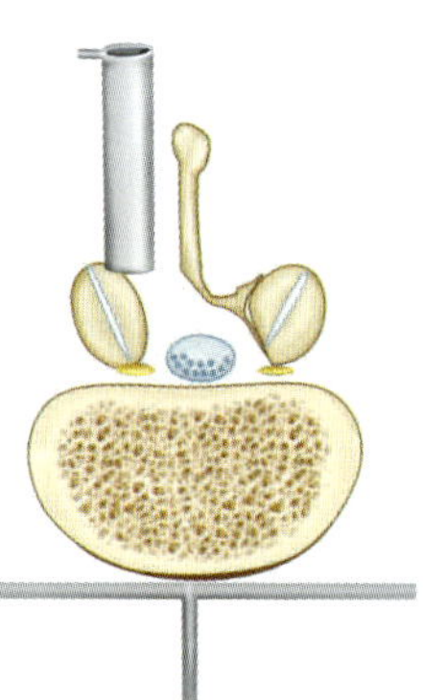

Figure 8: Ipsilateral nerve root decompression by under cutting

Table 1

Technical tips for contralateral decompression

1.	Patient should be tightly secured to the table to safely tilt the table to the right and left sides
2.	Adequate contralateral decompression can be achieved through a single ipsilateral incision
3.	L4–5 and L5–S1 levels may be approached through a single skin incision
4.	Too medial an incision, makes it difficult to achieve adequate medial tilting of the tubular retractor
5.	Too lateral an incision may block contralateral tilting of the retractor tube by a sagittally placed hypertrophied facet joint
6.	Adequate length of the tube is essential for it to sit on the lamina properly, so as to avoid muscle creep while allowing free angulation in all directions
7.	Long-bayonet instruments are required for an unobstructed visual field through the microscope.
8.	A cutting burr is used to drill the base of the spinous process and the undersurface of the contralateral lamina in order to approach the contralateral side
9.	An intact ligamentum flavum protects the dura during the drilling. Additionally, the suction cannula protects the dura from the drill
10.	Curved Kerrison rongeurs aid in opposite lateral recess decompression
11.	The nerve root must be traced from its origin to its exit through the neural foramen

light-duty work after 10 days and is not allowed to lift heavy weights. A gradual back strengthening program is started after 6 weeks. The scar usually shrinks to a size of 1.0–1.5 cm after healing (about 3 months).

Case Example: A 62-year-old lady had bilateral lower limb radiating pain for 6 months. Claudication distance was less than 500 meters with paresthesia in both lower limbs. Patient did not get adequate relief with conservative treatment. Preoperative images **(Figure 9)** revealed L4-L5 lumbar canal stenosis without instability. Patient was operated with Micro-Endoscopic Decompression [MED]. Intra operative images show docking of tubular retractor for decompression of ipsilateral and contralateral nerve roots [Over the top decompression] **(Figures 10 to 12)** Note the relative position of the retractor and patient with C-arm images). Adequate decompression of nerve roots on the contralateral and ipsilateral side can be seen. The procedure was done through a very small incision **(Figure 13)**. Patient was adequately relived of her symptoms at follow up with MRI images showing adequacy of decompression **(Figure 14)**.

COMPLICATIONS

The most commonly reported complication is durotomy. Other complications include neurological injuries, inadvertent facet violation, postoperative hematoma

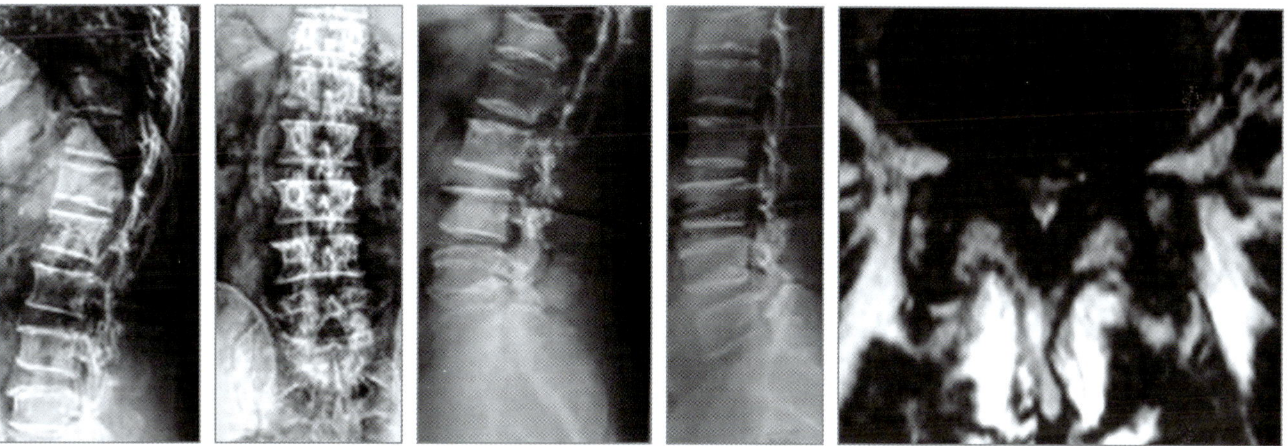

Figure 9: Case example: Preoperative radiological images

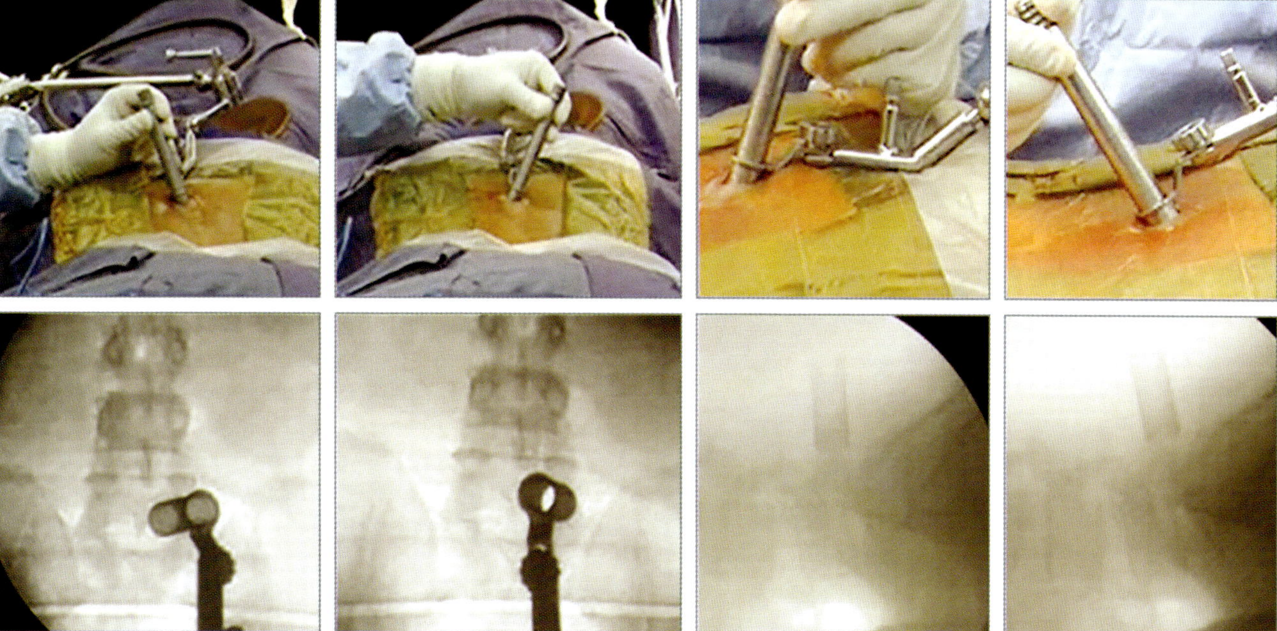

Figure 10: Case example: Docking of tubular retractor for ipsilateral and over the top decompression

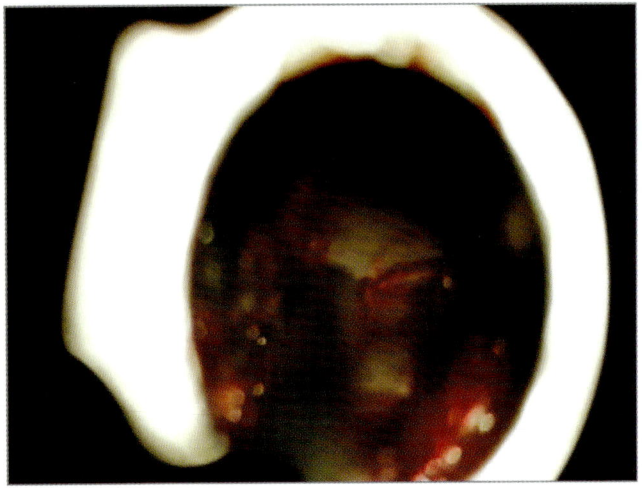

Figure 11: Case example: Contralateral nerve root decompression

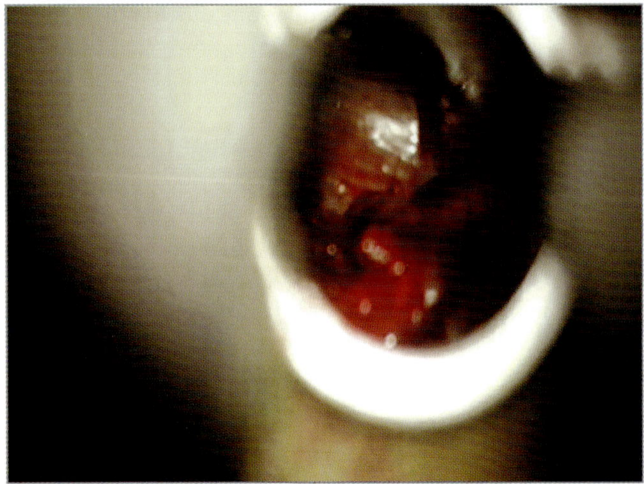

Figure 12: Case example: Ipsilateral nerve root decompression

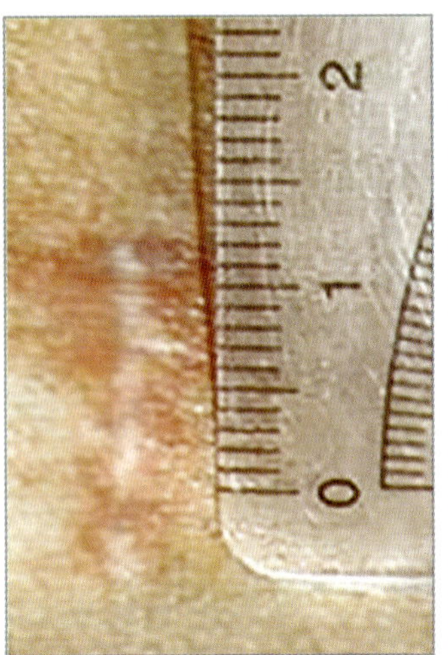

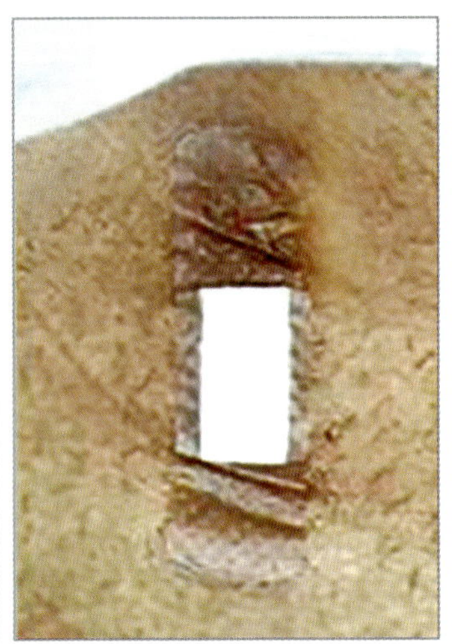

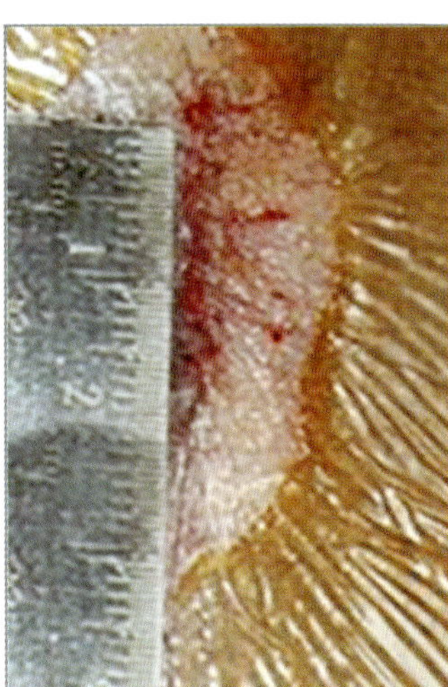

Figure 13: Skin incision

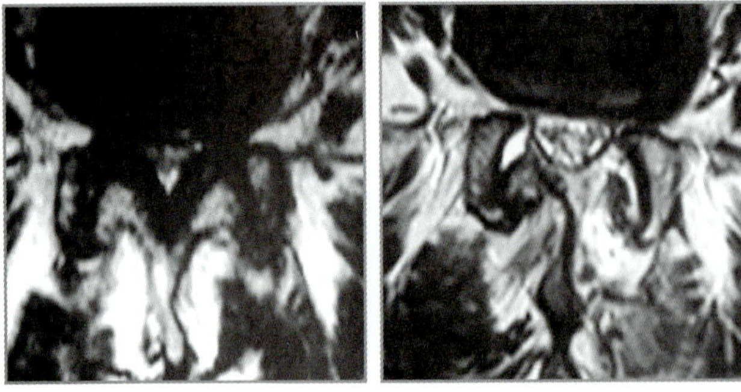

Figure 14: MRI shows adequate decompression

and wrong level surgeries.[16-18] Small dural tears can be managed with masterly inactivity.[19] but large tears may need the usage of fibrin glue to seal the tear. Use of sharp (Trocar tip) guidewires can lead to dural tears and neurological injuries and should be avoided. A laterally placed portal can lead to violation of the medial facet while executing ipsilateral decompression, requiring fusion. Spinous process fracture may occur while drilling the base. Inadequate decompression leading to an unfavorable outcome is a disappointing complication. One of the ways of avoiding this is to learn the technique from a master, by assisting a few simple and difficult cases. A good way of learning from mistakes is to perform a postoperative MRI and to keep a check on the locations of stenosis that one tends to miss and concentrate on them the next time.

Surgeon's anatomical knowledge and painstaking attention to details helps in reducing the complication rates. The author prefers to complete the bony decompression first, with the intact ligamentum serving as a shield reducing the risk of durotomy as well as neurological injury. The sharp ends of the instruments should be directed away from dura and suction tip can be used as effective protection for the neural structures. The spinous process and the inferior edge of the lamina can be used as anatomical landmarks to prevent injury to critical supporting structures, such as the facets. Meticulous hemostasis should be used to prevent postoperative hematoma. Intraoperative fluoroscopy and proper assessment of the preoperative films (especially in the presence of transitional vertebrae) can prevent surgeries at wrong levels.

Authors' Experience[20-28]

At authors' institution, almost all cases of single, two levels and occasionally 3-level lumbar canal stenosis without instability are operated with microendoscopic lumbar decompressive [MELD] technique. With vast experience in minimally invasive techniques, we found that MIS is associated with less postoperative infection rates[2] as compared to open techniques. In author's study of 1043 patients treated with MIS techniques, 763 underwent non-instrumented surgeries and 280 underwent instrumentation over a period of 8 years. The overall infection rate after MISS was 0.29% with surgical site infections of 0% in non-instrumented cases. Authors concluded that MISS can markedly reduce the SSI rate and can be an effective tool to minimize hospital costs.[14]

The use of tubular retractor system for decompression can be extended to numerous pathological conditions. The traditional approach for treatment of lumbar intra-spinal synovial cysts [LISC] is with decompression with or without fusion.[28, 29] The authors believe that stand-alone decompression is sufficient in selected patients unless associated with gross instability. In a total of 30 patients with LISCs treated with isolated microdecompression technique at author's institution over a period of 6 years and a minimum follow up of 3 years, all patients reported good to excellent results with no cases of recurrence or reoperation.[30]

Similarly, in patients with stable degenerative spondylolisthesis [DS], MELD has little influence on the natural history of DS and can be done as stand-alone procedure without adding fusion. Authors conducted a study[13] wherein patients with DS were divided into 2 groups [stable DS and unstable DS] based on multiple clinical, morphological factors and functional expectations. Out of 329 patients, 41 patients were classified as having stable DS and underwent stand-alone decompression. At a minimum follow-up of 3 years,[31] patients reported significant improvement in their symptoms. The author believes that this would have significant economic implications.

CONCLUSION

Tubular decompression technique for LSS has significant advantage of decreasing the collateral tissue damage reflecting clinically as decreased postoperative pain, less bleeding, less infection rate, early rehabilitation and early return to work. There is a learning curve associated with this technique but once the learning curve is overcome the results are better than traditional open decompression technique due to myriad of advantages as documented **(Table 2)**.

Table 2

Tubular decompression: Pearls and pitfalls

	Pearls	*Pitfall*
Preoperative evaluation	1. Thorough preoperative evaluation to identify and limit surgery to the symptomatic spinal segment 2. Contralateral approach is preferred in patients with synovial cysts, patients with unilateral symptoms due to one-sided lateral recess stenosis 3. Ipsilateral approach is preferred in patients with associated disk prolapse, severe stenosis. Patients with deg. Scoliosis are approached from the convexity	1. Failure to detect instability preoperatively, may compromise the clinical outcome. Vacuum sign within the disk, facet synovitis, mobile listhesis may indicate underlying instability 2. If the facets are extremely hypertrophic (kissing facets), docking of the tube is extremely difficult. Wanding can result in facet fractures 3. Since contralateral decompression is assessed by a tangential view, there are chances of incomplete decompression 4. Violation of the ipsilateral facet/ pars interarticularis during ipsilateral lateral recess decompression

Contd...

Contd...

	Pearls	*Pitfall*
Positioning	1. Decompression is performed with spine in extension, i.e. when there is maximum compression of neural elements	1. If the abdomen is not adequately free, especially in obese patients, back pressure may result in epidural venous congestion and troublesome intraoperative bleeding
Incision	1. Level confirmation must be done prior to making the skin incision 2. Incision is centered over the disk of the level to be decompressed 3. For 2 level decompressions, a single incision may be adequate in the lower lumbar spine, whereas separate incisions may be used in the upper lumbar spine 4. The incision is placed 1–1.5 cm from the midline so as to allow wanding for bilateral decompression	1. If the incision is too small, there can be difficulty in wanding, maceration of wound edges, and increased trauma to the paraspinal muscles 2. Incision is too medial, wanding for contralateral decompression becomes difficult and may fracture the base of the spinous process. 3. The incision is too lateral, a hypertrophied facet joint may get injured when docking and wanding
Tube docking	1. A perfect lateral image with parallel endplates helps guide the dilators 2. The first dilator is used to precisely feel the anatomical landmarks and clear the soft tissue 3. Adequate splitting of the paraspinal muscles is necessary when placing sequentially wider tubes, to prevent undue increase in intra-compartmental pressure 4. Proper docking: Inferior part of superior lamina superiorly, interlaminar space inferiorly, spinous process medially and facet joint laterally and the tube should be precisely in line with the surgical corridor 5. Length of the final tube should be long enough to prevent muscle from creeping into the surgical field	1. Sharp guidewire may penetrate the spinal canal and cause dural injury 2. Lateral docking may cause injury to pars or facetal violation 3. Since the entire process is performed under fluoroscopy, radiation exposure is high and hence all possible protection gears like the lead apron, thyroid shield and eye shields must be used
Decompression through the tube	1. Bony work must be completed bilaterally first, keeping flavum intact to protect the neural structures 2. Bilateral pedicle to pedicle decompression 3. Tilt the table and angulate tube for contralateral decompression 4. Use curved Kerrison rongeurs for decompression of difficult sites like the foramina 5. Use long and bayoneted instruments, specifically designed for MIS 6. The high speed drill must be used for contralateral decompression. Using the suction cannula to prevent plunging of the drill	1. Working through the tube requires orientation of 3D anatomy 2. Working through narrow portals requires working in different angles by manipulation of instruments 3. Ipsilateral foraminotomy is difficult with high risk of facet or pars fracture 4. In difficult situations like revision decompression/ severe stenosis/facetal cyst, the risk of inadvertent durotomy is high: precisely and patiently separate the tissues adherent to the dura 5. Dural punctures – difficult to suture 6. Limited dead space, so that even a small hematoma can result in pressure symptoms

REFERENCES

1. Atlas SJ, Keller RB, Robson D et al. Surgical and non-surgical management of lumbar spinal stenosis: four year outcomes from Maine Lumbar Spine Study. Spine 2000;25:556-62.
2. Hurri H, Slatis P, Soini K, et al. Lumbar spinal stenosis: Assessment of long-term outcome 12 years after operative and conservative treatment. J Spinal Disord. 1998;11:110-5.
3. Katz JN, Stucki G, Lipson SJ, et al. Predictors of surgical outcome in degenerative spinal stenosis. Spine. 1999;21:2229-33.
4. Houten JK, Tandon A. Comparison of postoperative values for C-reactive protein in minimally invasive and open lumbar spinal fusion surgery. Surg Neurol Int. 2011;2: 94
5. Schick U et al. Microendoscopic Lumbar Discectomy versus open surgery: an introp EMG study. European Spine J. 2002; 11,20-6.
6. Khoo LT, Fessler RG. Microendoscopic decompressive laminotomy for the treatment of lumbar stenosis. Neurosurgery. 2002;51: S146-S154.

7. Katayama Y, Matsuyama Y, Yoshihara H, Sakai Y, Nakamura H, Nakashima S, et al. Comparison of surgical outcomes between macro discectomy and micro discectomy for lumbar disc herniation: A prospective randomized study with surgery performed by the same spine surgeon. J Spinal Disord Tech. 2006;19: 344-7.
8. Larry Khoo, Fessler Richard. Microendoscopic Decompressive Laminotomy for the Treatment of Stenosis. Neurosurgery. 2002;Suppl 51:146-154.
9. David Rosen, John O, et al. Minimally invasive Lumbar Spinal Decompression in the Elderly. Outcomes of 50 patients aged 75 years and older. Neurosurgery. 2007; Suppl 60:503-10.
10. Sandhu FA1, Santiago P, Fessler RG, Palmer S. Minimally invasive surgical treatment of lumbar synovial cysts. Neurosurgery. 2004; 54(1):107-11; discussion 111-2.
11. Sehati N, Khoo LT, Holly LT. Treatment of lumbar synovial cysts using minimally invasive surgical techniques. Neurosurg Focus. 2006;20(3): E2.
12. James A, Laufer I, Parikh K, Nagineni VV, Saleh TO, Härtl R. J Lumbar juxtafacet cyst resection: the facet sparing contralateral minimally invasive surgical approach. Spinal Disord Tech. 2012;25:0-17.
13. Kulkarni AG et al. Degenerative spondylolisthesis. Is it always unstable? A new scoring system to aid decision making and apply value based spine care. Podium presentation at VTI gold medal session at Association of Spine Surgeons of India [ASSICON] Conference, 2017.
14. Kulkarni AG, et al. Does Minimally Invasive Spine Surgery Minimize Surgical Site Infections?Asian Spine J. 2016;10(6): 1000-6.
15. Kulkarni AG. The 'Nightmare' of Wrong Level In Spine Surgery: Is Minimally Invasive Spine Technique More Forgiving? (In Print JMISST, Korea).
16. Ikuta K, Tono O, Tanaka T, et al. Surgical complications of microendoscopic procedures for lumbar spinal stenosis. Minim Invasive Neurosurgery. 2007;50(3):145-9.
17. Jhala A, Mistry M. Endoscopic Lumbar discectomy: experience of first 100 cases. Indian J Orthop. 2010;44(2):184-90.
18. Podichetty VK, Spears J, Isaacs RE, et al. Complications assosiated with minimally invasive decompression fpr lumbar spinal stenosis. J Spinal Disord Tech. 2006:19(3):161-6
19. Kulkarni AG. Are Dural Tears in Minimal Invasive Spine Surgery of the Lumbar Spine More Forgiving than in Open Spine Surgery? Proceedings of the NASS 29th annual meeting/ The Spine Journal. 2014;14: IS183s.
20. Foley KT, Smith MM. Micro-endoscopic discectomy. Techniques in Neurosurgery. 1997;3:301-7.
21. Outpatient spine surgery. In: Perez-Cruet MJ, Fessler RG, editors 1stediction. St. Louis (MO): Quality Medical Publishing; 2002.
22. Guiot BH, Khoo LT, Fessler RG. A minimally invasive technique for decompression of the lumbar spine. Spine. 2002;27:432-8.
23. Stevens KJ, Spenciner DB, Griffiths KL, et al. Comparison of minimally invasive and conventional open posterolateral lumbar fusion using magnetic resonance imaging and retraction pressure studies. J Spinal Disord Tech. 2006;19: |77-86.
24. Kim KT, Lee SH, Suk KS, Bae SC. The quantitative analysis of tissue injury markers after mini open lumbar fusion. Spine (Phila Pa 1976). 2006;31:712-6.
25. Asgarzadie F, Khoo LT. Minimally invasive operative management for lumbar spinal stenosis: overview of early and long-term outcomes. OrthopClin North Am. 2007;38:387-99.
26. Palmer S, Turner R, Palmer R. Bilateral decompression of lumbar spinal stenosis involving a unilateral approach with microscope and tubular retractor system. J Neurosurg. 2002;97:213-7.
27. Nowitzke AM. Assessment of the learning curve for lumbar microendosopic discectomy. Neurosurgery. 2005;56:755-62.
28. Nancy E. Epstein, MD. Lumbar Laminectomy for the Resection of Synovial Cysts and Coexisting Lumbar Spinal Stenosis or Degenerative Spondylolisthesis. Spine 2004;29:1049-56.
29. Amir M Khan, Federico Girardi. Spinal lumbar synovial cysts. Diagnosis and management challenge. Eur Spine J 2006; 15: 1176-82.
30. Kulkarni AG, Dutta S, Dhruv A, Bassi A. Should we label all synovial cysts as unstable? In Pint, Global Spine Journal. 2017.
31. Kulkarni AG, Patel R, Dutta S, Patil V. Stand-alone Lateral Recess Decompression without Discectomy in Patients Presenting with Claudicant Radicular Pain and MRI Evidence of Lumbar Disc Herniation: A Prospective Study. In Print, Spine (Phila Pa 1976).

21

CHAPTER

Endoscopic Lumbar Canal Decompression in Degenerative Stenosis

Mohinder Kaushal

ABSTRACT

The main advantages of minimally invasive spine surgery is less tissue trauma, retention of all posterior elements, faster rehabilitation and lesser complications. The endoscopic access to the spine helps in achieving the goals and has become a boon to all spine surgeons. The procedure has gained increased popularity in recent past which aids in the treatment of wide range of spinal pathologies. This chapter deals with using endospine techniques in lumbar decompression.

INTRODUCTION

The traditional treatment of lumbar stenosis entails an extensive resection of posterior spinal elements, such as the interspinous ligaments, spinous processes, bilateral lamina, portions of the facet joints and capsule, and the ligamentum flavum. Additionally, wide muscular dissection and retraction is usually employed to achieve adequate surgical visualization. The extensive resection and injury of the posterior osseous and muscular complex can lead to significant iatrogenic pain, disability, and morbidity. The loss of the midline supra/interspinous ligament complex can cause a loss of flexion stability, thereby increasing the risk of delayed spinal instability.[1,2] Extensive laminectomy can also be associated with significant operative blood loss as well as prolonged postoperative pain and weakness secondary to the extensive surgical dissection and muscle detachment. Such iatrogenic injury can lead to paraspinal muscle denervation and atrophy, which may correlate with an increased incidence of "failed back syndrome" and chronic pain.[3,4] Because patients who have lumbar stenosis are usually elderly and medically frail, this delayed recovery often results in significant morbidity. Deep venous thrombosis, pulmonary embolism, pulmonary atelectasis, pneumonia, urinary tract infections, ileus, and narcotic dependency are examples of these potentially devastating sequelae

Over the last two decades, numerous surgeons have worked toward the goal of reducing the surgical morbidity of decompressive surgery for LCS. The ideal operation for LCS should simultaneously achieve an adequate decompression of the neural elements while at the same time minimizing damage to the posterior muscular, ligamentous, and bony complex. Because the pathologic changes typically are concentrated at the level of the interlaminar space, focal laminotomy was the nature first step in the evolution of surgical procedure for LCS. By sparing most of the lamina, spinous processes, and interspinous ligamentous complex, laminotomy helps to preserve the biomechanical integrity of the spine. Aryanpur and Duker,[5] in their description of multilevel open number laminotomies, reported longitudinal good outcomes rate of 79–85% at 2-year follow-up. As the use of operating microscope became increasingly common among spinal surgeons, unilateral microscopic hemilaminotomy was developed as a means of sparing the contralateral musculature as well. This procedure was characterized by unilateral multifidus retraction, ipsilateral decompression, and contralateral microscopic decompression performed under the midline bony and ligamentous structures. For this microscopic laminotomy as described by McCulloch[6] and Young et al.[7] and 80–95% improvement rate was reported over a short 9-month follow-up period. Despite this progressive movement toward a less extensive resection of the posterior bony elements, symptomatic outcomes have remained similar, regardless of the aggressiveness of the surgical procedure used to treat LCS.[8] It was observed, from one of the only studies correlating radiographic and clinical outcomes, that patients' satisfaction with the results of surgery (e.g. Oswestry score and walking capacity) was more important in surgical outcome than the degree of decompression as seen on a postoperative CT scan.[9]

In the last decade, significant strides in endoscopic visualization technology have been made. As such, endoscopy- assisted procedures have become increasingly popular for the treatment of a wide range of spinal pathologies, including hyperhydrosis, herniated disks, tumors, and fractures. In the lumbar spine, endoscopic diskectomies have been used to treat herniated disks successfully for the last 5 years. These procedures are particularly attractive for its small skin incision, gentle tissue dissection, excellent visualization, and ability to achieve results that are equivalent to open techniques. The endoscopic decompressive laminotomy (EDL) technique was thus developed as a synthesis of the unilateral hemilaminotomy (described previously) as endoscopic diskectomy technique. The EDL technique was initially validated in the series of cadaveric studies in which the equivalent bony decompression was achieved by way of either an open or endoscopic technique.[10] Since then, it has also been studied clinically with resultant good surgical outcomes, low morbidity, and a rapid postoperative functional recovery.[11] A bilateral decompression by way of a unilateral minimally invasive approach thus represents the next logical step in the evolution of modern surgical treatment for lumbar spinal stenosis.

CLINICAL PRESENTATION

The most common presentation of degenerative lumbar canal stenosis is an elderly patient with low back pain associated with neurogenic claudication brought on by standing or walking. Patients classically has stooped posture while walking and even during standing. the symptoms are relieved on sitting and supine positions. In lateral recess and padicle zone stenosis patients may have more unilateral leg symptoms at rest and during night and these are less disabling in terms of walking distance.

Neurogenic claudication should be differentiated from vascular claudication by history, examination and with appropriate investigations. Vascular claudication typically starts in calf and proceeds proximally and is brought on by walking, but not standing. Riding a bicycle elicits symptoms in vascular claudication while in neurological claudication the symptoms may not appear owing to the flexed posture of spine. In vascular claudication there are signs of decreased perfusion of the limb like absent pulses, trophic changes and discoloration of toe tips.

TREATMENT

Conservative

Initial treatment of **lumbar canal stenosis** should be conservative[12,13] master technology Patients with mild-to-moderate symptoms should be put on lumbar spinal flexion exercise program, to increase core muscle strength and and to avoid extension. Pain can be managed by NSAIDs and medications, such as gabapentin and amitryptylline. Amundsen et al in a 10-year follow- up study of 100 patients found that 70% of patients with mild to moderate symptoms had satisfactory result with conservative treatment. Role of epidural steroid injections is not clearly defined. Various studies show conflicting results.[14]

Surgical

Patients with debilitating symptoms and not responding to conservative treatment may be given option of endoscopic canal decompression. In Amundsen et al. series patients with severe symptoms underwent surgical treatment and 70% had excellent results with at 10-year follow-up.[15] Atlas et al. also reported good outcome in surgically treated patients at one year. Athiviraham and Yen reported that majority of patients who choose surgery will improve but may have residual symptoms.[16] Hence patient should be counseled about realistic expectations and gaurded prognosis of neurological deficits if any. Comorbid illness like diabetic peripheral neuropathy, peripheral vascular disease and parkinsonism may confound the diagnosis. Prior surgery at the same level significant epidural scarring and dense adhesions may make the endoscopic laminotomy technique particularly difficult, due to an increased risk of durotomy. Redo procedure should be attempted only by surgeons who have already gained experience with the MEDL technique in a good number of simple cases. Additionally, patients undergoing redo decompression with EDL should be clearly informed about the increased surgical risks and the possibility of conversion to an open procedure.

Indications

Patients undergoing endoscopic decompression of LSS should meet the same selection criteria as patients undergoing open decompressive laminectomy or laminotomy.

1. Patients with symptoms of neurological claudication with MRI demonstrating significant stenosis of ths spinal canal.
2. Failure of conservative treatment at least for a period of at least 3–6 months.
3. Acute neurological deficit. Chronic neurological deficit alone should be considered as relative indication for surgery.

When to Fuse?

With advent of endoscopic spinal canal decompression need for fusion has virtually become negligible. Fusion surgery in lumbar canal stenosis has been widely debated. Studies have shown that the choice of fusion along with decompression is highly surgeon dependant. Fox et al.[17] have shown that radiological instability does not imply a poor outcome when decompression without fusion is done. Fusion surgery increase the magnitude and complexity of surgery and hence should be carefully weighed against the benefits especially in the elderly. However, if there is intraoperative iatrogenic instability fusion may be considered.

Exclusion Criteria

1. Patients who have infection, tumor, arachnoiditis, pseudomeningocele, or cerebrospinal fluid fistula are generally not suitable for endoscopic canal decompression.
2. Radiological findings of stenosis in the absence of clinical symptoms should not be considered for surgical treatment.[14]

Surgical Technique: Endoscopic/Arthroscopic Canal Decompression (Endospine)

Because the endoscopic canal decompression technique is capable of decompressing the central canal, lateral recess, and proximal part of the ipsilateral neural foramen, symptoms of radiculopathy from either foraminal stenosis or disk herniation can also be successfully addressed by this method. When evidence of nerve compression is present, endoscopic canal decompression should ideally be performed on the same side as these symptoms to afford maximal surgical exposure.

Preoperative Preparation

Prior to surgery preanesthetic workup, including medical fitness for anaesthesia is obtained in Out patient department Patient is admitted day prior to surgery. Intravenous broad spectrum prophylatic antibiotic prior to start of surgery is recommended.

Anesthesia

This precedure can be done under general or spinal anesthesia but largely depends on choice of surgeon.

Position

We use and recommend knee chest position as this opens the interlaminar space and reduces the pressure over abdomen causing less venous engorgement thus reducing intraoperative bleeding. Surgeon operates from more symptomatic side, the instrument trolly is placed on right side of surgeon and imaging system is positioned opposite the surgeon to facilitate the viewing of procedure

Endoscopic Lumbar Canal Decompression Steps (Figures 1 to 9)

Under fluoroscopic guidance symptomatic level is marked with localizing devise, 15 mm skin and subcutaneous incision is given over marked level about 2 cm lateral to midline. Bleeding is controlled with bipolar coagulation. Fascia is incised with scissors or cutting diathermy. Paraspinal muscles are gently retracted from mid line subperiosteally with help of 15 mm chisel and interlaminar space is exposed. A special retractor blade can be used to prevent soft tissue interposition into mouth of tube. Endospine tube with opturator is inserted over interlaminar space and opturator is withdrawn. Any soft tissue coming into the tube is removed with disk rongeur till boundries of interlaminar window are clearly visible. Working insert with 0 degree scope is then fitted over tube. Suction canula is passed through suction port. The boundries of interlaminar window are defined under endoscopic vision. Endoscopic laminotomy comprises of nibbling of inferior margin of lamina to gain entry into the canal. At times interlaminar window is very narrow and covered with bone in that situation endoscopic burr or fine osteotome can be used to remove that bone to gain entry into the canal. This follows removal of ipsilateral ligamentum flavum and medial facetectomy to open foramina and to decompress ipsilateral nerve root, then attention is drawn to removal of contralateral ligamentum flavum and undercutting of facet to decompress contralateral nerve root by tilting the tube to opposite side. This results in good circumferential decompression. Both nerve roots and foramina are probed for adequacy of decompression. Cottonoid patties are used to control bleeding and to aid retraction. Diskectomy if indicated can be carried out by retracting dura and nerve root. Bleeding is controlled by endoscopic bipolar coagulation aided by cotton patties. Wound is closed in a subcuticular fashion followed by water impermeable

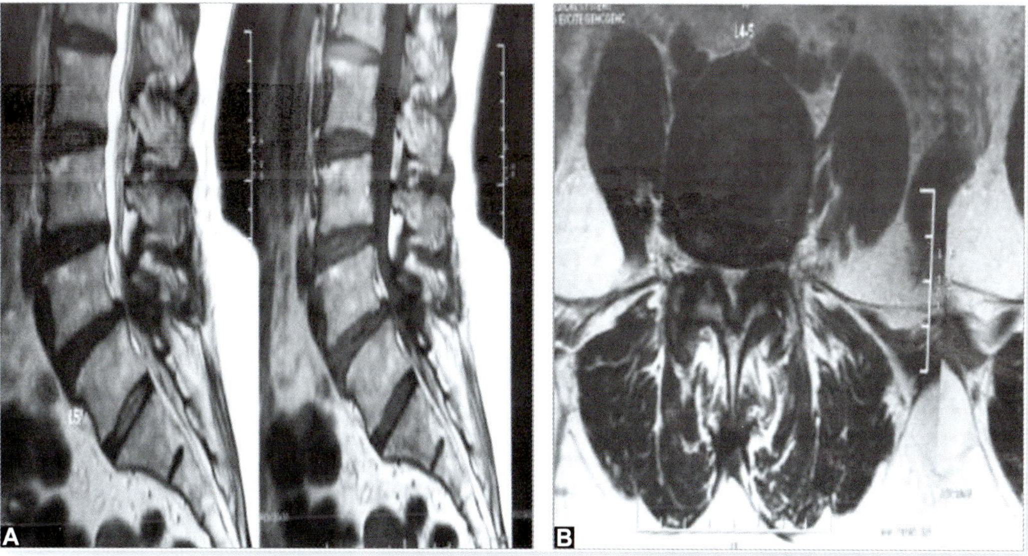

Figures 1A and B: Preoperative MRI LS spine. (A) Sagittal and (B) Axial views, showing lumbar canal stenosis

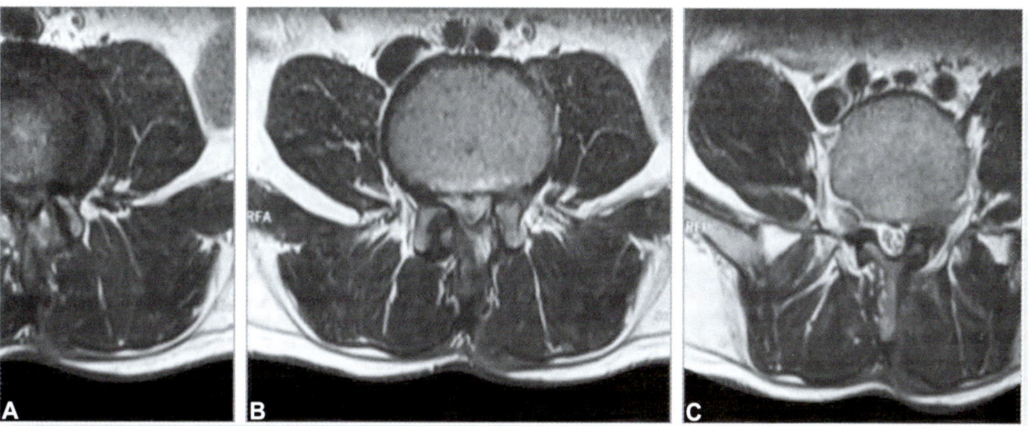

Figures 2A to C: Postoperative MRI axial showing extent of decompression

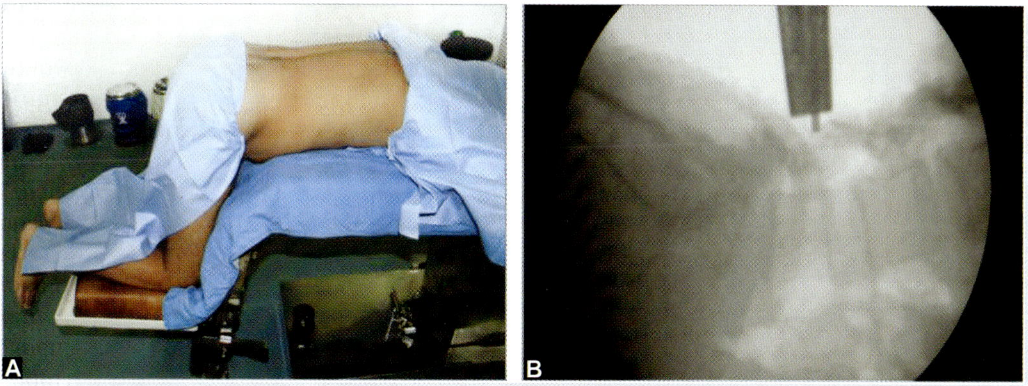

Figures 3A and B: (A) Patient positioning; (B) IITV confirmation of correct placement of tube

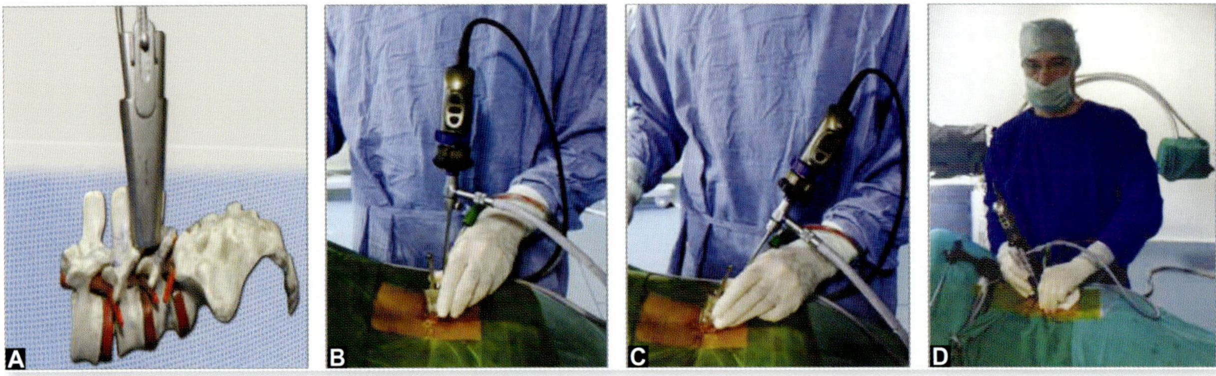

Figures 4A to D: Endospine tube in place and its mobility: (A) Vertical on model; (B) On patient; (C) Cephalad; (D) Side ways tilt to work on contralateral side

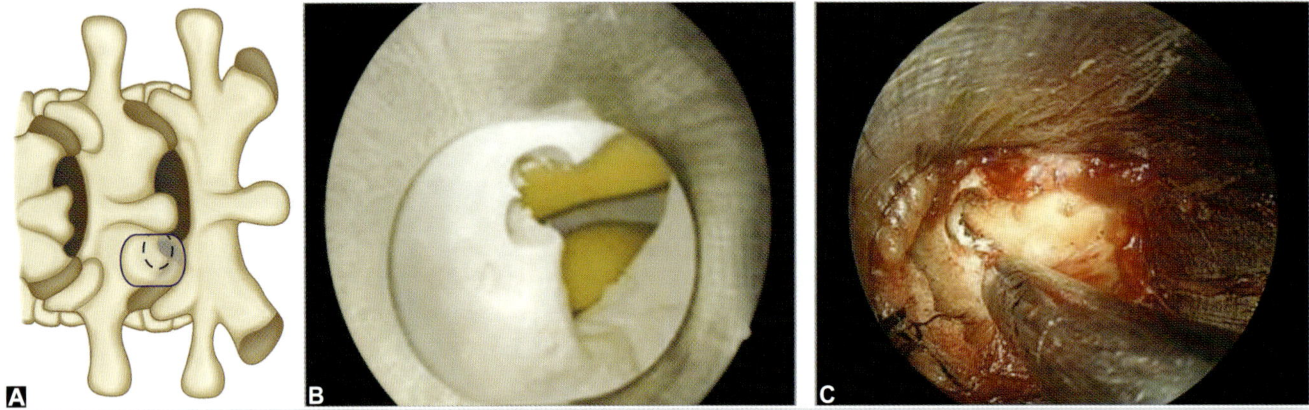

Figures 5A to C: Technique of ipsilateral decompression. (A) Diagrammatic; (B) Endoscopic on Mannequin; (C) On Patient

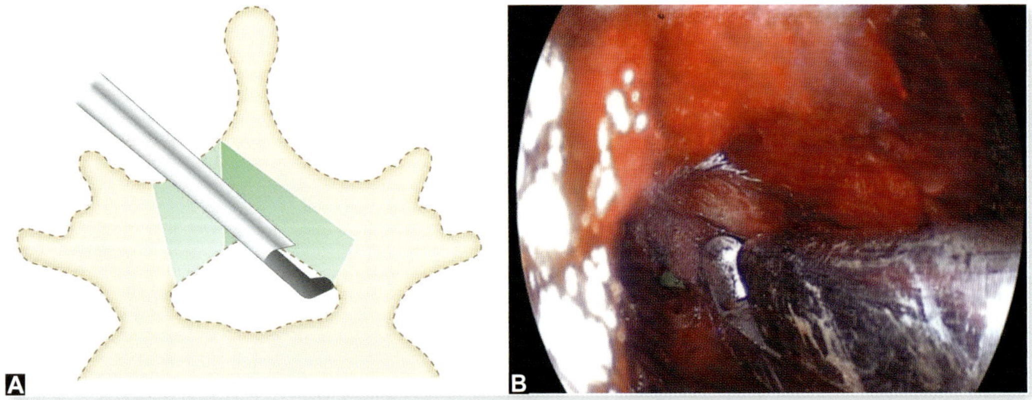

Figures 6A and B: (A) Diagram depicting technique of contralateral decompression; (B) Endoscopic view of removal of contralateral ligamentum flavum

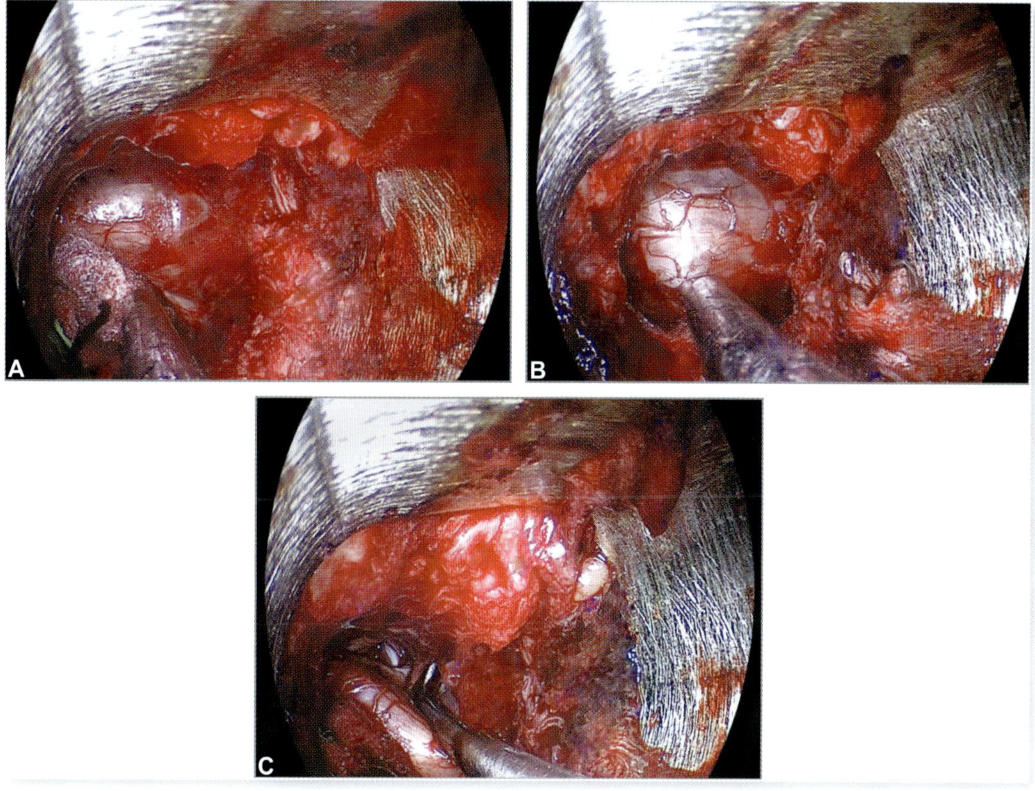

Figures 7A to C: Endoscopic view of decompressed dura. (A) Ipsi; (B) Midline; (C) Contralateral decompression and view of disk and nerve root

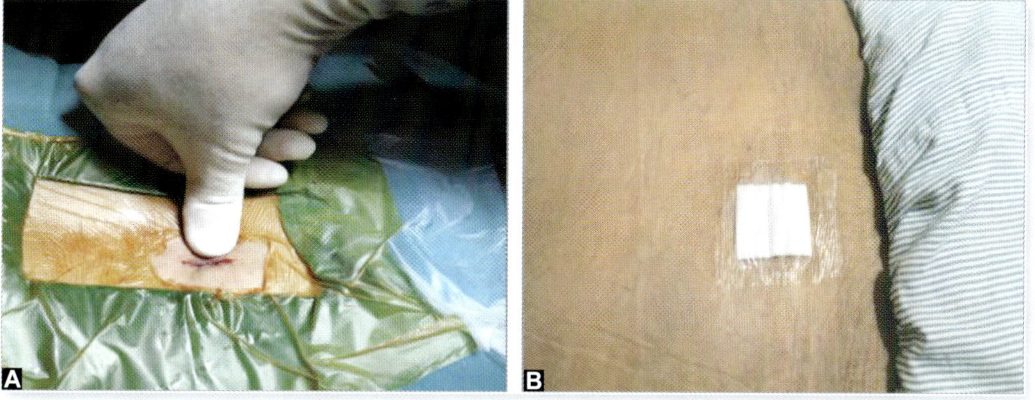

Figures 8A and B: (A) Subcuticular closure and incision size; (B) Water impermeable dressing

dressing. In cases of multiple adjacent level stenoses, the initial placement of endospine should be midway between the stenotic levels. In a patient with both L3/L4 and L4/L5 stenosis; for example, the endospine/arthrospine should be first docked on the L4 lamina and then swung caudad to decompress the L4/L5 level and cephalad to subsequently decompress the L3/L4 level.

Postoperative Care and Follow-up

Patients are mobilized out of bed on day of surgery in evening once effect of anesthesia is over. structured course of truncal stabilization and aerobic conditioning for these patients is started on first postoperative day. Shower is allowed same evening. Patients are followed up on 3rd day to

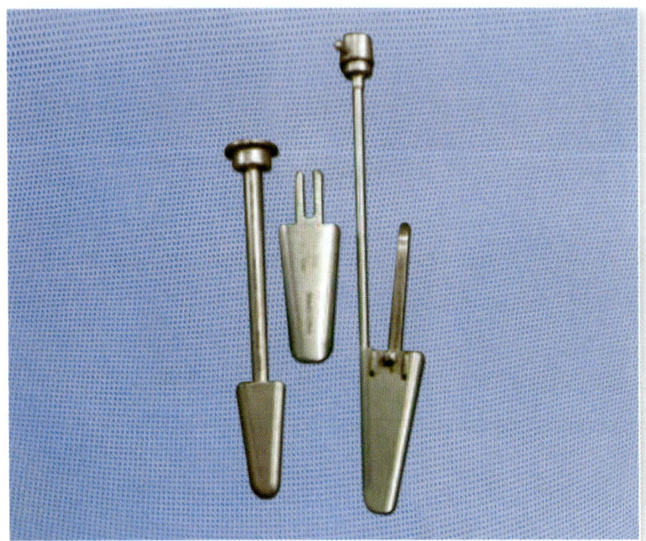

Figure 9: Endospine system

see any wound infection. Subsequently follow up is carried out at 6 weeks, 12 weeks, 6 months,12 months and 2 years. Light desk job is permitted within a week after surgery. Rehabilitation protocol may need to be varied depending upon individual patient's response.

Learning Curve

Like any endoscopic procedure, there is relatively steep learning curve in technique of endoscopic canal decompression. Surgeon should have patience and perseverance to work through narrow confines, should develop triangulation and hand eye coordination under 2D vision.It is strongly recommended that surgeon keen to learn these techniques must attend hands on models, cadaveric workshops and fellowships under trained surgeons before using them as treatment methods. If surgeon has difficulty in completing procedure during early phase of learning, he should not hesitate to convert to conventional open procedure. Properly done open spinal procedure is still better than poorly done endoscopic procedure.

CLINICAL OUTCOME AND COMPLICATIONS

As with all surgical procedures, the result of treatment with endoscopic canal decompression vary directly with the patient population and selection criteria of the surgeon. Additionally, operative times, blood loss, complication rates, and postoperative length of stay typically improve as a surgeon experience with these procedure grows.

Over last 10 years results of first 300 patients are presented here to serve as a useful guide for what to expect during the clinical follow up. 80% patients were relieved of neurological claudication and were satisfied with procedure. The patients had a mean age of 60.5 years. There was a male to female ratio of 3:2. The patients' clinical presentations were scored into four clinical categories: back pain, leg pain, gait limitation and distance, and urinary dysfunction. Patients who underwent fusion and patients with evidence of lumbar instability, severe deformity, spondyloptosis or severe spondylolisthesis, infection, tumor, and cauda equina syndrome were excluded from the study group. All patients had pain in their lower back; 80% of patients reported some degree of radiating leg pain and approximately 96% of patients had significant limitation in their ambulatory ability due to neurological claudication with about 16% of patients reporting symptoms of urinary dysfunction. Before surgery, all patients demonstrated compressive central canal stenosis, with or without lateral recess stenosis, on MRI.

Typically, the most clinically symptomatic side was chosen for the surgical approach. The operative time for a single-level endoscopic procedure averaged 50 minutes. The average blood loss per level decompressed was 25-50 mL. No intraoperative or postoperative transfusions were required. Our rate of minor dural violations and CSF fluid leak was 4% which did not require any additional procedure. The average length of hospital stay was 48 hours. All patients reported an increase in walking distance in immediate postoperative period, which was maintained in 80% of patients at a mean follow-up of 38 months. Patient satisfaction at 4 years was reported to be 78% of the patients, with 88% reporting improvement in symptoms. Overall, the Oswestry disability index scores were as follows: 46 preoperatively, 20 at 1 year, 21 at 2 years; 26 at 3 years.

SUMMARY

Endoscopic decompressive laminotomy combines advantages of minimal invasive spine surgery. The reduced dimension of access route minimizes muscular trauma and postoperative pain; this considerably facilitates the rapid resumption of physical activities in a aging population of patients. Better illumination and magnification provides improved visualization of operating field, facilitating the identification of the anatomical structures minimizing risk of neural complications. Like any endoscopic procedure, there is relatively steep learning curve in endoscopic canal decompression. However, for surgeons who are experienced with posterior approaches to the spine and have some experience with arthroscopy and microscope; it is relatively easier to graduate to endoscopic or arthroscopic decompressive laminotomy.

REFERENCES

1. Tsai RYC, Yang RS, Bray RS. Microscopic laminotomies for degenerative lumbar spinal stenosis. J. Spinal Disorders. 1998:11:389-94.
2. Tuite GF. Stern JD. Dran SE, et al. Outcome after laminectomy for lumbar spinal stenosis. part 1: clinical correlations. J Neurosurg 1994:81:699-706.
3. See DH, Kraft GH. Electromyography in paraspinal muscles following surgery for root compressions. Arch Phys Med Rehabil 1975:56:80-3.
4. Sihvonen T, Herno A, Paljarva L, et al. Local denervation atrophy of paraspinal muscles in post operative failed back syndrome. Spine (Phila Pa 1976). 1993;18(5):575-81.
5. Aryanpur J, Ducker T. Multilevel lumbar laminotomies: an alternative to laminectomy in treatment of lumbar stenosis. Neurosurgery 1990:26:429-33.
6. McCulloh JA. Microsurgical spinal laminitomies. In: Frymoyer JW, editor. The adult spine: priniciples and practice. New york: Raven press Ltd; 1991.pp 1765-84.
7. Young S, Veerapan R, O'Laire SA. Releif of lumbar canal stenosis using multilevel subarticular fenestrations as an alternative to wide laminectomy: preliminary report. Neurosurgery. 1988;23(5):628-33.
8. Turner JA, Ersek M, Herron L, et al. Surgery for lumbar spinal stenosis, attempted meta-analysis of the literature. Spine. 1992;17:1-8.
9. Herno A, Saari T, Suomalainen O, et al. The degree of decompressive relief and its relation to clinical outcome in patients undergoing surgery for lumbar spinal stenosis. Spine. 1999;24:1010-4.
10. Herron LD. Mangelsdorf C. Lumbar spinal results of surgical treatment. J Spinal Didord. 1991:4:26-33.
11. Khoo L, Fessler R. Microendoscopic decompressive laminotomy for the treeatment of lumbar stenosis. Neurosurgery. 2002:5(5 Suppl): S146-54.
12. Katz JN. Stucki G. Lipson SJ, et al. Predictors of surgical outcome in degenerative lumbar spinal stenosis. Spine 1999:21:2229-33.
13. Postacchini F. Spine update: surgical management of lumbar spinal stenosis. Spine 1999:24:1043-7.
14. Boden SD, Davis DO, Dina TS, et al. Abnormal magnetic -resonance scans of the lumbar spine in asymptomatic subjects. A prospective investigation. J Bone Joint Surg Am. 1990;72(3):403-8.
15. Amundsen T, Weber H, Nordal HJ, Magnaes B, Abdelnoor M, Lilleas F. Lumbar spinal stenosis: conservative or surgical management?: A prospective 10 year study. Spine (Philapa 1976). 2000:25(11):1424-35; discussion 1435-6.
16. Athiviraham A. Wali ZA, Yen D. Predictive factors influencing clinical outcome with operative management of lumbar spinal stenosis. Spine J. 2011 Apr 8. [Epub ahead of print].
17. White AH, Wiltse LL. Postoperative spondylolisthesis. In: Weinstein PR, Ehni G, Wilson CB, (Eds). Lumbar spondylosis: diagnosis, management and surgical treatment, St Louis: Mosby; 1977.

4

SECTION

MIS in Lumbar Spine—Instrumented

Section Outline

22

CHAPTER

MIS–TLIF Systems

Rajkumar Deshpande

ABSTRACT

The fusion technique has become one of the popular surgeries in the present day practice. Transforaminal lumbar interbody fusion (TLIF) is becoming increasingly popular because of its easier access , lesser complications and good union rates. The inclusion of minimal access (MIS) to TLIF procedure has indeed helped to achieve advantages of both the aspects and is gaining popularity in present day scenario. The chapter deals with the current available systems for MIS TLIF, indications and contraindications of the procedure.

INTRODUCTION

The spinal fusion procedure was introduced as a treatment option for chronic low back pain in degenerative disk disease more than 70 years ago.[1]

Albee and Hibbs are attributed to spinal fusion for stabilization for the first time in 1911.[2,3] Later, in 1923, Burns[4] described anterior lumbar interbody fusion (ALIF), following which in 1940 posterior lumbar interbody fusion (PLIF) was performed by Cloward[5] using a shaped spinous process autograft. He reported satisfactory results in more than 85% of 331 patients using this technique in 1951. Due to the high pseudoarthrosis rate with using stand-alone grafts, PLIF technique was augmented with instrumentation—initially Harrington rods[6] (1950s), Hartshill rectangle[7] and finally pedicle screws.

Transforaminal lumbar interbody fusion (TLIF) was popularized by Harms et al. as an alternative to PLIF.[8] TLIF offers several advantages including decreased retraction of the dural sac, lessening the risk of postoperative radiculitis. The major difference in the TLIF approach is that the operation is performed unilaterally, and the bone graft is inserted into the disk space through the side.[9]

A major inconvenience, however, with both PLIF and TLIF, was the surgical approach, in which a large midline skin incision had to be made with extensive muscle and aponeurosis detachment, resulting in significant iatrogenic soft-tissue damage. They are typically lengthy procedures and require a long exposure, which may result in ischemic necrosis of the paraspinal musculature, atrophy, and prolonged back pain.[9]

Foley et al.[10] described an alternative procedure minimally invasive transforaminal lumbar interbody fusion (MIS-TLIF), which decreased soft tissue injury but helped achieve the same desired surgical objective.

Minimally invasive surgery refers to any procedure that is less invasive than open surgery, used for the same purpose. The term was first coined by John EA Wickham[11] in 1984 for such procedures that would cause minimal damage to biological tissues at the point of instrument entrance. When compared to open cases, the minimally invasive procedure offers improved perioperative outcomes, improved or equivalent long-term effectiveness, and reduced rate of infection.[14]

A variety of minimally invasive procedures are being performed to achieve interbody fusion, such as anterior lumbar fusion (ALIF), posterior lumbar interbody fusion (PLIF), transforaminal lumbar interbody fusion (TLIF), lateral interbody fusion (e.g. extreme lateral interbody fusion [XLIF] or direct lateral interbody fusion [DLIF]), and para-axial interbody fusion (axial IF), with the intent of limiting iatrogenic damage to muscular, ligamentous, neural and vascular structures.

Due to the nature of the posterolateral extracanalicular diskectomy and fusion, MIS-TLIF has been reported as a safe technique, without the potential complications described when using combined ALIF and PLIF techniques.[8,12] Interbody fusion by conventional midline posterior approach has been reported to have a higher incidence of complications resulting from severe muscle damage and blood loss due to the dissection and retraction of broad muscular tissues as compared to MIS-TLIF.[8,15] Long-term results, however, may be similar to open surgery[13,14]

A review of the literature shows a large number of studies comparing open and minimally invasive transforaminal lumbar interbody fusion.

COMPLICATIONS

Decreased Blood Loss and Operative Time

Studies consistently report significantly less blood loss with minimally invasive TLIF than with open TLIF. In one of the studies, Issacs[16] showed that mean intraoperative blood loss for patients treated with open TLIF (1147 mL) was almost 2.5 times greater than the mean blood loss for MIS TLIF patients (226 mL). Even the operative time was shown to be better than if not similar to open surgeries, ranging from 2 hours for a single level fusion to 6 hours for multilevel fusions which was comparable with the available evidence in literature.[18]

Early Ambulation

Studies reveal that patients treated with minimally invasive TLIF ambulate significantly faster postoperatively than patients treated with open TLIF.[17] Earlier mobilization may be a result of diminished postoperative pain. In some studies[18] the average time to ambulation for patients treated with minimally invasive TLIF (1.2 days) was almost 2 days earlier than the average time to ambulation for patients treated with open TLIF (3.4 days).

Shorter Length of Stay

In most studies,[19,20] the length of hospitalization was significantly shorter for patients treated with minimally invasive TLIF than for patients treated with open TLIF. In fact, in one study[18] the mean length of stay for patients treated with minimally invasive TLIF was as short as 3.2 days-almost 3.5 days shorter than the length of stay for patients treated with open TLIF (6.8 days). Younger patients were discharged earlier as compared to the older adults.

Other Complications

Other complications, such as atelectasis, switch from percutaneous to open, neurological deficit, implant malposition, hematoma, anemia, cage migration, wound infection, deep venous thrombosis, ileus, nonunion, and any case requiring revision surgery are also reported in literature.[21] The quantitative analysis of back muscle degeneration after posterior lumbar fusion also done in some studies showed comparison of minimally invasive and conventional open surgery where significant muscle atrophy is replaced by fat which is evident in open surgery.[17]

Fusion Rates

The limited exposure inherent to minimally invasive fusion techniques has the potential to affect adequate bone grafting and graft site preparation to allow for arthrodesis to occur. Despite this concern, numerous studies have shown minimally invasive TLIF to deliver comparable fusion rates to conventional open surgical techniques—minimally invasive TLIF (93.4%) and open TLIF (93.8%).[22]

Pain Relief

The visual analogue scale (VAS) used to assess degree of pain in many studies has also revealed significantly reduced pain postoperatively as compared to the open counterparts.

INDICATIONS

Indications for surgery by MIS-TLIF are similar to that for open TLIF and are primarily determined by the surgeons' experience and comfort level. An adequate familiarity and competence is crucial prior to attempting any minimally invasive procedure. This skill level may be enhanced through cadaver courses, workshops and proper training, followed initially by rather simpler minimal-access procedures, such as MIS microdiskectomy through tubular retractors and then progressing toward MIS-TLIF.

Spondylolisthesis: Isthmic and Degenerative

Mechanical low-back and radicular pain associated with spondylolisthesis is one of the classical indications for MIS-TLIF. Grade I or II spondylolisthesis is usually suitable for minimally invasive applications; high grade slips are technically very challenging and are optimally treated by most surgeons via an open approach. The concept of fixation in such cases is primarily to stabilize and fuse the spinal deformity causing instability.[23-26]

Severe Degenerative Spinal Stenosis—Central and Foraminal (With Chronic Back Pain)

MIS-TLIF provides the ability to directly decompress both the ipsilateral exiting and traversing nerve roots. In cases of bilateral radiculopathy, contralateral decompression can be indirectly achieved following graft placement once foraminal height and sagittal balance have been restored. While treatment of degenerative lumbar stenosis without spondylolisthesis or deformity has traditionally included decompressive procedures, such as laminectomy with or without diskectomy, evidence of spinal instability should mandate a lumbar fusion as a recommended treatment option.[27,28]

Multiple Recurrent Disk Herniation

Patients with multiple (three or more) lumbar disk herniation with radiculopathy (with or without back pain) or those with only one recurrence but with significant mechanical back pain are also considered good candidates for the minimally invasive TLIF procedure, which can be a final definitive treatment. It can be repeated on the same side as the previous surgery because the transforaminal approach is usually lateral to the scar tissue. Usually, symptomatic herniated disk undergo diskectomy alone while routine use of lumbar fusion to augment the diskectomy is not justified. However, fusion may be used in cases where there may be evidence of preoperative spinal deformity. Since lumbar deformity, instability, or low back pain may result in the setting of a reoperative lumbar diskectomy, especially in cases where extensive bony removal is necessary for exposure of the disk fragments, fusion is often considered in such cases. Further, multiple diskectomies might lead to collapse of the interbody space post diskectomy with neuroforaminal stenosis and radiculopathy, in which case fusion might be a better alternative solution.[29,30]

Primary Degenerative Disk Disease Causing Diskogenic Low Back Pain (At One or More Lumbar Levels)

Another potential indication for MIS TLIF includes severe diskogenic low-back pain caused by degenerative disk disease. Since there a gamut of causes for mechanical low back pain, their etiology is not completely understood and hence, efforts to surgically treat these conditions also remain controversial. Various etiologies have been suggested, including lumbar segmental instability or facet joint syndrome, especially when no other objective signs of increased motion or spondylolisthesis could be explained. The intervertebral disk has also been implicated, along with the role of biochemical mediators, but ultimately, it may not be possible to pin-point any single factor alone in being able to generate the spinal tissue pathology. While most cases of low back pain may be managed by conservative measures along with lifestyle and activity modification, it remains ineffective in almost 5% of cases that can progress to more severe chronic and disabling forms requiring more aggressive treatment.[31,32]

Failed back syndrome

Treatment of pseudoarthrosis, postlaminectomy kyphosis, lumbar deformity with coronal and/or sagittal plane imbalance and failed previous lumbar fusions by other techniques, are some of the other indications that may represent the "failed back syndrome". These may also be successfully treated with MIS TLIF, when associated with chronic pain or instability.[33]

CONTRAINDICATIONS

Once again, there exist mostly similar contraindications for both open and minimally invasive posterior interbody fusion techniques.

Conjoined Nerve Roots

One of the few absolute contraindications is the presence of a conjoined nerve root within the foramen. Though this occurrence maybe extremely rare, this must be kept in mind and preoperative MRI images must be closely viewed to look for this. The conjoined root directly covers the desired entry point, and any attempt to retract or mobilize the root would have a very significantly high rate of neurological damage. If the conjoined root is discovered intraoperatively after complete facetectomy, it may be wiser to abort the procedure ipsilaterally. A contralateral TLIF could be considered at that point through a similar minimally invasive approach.[34]

Severe Osteoporosis

Poor bone quality unable to support an interbody construct due to attendant risk of graft subsidence through the endplates is also considered as potential contraindication. Risk of screw pullout is also high in such cases; however, alternate options are available, such as augmentation with PMMA cement.[35]

Other Relative Contraindications

Multilevel (> 3 levels) disk disease (in patients without lumbar spinal deformities) and single-level disk disease causing radicular pain without symptoms of mechanical low-back pain or instability.[36]

REFERENCES

1. Bick, Edgar M. An essay on the history of spine fusion operations. Clin Orthop Relat Res. 1964;35: 9-15.
2. Hibbs R A. An operation for progressive spinal deformities. New York Med J. 1911;21:1013-6.
3. Albee FH. Transplantation of a portion of the tibia into the spine for Pott's disease. JAMA. 1911;57:855.
4. Burns BH. An operation for spondylolisthesis. Lancet. 1933; 224:1233.
5. Cloward RB. The treatment of ruptured lumbar intervertebral disks by vertebral body fusion. I. Indications, operative technique, after care. J Neurosurg. 1953;10(2):154-68.
6. White A H, Zucherman JF, Hsu KY. Lumbosacral fusions with Harrington rods and intersegmental wiring. 1986; 203:185-90.
7. Dove J. Internal fixation of the lumbar spine. The Hartshill rectangle. Clin Orthop Relat Res. 1986; 203:135-40.
8. Harms J, Jeszenszky D. The unilateral transforaminal approach for posterior lumbar interbody fusion. Orthop Traumatol. 1998; 6:88-99.
9. Sait Naderi, Edward C. Benzel, Chap 1. History of Spine Surgery, 3rd Edition. Spine surgery -Techniques, Complication Avoidance and Management.
10. Foley KT, Holly LT, Schwender JD. Minimally invasive lumbar fusion. Spine (Phila Pa 1976). 2003; 28(15 Suppl):S26-35.
11. Wickham JE. The new surgery. Br Med J (Clin Res Ed). 1987; 295(6613): 1581-2.
12. Moskowitz A. Transforaminal lumbar interbody fusion. Orthop Clin North Am. 2002;33:359-66
13. Isaacs R, Podichetty V, Santiago P, Sandhu FA, Spears J, Kelly K, et al. Minimally invasive microendoscopy-assisted transforaminal lumbar interbody fusion with instrumentation. J Neurosurg: Spine. 2005;3:98-105.
14. Park Y, Won Ha J. Comparison of One-Level Posterior Lumbar Interbody Fusion Performed With a Minimally Invasive Approach or a Traditional Open Approach. Spine (Phila Pa 1976). 2007;32:537-43.
15. Potter BK, Freedman BA, Verwiebe EG, Hall JM, Polly DW Jr, Kuklo TR. Transforaminal lumbar interbody fusion: clinical and radiographic results and complications in 100 consecutive patients. J Spinal Disord Tech. 2005;18:337-46
16. Schwender JD, Holly LT, Rouben DP, Foley KT. Minimally invasive transforaminal lumbar interbody fusion (TLIF): technical feasibility and initial results. J Spinal Disord Tech 2005; 18: S1-S6.
17. Sang-Hyuk Min, Jae-Sung Yoo, The clinical and radiological outcomes of multilevel minimally invasive transforaminal lumbar interbody fusion. Eur Spine J. 2013, 22:1164-72.
18. Lee KH, Yue WM et al, Clinical and radiological outcomes of open versus minimally invasive transforaminal lumbar interbody fusion, Eur Spine J. 2012; 21(11):2265-70.
19. Park Y, Won Ha J. Comparison of One-Level Posterior Lumbar Interbody Fusion Performed With a Minimally Invasive Approach or a Traditional Open Approach. Spine (Phila Pa 1976). 2007; 32:537-43.
20. Wang M, Cummock M, Yu Y, et al. An analysis of the differences in the acute hospitalization charges following minimally invasive versus open posterior lumbar interbody fusion. J Neurosurg: Spine. 2010; 12:694-9.
21. Alphonse Lubansu MD With Kanna Gnanalingham MD, Paulo Pereira MD, Cornelius Wimmer MD. Evaluation of the complication rate after 500 minimally invasive spinal (MIS) procedures: a European multicenter prospective study - Presented at SMISS 2009 Annual Conference.
22. Moon-Chan Kim, Hung-Tae Chung et al, The Clinical and Radiological Outcomes of Minimally Invasive Transforaminal Lumbar Interbody Single Level Fusion, Asian Spine Journal. 2011;5(2):111-6.
23. Weinstein JN, Lurie JD, Tosteson TD, et al. Surgical versus nonsurgical treatment for lumbar degenerative spondylolisthesis. N Engl J Med. 2007; 356:2257-70.
24. Wang J, Zhou Y, Zheng Z, et al. Comparison of one-level minimally invasive and open transforaminal lumbar interbody fusion in degenerative and isthmic spondylolisthesis grades 1 and 2. Eur Spine J. 2010;19:1780-4.
25. Park P, Foley KT. Minimally invasive transforaminal lumbar interbody fusion with reduction of spondylolisthesis: technique and outcomes after a minimum of 2 years' follow-up. Neurosurg Focus. 2008;25:E16.
26. Resnick DK, Choudhri TF, Dailey AT, et al. Guidelines for the performance of fusion procedures for degenerative disease of the lumbar spine. Part 9: fusion in patients with stenosis and spondylolisthesis. J Neurosurg Spine. 2005;2:679-85
27. Scheufler KM, Dohmen H, Vougioukas VI. Percutaneous transforaminal lumbar interbody fusion for the treatment of degenerative lumbar instability. Neurosurgery. 2007;60(4 suppl 2):203–12; discussion 212-3.
28. Resnick DK, Choudhri TF, Dailey AT, et al. Guidelines for the performance of fusion procedures for degenerative disease of the lumbar spine. Part 10: fusion following decompression in patients with stenosis without spondylolisthesis. J Neurosurg Spine. 2005; 2:686-91.
29. Selznick LA, Shamji MF, Isaacs RE. Minimally invasive interbody fusion for revision lumbar surgery: technical feasibility and safety. J Spinal Disord Tech. 2009;22:207-13.
30. Resnick DK, Choudhri TF, Dailey AT, et al. Guidelines for the performance of fusion procedures for degenerative disease of the lumbar spine. Part 8: lumbar fusion for disk herniation and radiculopathy. J Neurosurg Spine. 2005;2:673-8
31. Shunwu F, Xing Z, Fengdong Z, et al. Minimally invasive transforaminal lumbar interbody fusion for the treatment of degenerative lumbar diseases. Spine. 2010;35:1615-20.
32. Resnick DK, Choudhri TF, Dailey AT, et al. Guidelines for the performance of fusion procedures for degenerative disease of the lumbar spine. Part 7: intractable low-back pain without stenosis or spondylolisthesis. J Neurosurg Spine. 2005;2:673-8
33. German JW, Foley KT. Minimal access surgical techniques in the management of the painful lumbar motion segment. Spine. 2005;30(suppl 16):S52-9.
34. Holly LT, Schwender JD, Rouben DP, Foley KT. Minimally invasive transforaminal lumbar interbody fusion: indications, technique, and complications. Neurosurg Focus. 2006;20(3):E6.
35. Karikari IO, Isaacs RE. Minimally invasive transforaminal lumbar interbody fusion: a review of techniques and outcomes. Spine (Phila Pa 1976). 2010;35(26 Suppl):S294-301.
36. Mummaneni PV, Haid RW, Rodts GE Jr: Lumbar interbody fusion: State-of-the-art technical advances. J Neurosurg. 2004;1[Suppl]:24-30.

23

CHAPTER

Minimally Invasive Surgery—Transforaminal Lumbar Interbody Fusion

Arvind G Kulkarni, Hussain Bohra, Vishwanath Patil

ABSTRACT

Minimal invasive surgery transforaminal lumbar interbody fusion (MIS–TLIF) has gained wide popularity because of its advantages over open TLIF. The lesser invasiveness of the procedure, less tissue trauma, faster rehabilitation, less postoperative complications are the main advantages over open TLIF. LIF has a steep learning curve and the instrumentation plays a special role in achieving satisfactory result. The procedure has wide indications, is especially helpful in obese patients and revision surgeries in which the extent of soft-tissue dissection is decreased and complications secondary to adhesions are reduced.

INTRODUCTION

Lumbar arthrodesis is a commonly performed surgical procedure for the treatment of degenerative spine, trauma, infection, neoplasm, and spinal instability. A posterolateral fusion with autologous on-lay bone graft has traditionally resulted in acceptable clinical results; however, reported fusion rates have been inconsistent. With the addition of internal fixation using pedicle screw instrumentation, fusion rates have improved significantly, especially in cases of instability.[1,2] Performing an interbody arthrodesis may further improve the clinical results by eliminating the disk as a potential pain generator, improving fusion rates, and restoring intervertebral height and lumbar lordosis.[3-8] Techniques to achieve anterior column interbody fusion include anterior lumbar interbody fusion (ALIF), posterior lumbar interbody fusion (PLIF), or transforaminal lumbar interbody fusion (TLIF).

Over the last decade, TLIF has become a popular technique for achieving interbody fusion. The TLIF approach may reduce the risk of iatrogenic neurologic injury when compared with PLIF; provide a circumferential arthrodesis; and avoid anterior spinal exposure and its associated complications.[9-14] Cole et al.[15] in 2009 compared posterior lumbar interbody fusion with transforaminal lumbar interbody fusion, and they found that the chief advantage of TLIF procedure compared to PLIF procedure included a decrease in potential neurological injury, improvement in lordotic alignment given graft placement within the anterior column, and preservation of posterior column integrity through minimizing lamina, facet, and pars dissection. Mura et al.[16] in 2011 did a retrospective analysis of 100 patients who underwent TLIF. They concluded that the TLIF procedure led to shortened surgical times, less neurologic injury, and improved overall outcomes. Audat et al.[17] in 2012 compared clinical and radiological results of PLF, PLIF and TLIF techniques in the treatment of degenerative lumbar spine. They concluded that surgical techniques, such as PLF, PLIF and TLIF are equally suitable for treating degenerative disk disease, with no differences observed in complications and clinical outcomes. However, the best radiological outcome was found in patients treated with TLIF.

With advances in minimal access technology, TLIF can now be performed through a minimally invasive, unilateral approach, providing an adequate decompression and circumferential fusion, and avoid many of the disadvantages of the traditional posterior open approach.[18,19] A study by Schwender et al.[20] reported clinically significant improvements in visual analog scale and Oswestry disability index scores along with a 100% fusion rate in a cohort of patients who underwent a minimally invasive TLIF procedure. A major break-through was achieved when intraoperative realtime navigation for placement of percutaneous pedicle screws answered the concerns of radiation hazard involved with any MIS procedure and led to substantial increase in accuracy of pedicle screw instrumentation.

ADVANTAGES

Traditional open posterior approaches to the lumbar spine provide access to the posterior spinal structures, including the lamina, facet joints, transverse processes, and to the intervertebral disk space. The posterior midline spinal exposure typically requires the subperiosteal dissection of the paraspinal muscles. The dissection is carried over the facet joints and laterally to the tips of the transverse processes when concomitant posterolateral arthrodesis is required. Although providing wide access to the spine, the disruption and retraction of the deep paraspinal musculature has been shown to cause localized denervation, which may lead to continued back pain and spasm after the procedure. [21] Multiple studies in this area have shown deleterious histologic effects, including regional ischemia from increased intramuscular pressure secondary to the use of retractor blades.[22,23] Kawaguchi et al.[24] demonstrated that the duration of muscle retraction during spinal surgery, pressure of the retractors, and the number of levels exposed, directly correlate with the postoperative elevation of serum creatinine phosphokinase isoenzymes, a marker of muscle injury. Blood loss (Intraoperative and postoperative) is far less compared to open TLIF hence, abolishing need for transfusion in most of the MIS-TLIFs. Minimal exposure of tissues to the exterior has been proven to reduce infection rates in MIS TLIF and fall-back of the dilated muscles in the tracts have been shown to aid management of dural leaks as well as hasten postoperative recovery and return to work status.

EVOLUTION

The development of minimally invasive techniques to address disease pathologies among several surgical specialties in place of traditional open surgery has become a noteworthy trend. Examples include the laparoscopic approach to gallbladder disease, urologic procedures, cardiac surgeries as well as knee and shoulder arthroscopy as a successor to open surgery for meniscal and rotator cuff disorders, respectively.

This shift toward minimally invasive or minimal-access technologies has also taken place in the specialty of spinal surgery. The goal of the procedure remains the same: to achieve outcomes equivalent to or better than that of traditional open surgery while trying to reduce overall postoperative pain, intraoperative blood loss, hospital stay, surgical scarring and long-term outcomes. Recently, minimally invasive spinal systems have been developed based on the principle of using a series of dilators of different lengths to create a path between muscle fascicles to access the posterior spinal elements.[25-28] This approach avoids stripping the paraspinal muscles and retains the midline ligamentous structures. A working channel is created through which spinal decompression and fusion can be accomplished. Initial surgeries using these access portals involved simple decompressive procedures; however, over the last decade, these systems have been expanded to facilitate interbody and posterolateral arthrodesis in addition to the placement of pedicle screws in a less invasive fashion in traumatic to deformity correction cases.[29-31]

Intraoperative navigation integrated with 2D or 3D-fluoroscopically generated Multiplanar reconstruction (MPR) images gives the surgeon an excellent opportunity to reduce the requirement of Fluoro imaging, dramatically improve the precision of screw placement, reduce the overall OR time and reduce the rates of revision surgeries and the resultant economic burden.

INDICATIONS

1. Grade I, II, III spondylolisthesis (degenerative/lytic) with or without neurological deficit.
2. Degenerative disk disease causing discogenic low back pain.
3. Recurrent lumbar disk herniation/large central disk prolapse with significant mechanical back pain.
4. Post-diskectomy collapse with neural foraminal stenosis and radiculopathy.
5. Treatment of pseudoarthrosis.
6. Treatment of post-laminectomy kyphosis.
7. Treatment of lumbar deformity with coronal and/or sagittal imbalance.

CONTRAINDICATIONS

1. Severe osteoporosis with potential of screw pull-out.
2. Revision of prior instrumented level.
3. Need to avoid Radiation exposure associated with Fluoro guided screw placements.
4. Tight anterior disk space with osteophyte formation in which there is no potential for disk space distraction. (We do it now).

PREOPERATIVE PREPARATIONS

Assessment

The presurgical evaluation should include a thorough history and physical examination. A detailed patient history, including the onset of complaints, aggravating and mitigating factors, and response to any treatments tried, should be entered into the medical record. A comprehensive review of the patient's medical comorbidities is necessary to assess and identify potential contraindications to spinal surgery. Nonorganic or psychological signs as described by Waddell et al.[32] should be noted during the examination.

DIAGNOSTIC TESTING

Radiography should be the initial imaging study. We advocate the use of *standing radiographs that include an anteroposterior (AP) view and lateral flexion and extension views.* The rationale is that most other diagnostic studies are performed in a supine position, which may not detect changes that occur in the spine in an erect position. Although no standard definition of radiographic instability exists, it is generally accepted that 3–4 mm of translation or greater than 11 degrees of angular motion is suggestive of segmental instability. Standing Flexion-extension radiographs allow for identification and quantification of abnormal motion as well as intradiskal vacuum sign.

Magnetic resonance imaging (MRI) has become the most commonly used modality for evaluating the disk, neural elements, surrounding soft tissue, marrow and deciding the surgical plan. Computed tomography with myelography (CT) can be considered when MRI is contraindicated. A CT scan allows for better delineation of osseous anatomy, which offers good picture of anatomy in cases of high-grade spondylolysis-listhesis and facet arthropathy.

Provocative diskography remains controversial in its value and approach. The role of diskography is that it may help differentiate painful disks from other causes of back pain.[33] Dual energy X-ray absorptiometry (DEXA) is an enhanced form of X-ray technology used to measure bone density. Although the reliability of results may be questionable, many surgeons have begun to include an osteoporosis evaluation as a part of the presurgical work-up, especially in postmenopausal women, as a guide for preoperative planning when fusion surgery with instrumentation is being considered.

SURGICAL TECHNIQUE

Anesthesia

General anesthesia is typically used for TLIF. However, when nerve monitoring is being performed, paralytic agents, muscle relaxants, or nitrous oxide, should be avoided, as these agents impede the direct monitoring of nerve-root stimulation.

Positioning

The patient is placed prone on a radiolucent operating table following intubation which allows tilting in all directions and is secured with tapes/belts. The elbows are placed at 90° to decrease traction on the brachial plexus. Pads are placed under the ulnar and peroneal nerves. In addition, pillows are placed under the lower extremities **(Figure 1)**. Prior to starting the case, ensure that the Foley catheter is mobile, endotracheal tube is secure, and the fluoroscopic machine is draped into the operative field. Reverse Trendelenburg position is given to make the involved level as vertical as possible to the floor and avoid prolonged abnormal postures with microscope usage.

SURGICAL PROCEDURE

Following standard skin preparation and sterile draping, AP fluoroscopic images should be obtained to locate the pedicles and relevant anatomy **(Figure 2)**. True lateral image

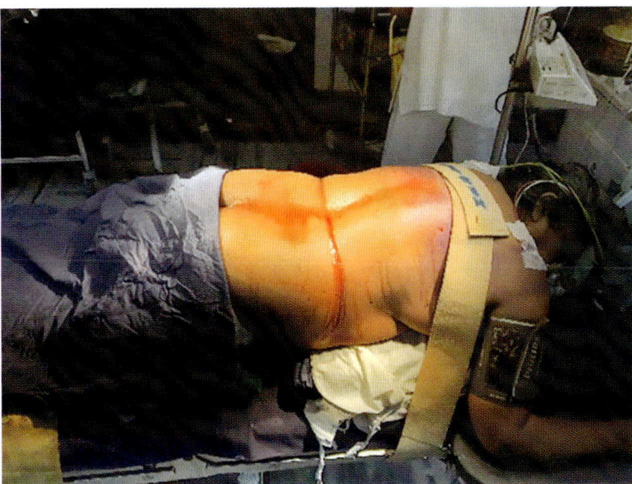

Figure 1: Positioning of the patient on a radiolucent operating table movable in all directions and secured by velcro-straps or adhesive tapes

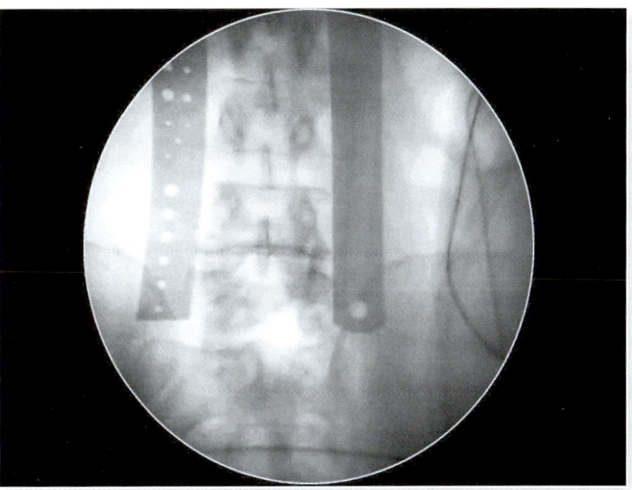

Figure 2: Marking of incision lateral to facet joint line in AP view

is also taken keeping the involved disk space in the center of fluoroimage **(Figure 3)**. (The authors prefer to place the pedicle guide wires first followed by interbody cage and finally pedicle screws with interconnecting rods). Ideal placement is generally 3–4 cm off the midline. After the correct pedicle is identified, a Jamshidi needle (11 G Cooks needle) is introduced, beginning at the outer-upper quadrant of the pedicle and advanced to just lateral of the medial pedicle wall in the inner quadrant **(Figure 4A)**. A lateral view is necessary to confirm correct placement within the pedicle. To overcome the effects of parallax, the fluoroscopy unit may have to be angled either cranially or caudally to be tangential to the end plates. Once optimal visualization is achieved, the Jamshidi needle is advanced through the isthmus of the pedicle, staying within a zone between the superior and inferior margins **(Figures 4B and C)**. The tip of the needle is advanced through the pedicle isthmus to the vertebral body. Once placement of the Jamshidi needle within the vertebral body at the appropriate orientation is confirmed, a blunt-tipped threaded guidewire is passed through the cannulated center of the entry needle. Care should be taken not to advance the guidewire to within 10 mm from the anterior wall of the vertebral body. Following confirmation by lateral fluoroscopic images of the tip of the guidewire, the Jamshidi needle is withdrawn. The steps are repeated for rest of the pedicles and all the guide wires bent away from the operative field securing them to the draping without introducing sharp bends into them **(Figures 5A and B)**.

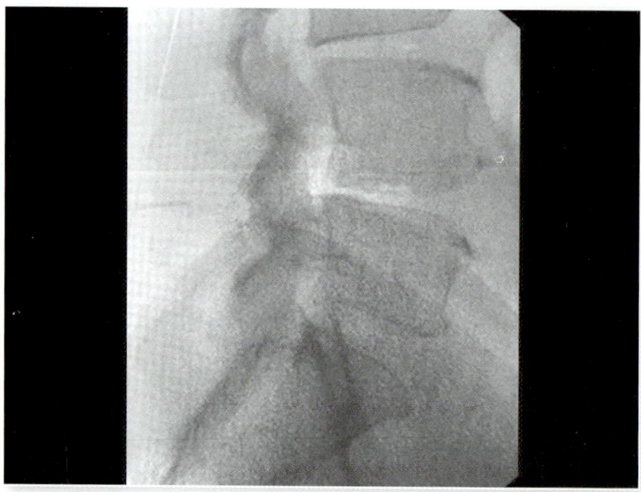

Figure 3: True lateral image of involved disk space to determine the superior and inferior margins of pedicles and depth of screw placement

Decompression and interbody cage placement is the next step for which a guide pin/22 G spinal needle is advanced onto the ipsilateral facet joint at a trajectory parallel to the disk space. A paramedian incision (3 cm) is made around the guide pin/22 G spinal needle and lateral to the facet joint to allow for medial direction of instruments in the disk space. The incision is then carried through the skin, soft tissue, and dorsal lumbar fascia. Often the incision lies between the two-pedicle guide-wire tracts and both can be connected to simplify the procedure and adding to the cosmesis. Under fluoroscopic guidance, serial dilators are placed docking on the facet joint and spreading the muscle fascicles. Once the largest dilator has been placed (22 mm outer diameter), a tubular retractor of appropriate length (5/6/7 cm) is placed over the dilator and locked in the correct position, position confirmed under C-arm **(Figure 6)**. The dilators are then removed. With certain systems, the final retractor is a fixed tube (METRx), whereas other systems have a split blade tubular retract or (QUADRANT, MARS 3 retractor) that can be expanded. The appropriate position of the retractor is on the facet joint and angled with a trajectory parallel to the intervertebral disk. Subsequently, microscope magnification can be used.

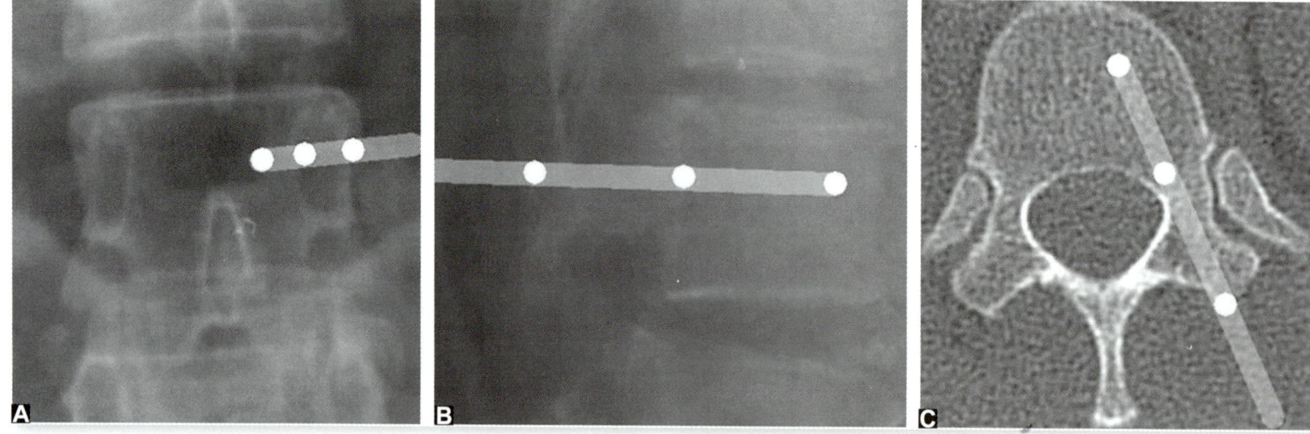

Figures 4A to C: (A) Anteroposterior view of pedicle illustrating needle entry point and path for needle advancement. Starting from outer wall of pedicle to medial wall of pedicle and beyond medial wall of pedicle; (B) Lateral view of pedicle corresponding to Figure 4A, showing the path for needle advancement.1, beginning point of pedicle, posterior margin of vertebral body and anterior 1/3rd of body; (C) Three points in axial view to achieve a pedicle screw without any breach

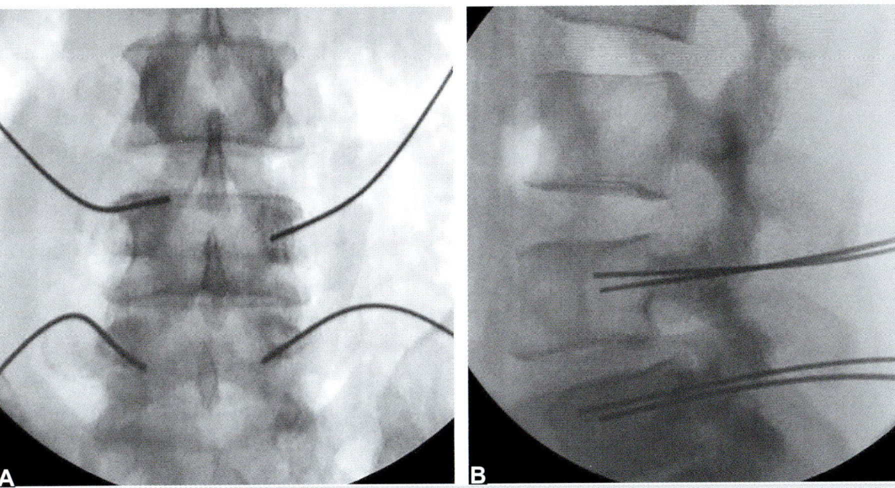

Figures 5A and B: Percutaneous placement of guidewires over Jamshidi needle. (A) AP view; (B) Lateral views

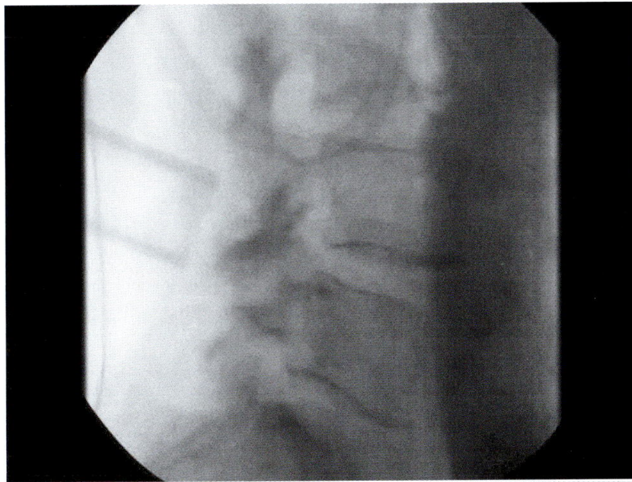

Figure 6: Placement of tube at desired level

The next step in the procedure is performing the facetectomy. The soft tissue over the facet is removed with a monopolar cautery and Kerrison rongeur. The facet–lamina junction is delineated using curettes. Using an angled curette, the space between the lamina and the ligamentum flavum is defined after thinning out the lamina with a high-speed burr. Using the Kerrison rongeur, the lamino-facet junction is removed. If there is no stenosis, then a small laminotomy can be done to allow the visualization of the neural elements in close proximity to the facet joint. If the patient has stenosis on the ipsilateral side, a complete laminectomy should be performed. In cases of bilateral stenosis, the spinous process can be undercut and a contralateral laminectomy and medial-facetectomy accomplished. If stenosis is severe or there is a significant foraminal component on the contralateral side, we suggest decompressing the lateral recess down to the exit zone by wanding the tube caudally. Using a combination of Kerrison rongeur and osteotomes, the facet joint is removed (the superior facet osteotomized flush to the superior end-plate) to be morcellated and used as interbody bone graft. A burr may be used to remove the facet joint, but this decreases the quantity of bone graft.

The next step involves identifying the disk space. If the laminectomy was already performed, dura and the nerve root are identified. If a laminectomy has not been done, remove the ligamentum flavum to expose the lateral edge of the dura and nerve root. In general, the traversing root is medial to the foramen and minimal if any retraction is required. The exiting nerve roots hug the pedicle as it exits the neural foramen and is generally cephalad to the level of the disk in the foramen. Although we do not necessarily dissect out the exiting root, it may be protected by placing a patty directed toward the cephalad pedicle in the foramen.

The annulus is incised with a bayonet long-handle mounted 15 no. blade directing the knife blade away from the nerve root and dura. A pituitary rongeur is used to initiate the discectomy. Subsequently, a series of curettes and disk shavers are used to loosen and remove the remainder of the disk from the endplates. Under lateral fluoroscopy a distractor and sizer are placed into the disk space **(Figure 7)**. An end-plate scraper is utilized to complete the disk-space preparation. A chisel can be used to remove osteophytes from the posterior vertebral body cortex that can impede the placement of the interbody device. Care must be taken to place the chisel parallel to the superior and inferior endplates preventing damage to the vertebral body.

The appropriate size trial interbody cage is then placed into the disk space. After confirming proper placement on fluoroscopy, the trial is removed and any fragment of bone and cartilage is removed. Autologous bone graft is then packed into the anterior disk space using a funnel.

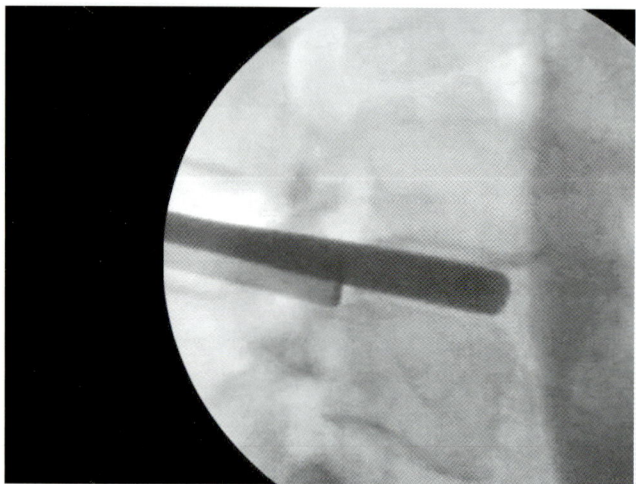

Figure 7: Cage size in the disk space after thorough diskectomy and end-plate preparation using an assortment of curettes

When bone morphogenic protein is used, we recommend placing this anterior to the interbody device to prevent posterior bony overgrowth toward the neural foramen. The interbody structural device (Cage filled with bone-graft) is then advanced into the disk space under fluoroscopy. An AP and lateral fluoroscopic X-ray is used to verify appropriate implant positioning **(Figures 8A and B)**.

Focus is now turned to placing percutaneous pedicle screws. Skin and underlying fascia are dilated by means of sequential dilators to create a pathway for the pedicle screw over the initially placed guidewires. The largest dilator is left in place to protect surrounding soft tissue and for measurement purposes. A cannulated tap is advanced over the guidewire down to the pedicle. Depth measurements located on the outside of the tissue dilator sleeve can help guide depth during tapping. Care should be taken to prevent the guidewire from advancing or backing-out. Once the pedicle is tapped, the tap and tissue dilator sleeve are withdrawn while the screwdriver and tower assembly are placed over the guidewire. The pedicle screw is advanced with the polyaxial screwdriver until the appropriate depth is achieved **(Figure 9)**. Anteroposterior and lateral fluoroscopic images are obtained to confirm the screw's placement within the pedicle, orientation, and overall depth. Care should be taken to avoid advancing the screw head to bone, which would limit the ability to seat the rod. The guidewire is withdrawn as the screw enters the pedicle inorder to avoid it getting bent ahead of screw tip and trapped. The screwdriver is withdrawn from the tower assembly. Subsequent pedicle screws are placed with this same technique. It is important to note that all screw tower assemblies should line up in the same orientation and height before the next step of the procedure. A rod measurement guide is placed to facilitate measurement of the rod size. The rod is passed percutaneously through a separate stab incision (SEXTANT) or placed free-hand in other designs leaving adequate lengths at both ends **(Figure 10)**. Once the rod is seated, a cap inserter is placed in the tower assembly. Subsequent screw caps are now placed. Compression can be achieved by system specific methods. Final tightening of the construct is performed with an antitorque stabilizer and torque-limited driver. The screw tower assemblies are loosened and removed. Final radiograph is obtained to confirm proper positioning of screws, cage and rod **(Figure 11)**. Dorsolumbar fascia is approximated with absorbable No. 2-0 vicryl and subcuticular running closure with monocryl 3-0 done.

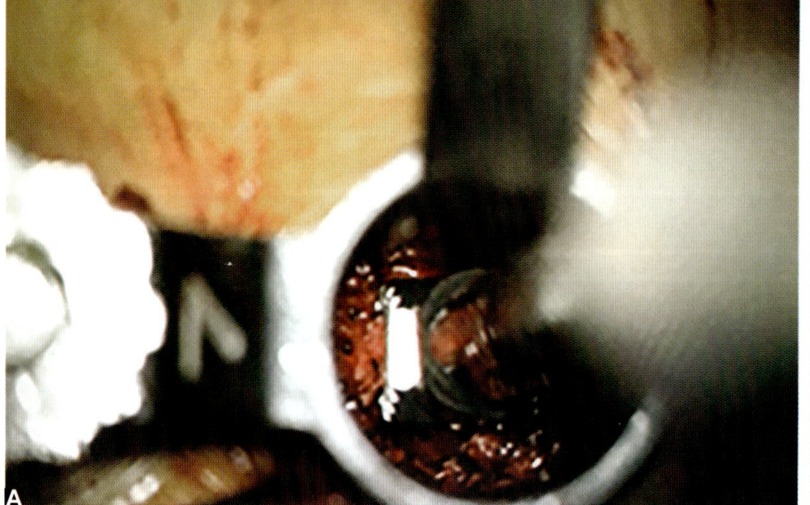

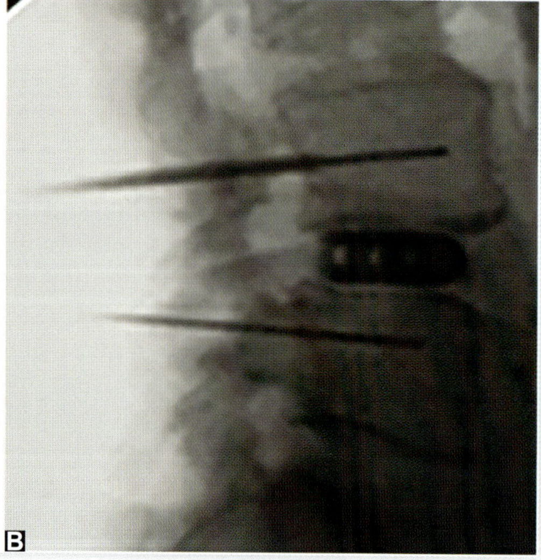

Figures 8A and B: Placement of appropriate cage through the tube under direct vision protecting the neural structures medially with a malleable retractor and confirmed under lateral fluoroscopy

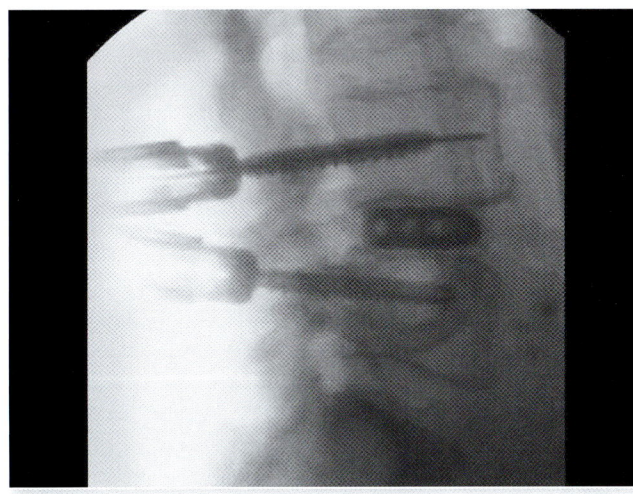

Figure 9: Percutaneous placement of pedicle screws with care taken to align the tulips at equal depth aiding easy placement of connecting rod

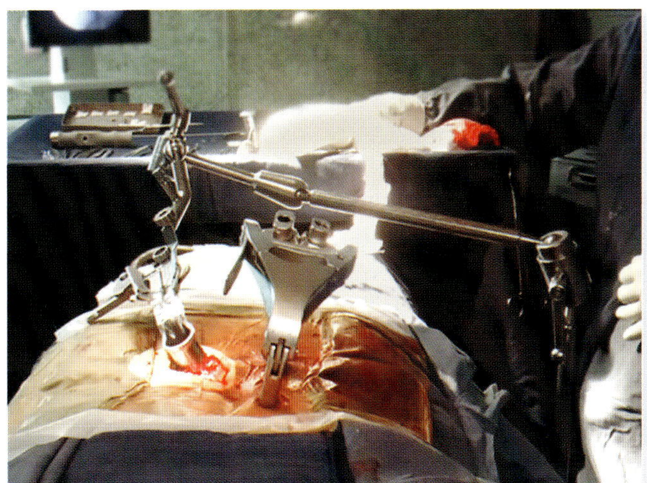

Figure 10: Percutaneous placement of connecting rod by SEXTANT assembly (Medtronic Inc). The METRx tube can be seen docked and medially angulated on the right side.

POSTOPERATIVE CARE

Postoperatively patients should be monitored with frequent neurologic assessments. Treatment for postoperative pain varies according to the clinical practice standards of the surgeon. Many surgeons do prescribe a lumbar orthosis after fusion surgery. Ambulation usually begins on postoperative day 1. The Foley catheter is removed and the patient is started on oral analgesics. Criteria for discharge from the hospital should include adequate pain control with oral analgesic medication, safe ambulation with the use of an assistive device (if needed), and medical stability. The hospital stay for minimally invasive lumbar fusion varies from an average of 2 days to longer for patients who have additional medical comorbidities. The usual precautions during the acute postoperative phase include avoidance of heavy lifting, bending, and high-impact activities. Generally, patients should be encouraged to ambulate to avoid deconditioning. Nonsteroidal anti-inflammatory medications should be avoided because they are known to decrease the fusion rate.[34] Instructions for surgical wound care should be given to and understood by the patient prior to discharge after a check dressing is done with transparent, nonpermeable (Tegaderm/OPsite) dressing. The scar at 6 weeks follow-up is cosmetic **(Figure 12)**.

APPLICATION OF MIS–TLIF IN SPECIAL SITUATIONS

MIS-TLIF can now be done in many different and previously thought difficult situations. These have been described in short with other steps remaining the same as mentioned previously.

Collapsed disk space: Patients having collapsed disk space usually have radicular symptoms. This is mainly due to decreased foraminal height which causes compression of

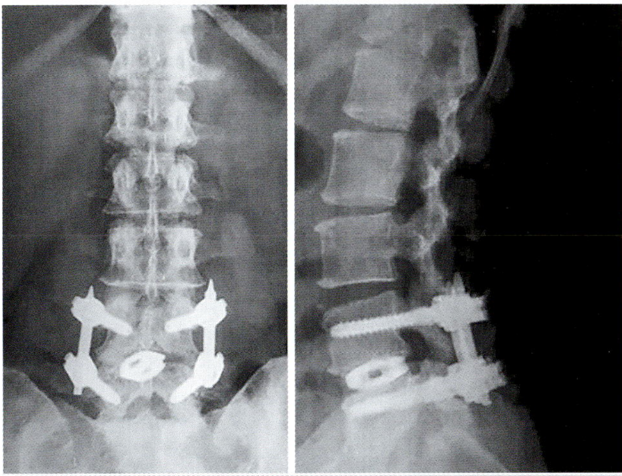

Figure 11: Final radiograph of MIS–TLIF

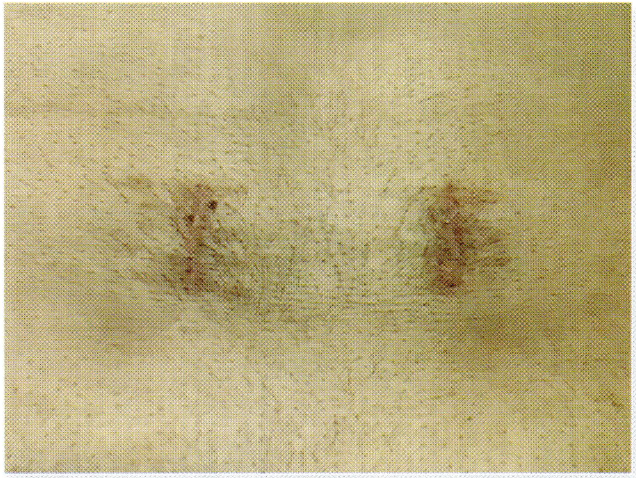

Figure 12: Scar at 6 weeks post-single level MIS–TLIF

the exiting nerve root. The minor changes in the technique to accomplish the aim, i.e. to jack up the disk height and relieve the symptoms are as follows: The disk space is mainly increased by two mechanisms. First, by application of unilateral percutaneous screws and rod. *Distraction* is applied across these to increase the disk space. Second is by *intradiskal distraction* **(Figure 13)**. Disc space is increased with application of increasing size of serial shavers/ smooth-edged spreaders after initial space is created with a special disk-opener of flat-blunt chisel. Finally, bone graft and interbody cage is inserted in this distracted position [resulting in better sagittal alignment] which also directly decompresses the nerve root and thus relieves the symptoms **(Figure 14)**.

High-grade spondylolisthesis: Patients having mobile high-grade anterolisthesis have exiting nerve root compression aggravated on load bearing. This is due to the compression caused by the pseudoarthrotic tissue around the cranial half of broken pars pressing on to the exiting nerve root. Technique of MIS–TLIF needs to be modified to partially/ completely reduce the listhesis, increase the effective foraminal dimensions by augmenting the disk height by getting a larger interbody cage and increase the bed available for solid fusion. Routine pedicle screws with special *reduction extenders* having capacity to pull the proximal pedicle screws help by seating the connecting rod into the tulip and avoid excessive stress on the implants. Using serially increasing sizes of disk space dilators/shavers also increases the ease of reduction and getting a better disc height **(Figure 13)**.

Hypertrophied facets with narrow canal: Special emphasis is given on this situation as proper docking of the tube in the presence of hypertrophied facets which are closely placed is a challenge. The tube gets a shallow docking **(Figure 15)** and may lead to higher chances of starting the facetectomy away from the region of interest. To avoid this, the authors, advise burring down on the facet **(Figure 16)** and removing the osteophytes encroaching the spinolaminar line during the first docking followed by sinking the METRx tube further down flush to the actual facet **(Figure 17)**. This helps in starting the facetectomy at a correct trajectory aiding further over-the-top decompression and interbody work later. Placement of the pedicle screws remains the same but getting an ideal facet-sparing entry-point for the proximal pedicle screw is essential.

3D Navigation guided MIS-TLIF: MIS–TLIF procedure has proven to be a boon for the patients but a bane for all the surgeon-staff involved in it on a routine basis. To answer this need for reduction in radiation exposure the technology of real-time intraoperative navigation was developed and has been extensively improvised over the past decade. 2-dimensional C-arm fluoroscopy based images give orientation in only the sagittal and coronal planes but the intraoperatively obtained 3D images with the help of a 3D capable C-arm or intraoperative CT scan takes this further by giving 1mm cuts in the axial plane in realtime **(Figure 18)**. This is possible due to the advancement of technology for quick integration of the multiplanar reconstruction (MPR) images with the optical navigation system used without adding much to the total operating time. Real advantage of this lies in the fact that precise facet joint sparing entry can be taken and optimal trajectory in axial plane can be made with maximal screw length to achieve a near perfect and extremely safe pedicle screw with the maximal possible pull-out strength **(Figures 19A to G)**. Detailed description of the procedure is out of the scope of this chapter.

At author's institution, almost all cases requiring fusion are operated with minimally invasive transforaminal lumbar interbody fusion [MIS–TLIF] technique. With vast experience in minimally invasive techniques, they find MIS to be associated with less postoperative infection rates as compared to open techniques. They believe that the muscle

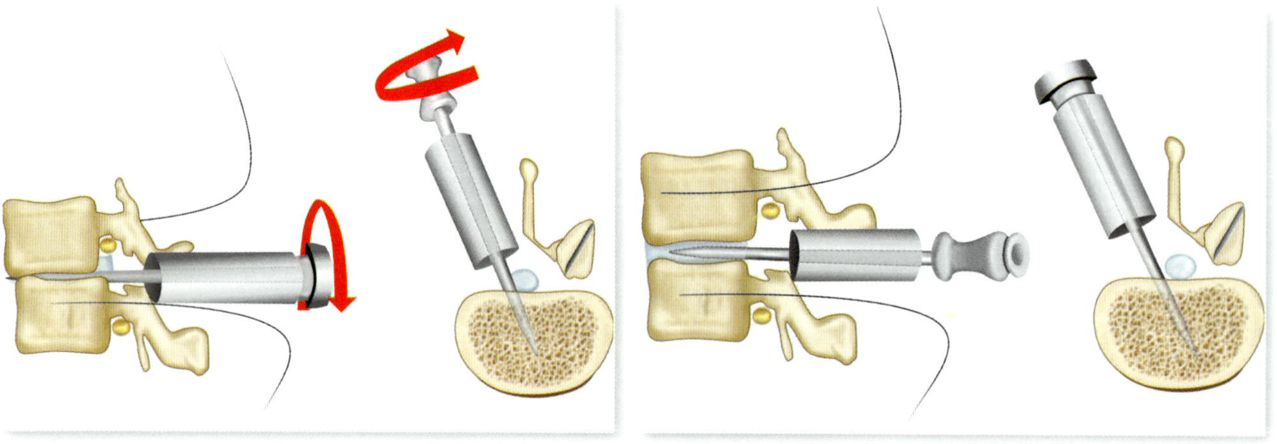

Figure 13: Opening up of collapsed disk space with blunt edged thin chisel and carefully rocking it avoiding end-plate fractures. This is followed by serial dilatation with incremental smooth edged shavers to achieve desired disk height

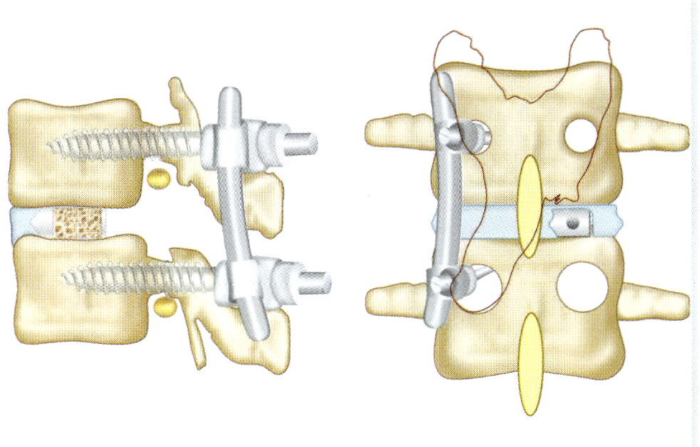

Figure 14: Placement of pedicle screws and compression over interbody cage

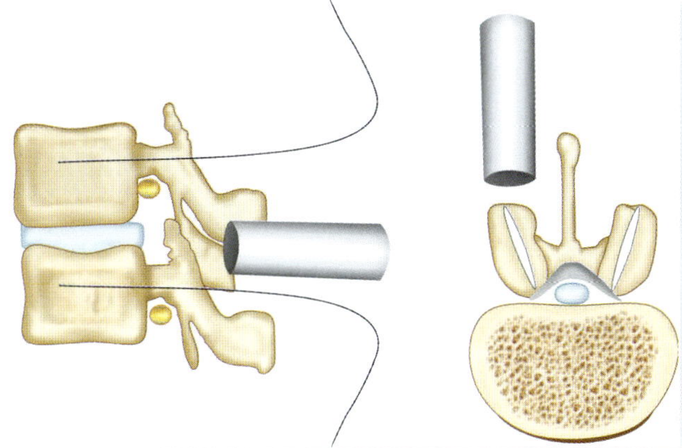

Figure 15: Shallow vertical docking over the hypertrophied facet joint

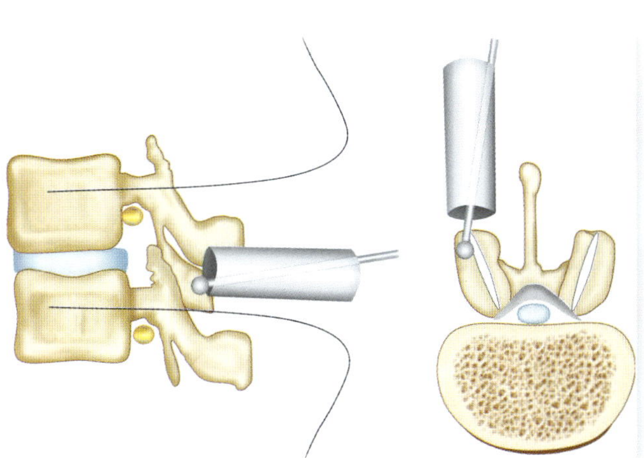

Figure 16: Burring down to remove osteophytes and delineate the spinolaminar line

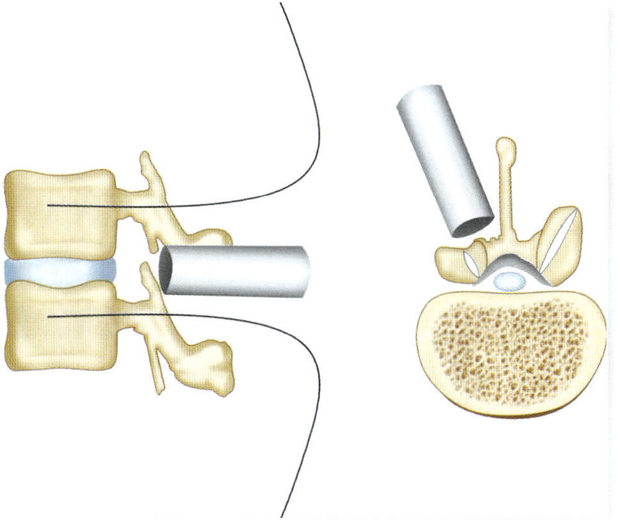

Figure 17: Medial angulation to facilitate the over-the-top decompression followed by ipsilateral facetectomy and disk space preparation

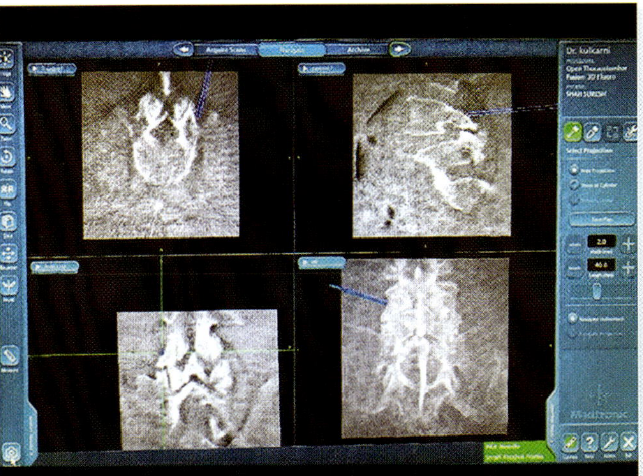

Figure 18: Intraoperative navigation with integrated 3D imaging in sagittal, coronal and axial planes

splitting approach causes fall back of the soft tissues after removal of tubular retractor, thus obliterating the dead space for development of postoperative hematoma and infection. In author's study of 1043 patients treated with MIS techniques,[35] 763 underwent non-instrumented surgeries and 280 underwent instrumentation over a period of 8 years. The overall infection rate after MISS was 0.29%, 0% in non-instrumented cases and 1.07% [3 out of 280 cases] in instrumented cases. Authors conclude that MISS can markedly reduce the surgical site infection (SSI) rates and can be an effective tool to minimize hospital costs.

COMPLICATIONS AND MANAGEMENT

Although offering certain advantages, minimally invasive lumbar spine surgery has several limitations and potential complications. There is a learning curve associated with

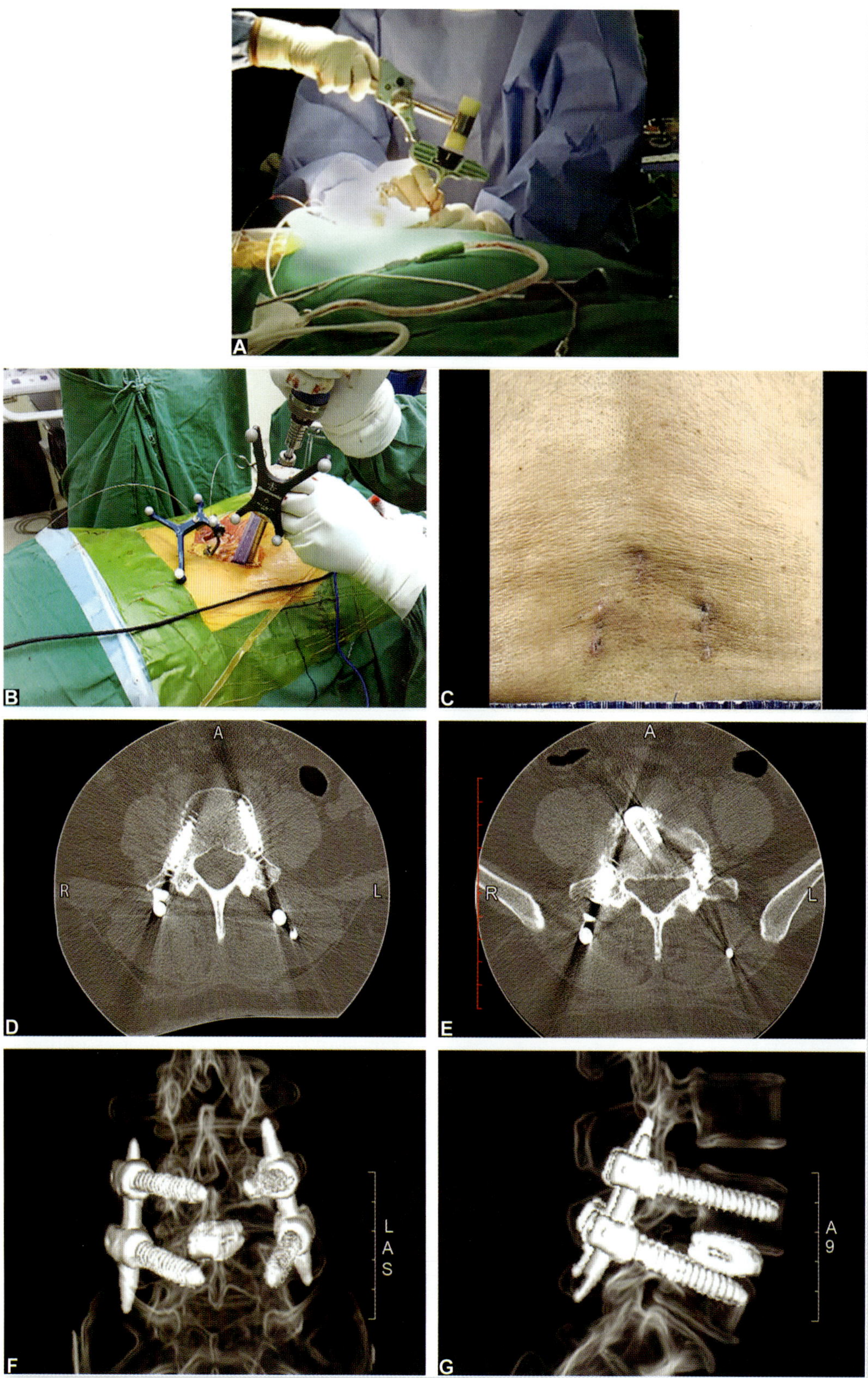

Figures 19A to G: (A and B) Set up of navigation apparatus; (B and C) Healed scar area; (D to G) CT scan showing good alignment of pedicle screws with interbody cage

the development of technical skills necessary to perform this procedure. In contrast to open procedures, minimally invasive exposures are limited to the area of surgical interest with a narrow field of view so that an appreciation of the underlying three-dimensional spinal anatomy is mandatory. Surgeons must become adept using longer instruments that are bayoneted. In addition, intraoperative fluoroscopic imaging is frequently utilized.[3,8,35] The ability to translate a two-dimensional radiographic image to three-dimensional anatomy can be challenging.

With the limited access intrinsic to minimally invasive surgery (MIS) approaches, the management of complications is more challenging. Inadvertent durotomy may occur and direct suture repair can be quite challenging down a tubular retractor. Dural sealants, such as Duragen, Durapatch and Tissel, may be used when direct repair is impossible.[28,30,31] Reported results from MIS-TLIF studies suggest a durotomy incidence of 0%–12.9% (average 2.9%).[36] Following precautions can be taken to decrease the risk of durotomy during MIS-TLIF: Before using a biting instrument, such as a Kerrison rongeur, a definitive and safe plane should be developed between the bony elements or ligaments and the thecal sac. This can be safely accomplished with a blunt dissector (e.g. nerve hook or Woodson elevator). The "biting window" of a Kerrison rongeur should always be turned 180° away from the thecal sac with gentle upward traction to avoid an inadvertent durotomy. Similarly, during a diskectomy, the thecal sac and nerve roots should be clearly identified before incision or resection of the annulus fibrosus. A blunt dissector (e.g. bayoneted Penfield No. 4 instrument) may be used to identify and separate the thecal sac from the underlying disko-ligamentous complex. A right-angle dissector can then be used for dissection ventral to the thecal sac to confirm a safe plane above the annulus. If there is significant resistance with the right-angle dissector, the plane between the ventral thecal sac and annulus needs to be more clearly dissected or there may be dense scarring, which may increase the risk of a durotomy. One of the advantages of MIS-TLIF over open approaches is the use of muscle-splitting tubular retractors, which minimizes the postoperative "surgical cavity" and helps tamponade against formation of a pseudomeningocele.

Percutaneous pedicle screw placement has been shown to be safe, with similar risks of misplacement to those reported for open-screw placement.[5,37,38] During percutaneous pedicle screw placement, care must be taken to ensure that the guide-wire does not advance through the anterior wall of the vertebral body where it might cause vascular or visceral injury. Here are few tips to avoid pedicle screw misplacement:[39] (i) depending on the patient's size, it may be necessary to modify the skin incision site by obtaining the proper distance lateral from the midline, measured from the preoperative axial images of an MRI; (ii) obtain a true anteroposterior fluoroscopic view of the target vertebrae to get a clear radiographic image; (iii) have sufficient time to get an appropriate medial to lateral trajectory of the guide needle until its tip appears at the lateral cortical margin of pedicle in the anteroposterior fluoroscopic view; (iv) spend time necessary to obtain a tactile feeling with the needle tip and try to palpate the bony junction between lateral facet wall and transverse process to select an optimal entry point; and (v) avoid driving screws too much deeper than necessary to prevent the screw tulip from resting on the facet joint.

Cage migration is also known to be a serious complication.[40] The migration can be classified as posterior, anterior, or sagittal. Posteriorly migrated cages could compress the nerve root or dura and might intensify neurological symptoms. The number, shape, size and implantation site of the cages could influence cage migration. Aoki et al.[41] reported that the use of lordotic bullet-shaped cages, higher posterior disk height, the presence of scoliotic curvature, and undersized fusion cages were possible risk factors for cage migration.

Nerve-root injury can be avoided by direct visualization of the working space during interbody fusion. The reported incidence of nerve-root injury is similar between open and minimally invasive TLIF procedures.[25,42]

A review of MIS-TLIF studies suggest an infection rate of 0–10%.[36] O'Toole et al.[43] found that the incidence of surgical wound infection was significantly lower after MIS-TLIF (0.6%) than after open TLIF (4.0%); To decrease the rate of infection with MIS-TLIF, it is recommended that one should avoid placing fingers into the surgical wound, which may increase the risk of surgical wound infection if there are microscopic breaks in the surgeons' gloves. Gerard et al.[44] also concluded that MIS-TLIF was associated with lower incidence of surgical site infection than open TLIF.

OUTCOMES

There are very few studies which directly compare MIS-TLIF with open procedure. Chusheng Seng et al.[45] concluded that MIS TLIF was comparable with open TLIF in terms of midterm (5 years) clinical outcomes and fusion rates with the additional benefits of less initial postoperative pain, less blood loss, earlier rehabilitation, and shorter hospitalization. The only drawback is an increase in both operative time and radiation exposure. Sulaiman et al.[46] concluded that MIS-TLIF is a more cost-effective treatment than open-TLIF for patients with degenerative spondylolisthesis and is equally effective as the conventional open-TLIF procedure. Phan et al.[47] concluded that MIS-TLIF appears to be a safe and efficacious approach compared to Open TLIF. MIS-TLIF is associated with lower blood loss and infection rates in patients, albeit at the risk of higher radiation exposure for the surgical team which now, is reduced with use of Navigation technology and better radiation exposure measures.

REFERENCES

1. Thomsen K, Christensen R. 1997 Volvo Award winner in clinical studies. The effect of pedicle screw instrumentation on functional outcome and fusion rates in posterolateral lumbar spinal fusion: a prospective, randomized clinical study. Spine. 1997;22(24):2813-22.
2. Dickman C, Fessler RG, MacMillan M. Transpedicular screw-rod fixation of the lumbar spine: operative technique and outcome in 104 cases. J Neurosurg. 1992; 77:860-70.
3. Brislin B, Vaccaro AR. Advances in posterior lumbar interbody fusion. Orthop Clin North Am. 2002;33(2):367-74.
4. Dewald CJ, Millikan, KW. An open, minimally invasive approach to the lumbar spine. Am Surg. 1999;65(1):61-8.
5. Figueiredo N, Martins JW. TLIF—transforaminal lumbar interbody fusion. Arq Neuropsiquiatr. 2004;62(3B):815-20.
6. Hackenberg L, Halm H. Transforaminal lumbar interbody fusion: a safe technique with satisfactory three to five-year results. Eur Spine J. 2005.
7. Harris BM, Hilibrand AS. Transforaminal lumbar interbody fusion: the effect of various instrumentation techniques on the flexibility of the lumbar spine. Spine. 2004;29(4): E65-70.
8. Javernick MA, Kuklo TR, Polly DW, Jr. Transforaminal lumbar interbody fusion: unilateral versus bilateral disk removal—an in vivo study. Am J Orthop. 2003;2(7):344-8. discussion 348.
9. Mayer HM. The ALIF concept. Eur Spine J 2000;9 (suppl 1): S35-43.
10. Moskowitz A. Transforaminal lumbar interbody fusion. Orthop Clin North Am. 2002;33(2):359-66.
11. Mummaneni PV, Haid RW, Rodts GE. Lumbar interbody fusion: state-of-the-art technical advances. Invited submission from the Joint Section Meeting on Disorders of the Spine and Peripheral Nerves, March 2004. J Neurosurg Spine. 2004;1(1):24-30.
12. Phillips FM, Cunningham B. Intertransverse lumbar interbody fusion. Spine. 2002;27(2): E37-41.
13. Rosenberg WS, Mummaneni PV. Transforaminal lumbar interbody fusion: technique, complications, and early results. Neurosurgery. 2001;48(3):569-74. discussion 574–575
14. Humphreys SC, Hodges SD, Comparison of posterior and transforaminal approaches to lumbar interbody fusion. Spine. 2001;26(5):567-71.
15. Chad D Cole, Todd D McCall, Meic H Schmidt, et al. Comparison of low back fusion techniques: transforaminal lumbar interbody fusion TLIF or posterior lumbar interbody fusion PLIF approaches. Curr Rev Musculoskelet Med. 2009;2(2):118-26.
16. Pier Paolo Mura, Mauro Costaglioli, Maurizio Piredda, et al. TLIF for symptomatic disc degeneration: a retrospective study of 100 patients. Eur Spine J 2011;20 (Suppl 1): S57–S60.
17. Audat Z, Moutasem O, Yousef K, et al. Comparison of clinical and radiological results of posterolateral fusion, posterior lumbar interbody fusion and transforaminal lumbar interbody fusion techniques in the treatment of degenerative lumbar spine. Singapore Med J. 2012;53(3):183-7.
18. An HS, Andersson G. Minimally invasive surgery for lumbar degenerative disorders: Part II. Degenerative disc disease and lumbar stenosis. Am J Orthop. 2000;29(12):937-42.
19. Deen HG, Fenton DS, Lamer TJ. Minimally invasive procedures for disorders of the lumbar spine. Mayo Clin Proc. 2003;78(10): 1249-56.
20. Schwender JD, Holly LT, Rouben DP, Foley KT. Minimally invasive transforaminal lumbar interbody fusion (TLIF): technical feasibility and initial results. J Spinal Disord Tech. 2005;18(Suppl.): S1-6.
21. Sihvonen T, Herno A, Paljärvi L, et al. Local denervation atrophy of paraspinal muscles in postoperative failed back syndrome. Spine. 1993; 18:575-81.
22. Styf JR, Willén J. The effects of external compression by three different retractors on pressure in the erector spine muscles during and after posterior lumbar spine surgery in humans. Spine. 1998; 23:354-8.
23. Gejo R, Matsui H, Kawaguchi Y, et al. Serial changes in trunk muscle performance after posterior lumbar surgery. Spine. 1999; 24:1023-8.
24. Kawaguchi Y, Matsui H, Tsuji H. Changes in serum creatine phosphokinase MM isoenzyme after lumbar spine surgery. Spine. 1997;22(9):1018-23.
25. Foley KT, Holly LT, Schwender JD. Minimally invasive lumbar fusion. Spine. 2003;28(15 suppl): S26-35.
26. Jahng TA, et al. Endoscopic instrumented posterolateral lumbar fusion with Healos and recombinant human growth/differentiation factor-5. Neurosurgery. 2004;54(1):171-80. discussion 180-181.
27. Kambin P, Foley KT, Holly LT, Schwender JD. Minimally invasive lumbar fusion. Spine 2003;28: S26-35; Spine. 2004;29(5):598-9.
28. Khoo LT, et al. Minimally invasive percutaneous posterior lumbar interbody fusion. Neurosurgery. 2002;51(5 suppl): S166-78.
29. Kim DH, Albert TJ. Update on use of instrumentation in lumbar spine disorders. Best Pract Res Clin Rheumatol. 2002;16(1):123-40.
30. Kim DH, Jaikumar S, Kam AC. Minimally invasive spine instrumentation. Neurosurgery. 2002;51(5 suppl): S15-25.
31. Mathews HH. Percutaneous interbody fusions. Orthop Clin North Am. 1998;29(4):647-53.
32. Waddell G, McCulloch JA, Kummel E, Venner RM. Nonorganic physical signs in low-back pain. Spine. 1980; 5:117-25.
33. Bini W, Yeung AT, Calatayud V, et al. The role of provocative discography in minimally invasive selective endoscopic discectomy. Neurocirugia (Astur) 2002; 13:27-31; discussion 32.
34. Deguchi M, Rapoff AJ, Zdeblick TA. Posterolateral fusion for isthmic spondylolisthesis in adults: analysis of fusion rate and clinical results. J Spinal Disord. 1998;11:459-64.
35. Kulkarni AG, Patel RS, Dutta S. Does minimally invasive spine surgery minimize surgical site infections? Asian Spine J 2016; 10(6): 1000-6.
36. Haaker RG, Senkal M. Percutaneous lumbar discectomy in the treatment of lumbar discitis. Eur Spine J. 1997;6(2):98-101.

37. Albert P. Wong, Zachary A. Smith, Alexander T. Nixon, et al. minimally invasive transforaminal lumbar interbody fusion: a review of 513 patients. J Neurosurg Spine. 2015; 22:487-95.
38. Beaubien BP, Mehbod AA. Posterior augmentation of an anterior lumbar interbody fusion: minimally invasive fixation versus pedicle screws in vitro. Spine. 2004;29(19): E406-12.
39. Folman Y, Lee SH. Posterior lumbar interbody fusion for degenerative disc disease using a minimally invasive B-twin expandable spinal spacer: a multicenter study. J Spinal Disord Tech. 2003;16(5):455-60.
40. Yung Park, Soo Bin Lee, Sang Ok Seok, et al. Perioperative Surgical Complications and Learning Curve Associated with Minimally Invasive Transforaminal Lumbar Interbody Fusion: A Single-Institute Experience. Clinics in Orthopedic Surgery. 2015; 7:91-6.
41. Aoki Y, Yamagata M, Nakajima F, et al. Examining risk factors for posterior migration of fusion cages following transforaminal lumbar interbody fusion: a possible limitation of unilateral pedicle screw fixation. J Neurosurg Spine. 2010;13(3):381-7.
42. Potter B, Freedman BA. Transforaminal lumbar interbody fusion: clinical and radiographic results and complications in 100 consecutive patients. J Spinal Disord. 2005;18(4):337-46.
43. O'Toole JE, Eichholz KM, Fessler RG. Surgical site infection rates after minimally invasive spinal surgery. J Neurosurg Spine. 2009; 11:471-6.
44. Wen Wei Gerard Ee, Wen Liang Joel Lau, William Yeo, et al. Does Minimally Invasive Surgery Have a Lower Risk of Surgical Site Infections Compared with Open Spinal Surgery? Clin Orthop Relat Res. 2014; 472:1718-24.
45. Chusheng Seng, Mashfiqul A. Siddiqui, Kenneth P.L.Wong, et al. Five-Year Outcomes Of Minimally Invasive Versus Open Transforaminal Lumbar Interbody Fusion. Spine. 2013;38(23):2049-55.
46. Wale AR. Sulaiman, Manish Singh. Minimally Invasive Versus Open Transforaminal Lumbar Interbody Fusion for Degenerative Spondylolisthesis Grades 1-2: Patient-Reported Clinical Outcomes and Cost-Utility Analysis. The Ochsner Journal. 2014; 14:32-7.
47. Kevin Phan, Prashanth J. Rao, Andrew C. Kam, Ralph J. Mobbs. Minimally invasive versus open transforaminal lumbar interbody fusion for treatment of degenerative lumbar disease: systematic review and meta-analysis.Eur Spine J. 2015;24:1017-30.

24 CHAPTER

Transforaminal Lumbar Interbody Fusion (TLIF): MISS/Mini-open

Vikas Gupte, Kumar Shetty

ABSTRACT

Traditional open spine surgery involves cutting or stripping of muscles from the spine. But today, TLIF may be performed using minimal invasive approach, involving small incision and muscle dilation, allowing surgeon to gently separate muscles surrounding the spine rather than cutting. MISS preserves surrounding muscular and vascular function and minimizes scarring. The advantage of interbody fusion over posterolateral fusion is increased surface area for bone contact and ability of graft to share load on anterior column. These factors translate to a more favorable fusion rate. TLIF avoids anterior access and associated complications, decreases manipulation of neural structures, reduces damage to ligamentous elements, minimizes excessive bone removal, enhances biomechanical stability and provides early mobilization.

HISTORICAL PERSPECTIVE

First described by Harms and Jeszensky in 1998 as an open procedure,[1] TLIF approaches the spine more laterally, thereby preserving more of the posterior ligamentous and bony complex, and certainly requires less retraction of the nerve root and thecal sac. In 1982, Magerl[2] mastered minimally invasive spinal instrumentation and used percutaneous pedicle screw insertion into the spine. In 1994, Foley and Smith[3] introduced a unique tubular retractor system which was initially designed for microdiskectomy, and that is composed of series of sequential dilators helping split the muscle in an atraumatic fashion, thereby allowing surgical access. Foley[4,5] came with a system for placing percutaneous screws and rods in submuscular plane, which was possible by using screw-extension sleeves and a unique rod insertion device. In 2003, adaptation of this non-expandable tubular retractor system and subsequent expandable tubes have led to the concept of minimally invasive TLIF.[6]

TERMINOLOGY

Mini-open approach to the spine utilize soft-tissue dilators and expandable tubular retractors. This internervous muscle splitting/Wiltse approach[7] reduces muscle trauma and allows direct visualization of up to two spinal motion segments. Also, this approach enables direct under -vision placement of pedicle screws, interbody cage and bone graft.

The percutaneous approach approach to the spine is more precisely a transmuscular approach, utilizing sequential dilators followed by extension screw sleeves and rod insertion device. The pedicle screw fixation is performed indirectly, i.e. without direct visualization of the target area, and entirely dependant on image-intensifier.

INDICATIONS, CONTRAINDICATIONS AND APPLICATIONS

Spinal arthrodesis is performed as a salvage procedure after a failed conservative trial.

Indications

- Primary DDD causing discogenic back pain with or without disk herniation
- Segmental instability causing low back pain with or without root compression
- Spondylolytic instability
- Degenerative spondylolisthesis with instability
- Recurrent disk herniation with significant back pain
- Short-segment degenerative scoliosis
- FBSS
- Treatment of pseudoarthrosis when interbody fusion is needed
- Post-laminectomy kyphosis
- For cases with unilateral stenosis with degenerative disk disease or spondylolisthesis, we use a unilateral

minimal invasive non-expandable tubular retractor with percutaneous pedicle screws.

- For cases with bilateral stenosis with DDD or spondylolisthesis, we use unilateral minimal invasive non-expandable tubular retractor with over the top ''In-out" technique for decompression of the other side along with percutaneous pedicle screws.

Contraindications

- Treatment of coronal and sagittal deformities of lumbar spine
  - Degenerative scoliosis/kyphosis
  - Deformity cases requiring 3-column osteotomies or SPOs at 3 or more levels (mini-open TLIF can be performed with SPOs at 1–2 levels)
- Multi-level involvement (>2 levels)
- Exposure deeper than 7 cm (maximum retractor depth
- Bleeding disorders
- Severe osteoporosis
- Active infection
- Distorted anatomical landmarks for pedicle screws
- Obesity.

Applications

- Using the tubular retractor systems (expandable or non-expandable), we can approach the spine posteriorly and achieve anterior interbody fusion at thoracic/ lumbar/ thoracolumbar level in cases such as spondylodiskitis eg. Pott's spine and augment with percutaneous transpedicular stabilization. In this way, midline structures of the spine are preserved and morbidity due to anterior approach is avoided.
- The non-expandable tubular retractor can be used for bilateral decompression by "over the top" technique wherein the tube is tilted by "Wanding maneuver" more medially and the operative table is tilted away from the surgeon. In this way, the dissection is carried out from under the base of spinous process to reach the other side; thereby, preserving the midline ligamentous and bony structures. This technique is also termed as intracanal approach "in-out" technique.
- Even in revision spine cases, where distorted anatomy is a concern, with the help of proper placement of the tubular retractor system, disscection is carried out from a virgin area to the scarred region. Safe and adequate neural decompression is achieved without damaging the midline structures, thereby reducing blood loss and neural injury.
- Using a non-expandable tubular retractor system in Mis-TLIF along with screw-extension sleeve with rod insertion device along with the cage is a costly affair. Unlike in mini-open TLIF, use of Indian-made screws and cage brings down the cost significantly, thereby cost-effective to the patient.
- Mis-TLIF requires good illumination and magnification along with long bayoneted instruments because the surgery is performed through a 18/22 mm diameter tube with a depth of 5–7 cm. Hence, for MIS-TLIF a good Microscope is a must which is most of the times available only in big hospitals. But in Mini-open TLIF one can operate using a surgical loupe with head light source thereby making it possible to operate in small set-up where microscope is not available.
- Not only interbody fusion fusion can be achieved, but facet and intertransverse fusion can be performed using expandable tubular retractor.

APPLIED ANATOMY AND TECHNIQUE

Preoperative Planning

Points to Look For

- Predominant axial back pain, radiculopathy or combination of symptoms
- Side of more symptoms/pain
- Instability
- Size of the patient
- Size of the spinal canal, amount of stenosis and amount of stenosis on other side
- Osteoporosis
- Local anatomical morphology.

X-rays of the Lumbar Spine

- Anteroposterior view
- Lateral view
- Lateral in flexion and extension (in standing)
- Oblique view.

Helps to Assess

- Instability
- Height of the disk space
- Facetal anatomy.

MRI

- Assess dural compression
- Assess root canal compromise
- Facetal pathology
- Assess foraminal stenosis
- Modic changes/disk pathology
- Measure cross-section area (CSA) of the multifidus muscle preoperatively and compare with postoperative measurment after 3 months.

CT Scan/CT-Myelo

- Assess size of spinal canal and lateral recess
- Plan entry points and trajectory for pedicle screw insertion

- Measure size and length of pedicle screw
- Assess topographical anatomy.

Anesthesia

As a routine general anaesthesia is given to the patient.

Position of the Patient

The patient is positioned prone on bholsters with no pressure on the abdomen and the operative table is Jack-knifed thereby flexing the spine. Most of the times, in mobile spondylolisthesis the vertebral slippage is partially corrected. The elbows are placed at 90° to avoid traction on the brachial plexus. Pads are placed under bony prominences, espacially ulna and peroneal. Pillows are placed under lower extremities. Prior to starting, it is ensured that the Foley's catheter is mobile and the endotracheal tube is secured. The C-arm is brought in and used in biplanar fashion. It is very important to confirm that both views are possible and the spinal anatomy is well visualized prior to prepping and draping. We usually do surface marking of the pedicles of the affected level on the patient under C-arm guidance **(Figure 1)**. Routine prepping and draping follows.

Mini-Open TLIF

The senior author prefers to start with the asymptomatic or less symptomatic side first. The skin incision is positioned 1.0–1.5 cm lateral to the lateral pedicular margin or 4.0–4.5 cm lateral to the midline.When using expandable retractor (MAST-Quadrant system), a 3–4 cm craniocaudal vertical incision for single level will suffice, and it should be extended to 5–6 cm for two-level surgery.

A medially oriented blunt digital dissection between multifidus and longissimus muscles is made according to the Wilste internervous muscle-splitting approach.[8] Then sequential soft-tissue dilators are docked accurately over the desired facet-joint complex, which is confirmed under C-arm. Appropriate length tubular retractors are firmly inserted and medially angulated for optimal trajectory. The dilators are removed and the working port is securely attached to the OT table frame and adjusted with a flexible clamp. The retractor is gently expanded as required in a cephalocaudal direction. Appropriate length medio-lateral distraction blades are adjusted providing maximum visualization of the working area.

The facet joint and transverse process are identified and decorticated. The pedicles are opened under direct visualization by introducing pedicle awl and finder, then palpated with pedicle feeler and tapped. The pedicle entry point is located at the mamillary process, corresponding to the midpoint junction where transverse process and the superior articulating process of the facet joint meets. The appropriate length, diameter and trajectory of the pedicle screws that have been preplanned on preoperative MRI or CT scan are inserted and confirmed under C-arm. Appropriate length rod is inserted and tightened temporarily in a distracted position thereby, opening up the interbody disk space.

The exact same steps are repeated on the contralateral affected side and the pedicle screws are inserted. Using Kerrison rongeurs, osteotomes a unilateral subtotal facetectomy is performed under direct visualization using head light source, surgical loupe or microscope. The extracanal "out-in" technique is used to perform decompression of the spinal canal and nerve root on the affected side. The "triangular working space" is made up of the exiting nerve root laterally, the dura alongside traversing nerve root medially, and the superior border of the inferior pedicle. The exiting nerve root is identified and protected with a cottonoid 'Patty'. Bleeding from the epidural veins is controlled by cauterization with bipolar forceps, thus exposing the posteromedial aspect of the intervertebral disk space.

Using a bayoneted dura retractor the neural structures are protected and a surgical blade number 15 used to incise the annulus fibrosus (box-cut) and as much of the disk material can be removed till bleeding endplates. The endplates are prepared methodically using a variety of bayoneted cartilage shavers, curettes and rasps. The disk space and lateral recess is examined with a nerve hook to remove any debri material.

Using a combination of enlarging trial implants and fixed distraction, the intervertebral disk space is enlarged to its natural size, thereby restoring normal lumbar lordosis and neuroforaminal diameter. The appropriate size of the implant is confirmed under C-arm in lateral view. Before placement of the cage close to anterior margin of the vertebral endplates, the disk space is packed with bone autograft (decompressed local bone) anteriorly. The cage is inserted making sure it is 3–4 mm inside the annular surface. Thorough wash is given, after which a nerve hook is used to confirm that the nerve roots are free of any soft tissue or bony compression **(Figure 2)**.

Finally, compression is applied on both sides and the screws are tightened. Final C-arm images are taken to see implants in position. Wounds are closed in layers and drain is generally not required.

MIS-TLIF (Figures 2 to 17)

Under C-arm guidance, Cook's biopsy needle position is confirmed at the lateral margin of the pedicle in the midpoint. The Cook's needle is taken 1 cm lateral and percutaneously penetrated into the skin over the target point for pedicle entry which is at the superior lateral border of the pedicle on perfect anteroposterior view of C-arm. The needle is inserted up to the posterior border of the vertebral body which is confirmed under lateral view of C-arm. The C-arm is positioned in AP view to confirm the needle placement in the pedicle not crossing the midline. Then the needle inserted 3/4th into the vertebral body under C-arm guidance in lateral view. A threaded guidewire is passed over the Cook's needle and in the vertebral body taking care not to penetrate too deeply as the anterior cortex could be violated and great vessel injury can occur. After the guidewire is secured, the Cook's biopsy needle is carefully withdrawn without moving the guidewire. In a similar manner all the guidewires are passed percutaneously and secured **(Figures 3 to 7)**.

The side which is least symptomatic or asymptomatic is stabilized first. Stab incision is taken where the guidewire is placed. Serial dilators are passed over the guidewire which is transmuscular (muscle-splitting) followed by cannulated tapping and the appropriate length of the polyaxial pedicle screw is measured and inserted with its extension sleeve. We routinely tap the pedicle 0.5 mm smaller than the anticipated screw diameter to achieve screw purchase in the pedicle. Cannulated polyaxial pedicle screw insertion is carried out under C-arm guidance taking care not to penetrate the anterior cortex of the vertebral body. Once all the screws are placed, subfascial rod insertion is carried out. The technique of rod insertion varies with the respective instrumentation manufacturer. At this point, distraction is applied to open up the interbody disk space and also to correct some anterolisthesis **(Figures 8 to 11)**.

Now we move on to the contralateral affected side. A K-wire is used to target the facet joint complex under C-arm guidance. Serial dilators are passed over the K-wire making sure that the dilators are docked onto the bone. The K-wire along with the dilators are removed after passing the working channel of appropriate length and securing it with the flexible clamp attached to the OT table.

At this point the microscope is brought in and unilateral subtotal facetectomy is performed **(Figure 12)**. Neural decompression by extracanal ''Out-In'' technique is performed. The exiting nerve root is identified and protected. The posteromedial aspect of the Intervertebral disk space is exposed and with a 15 number surgical knife mounted on a long handle is used to incise the annulus fibrosus. End-plates are prepared with routine bayoneted shavers, curettes and rasps. Trial cage of appropriate size is inserted and confirmed under C-arm in anteroposterior and lateral views. The disk space is packed with bone autograft using a funnel making sure good amount of bone graft is placed anteriorly. Final cage filled with bone graft is hammered into the disk space and disk height and lordosis is restored. Thorough wash is given, after which a nerve hook is used to confirm that the nerve roots are free of any soft tissue or bony compression.

Now polyaxial pedicle screws along with their extension sleeve's are inserted in the same manner as discussed above. After securing the pedicle screws, compression is applied on both sides providing compression of the bone graft in the middle column prior final tightening. Final C-arm images are taken to see the implants in position. Wound is closed in layers and drain is generally not required.

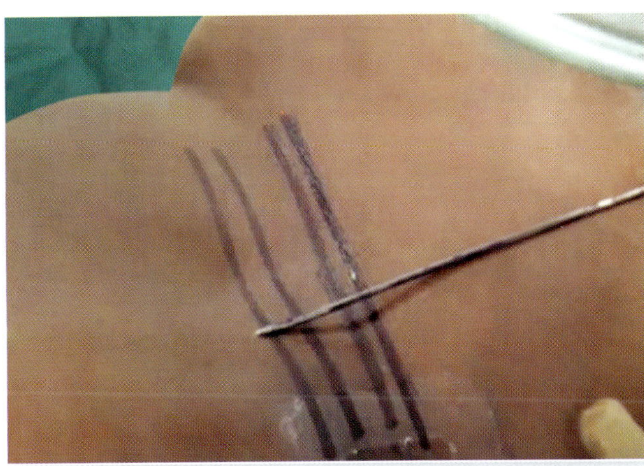

Figure 1: Surface marking of the pedicles

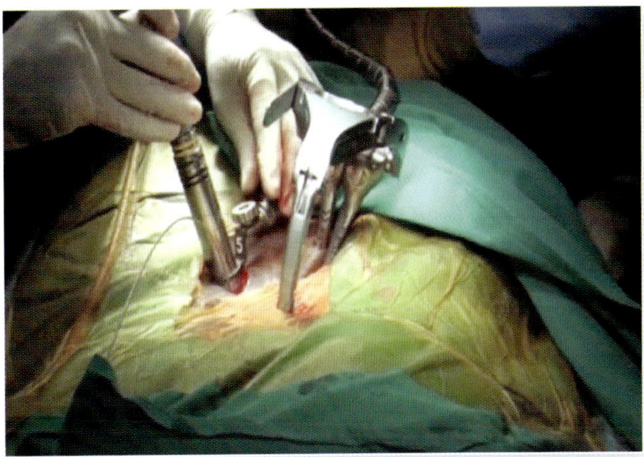

Figure 2: METRx tubular system with Flex-arm (Medtronics)

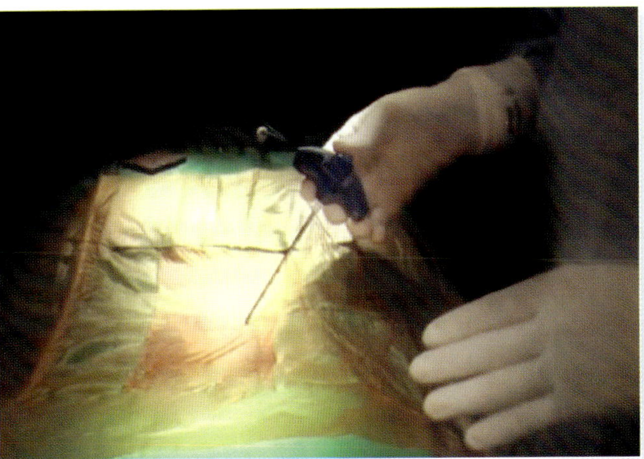

Figure 3: Percutaneous pedicular insertion of Cook's needle

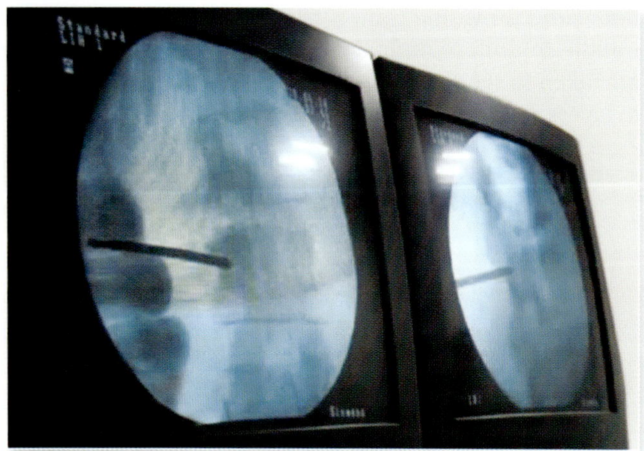

Figure 4: Cook's needle position confimed under C-arm

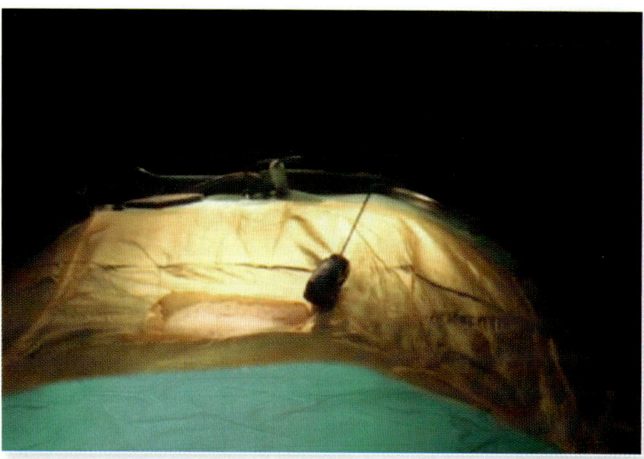

Figure 5: Insertion of threaded guidewire over Cook's needle

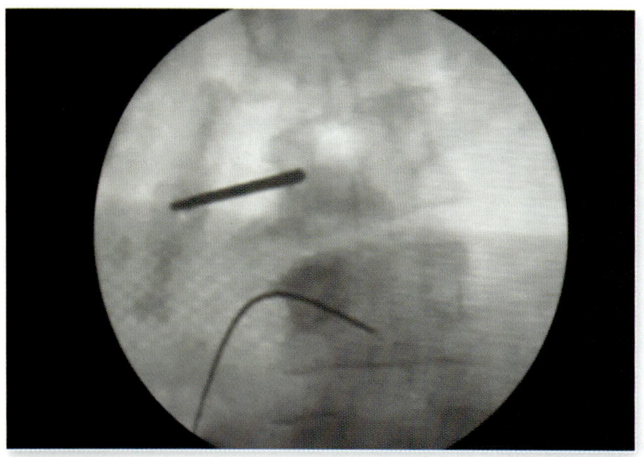

Figure 6: Guidewire position inside the pedicle

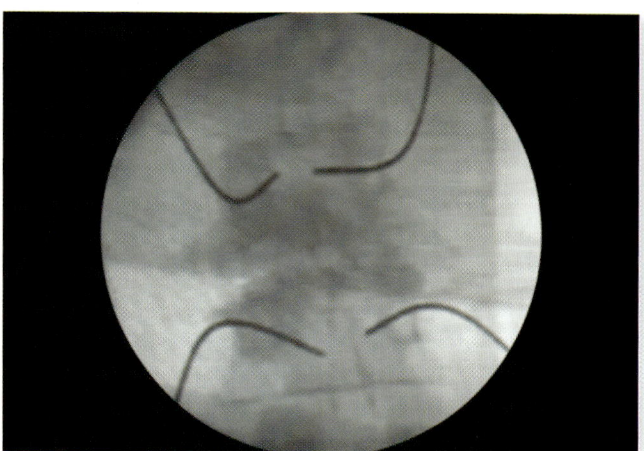

Figure 7: All 4 guidewires in position

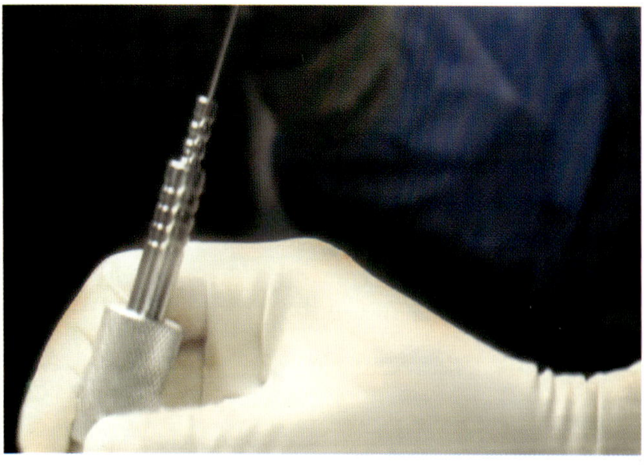

Figure 8: Serial muscle-splitting dilators for tapping/ screw insertion

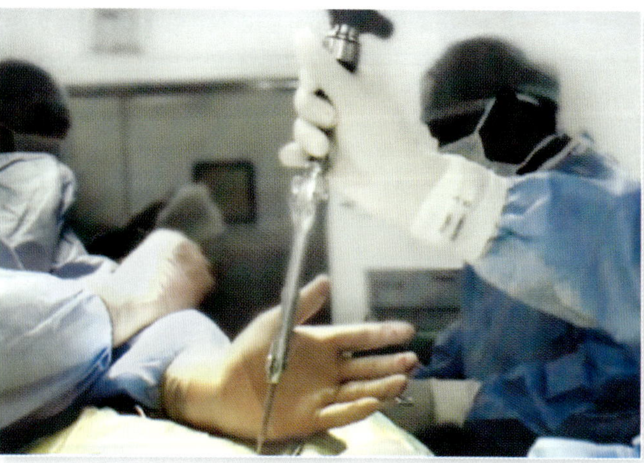

Figure 9: Insertion of cannulated polyaxial pedicle screw with extension sleeve

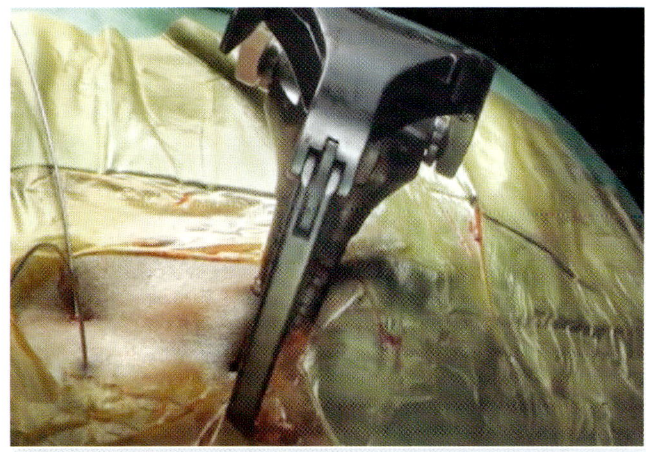

Figure 10: Jig for subfascial insertion of the precontoured rod

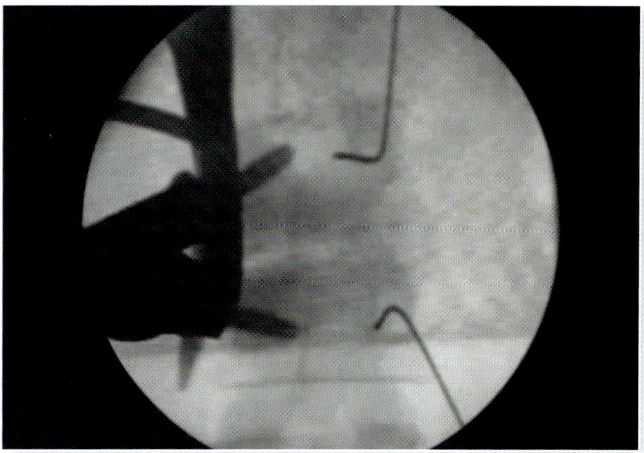

Figure 11: Asymptomatic side stabilized with screws and rod with distraction

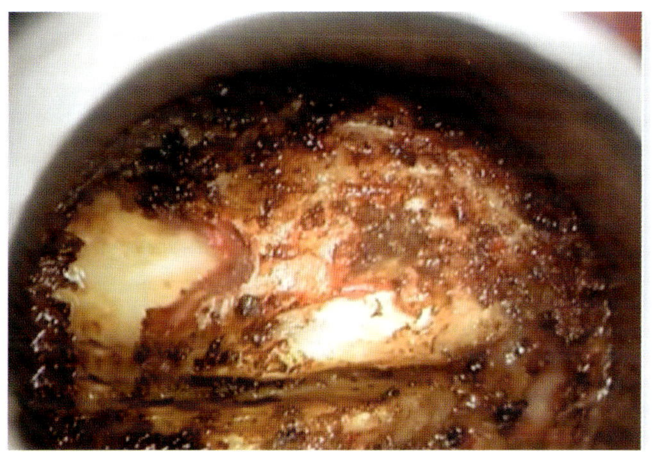

Figure 12: Microscopic subtotal facetectomy

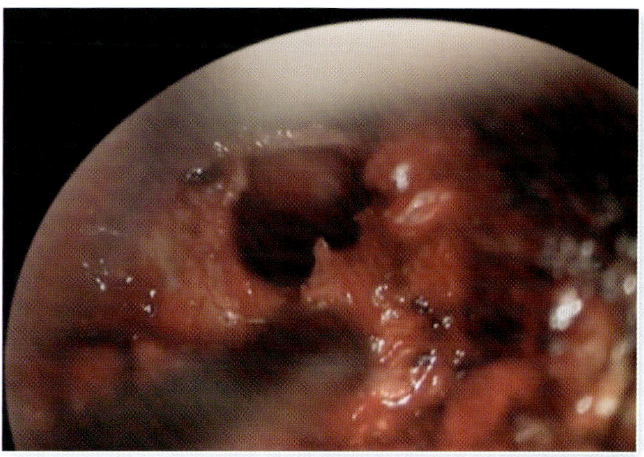

Figure 13: Box-cut of the annulus for disk space preparation for bone grafting

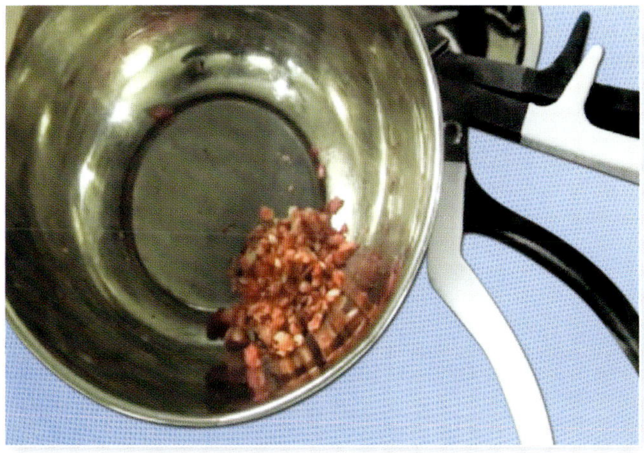

Figure 14: Autogenous bone graft

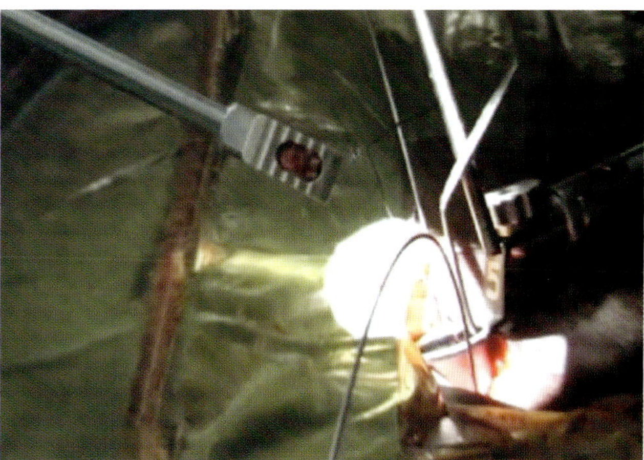

Figure 15: Peek cage filled with autogenous bone graft

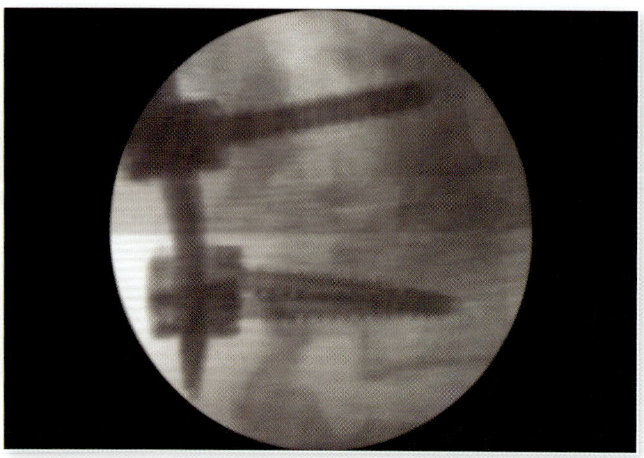

Figure 16: Position of the peek cage confirmed under C-arm

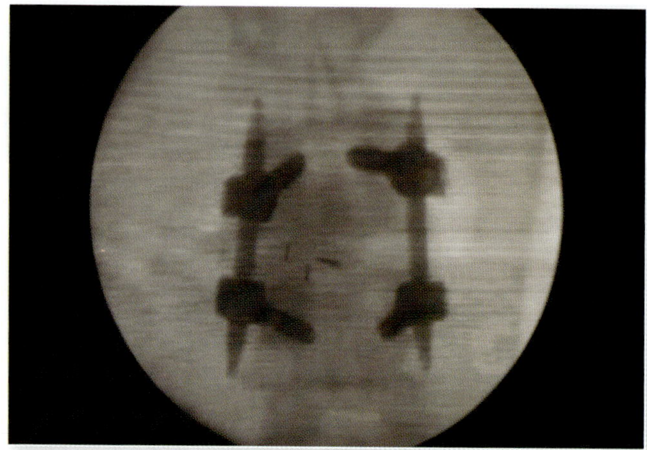

Figure 17: Final image after inserting screws and rods on the other side with bilateral compression applied

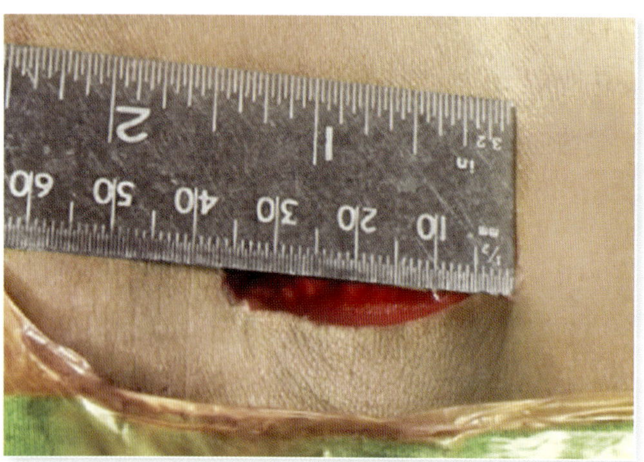

Figure 18: Small paramedian wounds

COMPLICATIONS

- Certain risks inherent to performing laminotomy, foraminotomy, diskectomy.
- Risk of bleeding and infection, though less than conventional approach.
- Getting lost in the minimal invasive anatomy can cause traouble
- Difficulty in controlling extensive bleeding or CSF leak in minimal invasive approach. Although since there is no ''dead-space" following the procedure, the soft-tiisue/ muscles fall back into anatomical position and creating a water-tight autoclosure, morbidity is greatly reduced.

25 CHAPTER

Outcomes of Lumbar Microendoscopic Decompression Surgery

Mehta Satyen, Jain Vikas

ABSTRACT

The minimally invasive techniques have theoretical advantages of minimizing lesser tissue trauma, less pain and faster rehabilitation compared to conventional open techniques. Microscopic-assisted tubular retactors has revolutionzed in the management of canal stenosis and disk prolapse patients. This chapter deals with the literature outcomes pertaining to the microendoscopic procedures, and complications of the procedure.

INTRODUCTION

Ever since the microendoscopic diskectomy system was introduced by Foley and Smith[1] in 1997 to decompress the lumbar nerve root, this technique has gradually been developed to decompress almost all kinds of lumbar spine pathologies. These lesser invasive operative options have the theoretical advantages of minimizing tissue injury thereby reducing the likelihood of adverse surgical stress response, including infections. It is also meant to preserve structural integrity of the spine leading to decreased incidence of post-surgical spinal instability.

MICROENDOSCOPIC DISKECTOMY

The philosophy behind minimally invasive spine surgery (MISS) is targeted pathology that is to focally address the spinal pathology and with the use of specially designed muscle-splitting serial dilators and retractors we can preserve the paraspinal muscle attachment especially the multifidus and cause minimal damage to the surrounding normal tissue.

Traditional surgical decompressive technique in the form of laminectomy with medial facetectomy and foraminotomy has stood its time and was a 'gold standard' approach in the treatment of lumbar canal stenosis. But this conventional approach also has a downfall of intraoperative bleeding, neural injury, infection, longer hospitalization, requiring long duration analgesics and a future course of chronic pain syndrome and iatrogenic spinal instability thereby needing fusion and stabilization.[2] The microlumbar diskectomy (MLD) by itself qualifies as a minimally invasive surgery and does not require the technical expertise of MED. However, lumbar diskectomy performed via microendoscopic tubular retractor carries the advantage of lower mean pressure applied at the muscles (30 mm Hg) as compared to MLD using a Caspar type retractor system (110 mm Hg). Ogata reported lesions in skeletal muscles at pressures as low as 30 mm of Hg studies have shown significantly lower levels of muscle injury markers phosphocreatine kinase, lactate dehydrogenase, C-reactive protein and interleukin-6 in microtubular procedures as compared to conventional MLD.

Studies published in literature involving case series and randomized control studies show similar results in terms of pain relief and functional scores with both these methods. Small case series like the one published by Kunert P et al. reported 100% good and excellent outcomes with MED. However, MED is shown to be associated with significantly lower requirement of postoperative analgesics when compared to conventional MLD. As expected, MED is associated with higher satisfaction rates and shorter hospital stay when compared to open diskectomy procedures.

Microendoscopic Decompression for Lumbar Stenosis

Many studies by multiple authors have shown similar outcomes with MISS techniques for lumbar decompression when compared to conventional open technique. Recent studies by multiple authors have shown similar patient outcomes with MISS approaches for lumbar decompression when these techniques are compared to the traditional open approach. Conventional lumbar decompression surgery involves a wide decompressive laminectomy, medial facetectomy and foraminotomy. This may potentially lead to mechanical instability/ failure of the spine and to chronic pain syndrome. Fenestration with minimal soft-tissue dissection and limited bone removal can potentially avoid these complications.[3]

In 2002, Khoo and Fessler[4] were the first authors to describe MEDS for lumbar stenosis. 25 consecutive patients were treated with MEDS and retrospectively compared to a historical control group of 25 consecutive patients treated with open laminectomies for lumbar decompression. For the MEDS group compared to the open laminectomy group, there was a statistical decrease intraoperative blood loss (68 cc versus 193 cc), postoperative narcotic requirement (31.8 eq versus 73.7 eq), and length of hospital stay (42 hr versus 94 hr).[4] After a one year follow-up, 90% of the patients in the microendoscopic decompression of stenosis (MEDS) group reported improved or complete resolution of their pain symptoms. Summary of recent papers, outcomes, and complications of MEDS for lumbar stenosis is shown in **Table 1**.

Improvement in Back pain, Leg Pain and Functional Scores

There are many longitudinal prospective studies published in literature providing results of lumbar decompression for

Table 1

Summary of recent papers, outcomes, and complications of MEDS for lumbar stenosis[2]

Authors	*Patients*	*Age*	*Functional outcome scores (VAS/ODI/ SF-36/JOA)*	*Follow-up (months)*	*EBL (cc)*	*OR TIME (mins)*	*Hospital (days)*	*Complications*
Khoo, 2002	25	68	No functional outcomes	12	68	109	1.8	4 durotomies
Ikuta, 2003	47	66	JOA 72%, VAS 70.6%	22	68	124	18	4 durotomies, 3 facet fractures, and 1 EDH
Ikuta, 2004	30	69	No functional outcomes	16	44	9	18	10 spinal EDH
Rahman, 2005	126	68	No functional outcomes	NR	50	108	0.75	1 durotomy
Castro, 2005	50	56	VAS 6.02, ODI 30.23	48	NR	94.3	3.16	5 durotomies, 2 infections, and 2 instabilities
Ikuta, 2005	114	67	JOA 9.4, VAS 38	28	NR	NR	NR	6 durotomies and 3 facet fractures
Rosen, 2005	57	80	VAS 2.4, ODI 21, SF-36 22	10	NR	NR	2.3	None
Ikuta, 2006	37	69	JOA 9.4, VAS 43, RMDQ	38	NR	NR	NR	1 durotomy
Asgarzadie, 2007	48	64	ODI 20, SF36 0.6	48	25	55	1.5	4% durotomies
Pao, 2007	53	62	JOA 14.8, ODI 47.6	15	104.5	126.7	NR	5 durotomies and 1 instability
Wada, 2008	15	72	JOA 6.3, dural CSA 408%	18	60	144.4	NR	1 EDH and 1 repeat operation
Yagi, 2009	20	73	JOA, VAS	18	37	71.1	3	Open:2 instability MEDS: None
Xu, 2009	32	65	MacNab: 21 Excellent, 11 Good	12	150	70	7	2 durotomies

Abbreviations: CSA, cross-sectional area; EDH, epidural hematoma; MEDS, microendoscopic decompression of stenosis; MISS, minimally invasive spine surgery; ODI, Oswestry disability index; RMDQ, Roland Morris disability questionnaire; SF-36, short form-36

stenosis using tubular retractors. All these studies show a significant improvement in back and leg pain scores in the short (<1 year) and medium (1–4 years) term. Good functional results have also been reported in these studies varying from 68% to 87% based on Oswestry Disability index (ODI) scores and Macnab functional scores. Weiner et al.[5], in 1999, showed good results in 87% patients in their prospective study of 30 patients. Similarly Khoo and Fessler[4] in 2002, Castro Menedez[3] in 2009 showed improvement in 68% and 72% respectively.

Oertel et al.[6] in 2006 and Mariconda et al.[7] in 2002 published medium term results showing good functional results in 85% and 68% patients respectively at 4 years follow-up. Similarly good improvements in ODI scores were also shown by Cavusoglu et al.[8] at 4 to 7 years follow up. Conventional lumbar decompression has given good outcomes in 62–70% patients in 4–7 years follow up.

While the main philosophy of MISS approaches is to preserve the majority of the native supportive anatomy, there are also many other beneficial results to MISS. In the majority of the MEDS articles reviewed, the authors have shown rapid improvement in their surgical skills after the initial steep learning curve and associated complications arising from a novel surgical technique. Shih et al. showed similar rates of clinical complications when comparing the open laminectomy to MEDS.[9] Since then, the authors have reported overall decreases in operative time, EBL, length of hospitalization, use of narcotics, incidence of symptomatic CSF leaks, incidence of wound infections, and minimal progression of postoperative spinal spondylolisthesis. In the senior author's experience, unintentional durotomies in MEDS have decreased with the use of a protective sleeve drill bit and preservation of the underlying ligamentum flavum during bony decompression. The use of a retractable, single-sided guard on the pneumatic drill bit protects the dura from inadvertent injury on one side while allowing visualization of the drill bit tip from the other side. In MEDS, the ligamentum flavum is kept intact until the bony decompression with the drill and Kerrison rongeurs is completed. The senior author recently showed a 4.5% incidence of durotomies in obese patients undergoing MEDS for lumbar stenosis.[2]

Another subpopulation of patients that would potentially benefit from MISS approaches to spinal pathology would be the elderly or medically frail patients.[10] Jansson et al.[11] discovered a four times increase in perioperative mortality in patients older than 80 years undergoing open laminectomy for lumbar stenosis. In contrast, Rosen et al. reported their success in treating elderly patients with MEDS for lumbar stenosis with minimal complications. They evaluated 57 patients with an average age of 80.8 years with multiple medical comorbidities. The elderly population demonstrated improved and sustained VAS, ODI, and short form-36 scores that reached statistical significance. Minimally invasive techniques may significantly decrease morbidity in the elderly, primarily due to decreases in blood loss, soft tissue injury, and physiological stress.

Another subpopulation of patients that may benefit from MISS approaches would be the obese patients.[12] Obese patients tend to have longer operative times, increased blood loss, larger incisions and soft-tissue dissection for exposure, and increased perioperative complications. MISS approaches would employ a small incision with minimal wound exposure and decreased soft-tissue trauma. Theoretically, there would be a decreased "potential space" for infection with overall decreased surgical trauma. Senker et al.[13] treated 72 patients with an MISS approach for a transforaminal lumbar interbody fusion and decompression.

COMPLICATIONS

Incidental durotomy is the most frequently reported complication with this technique. The incidence of this complication is reported as 3.5–16%. The incidence of this complication reduces as surgeons become more proficient in performing these procedures.

Rate of reoperation is reported as between 9% and 19%. The reasons for reoperations are usually infections, epidural fibrosis, epidural hematoma and preexisting spinal instability.

Prolonged wound healing is a significant complication associated with MED procedures when small skin incisions are made for aesthetic reasons, leading to wound edge necrosisd.[7] In order to avoid these it is recommended to make the skin incision slightly longer than the diameter of the tubular retractor used.

CONCLUSION

Technological advances have opened new doors for MISS approaches in treating spinal pathologies. While the MISS technique was originally designed for microdiskectomy, the paradigmshift of "less is more" has flourished in MISS approaches for diskectomies, foraminotomies, decompression for stenosis, instrumentation and fusion, spinal tumor resection, and deformity correction.[2,14]

MEDS is an effective technique for the treatment of lumbar spinal stenosis and is an alternative, minimally invasive technique that attempts to minimize the lesion of soft tissues and preserve the integrity and stability of the lumbar spine. Nevertheless, this technique involves some risks and, as in any other minimally invasive procedures, requires a learning curve. Hopefully, future studies will demonstrate the ultimate benefit of MEDS: preservation of native anatomic support structures leading to a decreased incidence of back pain and iatrogenic spinal instability and improved functional scores.

REFERENCES

1. Foley KT, Smith MM. Microendoscopic diskectomy. Tech Neurosurg. 1997;3:301-7.
2. Albert P Wong, Zachary A Smith, Rohan R Lall, et al. The Microendoscopic Decompression of Lumbar Stenosis: A Review of the Current Literature and Clinical Results. Minimally Invasive Surgery. 2012:
3. Manuel Castro-Menéndez, Jose A Bravo-Ricoy, Roberto Casal- Moro, et al. Midterm outcome after microendoscopic decompressive laminotomy for lumbar spinal stenosis: 4-year prospective study. Neurosurgery. 2009;65:100-10.
4. Khoo L, Fessler RG. Microendoscopic decompressive laminotomy for the treatment of lumbar stenosis. Neurosurgery. 2002;51:S146-S54.
5. Weiner BK, Walker M, Brower RS, et al. Microdecompression for lumbar spinal canal stenosis. Spine. 1999;24:2268-72.
6. Oertel M, Ryang Y, Korinth M, et al. Long-term results of microsurgical treatment of lumbar spinal stenosis by unilateral laminotomy for bilateral decompression. Neurosurgery. 2006;59:1264-70.
7. Mariconda M, Fava R, Gatto A. Unilateral laminectomy for bilateral decompression of lumbar spinal stenosis: A prospective comparative study with conservatively treated patients. J Spinal Disord Tech. 2002;15:39-46.
8. Cavusoglu H, Kaya RA, Turkmenoglu ON, et al. Midterm outcome after unilateral approach for bilateral decompression of lumbar spinal stenosis: 5-year prospective study. Eur Spine. J. 2007;16:2133-42.
9. Shih P, Wong AP, Smith TR, et al. "Complications of open compared to minimally invasive lumbar spine decompression," J Clini Neuroscience. 2011;18(10):1360-4.
10. Deyo RA, Cherkin DC, Loeser JD, et al. "Morbidity and mortality in association with operations on the lumbar spine. The influence of age, diagnosis, and procedure," J Bone Joint Surg. 1992;74(4):536-43.
11. Jansson KA, Blomqvist P, Granath F, et al. "Spinal stenosis surgery in Sweden 1987-1999," Euro Spine J. 2003;12(5):535-41.
12. Patel N, Bagan B, Vadera S, et al. Obesity and spine surgery: relation to perioperative complications. J Neurosurgery: Spine. 2007;6(4):291-7.
13. Senker W, Meznik C, Avian A, et al. Perioperative orbidity and complications in minimal access surgery techniques in obese patients with degenerative lumbar disease. Euro Spine J, 2011;20(7):1182-7.
14. Smith Z, Fessler RG. Concept and paradigm changes in spine surgery—minimally invasive spine surgery as the modern standard of care. In press.

26 CHAPTER

Outcomes in Minimally Invasive Spinal Surgery—Instrumented

Sreeharsha

ABSTRACT

Minimally invasive spinal surgeries are fast becoming an important tool for spinal surgeons and there is a great enthusiasm to adapt the technique and to use the technique for different indications. Although the technique is in use for more than a decade, recently there has been a dramatic increase in number of MISS surgeries. So, there is a need to look at the outcome of MISS surgeries. Being a relatively new technique not many long-term studies are available studying outcome of MISS surgeries. However, numerous short term studies and many medium-term results are currently available.

With the data available currently, minimal access surgeries do not have any clear advantages over conventional no fusion surgeries like decompression and diskectomies. The short-term outcome for fusion surgeries is in favor of minimally invasive surgeries with no clear advantage in the medium-term over conventional procedures. There may be some advantage of MISS surgery over conventional surgeries in special situations like elderly and obese patients.

INTRODUCTION

Minimally invasive spinal surgeries are gaining popularity among spine surgeons. With time, the indications are expanding as increasing number of surgeons are adopting the technique. From simple diskectomies to complex fusions and even deformity corrections are being increasingly done in minimally invasive fashion. The cited advantages of minimally invasive spine surgeries are reduction in soft-tissue injury, operative time, blood loss and risk of nerve root injury. The described disadvantages are increased operative time, increased radiation exposure, steep learning curve and increased costs. In addition, minimally invasive surgeries have been claimed to be advantageous in revision surgeries, obese individuals and in elderly patients.

Minimally invasive spinal surgeries are less disruptive surgeries utilizing serial dilators to develop the channel of approach followed by various types of retractors which will maintain the channel open to complete the proposed surgery. As the muscle cutting is kept to the minimum the bleeding during exposure will be naturally less. Unlike open surgery, in minimally invasive surgeries the exposure of bone is kept minimum enough to complete the fusion. As the amount of bone cut is minimum, subsequent ooze from the operative site is less. Similarly, after surgery, the dilated muscles fall back into place and no cavity is left behind for blood collection. All these factors effectively reduce the blood loss.

Less tissue damage also theoretically translates into less postoperative pain. Many studies have looked into postoperative analgesic requirement and have found significantly less analgesic requirement in MISS surgeries. Less postoperative pain leads to early mobilization, sometimes as early as same day of surgery. MIS diskectomies as daycare surgeries have become norm in some centers. When patients mobilize early, they are ready for discharge early which, in some countries may translate to significant cost saving for the hospitals. Early recovery may also lead to early return to work for the patient.

There are many studies describing the advantages of MIS spine surgeries in the short-term and medium-term. Long-term studies are still sparse and very long-term studies describing outcomes are currently unavailable.

MINIMALLY INVASIVE DECOMPRESSION SURGERIES

Surgeries for the lumbar radiculopathy caused by lumbar disk prolapse are the most successful interventions in spinal surgeries. Microdiskectomy and fenestration diskectomies have been the gold standard treatment for lumbar disk prolapse.[1-2] Similar procedures done with the help of tubular retractors might theoretically help improving the outcomes. On the contrary if too little disk material is removed there may be higher risk of persistant pain or recurrence.

Greg Anderson et al.[3] have reported on a matched cohort of patients undergoing surgery for lumbar disk prolapse 75 patients undergoing MIS diskectomies were matched with 20 patients undergoing traditional diskectomies. VAS, ODI and short form-12 (SF-12) were used to compare the outcome between the two groups. There was reduction in the blood loss and operative time in the minimally invasive group and there was decrease in hospitalization in traditional surgery group. The difference was not statistically significant. Both the groups showed significant improvement in SF-12, visual analog scal (VAS) and oswestry disability index (ODI) scores, and there was no statistically significant difference between the groups. Complication rate was11.9% in minimally invasive group and 15% in traditional surgery group.

In a similar retrospective study, Wu et al.[4] have reviewd 873 cases operated by tubular retractor with mean follow-up of 28 months. The authors used the ODI, VAS, and modified MacNab criteria to assess outcome and also studied a control group of 358 patients undergoing standard open diskectomy. VAS, ODI and modified Macnab scores were not found to be siginicantly different between the two groups.

Kamper et al.[5] did a meta-analysis and review of 29 studies comparing minimally invasive and conventional diskectomies. Out of these 16 were randomised studies and 13 nonrandomised studies. There was moderate-to-low quality evidence of no differences in clinical outcomes between MI surgery, using either the interlaminar or the transforaminal approach, and conventional microdiskectomy.

Other small studies have also demonstrated the lack of significnat differences between MIS and conventional diskectomies.[6] Therefore, MIS appears to be an alternative to traditional decompressive surgery, but there are no compelling reasons to favor MIS surgeries over traditional surgery for lumbar disk prolapse.

Surgeries performed for symptomatic lumbar canal stenosis are more extensive as the pathology is more frequently bilateral with often hypertrophic facets. Traditional surgeries have been laminectomy[7] or sometimes lamina splitting approach to prevent post-operative instabilities.[8] Both the surgeries involve extensive detachment of the paraspinal muscles unilaterally of bilaterally. So, MIS surgeries can be a safer alternative.[9,10] Apart from being able to perform unilateral decompression, the tubular retractor can be tilted to perform decompression on the opposite side over the dural sac. This preserves the muscles on the opposite side which are left untouched.

Pao et al.[11] in a prospective study evaluated outcomes in 53 patients undergoing MIS surgery for symptomatic lumbar canal stenosis with average follow up of 15.7 months. The clinical outcomes were evaluated with the ODI and the Japanese Orthopedic Association (JOA) score. Of the 50 patients providing sufficient data for analysis, the ODI improved from 64.3 ± 20.0 to 16.7 ± 20.0. The JOA score improved from 9.4 ± 6.1 to 24.2 ± 6.0. The improvement rate was 73.9 ± 30.7% and 40 patients (80%) had good or excellent results. There was no postoperative instability at the operated segment as evaluated with dynamic radiographs at final follow-up. The authors concluded that MIS decompression was a safe and very effective minimally invasive technique for degenerative LCS.

Minamide et al.[12] did a prospective study on 366 patients with single or double level stenosis. 310 patients were followed up for 2 years. The average recovery rate based on the JOA score was 61.3%. The overall results were excellent in 34.9% of the patients, good in 34.9%, fair in 21.7%, and poor in 8.5%. The mean RMDQ score significantly improved from 11.3 to 4.8 ($p < 0.001$). In all categories of both JOABPEQ and SF-36, scores at 2 years follow-up were significantly higher than those obtained before surgery. There were 12 surgery related complications but none of them serious. There were no post operative instabilities.

However, long-term reports specifically to determine the absence of postoperative instability are yet to come. So, it is safe to assume that MIS decompression is an alternative to open surgeries for lumbar canal stenosis. However, it would require considerably more surgical armamentarium in the form of flexible drills and visual aids to visualize and decompress the opposite side. The learning curve for such complex surgery is steep and can be attempted only after considerable surgical exposure to MIS techniques and instruments.

MINIMALLY INVASIVE FUSION SURGERIES

Minimally Invasive TLIF

Cloward[13] first described the technique of inter body fusion in the form of PLIF for lumbar fusion. PLIF and its variant TLIF described by Harms[14] remain one of the most common surgeries to be performed by spine surgeons. Minimally invasive TLIF was described by Schwender[15] and has become the number one MIS spine surgery by volumes. Extensive literature documenting the short- and medium-term outcome are becoming available now.

Seng et al.[16] in a matched paired study with 5 years follow-up demonstrated the difference in blood loss between open and minimal access surgeries, reduced morphine requirement in the postoperative period and reduced hospital stay. They studied 40 patients each of MIS and open fusion group. The patients were matched for age, sex, body mass index and level of surgery operated. MIS had less blood loss (127 mL) versus open (405 mL, $P < 0.001$) procedures. Morphine use for MIS cases (8.5 mg) was less compared with open (24.2 mg, $P = 0.006$). Patients who underwent MIS (1.5 d) ambulated earlier than those who underwent open fusion (3 d, $P < 0.001$). Patients who underwent MIS (3.6 d) had shorter hospitalization than those who underwent open fusion (5.9 d, $P < 0.001$). Postoperative scores for ODI, SF-36 and NSS at 6 months to 5 years showed no significant difference between the two groups. The overall complication rates were also comparable. The authors concluded that MIS TLIF is comparable to open TLIF in terms of midterm clinical outcomes and fusion rates.

Similar results have been reported by Peng et al.[17] They did a matched study of 29 patients each in open TLIF and MIS TlIF groups. At the end of two-year follow-up, they concluded that MIS TLIF has similar good long-term clinical outcomes and high fusion rates of open TLIF with the additional benefits of less initial postoperative pain, early rehabilitation, shorter hospitalization, and fesser complications.

Cheng et al.[18] in a retrospective study compared 25 patients of open TLIF with 25 patients of MIS TLIF. 41 of the 50 patients were operated for spondylolisthesis. Intra- operatively, compared with TLIF, MIS TLIF resulted in decreased lengths of operation, lower blood loss, and fewer complications ($p < 0.05$). Total administration of morphine-equivalent pain medication in the hospital also tended to be lower in the MIS TLIF than in the TLIF group. Functional assessment by physical therapy on postoperative Day 1 demonstrated higher function in the MITLIF patients for transfer-related tasks, ambulatory ability, and distance walked than in the TLIF patients ($p < 0.05$). Long-term fusion rates were 92% in the MITLIF group and 100% in the open TLIF group ($p = 0.09$). Preoperative VAS pain scores were 7.1 for the MITLIF patients and 7.6 for the TLIF patients ($p = 0.26$). At the last follow-up, the reported VAS pain score was 2.9 in the MITLIF patients and 3.5 in the open TLIF patients, but this difference was not statistically significant ($p = 0.25$).

One of the few prospective studies has been done by Lee et al.[19] They compared the radiological and clinical outcomes of 72 patients each in open TLIF and MIS TLIF group at 6 months and 2 years. Perioperative analysis revealed that MIS cases have comparable operative duration (open: 181.8 min, MIS: 166.4 min, $p < 0.05$), longer fluoroscopic time (open: 17.6 s, MIS: 49.0 s, $p < 0.05$), less intraoperative blood loss (open: 447.4 mL, MIS: 50.6 mL, $p < 0.05$) and no postoperative drainage (open: 528.9 mL, MIS: 0 mL, $p < 0.05$). MIS patients needed less morphine (open: 33.5 mg, MIS: 3.4 mg, $p < 0.05$) and were able to ambulate (open: 3.4 days, MIS: 1.2 days, $p < 0.05$) and be discharge from hospital earlier (open: 6.8 days, MIS: 3.2 days, $p < 0.05$). At 6 months, clinical outcome analysis showed both groups improving significantly (< 50.0%) and similarly in terms of VAS, ODI, SF-36, return to full function and patient rating ($p < 0.05$). Radiological analysis showed similar grade 1 fusion rates (open: 52.2%, MIS: 59.4%, p[0.05) with small percentage of patients developing asymptomatic cage migration (open: 8.7%, MIS: 5.8 %, $p < 0.05$). At 2 years, continued improvements were observed in both groups as compared to the preoperative state ($p < 0.05$), with 50.8% of open and 58% of MIS TLIF patients returning to full function ($p < 0.05$).

In another prospective study Perez-Cruet et al.[19] studied the outcome measures in 304 patients with mean follow-up of 47 months. The indications were mainly degenerative in nature and interestingly 23% patients had undergone previous lumbar spine surgery. Disability Index scores declined from 43.1 preoperatively to 28.2 at mean 47-month follow-up. Short-Form 36 mental component scores increased from 43.8 preoperatively to 49.7 at 47-month follow-up. Short-Form 36 physical component scores increased from 30.6 preoperatively, VAS scores decreased significantly from 7.0 preoperatively to 3.5 to 39.6 at 47-month follow-up ($P < 0.05$). Although authors did not have matched controls they compared their data with criterion set by Glasssman et al.[20] and concluded that their MIS TLIF patients compared well with open TLIF patients.

There is increasing evidence pointing towards advantages of MIS TLIF over Open TLIF in the short-term.[21] MIS surgeries seem to have a advantage in terms of reduced blood loss, decreased postoperative pain relief and early discharge from the hospital. Increased radiological exposure and steep learning curve seem to be downside. However, both these downsides tend to improve with incresing experience with the technique. Medium and long-term results have been comparable in each group in terms of clinical and radiological outcomes. However, prospective randomised control studies are lacking to clearly establish superiority of MIS TLIF over open TLIF in the long-term. Also any difference in outcome in terms of adjacent segment degeneration remains to be unravelled in long-term studies.

Other Interbody Fusion Surgeries

Alternatives to MIS TLIF for interbody fusion approaching spine either from lateral or anterior approach are also popular in some parts of the world. Anterior approaches in the form of laparoscopic anterior lumbar interbody fusion and mini open anterior lumbar interbody fusions have been described. Laparascopic surgeries have known to be associated with higher compliction rates. Mini open ALIF has demonstrated good clinical and radiological outcomes. But indications for such surgeries is largely limited to degenerative conditions requiring indirect decompression of spinal canal and restoration of spinal alignment.

Extreme lateral interbody fusion-XLIF, uses a lateral, retroperitoneal, transpsoas approach to the spine. The advantages of this surgery are decreased blood loss, least amount of damage to the spinal musculature and leaving the all important musculoligamentous structures intact.[22] Rodgers et al.[23] have reported largest series of XLIF patients. They described the outcomes in 600 patients undergoing XLIF at 741 levels. Interestingly nearly 40% patients were operated for adjacent segment degeneration following lumbar fusion surgeries. In addition to fusion procedure, 83% patient also had pedicle screw fixation. The authors used VAS scores to demonstrate the clinical outcome which was improved by 65% at one year follow-up. The authors noted that complication rates were less when compared to the open surgery.

Youseff et al.[24] retrospectively reviewed the outcome of 84 patients undergoing XLIF at 137 levels and also did a literature review. Supplementary pedicle fixation was done for 38 patients and lateral plates were used for 31 patients. Posterior decompression was also done when required. Average pain and function scores at 1-year follow-up were significantly improved over preoperative scores (VAS decrease from 58.9 to 13.7, a 77% improvement, $P < 0.0006$; ODI decrease from 39.7 to 17.3, a 56% improvement, $P < 0.0017$). Postoperative thigh pain was a common complaint but was transient. However, the XLIF with posterior fusion group had significantly higher operative time, blood loss and length of stay.

The technique has been proved to be more effective in correcting the coronal deformity. However, this is mostly achieved along with supplementary posterior fusion. This is a relatively new procedure and careful evaluation is required before deciding upon standalone XLIF. Additional studies are required to compare standalone XLIF with XLIF and posterior fusion to determine if supplementary procedures have any bearing on the outcome.

MIS AND SPECIAL CONSIDERATIONS

Obese patients have many risk factors that can jeopardize the outcome. Obese patients with comorbidities like diabetes mellitus, hypertension are prone to high rate of perioperative complications. Obese patients have a greater risk of wound infections, deep vein thrombosis and pulmonary embolism.[25,26] In addtion obese patients intraoperatively need bigger exposures to achieve desired trajectories, which itself increases blood loss. MIS surgeries do not dependent on traditional exposures. Usage of tubular retractors negates the went of extra-exposure and faster return to activity may also reduce the perioperative complication rates. Lau et al.[27] identified obese patients with BMI over 30 kg/m^2 undergoing single level lumbar fusion surgery. 41 patients underwent open TLIF and 78 underwent MIS TLIF. The intraoperative blood loss and hopsital stay was significantly lower in the MIS TLIF group. The complication rates were higher in the open TLIF group. On stratification of grade of obesity, the differences were more profound. Hence MIS surgeries can be of advantage in obese patients in reducing intraoperative difficulties and immediate postoperative complications.[28]

As the population ages, the number of elderly people requiring spinal surgery will rise.[29] Lumbar spinal fusions have traditionally been shown to have good results in elderly individuals as far as outcomes are considerd.[30,31] But increasing age is associated with increase in the rate of complications. Complication rates of 18–79.6% have been reported.[32] The complication rate generally increased with age, blood loss, operative time and number of level fused. Especially, intraopeartive blood loss has been associated with early postoperaative complications. Elderly patients are reluctant to undergo spine surgery in view of perceived increase in perioperative morbidity and mortality. Rodgers et al.[33] have looked into comparative outcome of patients over 80 years undergoing open PLIF surgery (20 patients) and XLIF surgery (80 patients). Patients were followed up for minimum 3 months follow-up. Intraoperative blood loss, transfusion rate and hospital stay were significantly shorter for XLIF group. More number of open PLIF patients weent to special rehab facilities. More importantly, there were 6 deaths in the PLIF group and only 1 in XLIF group.

It appears that all the intraoperative and short-term benefits of MIS surgeries translate into big advantages when the technique is applied to elderly people. There may be reason to consider MIS surgery in elderly individuals to improve the quality of life rather than discouraging them in view of high rate of complications.

Increase in the number of lumbar spinal surgeries translates into potential increase in the number of revision surgeries. Revision surgeries are associated with increased complications in the form of increased blood loss, dural tears, increased operative time and neurological injuries. Using tubular retractors in para midline approach bypasses the previously used midline approach. Avoiding the scar tissue reduces blood loss and reduces the chances of neurological injury. Wang et al.[34] have done prospective study on patients undergoing revision lumbar fusion surgery. All patients had undergone previous surgery for disk prolapse or stenosis. 25 patients underwent MIS TLIF and 27 patients underwent open TLIF procedure. The authors found significant reduction in intraoperative and postoperative blood loss and less back pain in MIS TLIF group. There were three instances of dural tear in MIS TLIF group which did not require repair. 5 cases of dural tear occurred in open TLIF group which required repair. In addition there were two cases of superficial wound infection in open TLIF group.

MIS and Learning Curve

MIS techniques are technically demanding procedures and considerable experience and skill is necessary before optimum results are abtained. Increased operative time during intial cases may increase the chances of infection. Lee et al.[35] have studied their single surgeon experience in determinig the effect of learning curve. 60 patients were studied. The learning curve was assessed using logarithmic curve fit regression analysis. Using these, first 22 patients were considered early cases. In the single-level TLIF series, operative time was significantly shorter in the late group (183 ± 23 min) than the early group (254 ± 44 min), and blood loss during the operation was significantly reduced in the late group (292 ± 280 mL) compared with the early group (508 ± 278 mL). Ambulation recovery time significantly decreased from 2.4 ± 0.6 days in the early group to 2.0 ± 0.5 in the late group. ODI and VAS scores for lower back pain and radiating pain did not differ between the 2 groups. Few authors have also had similar experiences wherein the outcome improved with increasing experience. Adequate training in the form of cadaveric surgery is necessary before embarking on MIS spinal surgeries. During initial few surgeries it is prudent to concentrate on technique and prevention of dural injuries even if it means increase in the operative time and radiological exposure. With experience both these parameters can be brought down to comparable levels to open surgeries and the advantages of MIS surgeries become reality to the patient.

MIS Surgeries and Cost Effectiveness

MIS surgeries apart from being technically demanding procedures, they are also costly procedures. As the complexity of surgeries increase the need for expensive equipment increases. In developing countries, including India, procuring of such equipments when already not available can be costly affair. The special implants and instrumentation used are recurring costs which have to be borne by the patients. Many western studies have tried to justify the increased costs by concluding that more money is saved by early discharge of patients to home than what is spent on the implants. Al-Khouja et al.[36] reviewed papers mentioning the cost factor in minimally invasive surgery. They found that the minimally invasive surgerires were better in outcome and cost effective. In a contradicting study Akker et al.[6] did a double blinded randomized prospective study wherein cost utility analysis was done between conventional microdiskectomy and tubular diskectomy. They found there was no cost advantage of tubular diskectomy over conventional diskectomies.

There are huge cultural differences between countries and in many countries, early discharge home is not possible and when possible, does not necessarily negate the escalated cost of implants. In underdeveloped and developing world where most of the patients pay for themselves for medical care or are dependent on various subsidized healthcare schemes, financial factors will play a major role in the advancement and acceptance of MIS surgeries irrespective of better outcomes. In this regard development of indigenous techniques to bring down the cost of surgery will help in bringing MIS surgeries within the reach of majority population.

CONCLUSION

MIS spine surgeries promise what every surgeon always wishes for reduction in complication rates and improving clinical outcome. Existing evidence shows MIS fusion surgeries to be of advantageous in the short-term outcome. Patients are more comfortable and go home early. Medium-term outcomes have been comparable to open surgeries in terms of clinical outcome and fusion rates. MIS surgeries are still evolving technique and all the reports available include patients involved in learning curve of the surgeons. Results may improve as surgeons get more experience. There is considerable lack of prospective randomized studies. The long-term reports are awaited to know which way the results will evolve, especially in relation to adjacent segment degeneration.

REFERENCES

1. Tureyen K. One-level one-sided lumbar disk surgery with and without microscopic assistance: 1-year outcome in 114 consecutive patients. J Neurosurg. 2003;99:247-50.
2. Weinstein JN, Lurie JD, Tosteson TD, et al. Surgical versus nonoperative treatment for lumbar disk herniation: four-year results for the Spine Patient Outcomes Research Trial (SPORT). Spine. 2008;33:2789-800.
3. Greg Anderson D, Amar Patel, Mitchell Maltenfort,et al. Lumbar Decompression Using a Traditional Midline Approach Versus a Tubular Retractor System. Comparison of Patient-Based Clinical Outcomes. Spine. 2011;36:E320-5.
4. Xiaotao Wu, Suyang Zhuang, Zubin Mao, et al. Microendoscopic diskectomy for lumbar disk herniation Surgical Technique and Outcome in 873 Consecutive Cases. Spine. 2006;31:2689-94.
5. Kamper SJ, Ostelo WJGR, Rubinstein SM, et al. Minimally invasive surgery for lumbar disk herniation: Asystematic review and meta-analysis. Eur Spine J. 2014;23:1021-104.
6. Van Den Akker ME, Arts MP, van den Hout WB et al. Tubular diskectomy vs conventional microdiskectomy for the treatment of lumbar disk-related sciatica: cost utility analysis alongside a double-blind randomized controlled trial. Neurosurgery 2011;69(4):829-35. discussion 829-36.
7. Wiltse LL, Kirkaldy-Willis WH, McIvor GW .The treatment of spinal stenosis. Clin Orthop Relat Res. 1976;115:83-91.
8. Niggemeyer O, Strauss JM, Schulitz KP. Comparison of surgical procedures for degenerative lumbar spinal stenosis: a meta-analysis of the literature from 1975 to 1995. Eur Spine J. 1997; 6:423-9.

9. Palmer S, Turner R, Palmer R Bilateral decompression of lumbar spinal stenosis involving a unilateral approach with microscope and tubular retractor system. J Neurosurg. 2002;97:213-7.
10. Khoo LT, Fessler RG Microendoscopic decompressive laminotomy for the treatment of lumbar stenosis. Neurosurgery 2002; 51:S146-54.
11. Pao JL, Chen WC, Chen PQ. Clinical outcomes of microendoscopic decompressive laminotomy for degenerative lumbar spinal stenosis. Eur Spine J. 2009; 18:672-8.
12. Minamide A, Yoshida M, Yamada H. Endoscope-assisted spinal decompression surgery for lumbar spinal stenosis Technical note. J Neurosurg Spine. 2013;19:664-71.
13. Cloward RB. The treatment of ruptured intervertebral disks by vertebral body fusion. Indications, operative technique, after care. J Neurosurg. 1953;10:154-68.
14. Harms JG, Jeszenszky D .The unilateral transforaminal approach for posterior lumbar interbody fusion. Orthop Traumatol. 1998; 6:88-99.
15. Schwender JD, Holly LT, Rouben DP, Foley KT. Minimally invasive transforaminal lumbar interbody fusion (TLIF): Technical feasibility and initial results. J Spinal Disord Tech 2005;18 Suppl:S1-6.
16. Seng C, Siddiqui MA, Wong KPL et al. Five year outcomes of minimally invasive versus open transforaminal lumbar interbody fusion: A matched-pair comparison study. Spine. 2013; 38:2049-55.
17. Peng CWB, Yue WM, Poh SY et al. Clinical and radiological outcomes of minimally invasive versus open transforaminal lumbar interbody fusion. Spine. 2009;34:1385-9.
18. Cruet MJP, Hussain NS, White GZ. Quality-of-life outcomes with Minimally Invasive Transforaminal Lumbar Interbody Fusion Based on Long-Term Analysis of 304 Consecutive Patients. Spine. 2014;39:E191-8.
19. Lee KH , Yue WM , Yeo W, et al. Clinical and radiological outcomes of open versus minimally invasive transforaminal lumbar interbody fusion. Eur Spine J. 2012;21:2265-70.
20. Glassman, Copay A , Berven S, et al. Defining substantial clinical benefit following lumbar spine arthrodesis. J Bone Joint Surg Am. 2008;90:1839-47.
21. Brodano GB, K. Martikos K, Lolli F, et al. Transforaminal lumbar interbody fusion in degenerative disk disease and spondylolisthesis grade I: minimally invasive versus open surgery. J Spinal Disord Tech. 2013.
22. Ozgur BM, Aryan HE, Pimenta L, et al. Extreme Lateral Interbody Fusion (XLIF): a novel surgical technique for anterior lumbar interbody fusion. Spine J. 2006;6:435-43.
23. Rodgers WB, Gerber EJ, Patterson JR. Intraoperative and early postoperative complications in extreme lateral interbody fusion (XLIF): an analysis of 600 cases. Spine. 2011;36:26-32.
24. Youssef JA, McAfee P C, Patty C A, et al. Minimally Invasive Surgery: Lateral Approach Interbody Fusion Results and Review. Spine. 2010;35:S302-S311
25. KnutssonB, Michaëlsson K,SandénB: Obesity is associated with inferior results after surgery for lumbar spinal stenosis: a study of 2633 patients from the Swedish spine register. Spine.1976; 38:435-41.
26. Espejo B, Torres A, Valentín M et al. Obesity favors surgical and infectious complications after renal transplantation. Transplant Proc. 2003;35:1762-3.
27. Lau D, Khan A, Terma SW et al. Comparison of perioperative outcomes following open versus minimally invasive transforaminal lumbar interbody fusion in obese patients. Neurosurg Focus. 2013;35(2):E10.
28. Wang J, Zhou Y, Feng Zhang Z et al. Comparison of clinical outcome in overweight orobese patients after minimally invasive versus open transforaminal lumbar interbody fusion. J Spinal Disord Tech. 2012;27(4)202-6.
29. Deyo RA, Gray DT, Kreuter W, et al. United States trends in lumbar fusion surgery for degenerative conditions. Spine. 2005; 30:1441-5.
30. Cassinelli EH, Eubanks J, Vogt M, et al. Risk factors for the development of perioperative complications in elderly patients undergoing lumbar decompression and arthrodesis for spinal stenosis. Spine. 2007;32:230-5.
31. Kilincer C, Steinmetz MP, Sohn MJ, et al. Effects of age on the perioperative characteristics and short-term outcome of posterior lumbar fusion surgery. J Neurosurg Spine. 2005; 3:34-9.
32. Carreon LY, Puno RM, Dimar JR, et al. Perioperative complications of posterior lumbar decompression and arthrodesis in older adults.JBoneJoint Surg [Am]. 2003;85:2089-92.
33. Rodgers WB, Gerber EJ, Rodgers JA. Lumbar fusion in octogenarians the promise of minimally invasive Surgery. Spine. 2010;35:S355-60.
34. Wang J, Zhou Y, Zhang ZF et al. Minimally invasive or open transforaminal lumbar interbody fusion as revision surgery for patients previously treated by open diskectomy and decompression of the lumbar spine. Eur Spine J. 2011;20:623-8.
35. Lee JC, Jang HD, Shin BJ. Learning curve and clinical outcomes of minimally invasive transforaminal lumbar interbody fusion our experience in 86 consecutive cases. Spine. 2012;37:1548- 57.
36. Al-Khouja LT, Baron EM, Jhopson JP, et al. Cost-effectiveness analysis in minimally invasive spine surgery. Neurosurg Focus. 2014;36(6).

27

CHAPTER

Management of Surgical Site Infection after Minimally Invasive Spine Surgery

Arvind G Kulkarni, Ravish Patel

ABSTRACT

Surgical site infections can lead to profound physical, psychological and financial implications. It can increase postoperative morbidity, prolongs hospital stay, leads to repeated surgeries and increases healthcare costs. During last two decades, the minimally invasive surgical techniques have evolved enormously and there is a widespread acceptance of these techniques. Several authors have demonstrated that there is a significant reduction in the risk of infection after primary minimally invasive surgery. However, there is a paucity of literature on the management of infections after the minimally invasive techniques. This chapter describes the approach a spine surgeon should adopt for surgical site infection after minimally invasive spine surgery. Also, the chapter highlights the fact that the risk of infection is reduced and the management of infection is simplified, if a patient has undergone a primary minimal invasive surgery.

INTRODUCTION

Infections after spine surgery are one of the most challenging complications and require special care and attention. It results in physical suffering, mental agony and huge financial burden to the patients. It also brings disrepute to the treating doctors and their organizations. The neural tissues and the added implants in the vicinity add to the detrimental consequences.

As a result of advances in medical science, a large number of immunocompromised patients, patients with medical comorbidities and chronic diseases are able to live a longer life than before. Such patients will be prone to infections if they undergo spine surgery. Also, the spinal instrumentation has evolved enormously over last few decades from Harrington rods to complex spinal fixations devices like pedicle screw systems. More and more patients are receiving spinal instrumentation. Even though these can be more helpful than harmful but wider application of instrumentation has increased the rate of infection and made the management of infections more difficult. There is a risk of biofilm formation and adhesion of offending organisms to the implants.[1] Antibiotics cannot be delivered in the required concentrations to these organisms.

A spine surgeon should always keep on revisiting their operative strategies and should utilize the advances in the field to the fullest to curb this deep-rooted adversary. Minimal invasive spine surgeries (MISS) reduce the rate of surgical site infections (SSI) significantly.[2-6] Adoption of the minimally invasive techniques would thereby improve the patient care considerably. At the same time, it should be noted that it does not eliminate infection completely. Hence, obligatory steps to minimize SSI should always be practiced even by minimal invasive surgeons. Early detection and prompt but structured treatment plan are crucial for successful outcome following SSI. This chapter illustrates how the basic principles of managing infections should be applied for infection following MISS. It also infers that minimal access primary surgery simplifies and facilities the management of SSI.

EPIDEMIOLOGY

The overall incidence of infection after spine surgery **(Table 1)** is reported to range from 0.07 to 16%.[1-18] Age-old technique of open spine surgery has infection rates reported from 0.5% to 16%.[1,7-18] With minimally invasive spine surgeries the infection rates range from 0.07% to 7%.[2-6] Minimal tissue destruction, smaller dead space, lesser blood loss and shorter hospital stay are the main reasons for reduced infection rates following MISS.[2-4] There is a reduction in the surface area exposed to the pathogenic organisms due to a reduction in the width of the surgical corridor. The

Table 1

Comparison of infection rates between open surgery and MISS

Parameters	Open srgery[1,7-18] (%)	MISS[2-6] (%)
Overall infection rate	0.5–16	0.07–7
Noninstrumented surgeries	0.5–5	0.07–0.4
Instrumented surgeries	2.9–16	1.3–7
Single V/S two-level procedures 1 level 2 levels	 4.8–6.3 5.1–7	 1.6–4.5 0–4.6

invasiveness and the soft-tissue destruction are much less as observed by Sasaoka et al.[19] Also, the amount of back muscle degeneration and destruction is less after minimally invasive procedures.[20,21] It is important to note that the difference in infection rates between MISS and open surgery is mainly because of reduction in deep/organ spaced infection with MISS as observed by Smith et al.[22] Reduced infection rates after MISS also lead to significant reduction in the overall health care costs.[5,23,24] Infections after open spine surgery increase the healthcare utilization cost by fourfold whereas infection following MIS increases the cost by 1.5-fold.[23,25]

Risk Factors

Risk factors for infection following spine surgery **(Table 2)** can be either patient-related or surgery-related. Careful attention should be made to patient-related risk factors during preoperative examination and necessary steps should be taken to control or obviate them before elective surgeries. Surgery-related risk factors can be analyzed on an individual basis, and it should be kept in mind that selection of surgery, duration of surgery and approach or technique used can influence the risk of encountering an infection.

Table 2

Risk factors

Patient related	Surgery related[26-29]
Diabetes mellitus (blood sugar >200mg/dL)[15]	Duration of surgery (>3 hours)
Malnutrition[30]	Blood loss (>1 L)/blood transfusion
Smoking	Length of hospital stay
Obesity[27,29,31]	Multi-level procedures
Immunocompromised patients	Revision surgeries
Patients on radiotherapy and immune modulators, steroids (RA, cancer)[28,29]	Fusion extending to sacrum
Preoperative sepsis	Posterior surgeries/posterior osteotomies

Obesity is a known risk factor for infection following spine surgery, but there are many advantages for obese patients undergoing minimally invasive surgeries. MISS causes lesser soft tissue dissection, lesser fat destruction, and lesser blood loss than the conventional open surgery. So, obese patients have fewer infections after MISS compared to that after open surgeries.[31] Similarly, patients with diabetes have lesser infection rate with MISS than that of the similar open surgery cohort.

Cessation of smoking, discontinuation of antimetabolites, prior treatment of septic foci and cessation of radiotherapy (a week prior to surgery and for three weeks postoperatively) needs to be practiced even for MISS.

Clinical Features

One must initiate thorough diagnostic workup and detailed clinical examination in presence of slightest suspicion of SSI. A high index of suspicion helps in early diagnosis and prompt treatment. Infections have a varied clinical presentation and sometimes the results of diagnostic modalities are difficult to interpret. Clinical Presentation may be early (<3 months) or late (>3 months).

Local Features

The most consistent finding in the clinical presentation of infection is operative site pain. Pain is typically out of proportion to the surgical invasiveness and may be associated with systemic features. The resurgence of pain after a relatively pain-free interval may indicate infection, especially in the early postoperative period.

Another finding that provides a valuable diagnostic clue is discharge from the surgical site. Usual blood stained discharge/collection following MISS do not persist for more than a day or two.[2-6] Discharge from wound especially serosanguinous, seropurulent and purulent are suggestive of infection. Serous/ serosanguinous discharge may also be present in patients with hematoma formation or due to fat necrosis in obese patients.

On examination infection in usually associated with erythema, warmth and tenderness. There can be a severe restriction of movements due to painful spasm. In obese patients, excessive fat necrosis may mimic infection. Although, the absence of systemic features and normal laboratory parameters help differentiate between them. In patients presenting as superficial infection, the presence of systemic features, failure respond to antibiotics and increasing operative site pain should alert the surgeon of the possibility of underlying deep seated infection.

Infections presenting after 3 months of the postoperative period usually present with a vague clinical picture. The surgical incision site is healed and hence may not have obvious discharge. In such situation, local features of disproportionate pain, erythema, and redness with systemic features should raise suspicion of infection. In patients with late infections, raised laboratory parameters (in absence of septic foci elsewhere) indicate the presence of infection.

Systemic Features

Systemic features are less commonly observed in cases of SSI following MISS. They can be divided into two broad categories as under.

The first category consists of symptoms that are secondary to involvement of neural tissues. This includes radicular pain, neurological deficit, myelopathic symptoms, cauda equina syndrome. These symptoms occur due to space occupying lesions like epidural abscess, granuloma or due to spinal instability.[32]

The second category consists of constitutional symptoms like fever, chills, malaise and anorexia. These symptoms point towards the existence of deep-seated organ-spaced infections or infections with multi-system involvement. Life-threatening infections with signs and symptoms of sepsis are rare after MISS. In presence of comorbid conditions and chronic illnesses, patients may present with a confusing clinical picture. The systemic symptoms may be absent if the infection is picked up early and treated promptly.

Diagnostic Workup

Common laboratory parameters like Total leukocyte count (TLC), ESR and CRP are acute phase reactants suggesting the presence of inflammation in the body. Most of the times, it is difficult to detect infection before seven days with these parameters as an incubation period of around four days is required for the immune system to get activated against the offending organism. Moreover, rise due to surgical invasiveness and rise due to infection cannot be differentiated in this initial period. It has been observed by several authors that the peak measurements in non-infective patients are much less after MISS when compared to open surgeries due to lesser tissue trauma.[19] This may increase the sensitivity of these parameters to detect infections after MISS.

A persistent rise in leucocyte (particularly neutrophil count) on 7th postoperative day or a fall in lymphocyte count below 1000 cells/μL (10% or less) on 4th postoperative day suggest infection.[33] In a recent unpublished data, the sensitivity and specificity of lymphocyte count are 65.4% to 90.9% on 4th postoperative (cutoff 1180 cells/μL) and 63.3% to 78.5% on 7th postoperative day (cutoff 1090 cells/μL).[34] It is worthy to note that infection elsewhere in the body can also give rise to raised leukocyte count. Moreover, leukocytes may fail to rise after infection in immunocompromised patients.

After surgery, ESR (0–15 mm/hr) peaks on the seventh or eighth day and usually takes three to six weeks to return to baseline. It is usually less than 25 mm/hour in the post-operative period. Any deviation from above measurements should raise suspicion of infection. However, ESR is non-specific and nonsensitive. It can be normal in case of occult infections with low virulent organisms and may be raised due to inflammation elsewhere in the body. Once the diagnosis is established, ESR is not preferred for monitoring treatment response as even after successful treatment ESR takes a longer time to return to baseline than CRP.

C-reactive proteins (CRP) has a half-life of 2.6 days and it peaks usually on third postoperative period and remains elevated for 10–14 days.[35] The presence of the second rise of CRP or failure of CRP to return to normal level within two weeks usually suggests an infection. The second rise of CRP was defined as a measurement taken after the postoperative peak had occurred and with a value that exceeded the previous measurement by at least 2.33% for CRP.[35] CRP has a sensitivity of 80.9% and specificity of 90.2%.[34] The rise is CRP is much higher (10000 folds) and short-lived compared to ESR (10–100-fold). Not being an expensive test, it is among the first-line investigations which are carried out in suspected cases of postoperative infections. It is most commonly used parameter for monitoring treatment response.

Serum procalcitonin has been suggested by several authors for early detection of infection. It has comparable postoperative spectrum to CRP. In presence of raised serum procalcitonin, one should rule out infection elsewhere in the body before suspecting SSI.[36] It can also be helpful in guiding continuation/discontinuation of antibiotic therapy.

The aspirate, wound swab or pus specimen from the wound sent for the culture and sensitivity will not only confirm the presence of infection, but it will also help initiate targeted antibiotic therapy as soon as possible. Intraoperative specimens are more reliable then the wound sample as the risk of contamination from the skin flora is less. However, it is important to note that cultures may not be positive in all suspected cases of infection or even in patients with frank infections. As a surgeon, it is important to guide the treatment based on clinical experience and evidence from other investigations. Blood cultures are rarely positive but can be useful to advice appropriate antibiotic therapy as the organisms isolated with blood culture correlates with the organism obtained from surgical site.[37]

MICROBIOLOGY

Acute infections occurring in the early postoperative period are usually caused by high virulent organisms like *Staphylococcus aureus* (>50%), *Klebsiella pneumoniae,*

Pseudomonas aeruginosa, etc. Surgeries in lumbosacral regions are more prone to infection by gram-negative organisms. For gram-negative infections, it is unclear whether this infection is from primary inoculation or by contamination from fecal or urinary flora.[38] Bloodborne infections are also due to highly virulence organism, and systemic features are more pronounced in such infections.

Late infections are usually caused by low-virulence organisms like *Propionibacterium acnes*, coagulase-negative staphylococci, *Staphylococcus epidermidis* etc.[38] These organisms can be present in normal skin flora and prolonged open wounds. Chronic inflammation may predispose to infections from these organisms.

IMAGING

The sensitivity (82%) and the specificity (57%) of plain radiography are very low, especially in an early stage infection.[39] Initial radiographs may be normal, but they do provide a benchmark for comparison with further X-rays. It takes at least four weeks to show some substantial changes in radiographs. Usual radiological signs are lysis around implants, narrowing of the disk space, paravertebral soft tissue shadows, endplate changes, reactive bone formation, kyphotic deformity, and collapse.

The utility of CT scan is limited by the presence of implant related artefacts but the changes occurring in the end plates, bone lysis, and soft tissue collections can easily be noted in CT scan. These are the early indicators of infection.

Nuclear magnetic studies like gallium-67 scans, technetium-99 scans or indium 111 labeled WBC scans were used previously but lacked sensitivity in SSI after instrumented spinal surgeries.[40] Recently, studies have shown that FDG-PET scan has 100% sensitivity and 47–95% specificity for detecting postoperative infections after instrumented surgeries.[40] It provides rapid results (2 hours) and high-resolution images (4–5 mm) even in presence of metallic implants. FDG-PET can help localize the exact focus of infection so that selective implants can be removed and salvage surgeries can be avoided.[40] F-18 FDG PET/CT is also useful for discrimination of residual and nonresidual SSI after treatment.[41]

MRI is currently the imaging modality of choice. MRI is highly sensitive (93%) and specific (96%) in evaluating spinal infections.[39] It gives more information than nuclear imaging and helps differentiate nonpathological and degenerative changes from postoperative infections.[39] For patients with implants in-situ specialized metal artefact suppression sequence as described by Chang et al. is useful.[42] In early postoperative period, it may be difficult to differentiate normal postoperative changes from infection. **Table 3** shows the MRI features indicative of postoperative infections.

Table 3

MRI features suggestive of surgical site infections

	T1-weighted images	*T2-weighted images*	*Contrast*
Diskitis (earliest) (D/D Modic type I)	Hypointensity disk changes with adjacent vertebral marrow edema (hyper-intense body changes)	Hyperintensity in disk space and adjacent bone marrow	Disk signal enhancement with addition of contrast
Epidural abscess	Isointense signal compressing the neural elements.	Hyperintense signals	Ring enhancement on T1 images with IV gadolinium
Osteomyelitis	Hypointense body changes with loss of demarcation between body and disk space.	Hyperintense signals form vertebral body	

CLASSIFICATIONS

CDC Classification for SSI[43]

This classification classifies SSI in to superficial or deep incisional SSI or organ-spaced SSI.

Superficial SSI is defined as an infection occurring within thirty days of surgery and involving skin and subcutaneous tissues at the incision site with a purulent discharge or positive culture from aseptically obtained specimen or diagnosis of a superficial incisional SSI by the surgeon or attending physician.

Deep incisional SSI is an infection occurring within ninety days of surgery, involving deep soft tissues of the incision (e.g. fascial and muscle layers) with one of the following:

a. Purulent drainage from the deep incision.
b. The deep incision that spontaneously or deliberately opened or aspirated by a surgeon. And organism is identified or the patient has at least any of the signs or symptoms like fever (>38°C), localized pain or tenderness.
c. Evidence of infection involving the deep incision which is detected on gross anatomical or histopathology examination or imaging test.

Organ-spaced SSI is an infection occurring within ninety days after surgery and involving any part of the body deeper than the fascial or muscle layers (that is opened or manipulated during the operative procedure) with at least one of the following:

a. Purulent drainage from a drain that is placed into the organ/space.
b. Organisms are identified from an aseptically obtained fluid or tissue in the organ/space by culture or non-culture based microbiologic testing method.
c. Evidence of infection which is detected on gross anatomical or histopathologic exam, or imaging test.

Thalgott[44] proposed a classification to guide towards the treatment of postoperative spine wound infections. Classification is based on host response and severity of the infection.

Class A patients have normal host systemic defenses and local conditions.

Class B patients have local or multiple systemic diseases.

Class C has an immunocompromised or severely malnourished host.

Classes B and C are at high risk for developing a postoperative wound infection.

He also suggested three groups.

Group 1, which represents a single-organism infection, either superficial or deep, can usually be effectively treated with single irrigation and debridement, and closure over suction drainage tubes.

Group 2, deep and multiple-organism infection, requires an average of three irrigation debridement and closure with closed inflow-outflow suction irrigation system.

Group 3 infections (multiple-organism infections with myonecrosis) are exceedingly difficult to manage and predict a poor outcome. These patients require an average of six debridements followed by flap reconstruction for wound closure.

PREVENTIVE STRATEGIES

Antibiotic prophylaxis given ½ to 1 hour before surgery has shown to reduce infection with almost all types of spinal surgeries.[45] The choice of antibiotic depends on the local prevalence of resistant organisms, pharmacokinetic and pharmacodynamics profile of the antibiotics and allergic sensitivity of the patients. Third generation cephalosporins are usually preferred as they are relatively safe and are effective against some gram-negative organisms along with many gram-positive organisms. There are no evidence to support multiple antibiotics for prophylaxis.[45] But, it is preferred to combine third-generation cephalosporin with an aminoglycoside for instrumented surgeries. Gentamicin and vancomycin are positively charged antibiotics and have better diffusion profile, especially in the annulus and nucleus pulposus.[46] Since the serum concentration of antibiotics falls over a period of time, several authors have suggested repeating antibiotics every 4 hourly during the surgery. Usually, it is not advisable to continue antibiotics postoperatively for more than 24 hours. However, authors prefer to continue antibiotics for 48 hrs in cases of instrumented surgeries. A wound wash with dilute povidone-iodine (3.5%) at the end of procedure has shown to reduce infection rates.[47]

Adherence to strict aseptic precaution is of paramount significance. Various studies have shown that handling of microscope and image intensifier is crucial and failing which can increase infection rate. Microscope drapes and C-arm drapes should be used. It is advisable not to touch the optical piece and any portion of microscope drape above the optical piece during surgery.[48] The portion of image intensifier that goes below the table must be draped again every time it is positioned for lateral exposure. Laminar air-flow systems have been shown in several studies to reduce the infection rates.[49]

MANAGEMENT

Early diagnosis and prompt management are the key parameters for successful outcome following spinal infections. Management goals include:

1. Extermination of the infecting organism.
2. Maintenance of spinal stability and protection of neural tissues.
3. Achieving adequate soft tissue coverage.
4. Obtaining good functional outcome.

The first step in the management of suspected or definitive infection after a minimally invasive surgery is to decide whether to treat the patient conservatively or to offer surgical intervention. **Flowchart 1** shows management algorithm for SSI.

Conservative Treatment

For superficial infections and selected cases of deep infections after non-instrumented surgeries, conservative treatment may be attempted. The progress of treatment is to be monitored by repeated ESR, CRP estimation, and clinical improvement. Indications of surgical intervention in such cases would be an uncontrolled pain, neurological deficit, failure of the patient to respond to conservative treatment, the presence of an epidural abscess or large paravertebral abscess, the progression of deformity and instability.[50]

Superficial infection, such as stitch abscess or cellulitis can usually be treated with two weeks of oral antibiotics with or without a bedside local incision and drainage. Deep (subfascial) infections usually require six weeks of intravenous antibiotics followed by at least six weeks of oral antibiotics. Antibiotics should be continued for one month

Flowchart 1: Management algorithm for SSI

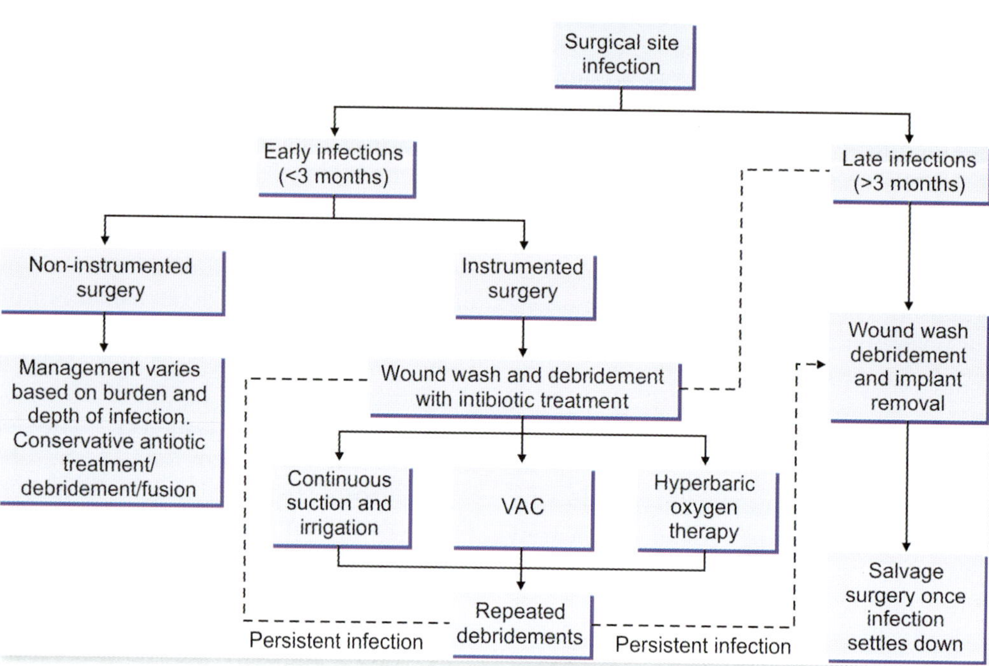

after CRP returns to normal.[51] Postprocedure diskitis that presents with a history of increasing low back pain after surgery can be treated with image-guided percutaneous aspiration and guided antibiotics in about 60% of diskitis patients.[52] Most of the patients that responded to this form of treatment would land up with fusion at that level. Elderly patients, immunocompromised patients, patients with large epidural abscess should be treated by surgical intervention at the earliest as poor outcomes have been reported.[52]

In instrumented surgeries, one should be very cautious in subjecting a patient to conservative management. If the infection is not eradicated completely, it may lead to widespread seeding of the offending organisms along the wound. The patient may land up undergoing repeated debridements and may end up with an implant removal.

For antibiotic treatment, one needs to have definitive bacteriological diagnosis along with culture and sensitivity assay. Swabs from infected wounds may get contaminated with normal skin flora. Hence, for accurate identification of organisms, intraoperative samples during debridement are the most appropriate specimen. If multiple layers are infected, swab/pus needs to be taken from all the layers and should be sent separately. CT-guided biopsies can be helpful in presence of spondylodiscitis. Aerobic culture and sensitivity, histopathological examination with Gram staining and AFB staining should be performed on all the samples. Anaerobic culture, gene expert, tubercular culture and fungal culture are to be performed in special circumstances like atypical presentations, immunocompromised patients, malnourishment, and failure to respond to antibiotics.

SURGICAL TREATMENT

Infections after non-instrumented MISS can be treated with wound wash and debridement through the same incision used for primary surgery. The goal of debridement is to (i) reduce the load of organisms, (ii) provide culture sample to guide antibiotic treatment and (iii) to remove debris and avascular disk components. Early postoperative diskitis following minimal invasive surgeries can be effectively treated with a percutaneous transforaminal endoscopic debridement with immediate pain relief and good clinical outcomes.[53] Interlaminar endoscopic debridement or tubular retractor system assisted debridement are also useful. Certain antibiotics or antiseptic agents that are not harmful to the neural tissues can be instilled during the endoscopic debridement. In presence of a large epidural abscess, severe neurological deficit, infection by highly virulent organisms and spinal instability an open debridement with or without fusion is preferred.

In instrumented surgeries, the previous incision may have to be extended in order to visualize the wound entirely and to avoid leaving pus pockets in its vicinity. Separate midline incision exposing spinous process and/or the neural tissue is not advocated if not performed primarily.[2-6] All deep and organ-spaced infections following instrumented surgeries require surgical debridement in addition to intravenous antibiotics. All loose tissues and necrotic materials should be removed. Loose particles of bone graft should also be removed as dead bone can serve as a nidus for the growth of organisms. Aggressive surgical debridement exposing all the planes till bone and implants is advocated. It is a good practice to stain the track with methylene blue or other staining material after obtaining a culture specimen so that the exact source of infection can be reached. Some authors believe that deeper planes are to be explored only when such layers are suspected to foster infection.[54] However, in our experience thorough exploration and debridement is preferred to prevent missing a potentially disastrous deep infection. In selected cases of minimally invasive surgery with two paraspinal incisions, only the infected side can be explored and debrided. But the patients should be investigated thoroughly and there should not be any septic foci reaching the contralateral side.

In the literature, authors share divided opinion on whether to retain or remove well-fixed implants. But certain conclusions can be made. Implants can be retained usually in the case of the acute infections.[55-57] Titanium implants that are used today give better outcomes compared to previously used stainless steel implants in infections with implants in-situ.[58] Implants may not be the source of infection but provide a scaffold for glycocalyx formation and serve as a nidus for the growth of microorganisms in its vicinity. Removal of implants is necessary for certain conditions. The indications of implant removal are as follows:

1. Infection caused by low virulent organisms or with delayed presentation (>3 months). In such infections, glycocalyx formation helps organisms grow and spread close to the implant surface. Antibiotics are usually not able to reach the desired concentration in the vicinity of these offending organisms.
2. In presence of clinical or radiological signs of instability (radiographs/CT scan showing lysis around implants or abnormal mobility). Reimplantation should be performed only when the infection is convincingly resolved. Patients should be provided with brace and allowed strict bed rest during the interval period. The midline corridor of soft tissues which is preserved in case of the minimally invasive spine surgery allows ipsilateral removal of the implants in selected unilateral deep infections. Thus secondary salvage procedures to maintain spinal stability can be avoided.
3. Failure of repeated debridement (>3 debridements) and long-term antibiotic treatment.[55]
4. Once vertebral osteomyelitis and/or intervertebral abscess were evident in MR images, all the hardware should be removed.[58] Failing this will result in multiple failed debridement and pseudoarthrosis.

After thorough debridement, a plan for closure of the surgical wound must be decided. Primary closure is usually feasible and preferred in patients undergoing debridement after primary MISS as the soft-tissues destruction after minimally invasive surgery was minimal. Wounds if kept open are susceptible to superinfection and wound contracture.

In cases infected by multiple organisms and in patients undergoing repeated debridements, the primary closure can be combined with continuous suction irrigation or hyperbaric oxygen therapy.[59,60]

1. Usually, three deep drains one for irrigation cranially and two for collection caudally (one subfacial and one deep) are used for continuous suction-irrigation. The duration of suction-irrigation can vary from 5 to 14 days depending on the severity of the infection. Antibiotics used for irrigation depends on the culture sensitivity assay.
2. Hyperbaric oxygen therapy is indicated when there is no significant drop in ESR and CRP after 3 weeks of starting antibiotic therapy. Duration of HBO therapy and number of sessions (range: 10–40 sessions) depends on type and depth of the infections. Its mechanism of action was attributed to an increase in the oxygen saturation in the ischemic tissue, with a resultant increase in microcirculation, and direct antimicrobial effect against microorganisms.[61]
3. Negative pressure VAC dressing act by continuous removal of wound fluid which inhibits mitosis, protein synthesis, and fibroblast collagen synthesis. Reduced interstitial pressure, increasing blood flow and a lesser number of debridement (2.2 vs. 4.7) are touted advantages.[62]

When primary closure is not possible then the wound can be closed as under

1. Closed with a coverage procedure.
2. Closed primarily or gradually over a vacuum suction system.[62]
3. Delayed closure with intermittent debridement.

The possibility of not achieving primary closure is rare with SSI after MISS.

The surgical debridement should be followed by a six weeks of intravenous antibiotics. Initially, empirical broad spectrum antibiotics can be initiated and later on can be modified as per culture sensitivity reports. It is recommended to continue IV antibiotics for patients with infection by resistant organisms such as MRSA.[63] Intravenous antibiotics should be followed by a six weeks course of oral antibiotics selected as per susceptibility of the offending organism. It is recommended that patients should be monitored by laboratory and radiological investigations during this period.

AUTHORS' EXPERIENCE[23]

We encountered three deep infections following over a thousand MISS and all of them were following instrumented surgery. The patients presented early with typical clinical features, raised laboratory markers and culture proven organisms. The infections resolved with single debridement and wound wash extending the previous incision in all patients. In one of the three cases unilateral implant had to be removed and contralateral implants were retained. None of the infected patients required repeated debridement or salvage surgery and fusion was achieved in all without any adverse sequelae on long-term follow-up.

REFERENCES

1. Pappou IP, Papadopoulos EC, Sama AA, et al. Postoperative infections in interbody fusion for degenerative spinal disease. Clin Orthop Relat Res. 2006;444:120-8.
2. Ee WW, Lau WL, Yeo W, et al. Does minimally invasive surgery have a lower risk of surgical site infections compared with open spinal surgery? Clin Orthop Relat Res. 2014;472:1718-24.
3. McGirt MJ, Parker SL, Lerner J, et al. Comparative analysis of perioperative surgical site infection after minimally invasive versus open posterior/transforaminal lumbar interbody fusion: analysis of hospital billing and discharge data from 5170 patients. J Neurosurg Spine. 2011;14:771-8.
4. O'Toole JE, Eichholz KM, Fessler RG. Surgical site infection rates after minimally invasive spinal surgery. J Neurosurg Spine. 2009;11:471-6.
5. Parker SL, Adogwa O, Witham TF, et al. Post-operative infection after minimally invasive versus open transforaminal lumbar interbody fusion (TLIF): literature review and cost analysis. Minim Invasive Neurosurg. 2011;54:33-7.
6. Shousha M, Cirovic D, Boehm H. Infection rate after minimally invasive noninstrumented spinal surgery based on 4350 procedures. Spine (Phila Pa 1976). 2015;40:201-5.
7. Beiner JM, Grauer J, Kwon BK, et al. Postoperative wound infections of the spine. Neurosurg Focus. 2003;15:E14.
8. Collins I, Wilson-MacDonald J, Chami G, et al. The diagnosis and management of infection following instrumented spinal fusion. Eur Spine J. 2008;17:445-50.
9. Fang A, Hu SS, Endres N, et al. Risk factors for infection after spinal surgery. Spine (Phila Pa 1976). 2005;30:1460-5.
10. Friedman ND, Sexton DJ, Connelly SM, et al. Risk factors for surgical site infection complicating laminectomy. Infect Control Hosp Epidemiol. 2007;28:1060-5.
11. Gaynes RP, Culver DH, Horan TC, et al. Surgical site infection (SSI) rates in the United States, 1992-1998: the National Nosocomial Infections Surveillance System basic SSI risk index. Clin Infect Dis. 2001;33 Suppl 2:S69-77.
12. Kanayama M, Hashimoto T, Shigenobu K, et al. Effective prevention of surgical site infection using a Centers for Disease Control and Prevention guideline-based antimicrobial prophylaxis in lumbar spine surgery. J Neurosurg Spine. 2007;6:327-9.
13. Mirovsky Y, Floman Y, Smorgick Y, et al. Management of deep wound infection after posterior lumbar interbody fusion with cages. J Spinal Disord Tech. 2007;20:127-31.
14. Olsen MA, Mayfield J, Lauryssen C, et al. Risk factors for surgical site infection in spinal surgery. J Neurosurg. 2003;98:149-55.
15. Olsen MA, Nepple JJ, Riew KD, et al. Risk factors for surgical site infection following orthopaedic spinal operations. J Bone Joint Surg Am. 2008;90:62-9.
16. Picada R, Winter RB, Lonstein JE, et al. Postoperative deep wound infection in adults after posterior lumbosacral spine fusion with instrumentation: incidence and management. J Spinal Disord. 2000;13:42-5.
17. Valentini LG, Casali C, Chatenoud L, et al. Surgical site infections after elective neurosurgery: a survey of 1747 patients. Neurosurgery. 2008;62:88-95; discussion -6.
18. Weinstein MA, McCabe JP, Cammisa FP, Jr. Postoperative spinal wound infection: a review of 2,391 consecutive index procedures. J Spinal Disord. 2000;13:422-6.
19. Sasaoka R, Nakamura H, Konishi S, et al. Objective assessment of reduced invasiveness in MED. Compared with conventional one-level laminotomy. Eur Spine J. 2006;15:577-82.
20. Min SH, Kim MH, Seo JB, et al. The quantitative analysis of back muscle degeneration after posterior lumbar fusion: comparison of minimally invasive and conventional open surgery. Asian Spine J. 2009;3:89-95.
21. Stevens KJ, Spenciner DB, Griffiths KL, et al. Comparison of minimally invasive and conventional open posterolateral lumbar fusion using magnetic resonance imaging and retraction pressure studies. J Spinal Disord Tech. 2006;19:77-86.
22. Smith JS, Shaffrey CI, Sansur CA, et al. Rates of infection after spine surgery based on 108,419 procedures: a report from the Scoliosis Research Society Morbidity and Mortality Committee. Spine (Phila Pa 1976). 2011;36:556-63.
23. Kulkarni AG, Patel RS, Dutta S. Does Minimally Invasive Spine Surgery Minimize Surgical Site Infections? Asian Spine J. 2016;10:1000-6.
24. Al-Khouja LT, Baron EM, Johnson JP, et al. Cost-effectiveness analysis in minimally invasive spine surgery. Neurosurg Focus. 2014;36:E4.
25. Calderone RR, Garland DE, Capen DA, et al. Cost of medical care for postoperative spinal infections. Orthop Clin North Am. 1996;27:171-82.
26. Mikhael MM, Huddleston PM, Nassr A. Postoperative culture positive surgical site infections after the use of irradiated allograft, nonirradiated allograft, or autograft for spinal fusion. Spine (Phila Pa 1976). 2009;34:2466-8.
27. Pull ter Gunne AF, Cohen DB. Incidence, prevalence, and analysis of risk factors for surgical site infection following adult spinal surgery. Spine (Phila Pa 1976). 2009;34:1422-8.
28. Schuster JM, Rechtine G, Norvell DC, et al. The influence of perioperative risk factors and therapeutic interventions on infection rates after spine surgery: a systematic review. Spine (Phila Pa 1976). 2010;35:S125-37.
29. Veeravagu A, Patil CG, Lad SP, et al. Risk factors for postoperative spinal wound infections after spinal decompression and fusion surgeries. Spine (Phila Pa 1976). 2009;34:1869-72.
30. Klein JD, Hey LA, Yu CS, et al. Perioperative nutrition and postoperative complications in patients undergoing spinal surgery. Spine (Phila Pa 1976). 1996;21:2676-82.

31. McGuire KJ, Khaleel MA, Rihn JA, et al. The effect of high obesity on outcomes of treatment for lumbar spinal conditions: subgroup analysis of the spine patient outcomes research trial. Spine (Phila Pa 1976). 2014;39:1975-80.
32. Rawlings CE, 3rd, Wilkins RH, Gallis HA, et al. Postoperative intervertebral disc space infection. Neurosurgery. 1983;13:371-6.
33. Takahashi J, Shono Y, Hirabayashi H, et al. Usefulness of white blood cell differential for early diagnosis of surgical wound infection following spinal instrumentation surgery. Spine (Phila Pa 1976). 2006;31:1020-5.
34. Iwata E, Shigematsu H, Koizumi M, et al. Lymphocyte Count at 4 Days Postoperatively and CRP Level at 7 Days Postoperatively: Reliable and Useful Markers for Surgical Site Infection Following Instrumented Spinal Fusion. Spine (Phila Pa 1976). 2016;41:1173-8.
35. Mok JM, Pekmezci M, Piper SL, et al. Use of C-reactive protein after spinal surgery: comparison with erythrocyte sedimentation rate as predictor of early postoperative infectious complications. Spine (Phila Pa 1976). 2008;33:415-21.
36. Chung YG, Won YS, Kwon YJ, et al. Comparison of Serum CRP and Procalcitonin in Patients after Spine Surgery. J Korean Neurosurg Soc. 2011;49:43-8.
37. O'Daly BJ, Morris SF, O'Rourke SK. Long-term functional outcome in pyogenic spinal infection. Spine (Phila Pa 1976). 2008;33:E246-53.
38. Abdul-Jabbar A, Berven SH, Hu SS, et al. Surgical site infections in spine surgery: identification of microbiologic and surgical characteristics in 239 cases. Spine (Phila Pa 1976). 2013;38:E1425-31.
39. Rothman SL. The diagnosis of infections of the spine by modern imaging techniques. Orthop Clin North Am. 1996;27:15-31.
40. Inanami H, Oshima Y, Iwahori T, et al. Role of 18F-fluoro-D-deoxyglucose PET/CT in diagnosing surgical site infection after spine surgery with instrumentation. Spine (Phila Pa 1976). 2015;40:109-13.
41. Kim SJ, Kim IJ, Suh KT, et al. Prediction of residual disease of spine infection using F-18 FDG PET/CT. Spine (Phila Pa 1976). 2009;34:2424-30.
42. Chang SD, Lee MJ, Munk PL, et al. MRI of spinal hardware: comparison of conventional T1-weighted sequence with a new metal artifact reduction sequence. Skeletal Radiol. 2001;30:213-8.
43. Horan TC, Gaynes RP, Martone WJ, et al. CDC definitions of nosocomial surgical site infections, 1992: a modification of CDC definitions of surgical wound infections. Infect Control Hosp Epidemiol. 1992;13:606-8.
44. Thalgott JS, Cotler HB, Sasso RC, et al. Postoperative infections in spinal implants. Classification and analysis--a multicenter study. Spine (Phila Pa 1976). 1991;16:981-4.
45. Dobzyniak MA, Fischgrund JS, Hankins S, et al. Single versus multiple dose antibiotic prophylaxis in lumbar disc surgery. Spine (Phila Pa 1976). 2003;28:E453-5.
46. Boscardin JB, Ringus JC, Feingold DJ, et al. Human intradiscal levels with cefazolin. Spine (Phila Pa 1976). 1992;17:S145-8.
47. Cheng MT, Chang MC, Wang ST, et al. Efficacy of dilute betadine solution irrigation in the prevention of postoperative infection of spinal surgery. Spine (Phila Pa 1976). 2005;30:1689-93.
48. Bible JE, O'Neill KR, Crosby CG, et al. Microscope sterility during spine surgery. Spine (Phila Pa 1976). 2012;37:623-7.
49. Erichsen Andersson A, Petzold M, Bergh I, et al. Comparison between mixed and laminar airflow systems in operating rooms and the influence of human factors: experiences from a Swedish orthopedic center. Am J Infect Control. 2014;42:665-9.
50. Duarte RM, Vaccaro AR. Spinal infection: state of the art and management algorithm. Eur Spine J. 2013;22:2787-99.
51. Hong HS, Chang MC, Liu CL, et al. Is aggressive surgery necessary for acute postoperative deep spinal wound infection? Spine (Phila Pa 1976). 2008;33:2473-8.
52. Carragee EJ. Pyogenic vertebral osteomyelitis. J Bone Joint Surg Am. 1997;79:874-80.
53. Ito M, Abumi K, Kotani Y, et al. Clinical outcome of posterolateral endoscopic surgery for pyogenic spondylodiscitis: results of 15 patients with serious comorbid conditions. Spine (Phila Pa 1976). 2007;32:200-6.
54. Perry JW, Montgomerie JZ, Swank S, et al. Wound infections following spinal fusion with posterior segmental spinal instrumentation. Clinical Infectious Diseases. 1997;24:558-61.
55. Hedequist D, Haugen A, Hresko T, et al. Failure of Attempted Implant Retention in Spinal Deformity Delayed Surgical Site Infections. Spine. 2009;34:60-4.
56. Kanayama M, Hashimoto T, Shigenobu K, et al. MRI-based Decision-making of Implant Removal in Deep Wound Infection After Instrumented Lumbar Fusion. Clin Spine Surg. 2016.
57. Kowalski TJ, Berbari EF, Huddleston PM, et al. The management and outcome of spinal implant infections: Contemporary retrospective cohort study. Clinical Infectious Diseases. 2007;44:913-20.
58. Ahmed R, Greenlee JDW, Traynelis VC. Preservation of Spinal Instrumentation After Development of Postoperative Bacterial Infections in Patients Undergoing Spinal Arthrodesis. Journal of Spinal Disorders & Techniques. 2012;25:299-302.
59. Onen MR, Yuvruk E, Karagoz G, et al. Efficiency of Hyperbaric Oxygen Therapy in Iatrogenic Spinal Infections. Spine (Phila Pa 1976). 2015;40:1743-8.
60. Rohmiller MT, Akbarnia BA, Raiszadeh K, et al. Closed suction irrigation for the treatment of postoperative wound infections following posterior spinal fusion and instrumentation. Spine (Phila Pa 1976). 2010;35:642-6.
61. Mehbod AA, Ogilvie JW, Pinto MR, et al. Postoperative deep wound infections in adults after spinal fusion: management with vacuum-assisted wound closure. J Spinal Disord Tech. 2005;18:14-7.
62. Canavese F, Gupta S, Krajbich JI, et al. Vacuum-assisted closure for deep infection after spinal instrumentation for scoliosis. J Bone Joint Surg Br. 2008;90:377-81.
63. Liu C, Bayer A, Cosgrove SE, et al. Clinical practice guidelines by the infectious diseases society of america for the treatment of methicillin-resistant Staphylococcus aureus infections in adults and children: executive summary. Clin Infect Dis. 2011;52:285-92.

5

SECTION

Tumors, Infections and Osteoporosis

Section Outline

28
CHAPTER

Vertebroplasty and Vesselplasty

Arvind Bhave

ABSTRACT

Osteoporotic vertebral compression fractures are one of the most common fractures in elderly which results in disability affecting the quality of life and morbidity. In cases of failed conservative treatment and with persistence of back pain , minimally invasive techniques like vertebroplasty and vesselplasty has got a definitive role. The ease of the procedure and promising results of lesser complications, faster rehabilitation in elderly are all the major advantages of these two techniques.

VERTEBROPLASTY

INTRODUCTION

Vertebral compression fractures is most common complic-ations of osteoporosis. It causes progressive pain, deformity, disability finally affecting the quality of life and morbidity.[1,2] The quality of life is further affected by increased pain leading to depression, subsequent fractures resulting in much more disability and loss of social life.[2] Standard conservative treatment consists of analgesics, bed rest, and use of braces. It temporarily reduces pains, but dependence of drugs and narcotics progressively increases. Also lying in bed causes further bone loss, and kyphotic deformity leading to substantial limitation of activities of life. Surgical treatment is mostly considered in cases of neurological deficits, it has its own problems of extensive surgery, morbidity and implant loosening.[3]

Vertebroplasty is currently accepted minimally invasive treatment of stabilizing the fractured vertebra with Cementing material usually methyl methacrylate cement (PMMA). It was initially done in France and published in 1987 for hemangioma.[4] Later on, it was widely popularized in United States.[5-8] Vertebroplasty is a very good surgical choice for patients with vertebral compression fractures, as it eliminates the risk of major spinal surgery, and through prompt pain relief, may provide early mobilization and rehabilitation for elderly multimorbid patients.

DIAGNOSIS

Fractures by Imaging for Identification of Symptomatic

Xrays of Spine: AP/Lateral Views in the Affected Region

Plain radiographs: Preferable in standing position will give more information in addition to than the routine. X-rays in AP and Lateral views. Thoracolumbar fractures are easily diagnosed but sacral fractures may require CT scans.

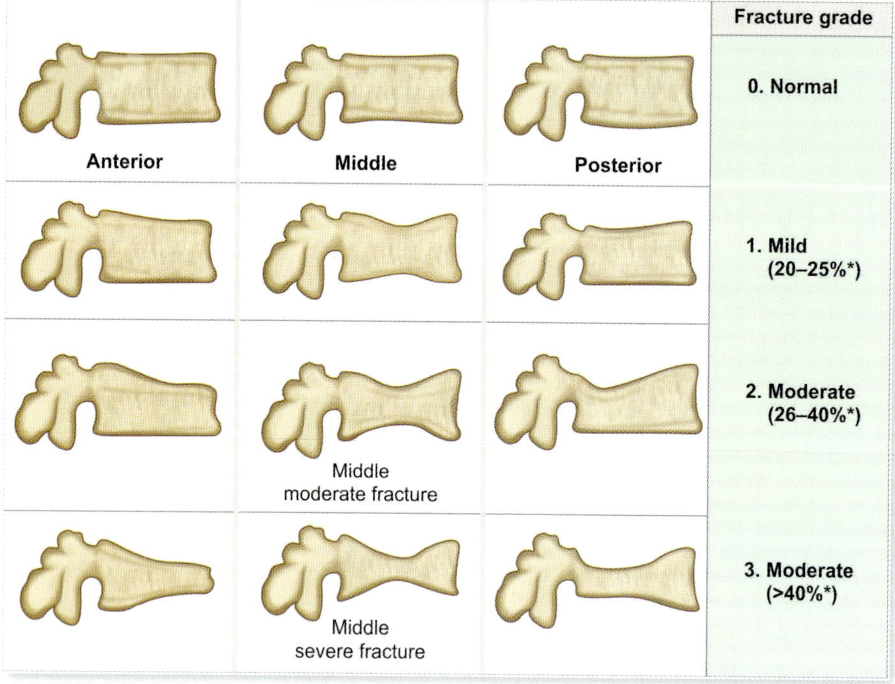

Figure 1: Classification of vertebral compression fractures

X-rays will show:

a. Extent of the vertebral collapse, location and extent of the fractures.
b. The posterior cortical collapse will be evident by increase in bipedicular distance. Another thing to look for is 50% or more compression of the posterior wall.

CT Scans and 3D Reconstruction

CT scan gives information about the intactness of the posterior cortex of the vertebral body. The CT scanning with 3D, sagittal and coronal reconstructions are helpful in assessing the complex vertebral fractures **(Figure 1)**. Thin reconstructed sections show the fracture and the integrity of the posterior vertebral wall Intact posterior verterbal wall, is favorable condition for vertebroplasty.

Magnetic Resonance Imaging modality of choice is MRI of spine as it is highly sensitive. Increased signals in T2 sequence shows acute fracture because of bone edema. Increased signal T1 STIR T2 enhanced signals is mostly diagnostic of acute vertebral fracture.[9] Avascular necrosis is seen in chronic unhealing fractures, characterized by 'double line sign' as areas of discrete fluid collections within the vacuum with reduced areas of signals on T2 scans **(Figure 2)**.

STIR sequence is the most sensitive in bone marrow edema due to trauma or inflammation.

High intensity signal on STIR MRI has been shown 100% association with OVCF correction predictor for the vertebral body fracture correction.

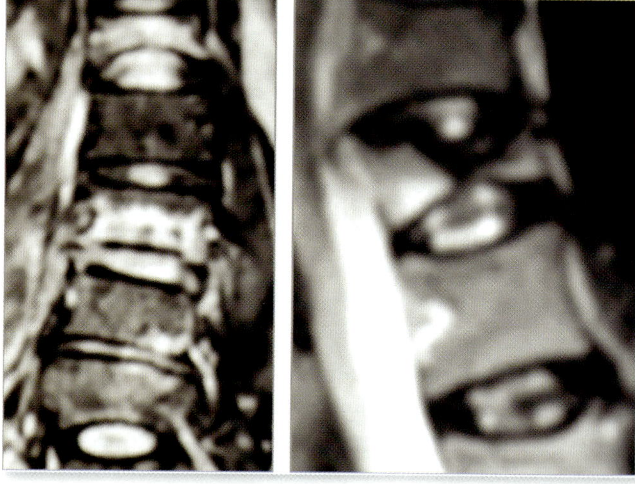

Figure 2: Unhealing fracture

Duration of Pain Prior to Vertebroplasty

The indications from the Consensus Guidelines for Vertebroplasty developed by the Standards of Practice Committee of the Society of Interventional Radiology are:

1. Painful primary and secondary osteoporotic vertebral compression fractures refractory to medical therapy.
2. Painful vertebrae with extensive osteolysis or invasion secondary to benign or malignant tumors.
3. Painful vertebral fracture associated with osteonecrosis.[10]

Contraindications to Vertebroplasty

1. Unmanageable bleeding disorder.
2. Improvement of symptoms with conservative management.
3. Asymptomatic vertebral body fracture.
4. Local or generalized infection.
5. Allergy to bone cement, and
6. Tumor mass with involvement of the spinal canal.[11]

*Retropulsion of a fragment into the spinal canal is no longer considered a contraindication if no neurologic sign exists before surgery.[12,13] The risk of nerve compression and cement leakage is theoretically higher. Only a skillful and experienced surgeon should perform a vertebroplasty on these patients.

PHYSICAL EXAMINATION

Patient having back pains, paraspinal tenderness makes one strongly suspect fracture [#]. Localized bony tenderness over the spinous process is the characteristic clinical significance of the vertebral pathology. Additional kyphosis may indicate severity of the collapse.

Neurological examination of sensory, motor system and reflexes need to be accessed to rule out neurogical deficit. Vertebroplasty alone without decompression is contraindicated in case of neurological deficit.

TECHNICAL CONSIDERATIONS: IMAGE-GUIDED APPROACH

The most important factor in achieving a low incidence of complications, is visualization of needle insertion and bone cement injection.[14] Vertebroplasty can be performed by single-plane or biplanar fluoroscopy. Monitoring cement distribution under direct fluoroscopic control is crucial to detect leakage. If cement leakage occurs, the procedure should be immediately stopped. Some clinicians have advocated the use of CT to reduce the operative time and facilitate accurate visualization of the needle position and bone cement distribution.[15]

Vertebroplasty Technique: Vertebroplasty with PMMA

Anesthesia: General Anesthesia Versus Local Anesthesia

Vertebroplasty can be performed under local anesthesia.[16] It is particularly useful in patients with risks for general anesthesia. However, some surgeons prefer general anesthesia so that the surgery will cause less stress and pain for the patients.

Postural reduction: Postural reduction, which is done by placing the patient in the prone position with support at the chest and pelvis, can help restore the vertebral height of fractured vertebra. Closed reduction of the fractured and kyphotic spine can be achieved by extending the table to restore the kyphotic angle and vertebral body height.[17]

Uni/bipedicular approach: mostly it is surgeons preference. There is no difference of result with uni- or bipedicular Vertebroplasty. In case of vertebral osteonecrosis with intraosseous vacuum clefts, such as Kummel's disease, percutaneous vertebroplasty can be done successfully via a single pedicle approach.[18]

Venogram: Some clinicians advocate the use of venography to evaluate the vertebral venous system before cement injection to identify potential routes of bone cement extravasations into the vein, but its effectiveness is still debated.[19-21]

Material: The high-viscosity PMMA system is safe and effective for clinical use, allowing a significant reduction of the extravasation rate and, thus, leakage-related complications.[22] For both short and intermediate time periods, the injection of absorbable calcium phosphate cement has shown to be an effective method to treat large vertebral defects. Early results indicate that calcium phosphate remodeling might result in the resorption of the majority of the cement with replacement by lamellar bone. However, some clinicians have warned about the risk of early collapse after injection of absorbable cement. Lewis et al. reported that bioactive glass is compatible with PMMA bone cement in terms of axial compressive strength.[23,24] A biomechanical study showed that about 3.5 cm of PMMA largely restored normal stress distributions to fractured and adjacent vertebral bodies.

Injection Devices

Many devices for doing vertebroplasty are available. The author has devised a device termed 'AB needle'.[25,26] **(Figure 3)**.

Advantages of the Needle Assembly

1. The design of the Vertebroplasty needle in such a way that gives better spreadability of the cementing materials through multiple portals **(Figure 4)**.
2. It possesses a unique locking system at the neck of the vertebroplasty needle, which prohibits or restricts the movement of the vertebroplasty needle while hammering it, at the time of operation. The Luer locking knob of the stylet and groove in it aligns the direction of the flanged tip of the needle; deep inside the body at the time of surgery.
3. The vertebroplasty needle that possesses a unique system at the proximal end, which can accept any syringe or cement delivery system available for the delivery of the cementing material.

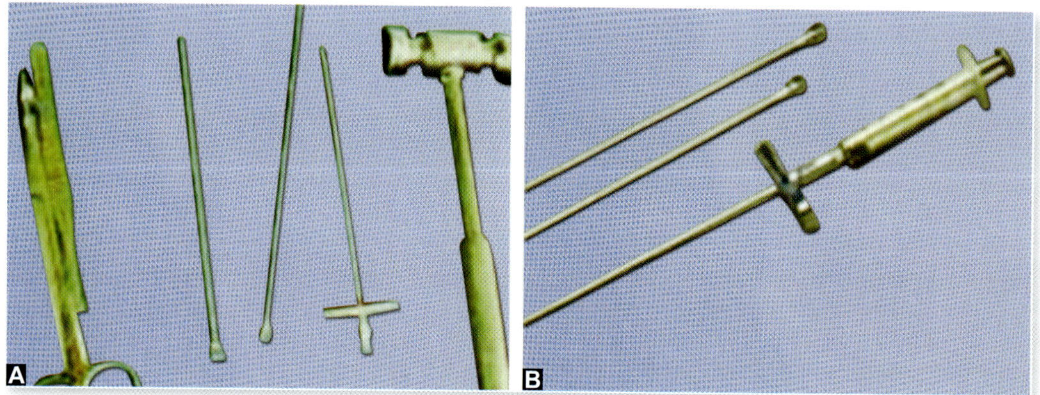

Figure 3: (A) Assembly of 'AB needle' for vertebroplasty; (B) Other instruments required for vertebroplasty

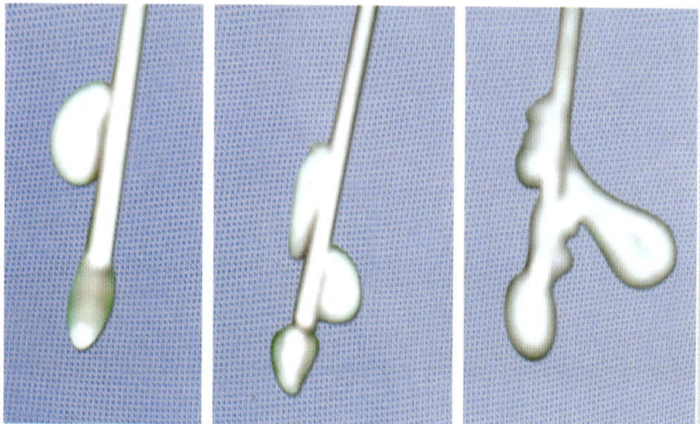

Figure 4: Use of multiple channels for proper multidirectional delivery of the cement

The multiple channels of the needle are important for 360 degrees filling of the bone cement in a cavity, rather than only in unidirectional way, as in any other needle.

If one channel gets blocked the other channels may work for you, one need not change the needle or terminate the procedure.

Other devices for doing vertebroplasty: Many companies have come out with devices having long connecting tubings connecting to cement mixing chamber. The major advantage of it is the operator can stand away from the X-ray exposure. Major disadvantage of these systems is the operator has less control over the cement which has already escaped into the delivery tubes and in the vertebroplasty needle. Hence, if the operator identifies a cement leak then it is difficult to control it, as the cement in the tube is more liquid than directly injecting in the vertebroplasty needle.

Most Important Commandments to Do Vertebroplasty

1. Must be trained surgeon. They should know when to stop injection the cement and in case of cement leak how to deal with it.
2. Should use good imaging equipment, continuous monitoring while injecting cement is must .
3. Must have proper indication for the procedure.

COMPLICATIONS OF VERTEBROPLASTY[27-44]

Neurological injury due to compression: Neurological complications can occur because of cement leakage into the spinal canal and less exceptionally into the intervertebral foramen[27] The incidence of cement extravasation is up to 40%, however major adverse events occur in less than 1% of patients.[17]

Thermal injury: Thermal damage to the intraosseous neural tissue caused by cement polymerization cannot be ruled out as a potential mechanism for pain relief after vertebroplasty.[28,41] In addition, an exothermic reaction from the bone cement may cause thermal damage to surrounding tissue.[29,42]

Embolism: Clinical studies have shown extravasation of bone cement into the vena cava,[30,43] lung,[31,44] heart, and kidney.[32] Rarely, cement leakage into the paravertebral venous system may result in embolization of particles into the right cardiac chambers and pulmonary artery.[9] One systematic literature search revealed that the risk of a pulmonary embolism ranged from 3.5% to 23% for osteoporotic fractures.[33]

Adjacent fracture and refracture: An increased fracture rate has been observed in adjacent vertebrae after vertebroplasty. Decreased failure strength has been noted in a laboratory study of augmented functional spine units where the adjacent,non-augmented vertebral body always failed.[34] This may provide evidence that rigid cement augmentation may facilitate the subsequent collapse of adjacent vertebrae. In one study, new fractures occurred in 18.9% of 106 patients at 22 adjacent vertebral bodies after percutaneous vertebroplasty during at least 24 months of follow-up.[35] Refractures of cemented vertebrae after Vertebroplasty occur in up to 63% of osteoporotic patients.[36]

Outcomes

Hulme et al.[37] conducted a systematic literature review to evaluate the safety and efficacy of kyphoplasty and vertebroplasty in terms of pain relief,restoration of vertebral body height, complications and incidence of new adjacent vertebral fractures. Effective pain relief was achieved in 87% of patients with Vertebroplasty. Cement leakage was found 41% and 9% of patients with vertebroplasty and kyphoplasty, respectively.

Risk of Subsequent Fracture

Long-term Follow-up of Cement: An increased fracture rate has been observed in adjacent vertebrae after vertebroplasty. Decreased failure strength has been noted in a laboratory study of augmented functional spine units where the adjacent, non-augmented vertebral body always failed. This may provide evidence that rigid cement augmentation may facilitate the subsequent collapse of adjacent vertebrae. In one study, new fractures occurred in 18.9% of 106 patients at 22 adjacent vertebral bodies after percutaneous vertebroplasty during at least 24 months of follow-up.[38-40] Bone cement leakage into the intervertebral disc may cause adjacent vertebral fractures. One study showed that patients with acute or subacute vertebral fractures who underwent vertebroplasty experienced more and earlier new fractures than those who did not, but the observed differences failed to reach statistical significance.[41] Refractures of cemented vertebrae after vertebroplasty occur in up to 63% of osteoporotic patients.[36] Significant anterior vertebral height restoration increases the risk of subsequent fracture in cemented vertebrae. Successful treatment of painful refractures can be achieved by repeating the vertebroplasty. Vertebroplasty with low viscocity cement is found to have more leakage problems.[42] In most of the studies on vertebroplasty showed cement leakage from 2% to 67%.

OUTCOMES MEASURES

Vertebroplasty can improve quality of life and physical activity, because pain can be relieved significantly, which reduces the demand for analgesics. Mechanical stabilization of fractured vertebra and thermal necrosis of nerve endings are the main reasons for postoperative pain relief. Even though vertebroplasty has a low incidence of complications, some potentially serious squeal should be discussed with patients and their families before surgery.

CASE STUDIES

Case 1: 68 years male X-ray showing # L1 of 4 months duration **(Figures 5 to 8)**

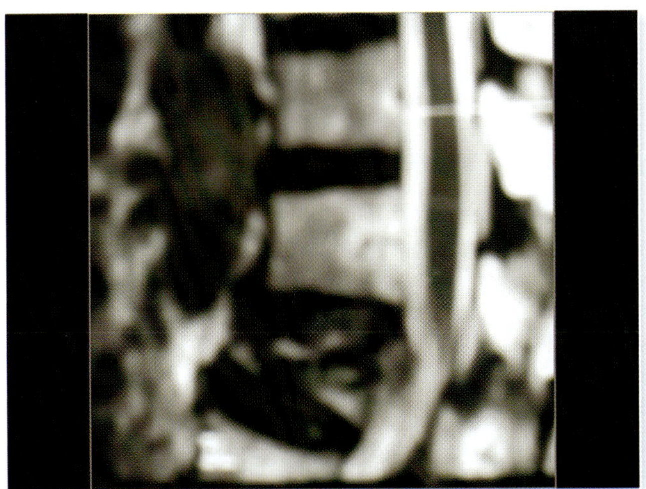

Figure 5: X-ray shows L1 fracture

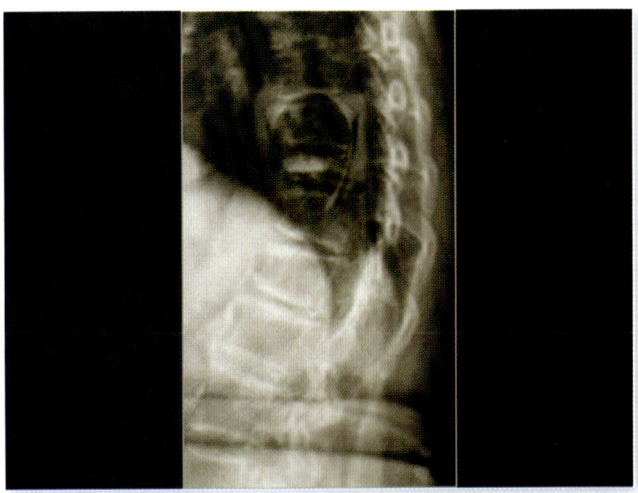

Figure 6: X-ray (lateral view)

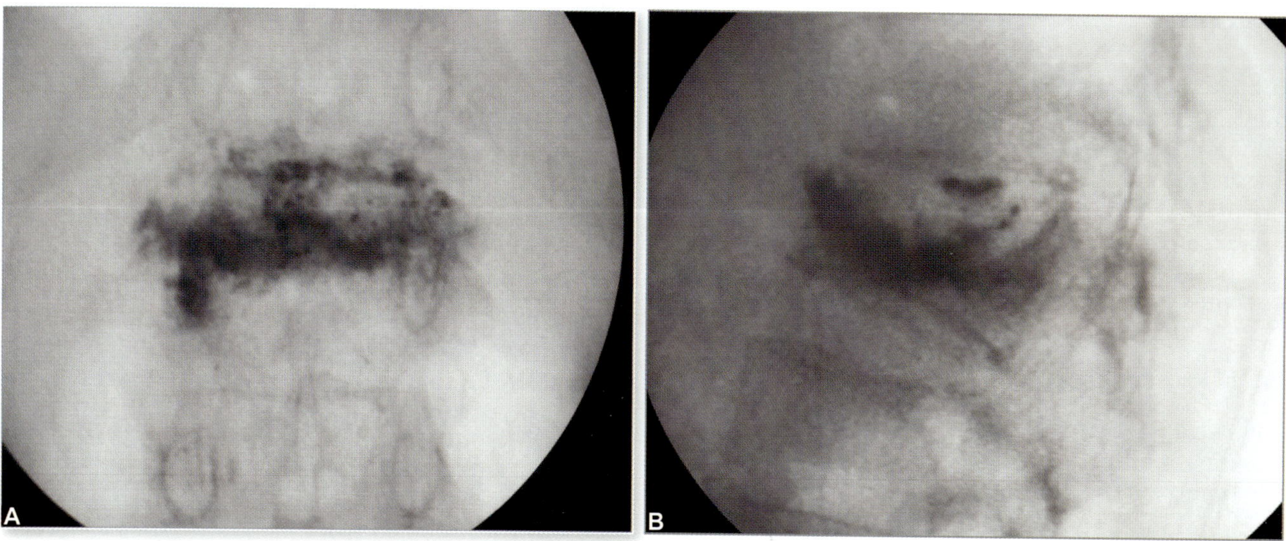

Figure 7: Intraoperative C-arm picture at the end of surgery

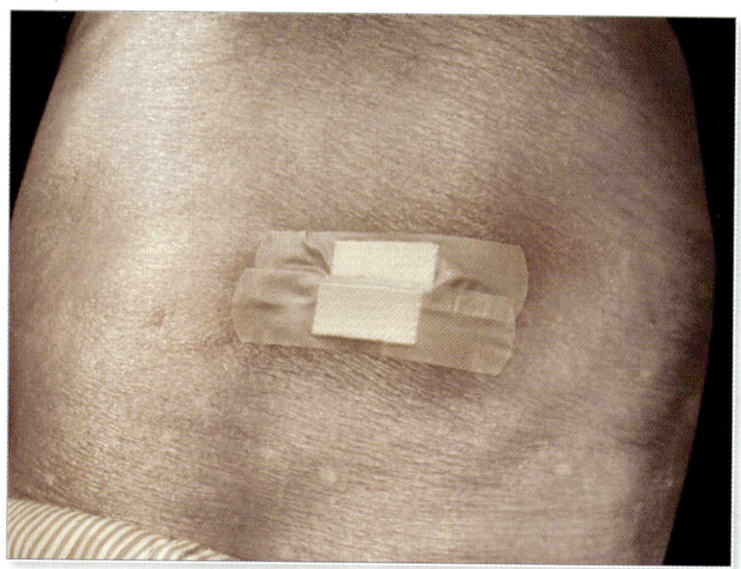

Figure 8: Band aid dressing

Case 2: 68 years male with lymphoma—painful pathological # L2 **(Figures 9 to 12)**

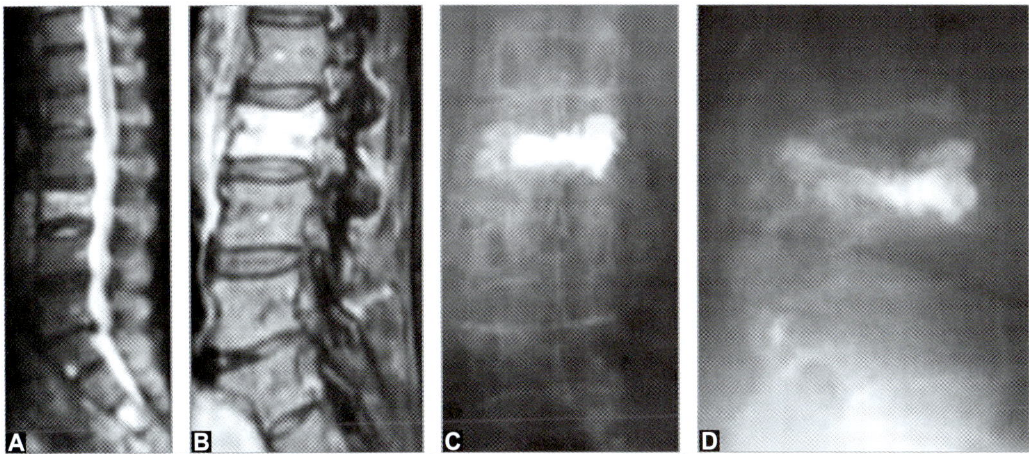

Figure 9: Painful pathological L2 fracture

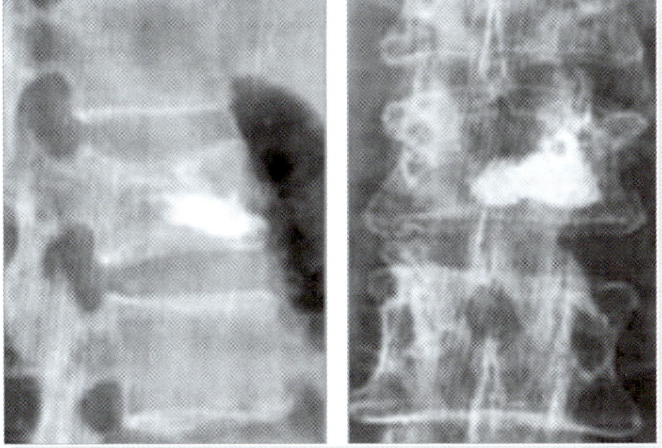

Figure 10: 9-months post-PVP

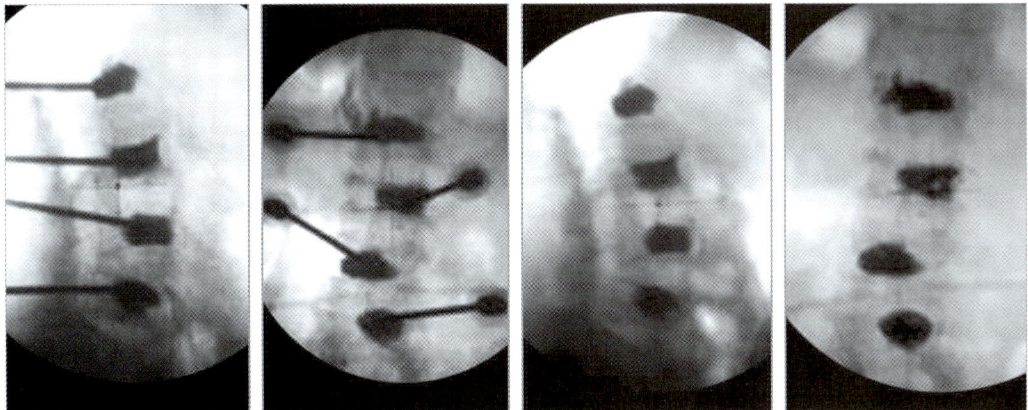

Figure 11: Multilevel vertebroplasty: Intraoperative and postoperative 'C' arm pictures

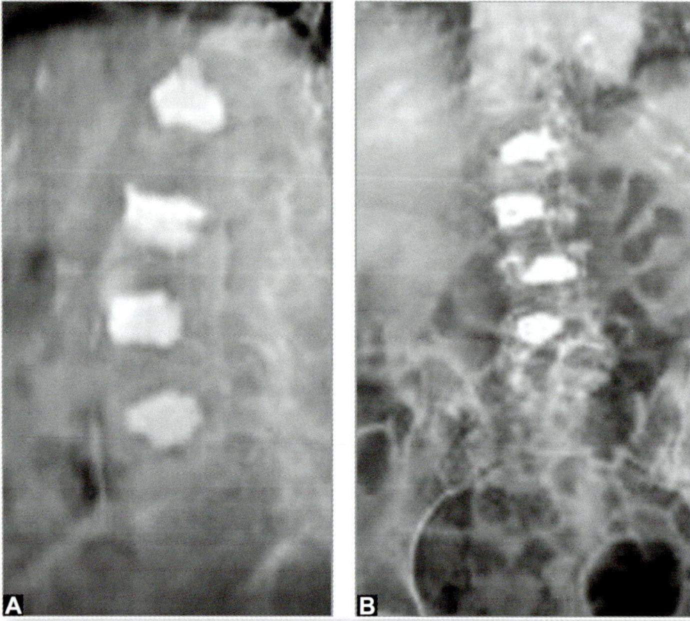

Figure 12: Postoperative 6 months follow-up X-rays: (A) AP view; (B) Lateral view

VESSELPLASTY

INTRODUCTION

Vesselplasty is a new intriguing alternative to vertebroplasty and kyphoplasty.

It was devised to obtain:

1. Control of the volume of void created in the vertebral body,
2. Prevent the leakage of bone filler material,
3. Restore vertebral body height.

Designed by Jerry Lin, the chairman of A-Spine Holding Group Corporation (Taipei, Taiwan), Vesselplasty was first performed in 2004 by Darwono.[43] Instead of using a balloon to create a cavity, vesselplasty uses a polyethylene terephthalate (PET) balloon container (Vessel-X, A-Spine Holding Group Corporation) to restore the height of the vertebral body. This receptacle serves as both a vertebral body expander and a bone cement container. It is introduced into the vertebra in its reduced configuration and, once positioned within the vertebra, is expanded by the injection of PMMA. Then, owing to the porous structure comprising the fibers of the PET vessel, a small amount of bone cement permeates through its wall and interdigitates within the vertebral body to increase its stability. Theoretically, this technique solves the problem of leakage of cement from the vertebral body because most of the cement is contained by the expandable artificial vessel, providing a safe method to treat VCFs. The incidence of cement extrusion with kyphoplasty is 8.6–33%.[1,44] Vesselplasty adds to this advantage by controlling cement extrusion through the utilization of the PET artificial vessel.

PROCEDURE

Vesselplasty procedures were performed at our institution using the Vessel-X Bone Filling Container System (A-Spine Holding Group Corporation) with CE mark (certifying product has met European Union consumer requirements) and current good manufacturing practice approval. The system consists of the following items **(Figure 13)**: bone access needle (10-gauge), composed of a cannula tube and stylet, used for initial access into the vertebra; precision drill, used to create a working channel; controllable cement delivery system with an extension tube, available to deliver the high-viscosity cement; and vessel-X bone filling container. The last item comprised a Vessel-X introducer (with a bone filling container, the PET container) and a pushing rod. The vessel-X introducer, available in two diameters (20 or 25 mm) depending on vertebral body size, is used for the injection and containment of bone cement within the created void. The pushing rod serves as a fluoroscopic reference of the tip of the vessel and gives stability to the PET container during introduction in the vertebral body; it also avoids the leakage through the cannula and introducer throughout the cement injection.

The bone cement used was PMMA.

The procedures were performed in a consistent manner each patient was placed in the prone position on a routine radiolucent top operation table for the procedure, which we describe in eight steps:

First: The fractured vertebral body was localized under fluoroscopic control in both the anteroposterior and lateral planes. The pedicle was isolated on the lateral plane for positioning in the cranio-caudal plane and anteroposterior oblique plane for a lateral to medial approach.

Second: Conscious sedation (IV fentanyl and midazolam) and local anesthetic in the skin over the pedicle (0.25% bupivacaine) were administered to the patient. A small skin incision was made, and the bone access needle (10-gauge needle with an inner stylet) was advanced into the fractured vertebral body creating a path through the pedicle **(Figure 14A)**. The bone access needle was halted 2–3 mm anterior to the posterior wall of the vertebral body. This transpedicular approach, which was either uni- or bipedicular, was empirically chosen to avoid the risk of leakage outside the

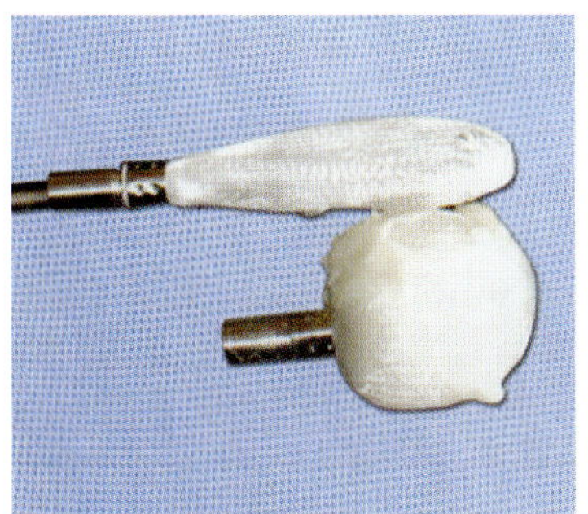
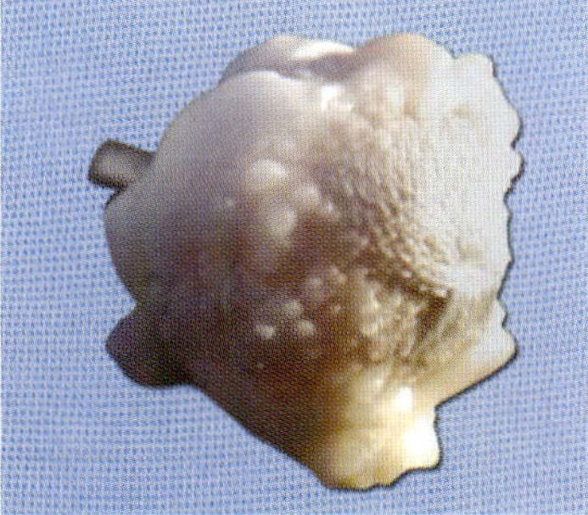
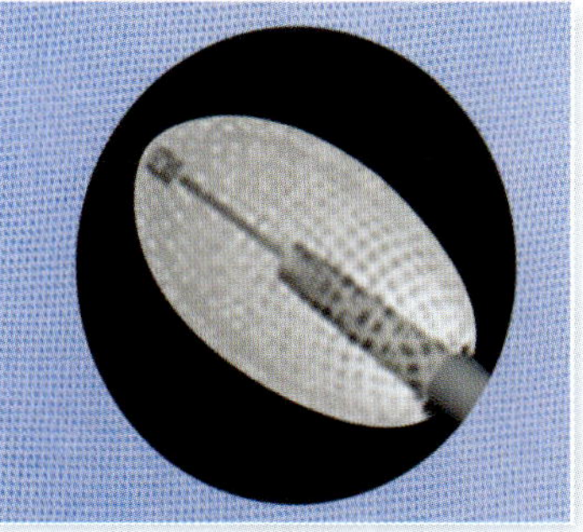

Figure 13: Instrumentation in vesseplasty

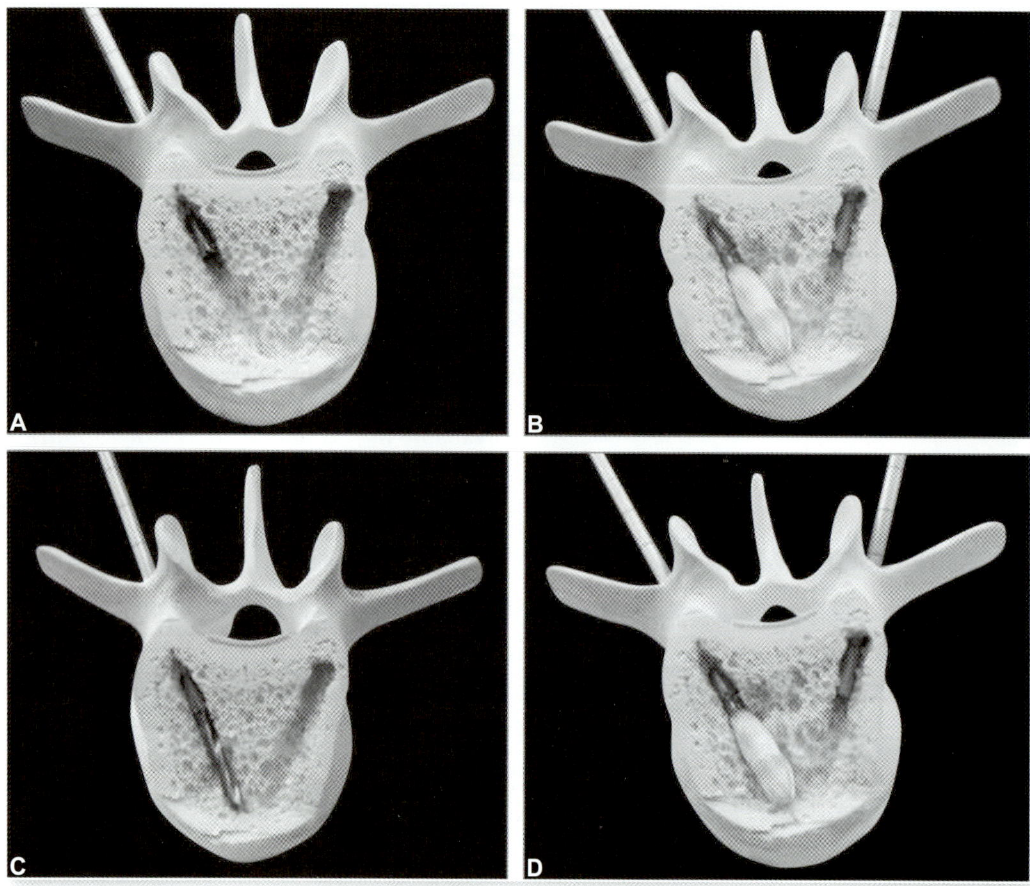

Figures 14A to D: Vesselplasty procedure using vessel-X bone filling container system. (Courtesy: A-Spine Holding Group Corporation). (A) Bone access needle is introduced through pedicle, retaining it 2–3 mm anterior to posterior wall of vertebra body; (B) Precision drill is introduced through cannula tube until tip of drill is positioned 2–3 mm posterior to anterior wall of vertebra; (C) Precision drill is removed, and vessel-X bone filling container (balloon catheter) is inserted into cannula tube; (D) Controlled cement extrusion. Process is repeated through contralateral pedicle

vertebral body throughout the needle tract. Although a unipedicular approach does require a more oblique route, it was used because correct expansion of the vertebral body can be achieved with the placement of the needle tip in a middle position. Due to technical characteristics of the equipment used, a left transpedicular approach was selected.

An alternative approach is the parapedicular route, which is most often used to access the thoracic spine. The parapedicular route involves inserting the needle between the lateral margin of the pedicle and the head of the rib.

Third: The stylet was then removed, leaving the cannula tube in the vertebral body.

Fourth: The precision drill was introduced into the vertebral body through the cannula tube forging a path through the pedicle until the tip of the drill was 2-3 mm posterior to the anterior wall of the vertebra **(Figure 14B)**.

Fifth: The precision drill was removed.

Sixth: The vessel-X bone filling container was next inserted into the cannula tube and the introducer sheath was firmly pushed, lodging it 2-3 mm posterior to the anterior wall **(Figure 14C)**.

Seventh: The cement delivery system was connected, and the bone cement was progressively filled in. Injection of PMMA was performed under fluoroscopic guidance and continued until maximal expansion of the PET vessel (20 or 25 mm) was achieved, no more material could be injected, or extravasation was noted. Controlled-cement extrusion through the walls of the vessel X for interdigitation with the bone marrow is seen with injection of additional cementing material **(Figure 14D)**.

Eighth: The Vessel-X introducer and the pushing rod were then removed, followed by the cannula tube. Once these elements had been removed, the posterior opening of the PET container was mostly sealed because of the cement's short solidification time.

At the end of the procedure, IV methyl prednisolone (1 mg/kg) was administered empirically to all patients to reduce the local inflammatory response associated with the procedure. After a 24-hour hospital stay, all patients were discherged from the hospital.

CASE STUDIES

Case 1: 75-year-female patient suffering from # spine D12 treated conservatively with rest, brace, NSAIDs. She developed renal and hepatic failure for 3 months. Pains increased, resulting in severe pains at rest. X-rays showed further collapse of the vertebral body. She was subjected to vesselplasty and had good pain relief immediately after surgery and mobilized on the same day **(Figures 15 to 24)**.

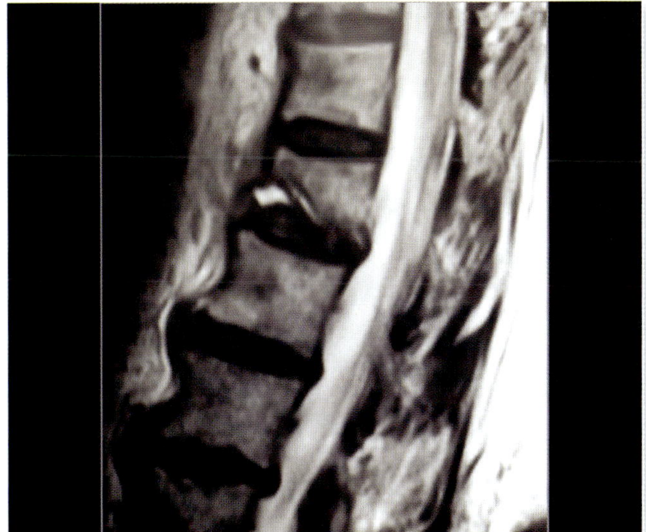

Figure 15: MRI showing compression # D12

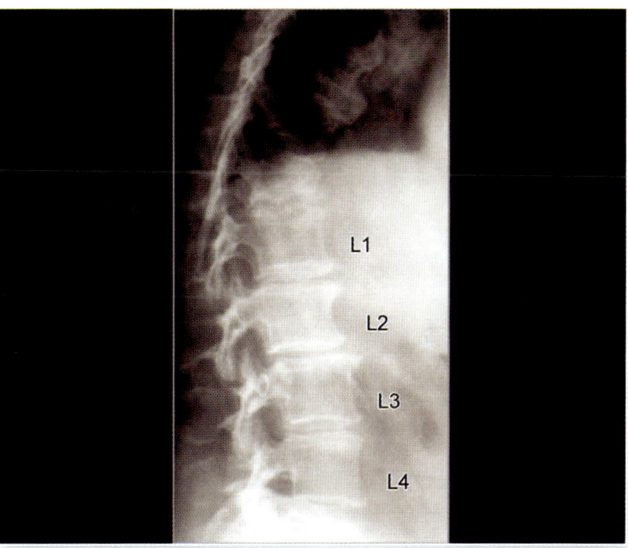

Figure 16: Standing X-rays T-L spine lateral view showing further collapse of D12 vertebra

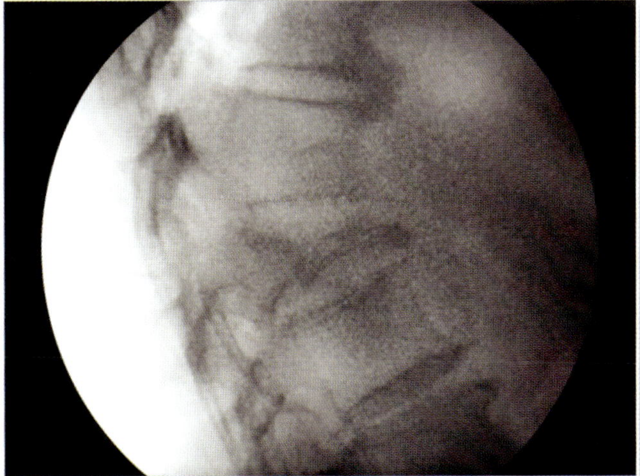

Figure 17: 'C' arm picture showing collapse and kyphotic deformity at the beginning of the procedure

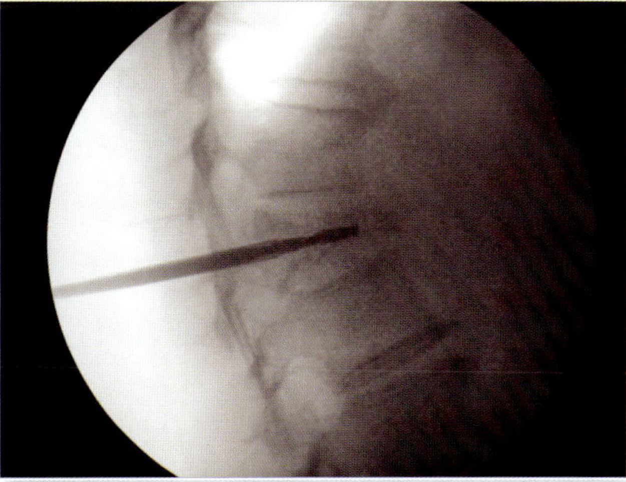

Figure 18: Insertion of bone biopsy needle and bone drill

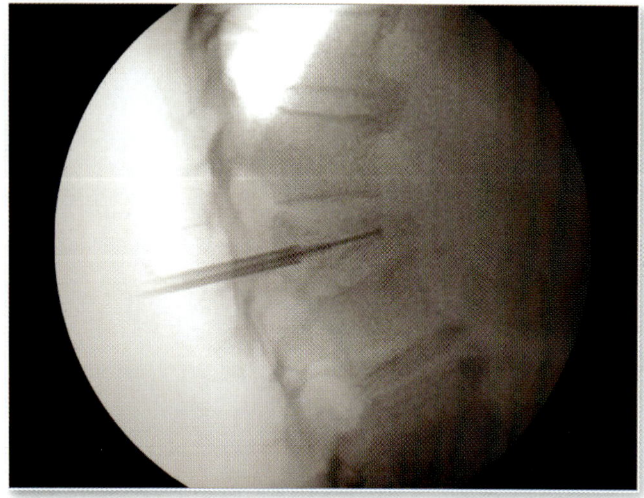

Figure 19: Insertion of the 'vessel X' implant

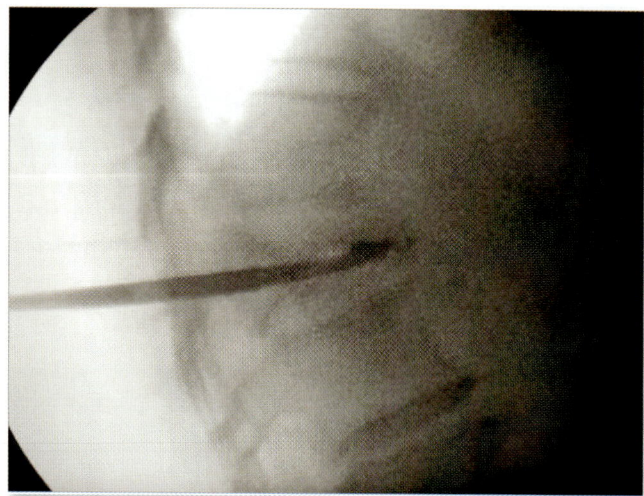

Figure 20: Bone filler material/cement injection and opening up of the implant

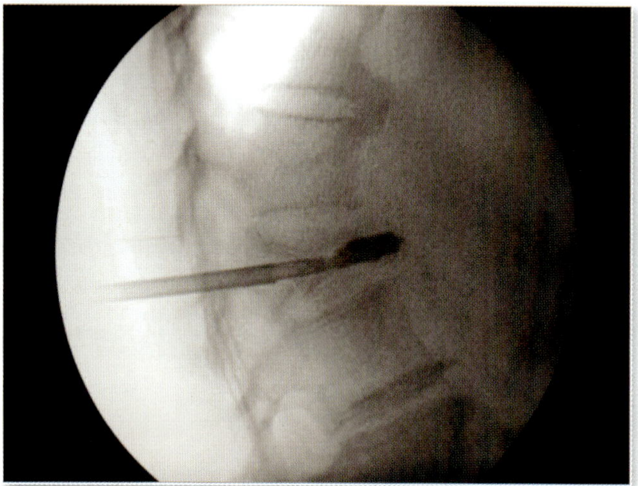

Figure 21: Implant opening up

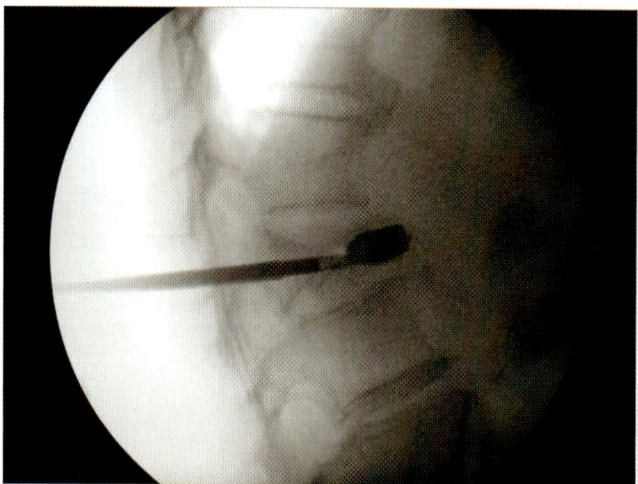

Figure 22: Kyphosis getting corrected

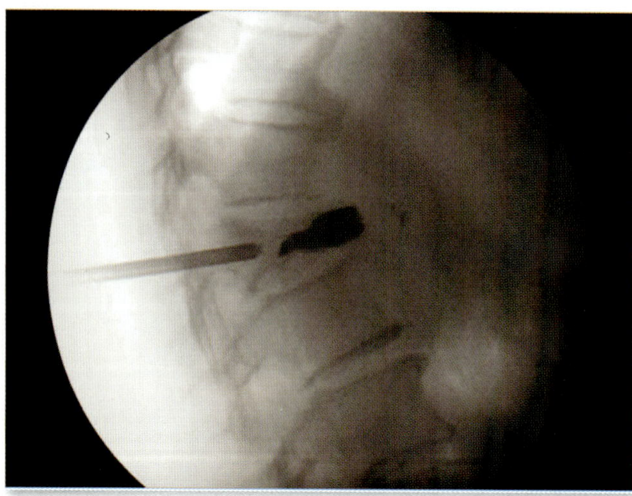

Figure 23: Implant detached

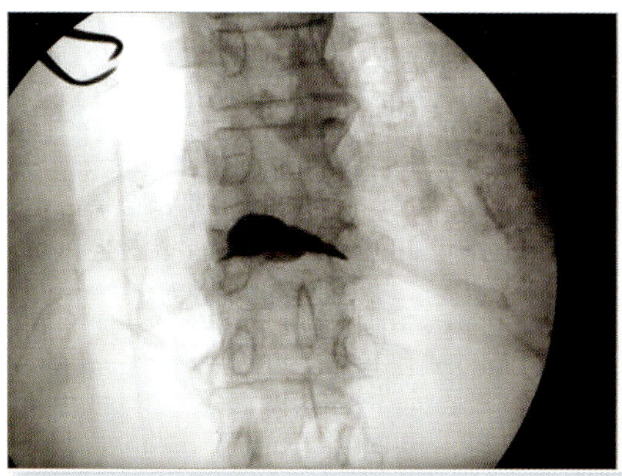
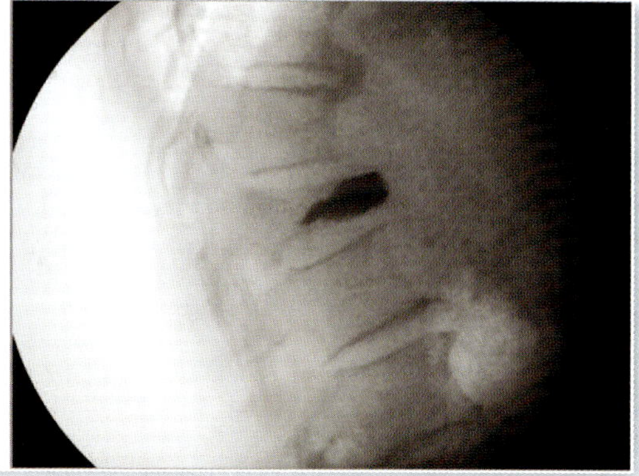

Figure 24: Final position in AP/lateral views of implant with cement interdigitation with vertebral marrow

REFERENCES

1. Silvarmann SL. The clinical consequences of vertebral compression fracture. Bone. 1992;13:27-31.
2. Gold DT. The clinical impact of vertebral fractures: quality of life in women with osteoporosis. Bone. 1996;18:185S-9S.
3. Dickman CA FR, MacMillan M, Haid RW. Transpedicular screw-rod fixation of the lumbar spine: operative technique and outcome in 104 cases. J Neurosurg. 1992;77:860-70.
4. Galibert P, Rosat P, Le Gars D. Preliminary note on the treatment of vertebral angioma by percutaneous acrylic vertebroplasty. Neurochirurgie. 1987;33:166-8.
5. Yu SW, Kao YH, Yen CY, et al. Clinical evaluation of vertebroplasty for multiple-level osteoporotic spinal compression fracture in the elderly. Arch Orthop Trauma Surg. 2008;128:97-101.
6. Zampini JM, McGuire KJ. Comparison of 5766 vertebral compression fractures treated with or without kyphoplasty. Clin Orthop Relat Res. 2010;468:1773-80.
7. Zoarski GH, Olan WJ, Stallmeyer MJB, Dick BW, Hebel JR, De Deyne M. Percutaneous vertebroplasty for osteoporotic compression fractures: quantitative prospective evaluation of long-term outcomes. J Vasc Interv Radiol. 2002;13:139-48.
8. Chen LH, Yu SW, Fu TS, et al. Minimally invasive treatment of osteoporotic vertebral compression fracture. Gung Med J. 2004;27:261-7.
9. Qaiyum M, McCall PN, Cassar-Pullicino IW, Germany VN. MRI detection of unsuspected vertebral injury in acute spinal trauma: incidence and significance. Skeletal Radiol. 2001;30:(6): 299-304.
10. McGraw JK, Barr JD, Mathis JM, Sanchez O, Schwartzberg MS, Swan et al. Society of Interventional Radiology quality improvement guidelines for percutaneous vertebroplasty. J Vasc Interv Radiol. 2003;14:827-31.
11. Denaro L, Denaro V. Vertebroplasty and kyphoplasty: reasons for concern? Orthop Clin North Am. 2009;40:465-71.
12. Chen JF. Percutaneous vertebroplasty for treatment of thoracolumbar spine bursting fracture. Surg Neurol. 2004;62::494-500.
13. Denaro L, Denaro V. Vertebroplasty and kyphoplasty: reasons for concern? Orthop Clin North Am. 2009(40):465-71.
14. Laredo JD HB. Complications of percutaneous vertebroplasty and their prevention. Skeletal Radiol. 2004;33:493-505.
15. Tam AL MA, Pfister M, Chinndurai P, Rohm E, Hall AF, Wallace MJ. C-arm cone beam computed tomography needle path overlay for fluoroscopic guided vertebroplasty. Spine. 2010;35:1095-9.
16. Gangi A, Imbert JP, Marin H, Dietemann JL. Percutaneous vertebroplasty: indications, technique, and results. Radiographics. 2003;23(10).
17. Lee ST. Closed reduction vertebroplasty for the treatment of osteoporotic vertebral compression fractures.Technical note. J Neurosurg. 2004;100:392-6.
18. Chen LH, Chen WJ. Unipedicle percutaneous vertebroplasty for spinal intraosseous vacuum cleft. Clin I Orthop Relat Res. 2005;435:148-53.
19. Mathis JM. Percutaneous vertebroplasty: complication avoidance and technique optimization. AJNR Am J Neuroradiol. 2003;24:1697-706.
20. Vasconcelos C, Guilloud P, Beauchamp NJ, et al. Is percutaneous vertebroplasty without pretreatment venography safe? Evaluation of 205 consecutives procedures. AJNR Am J Neuroradiol. 2002;23:913-7.
21. Deramond H, Depriester C, Galibert P, Le Gars D. Percutaneous vertebroplasty with polymethylmethacrylate.Technique, indications, and results. Radiol Clin North Am. 1998;36:533-46.
22. Anselmetti GC Zoarski G, Manca A, Masala S, Eminefendic H, Russo F, et al. Percutaneous Vertebroplasty and bone cement leakage: clinical experience with a new high-viscosity bone cement and delivery system for vertebral augmentation in benign and malignant compression fractures. Cardiovasc Intervent Radiol. 2008;31:937-47.

23. Turner TM, Singh K, Hall DJ, Renner SM, Lim TH, Tomlinson MJ, An HS. Vertebroplasty comparing injectable calcium phosphate cement compared with polymethylmethacrylate in a unique canine vertebral body large defect model. Spine J. 8:482-7.
24. Lewis G, Boyd D, German MJ, Wren AW,Clarkin OM, Yates A. Evaluation of two novel aluminumfree, zinc-based glass polyalkenoate cements as alternatives to PMMA bone cement for use in vertebroplasty and balloon kyphoplasty. J Mater Sci Mater Med. 2010;21:59-66.
25. Bhave A. Vertebroplasty for special situations. New Delhi: Jaypee Brothers Medical Publishers; 2008.
26. Bhave A. Vertebroplasty. New Delhi: Jaypee Brothers Medical Publishers; 2009.
27. Laredo JD. Complications of percutaneous vertebroplasty and their prevention. Skeletal Radiol 2004;33:493-505.
28. Lee BJ LS, Yoo TY. Paraplegia as a complication of percutaneous vertebroplasty with polymethylmethacrylate: a case report. Spine. 2002;27:419-22.
29. Deramond H, Belkoff S. Temperature elevation caused by bone cement polymerization during vertebroplasty. Bone 1999;25.
30. Kao FC, Lai PL, Yu SW, et al. Inferior vena cava syndrome following percutaneous Vertebroplasty with polymethylmethacrylate. Spine. 2008;33:329-33.
31. Kim YJ, Park KW, Yeom JS, Jeong HS, Park JM,Kang HS. Pulmonary cement embolism after percutaneous vertebroplasty in osteoporotic vertebral compression fractures: incidence, characteristics, and risk factors. Radiology. 2009;251:250-9.
32. Chung SE, Kim TH, Yoo KH, et al. Renal cement embolism during percutaneous vertebroplasty. Eur Spine J. 2006;15:590-4.
33. Caynak B, Sagbas E, Duran C, et al. Cardiac tamponade and pulmonary embolism as a complication of percutaneous vertebroplasty. Ann Thorac Surg. 2009;87:299-301.
34. Boger A, Windolf M, Schneider E. Adjacent vertebral failure after vertebroplasty: a biomechanical study of low-modulus PMMA cement. Eur Spine J. 2007;16:2118-25.
35. Chen WJ, Yang SC, Yu SW, Tu YK, Chung KC. Impact of cement leakage into disks on the development of adjacent vertebral compression fractures. J Spinal Disord Tech. 2010;23:35-9.
36. Lin WC, Lee CH, Kuo YL, Cheng YF, Lui CC, Cheng TT. Refractures in cemented vertebrae after percutaneous vertebroplasty: a retrospective analysis. Eur Spine J. 2008;17:592-9.
37. Hulme PA, Ferguson SJ, Berlemann U. Vertebroplasty and kyphoplasty: a systematic review of 69 clinical studies. Spine. 2006;31:1983-2001.
38. Chen WJ, Yang SC, Yu SW, et al. Impact of cement leakage into disks on the development of adjacent vertebral compression fractures. J Spinal Disord Tech. 2010;23:35-9.
39. Lih-Hui Chen EA. VP for osteoporotic spine fracture. Chang Gung Med J. 2011; 34(4):356.
40. Lo YP, Chen LH, Lai PL. New vertebral fracture after vertebroplasty. J Trauma. 2008;65:1439-45.
41. Ehteshami Rad GAL, Kallmes DF. Incident vertebral fractures in patients not undergoing vertebroplasty. J Vasc Interv Radiol. 2010;21:856-60.
42. Phillips FM TWF, Lieberman I, Campbell-Hupp M. An in vivo comparison of the potential for extravertebral cement leak after vertebroplasty and kyphoplasty. Spine. 2002;27:2173-8.
43. Darwono B. Vesselplasty. A novel concept of percutaneous treatment for stabilization and height restoration of Vertebral compression fractures-technical considerations. 1st ed. Bhave A, editor. New Delhi, India: Jaypee Brothers Medical Publishers; 2009.
44. Lieberman IH, Reinhardt MK, et al. Initial outcome and efficacy of "kyphoplasty" in the treatment of painful osteoporotic vertebral compression fractures. Spine. 2001;26:1631-8.

29

CHAPTER

Kyphoplasty

Abhay Nene, Manish Kothari, Kunal Shah

ABSTRACT

The kyphoplasty is and minimally invasive technique in the management of osteoporotic vertebral compression fractures.The fractures in elderly are usually associated with pain and deformity of the affected segment. This technique is being developed advanced to vetebroplasty and helps in effective relief of pain, lesser complications like cement leakage and helps in correction of deformity.

INTRODUCTION

Balloon kyphoplasty is a minimally invasive percutaneous technique for vertebral augmentation in compression fractures. Kyphoplasty was first performed in California by an orthopedic surgeon MA. Reiley in 1998. It was been developed as an advanced procedure to vertebroplasty. Main advantages over vertebroplasty were less chances of cement leakage and possibility of deformity correction. The goal of kyphoplasty is to achieve rapid pain relief and restoration of vertebral height and reduction of kyphosis.

INDICATIONS

1. Osteoporotic vertebral compression fractures:
   a. Compression fracture (AO type A1) (MRI showing edema).
   b. Failure of conservative treatment (2–6 weeks).
   c. Pain on visual analogous scale (VAS) above 4 out of 10.
2. Instrumention associated adjacent segment vertebral fractures (as prophylaxis and treatment).
3. Compression fractures due to plasmacytoma, painful hemangiomas and osteolytic metastasis.[1]
4. Certain types of burst fractures (A3.1) have also been treated with kyphoplasty with posterior instrumentation.[2]
5. Its use in compression fractures in osteogenesis imperfecta is also described.[3]

CONTRAINDICATIONS

1. **Absolute contraindications**
   a. Coagulation disorders
   b. Infection in the proposed site of entry
   c. Burst fractures, AO type B, type C. Unstable fractures with involvement of the posterior vertebral wall and accompanying spinal canal compromise.
   d. Vertebra plana not opening up on prone lateral films.
2. **Relative contraindications**
   a. Severely collapsed vertebra
   b. Fractured pedicles
   c. Tumor invasion into the spinal canal, making any potential leakage of even a small amount of cement into the already compromised spinal canal.
   d. More than 3 levels at a time.

APPLIED ANATOMY

Vertebral Anatomy (Figure 1)

For precise placement of the needle, one has to understand the 3D bony anatomy of the vertebral body as well as the pedicles. Vertebral bodies in thoracic region are wedge-shaped with anterior height being shorter than the posterior height. In the lumbar spine, anterior and posterior heights are generally equal. The vertebral body cross-sectional area gradually increases from the thoracic spine to the midlumbar spine, from whereon it

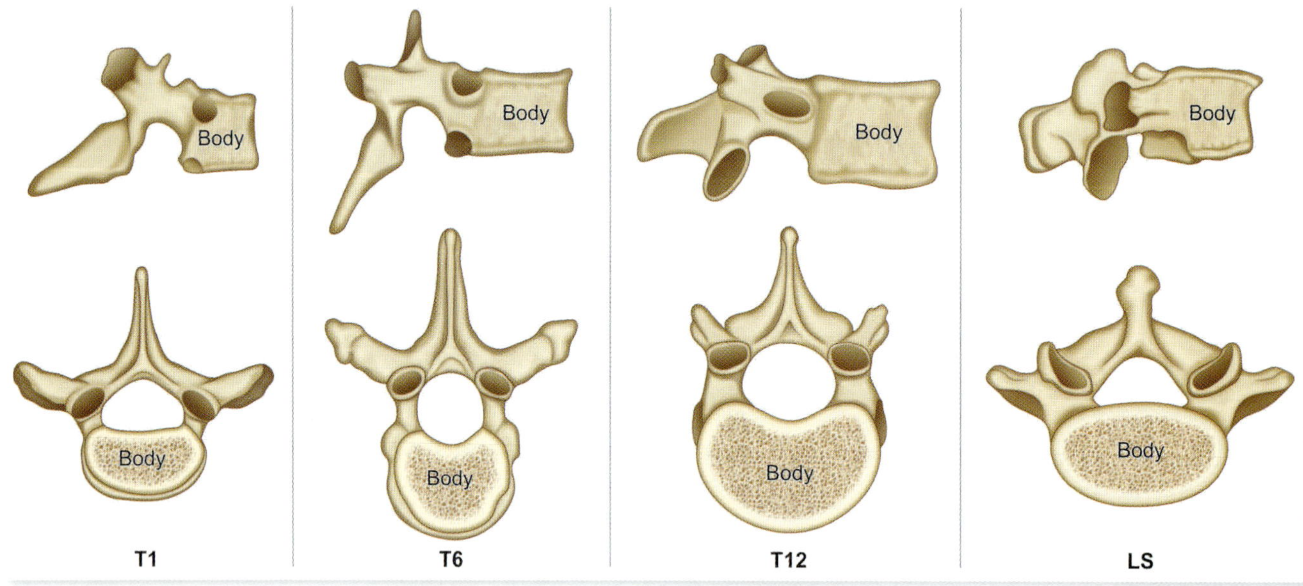

Figure 1: Anatomy of vertebrae at different levels

is stable till L5. Thus smaller balloon size is needed for mid and upper thoracicspine. In the thoracic vertebrae, the pedicle is angled caudad to meet the vertebral body. From cranial to rostral, this angle progressively decreases. In the lumbar region, the pedicle is coplanar with the vertebral body. The pedicle angle and fracture location has to be considered for the needle trajectory. Pedicle width is narrowest in the region of T4–6, which gradually increases cranially and caudally. Transverse pedicle angle decreases from upper thoracic spine steadily as one proceeds down till the thoracolumbar junction where the pedicles are straight. In the lumbar spine this angle rapidly increases such that at L5 it is 25 to 30 degrees. Thus, in the lower thoracic spine two balloons are usually necessary as the needle cannot be placed across the midline by a transpedicular route.

Venous Anatomy (Figure 2)

Due to high incidence of cement leakage into the local venous system, it is important to know the venous anatomy. The vertebral venous system, popularly called as Batson plexus, is divided into three parts, the external venous system, internal venous system and basivertebral system. These veins typically are valveless and their volume is atleast 20 times more than arterial volume. This allows the blood to flow in either direction based on intrathoracic and intra-abdominal pressure. Such typical anatomy of venous system predisposes to leakage of cement or marrow into the system if they are punctured. This causes potentially fatal complications like pulmonary embolism. The prone position of patient is also important in view that increased abdominal pressure (thus increased caval pressure) diverts blood flow through vertebral veins which increases the chance of embolism. Thus, optimum positioning with abdomen free can minimize embolism.

PREOPERATIVE WORKUP

1. MRI scan should be done to confirm the diagnosis. Sometimes, early infection can mimic osteoporotic fractures. Pre- and paraverebral soft tissues should be looked for. On the other hand, fracture hematoma also appears as paravertebral soft tissue shadow. In such cases, it is better to discuss with the radiologists and ask for a contrast scan. Also, it is not uncommon to see fresh uncollapsed fractures adjacent to collapsed old healed fractures **(Figure 3)**. MRI helps identify the fresh lesion and even multiple level fractures. This avoids wrong level/missed level procedures. MRI will also show posterior ligamentous complex (PLC) injury which will mandate posterior instrumentation **(Figure 4)**. If MRI is contraindicated, CT should be done.

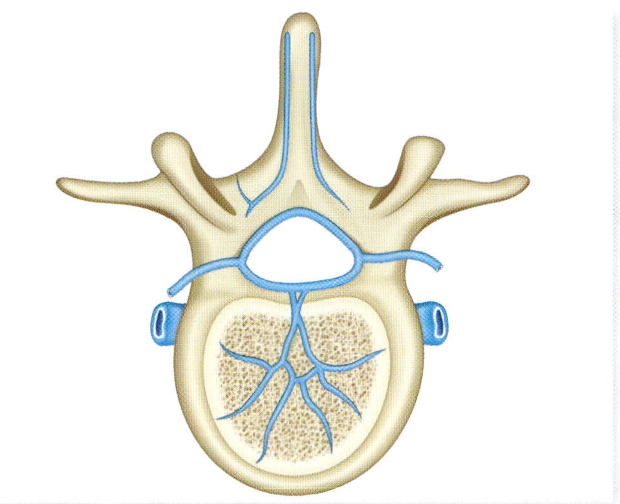

Figure 2: Venous system anatomy around the vertebrae

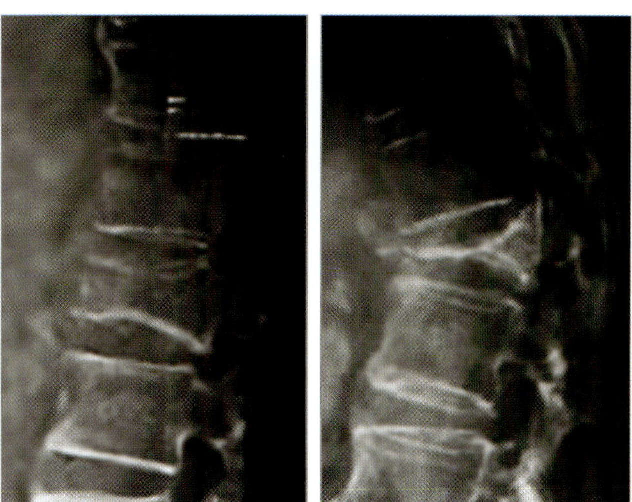

Figure 5: Sitting supine X-rays showing gross instability suggestive of posterior tension band insufficiency

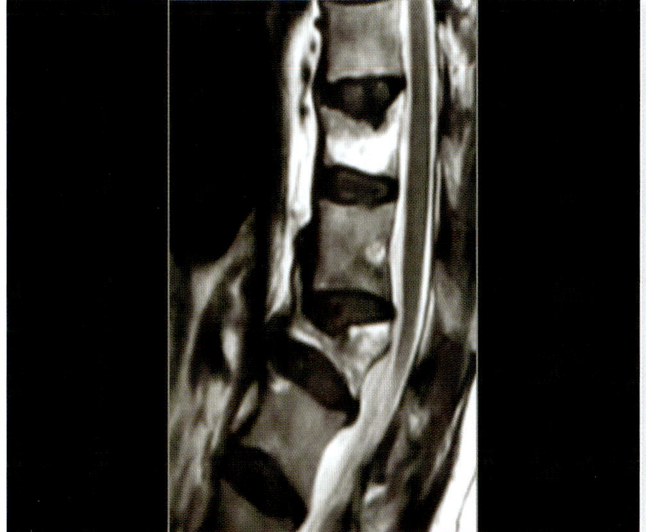

Figure 3: MRI shows that L1 is old fracture and D11 is fresh fracture

Figure 4: Radiograph shows osteoporotic fracture but MRI shows PLC injury also

2. AP and lateral x rays with supine lateral and sitting lateral.
   a. AP view: to look for pedicle destruction in case of metastasis. To look whether the pedicles of the fractured vertebrae are clearly visible. In case of difficulty in defining the pedicles then high definition fluoroscopy or CT guidance should be used for kyphoplasty.
   b. The supine and sitting lateral view will reveal the mobility of the fracture and can predict the vertebral body height restoration by positioning the patient. In case of gross mobility indicating posterior tension band disruption, it may be prudent to add posterior instrumentation **(Figure 5)**.
3. CT scan is not always required. In case of malignancies or select burst fracture types (A3.1), CT scan will be required to define the integrity of the vertebral body walls, define fracture type and can also help decide the side to be chosen in unipedicular techniques.
4. Physician assessment is required for GA fitness (even if planning under LA) and anticoagulant/antiplatelet therapy management.

TECHNIQUE

A Set of Instruments (Figure 6)

1. Basic instruments: Kirschner wires, Jamshidi needle, working cannula, drill, mallet and cement preparation set and syringes.
2. Special instruments: Inflatable bone tamps and pressure syringes.
3. Bone cement (monomer and polymer), bone filler devices.

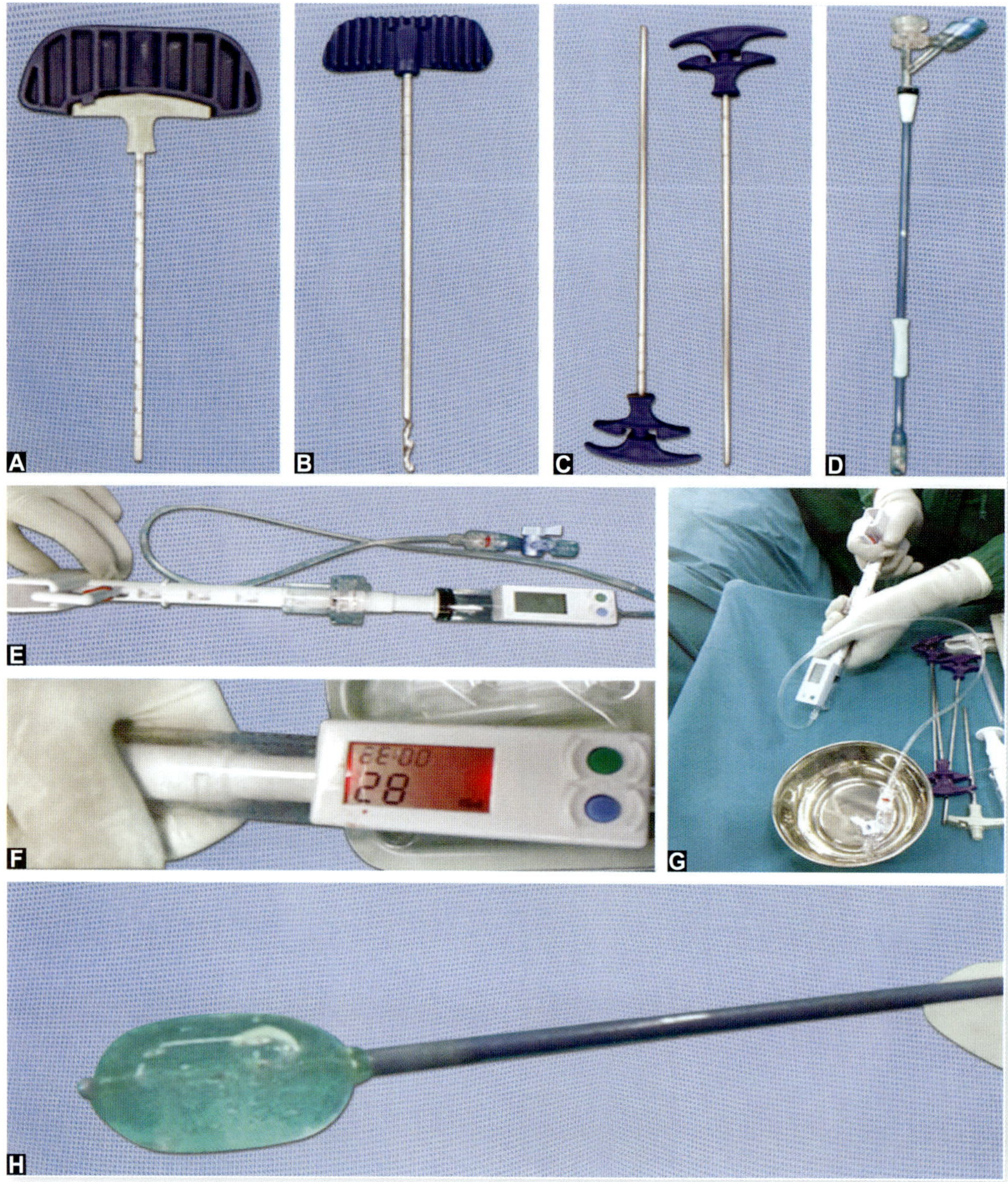

Figures 6A to H: A set of instruments for kyphoplasty: (A) Working cannula; (B) Bone drill; (C) Bone filler device; (D) Inflatable bone tamp; (E) Pressure syringe with gauge; (F) Pressure monitor; (G) Filling of pressure syringe with contrast; (H) Balloon inflation

Inflatable Bone Tamps (Balloon Catheter) and Pressure Syringe

Conventionally there are three parts of an IBT, namely balloon, shaft and two adapters.

The balloons length comes in various sizes 10 mm, 15 mm and 20 mm depending on the size of the vertebra. The shaft length also varies. The maximum volume of the balloon varies according to the maximum pressure possible for each balloon. The content capacity can vary from 3mL to 6 mL depending on different systems. The pressure syringe is used to fill cement and indicates pressure in pounds/inch^2 (psi). The maximum pressure varies from 300 psi to 400 psi depending on cement volume in various systems.

Bone Cements

The polymethylmethacrylate (PMMA) and calcium phosphate cement (CPC) are used for vertebral augmentation procedure. PMMA is more commonly used. There are few clinically important differences between the two cements, which surgeons should know. The CPC is hydrophilic while PMMA cement is hydrophobic. Thus the setting reaction is hardly affected by surrounding body fluids in case of PMMA. However, the CPC cement can disintegrate and microparticulate matter can spread in blood. The setting reaction and heat released is faster in case of PMMA as compared to CPC. The PMMA cement has shown better resilience to compressive, tensile and shear forces while CPC shows resilience to only compressive forces. Thus, leading to cement cracking within the bone with movement within the fractured fragments of the vertebra. In contrast to PMMA, the CPC are resorbable and can get replaced by bone. However, the exact mechanism and duration of it is unknown. The bone cement integration is excellent in cases of CPC, compared to PMMA.

Type of Approaches

1. Transpedicular bilateral (most commonly used).
2. Extrapedicular unilateral (used for high thoracic fractures).
3. Open interlaminary (along with thecal decompression).

Preparation and Positioning of the Patient

Anesthesia: Local infiltration plus intravenous(iv) sedation or GA. Single dose of prophylactic iv antibiotic is given at this time.

Positioning: When performing the procedure under LA, the surgeon should make sure that all the requirements are ready on the trolley and the staff nurse has scrubbed before positioning. The patient is positioned prone **(Figure 7A)** on radiolucent operating table making sure all bony points well cushioned and abdomen is free (decreases venous pressure and chances of embolism). The patient should be positioned in a lordotic fashion to aid in ligamentotaxic restoration of vertebral height. (*Tip:* Placing the bolsters horizontally helps). Before painting, a C-arm image is taken to check for the visibility of the pedicles as well as to look for the amount of verterbral body height restoration. On occasions, the pedicles may not be clearly visible on AP image despite high resolution fluoroscopy due to severe osteoporosis. (*Tip:* this embarrassing situation can be avoided by preoperative evaluation). In such cases one has to decide for alternate approaches (CT guided/in DSA suite). This will also serve to check for 'squaring' of the vertebra to be treated. This assumes great importance in a deformed spine especially degenerative scoliosis. Any changes in the patient positioning can be done now (*Tip:* Tilting the table rather than rotating the C-arm makes the procedure easier). The back is prepared and draped in an aseptic manner. The draping should be wide when using extrapedicular approach. (*Caution:* Do not use adhesive plastic drapes at the operative site.

C-arm management: Ideally a two C-arm set up (one for AP and one for lateral) saves time and radiation **(Figure 7C)**. However, most commonly single C-arm is available. *Tip:* Keep the height of the operating table constant. The surgeon may elevate himself on a platform rather than changing the height of the table repeatedly to accommodate the C-arm. The C-arm technician should be asked to note the vertical elevation (for lateral image) and location on the floor (for AP image) to save time and unnecessary radiation exposure.

Surface Marking and Skin Incision

The fractured vertebra is squared under C-arm **(Figure 8)**. The vertebra is called "squared" when the superior and inferior endplates are seen superimposed without a double shadow and are parallel to each other (true AP). The pedicles should appear at upper third of the body and pedicle ring should represent the narrowest part of the pedicle in anteroposterior (AP) view. In case of scoliotic vertebrae, the image intensifier should be rotated so as to get the end on view of the pedicle (in AP view) which is chosen for the procedure. In lateral view, both the pedicles should be superimposed without any double shadow. The pedicle is marked over the surface of the skin **(Figure 7B)**. The stab incision is marked about 5 mm lateral to the marked pedicle on the skin in transpedicular approach. In extrapedicular approach, the skin incision will be much lateral and proximal to the marked pedicle. This helps in getting the convergence and trajectory required to place the needle in the center of the body. **Figure 9** shows stepwise procedure of kyphoplasty performed.

Procedure of Balloon Kyphoplasty (Percutaneous Bilateral Transpedicular)

When performing the procedure under LA, sedation should also be given. A cocktail containing 10 mL of 2% Lignocaine with Epinephrine and 10 mL of 0.5% Bupivacaine (preservative free) is used by the authors. (*Tip:* We first infiltrate subdermal and subcutaneous tissue with 26 G needle. We then use the 21 G needle for localization of the bony entry point under C-arm and infiltrate generously in the deeper tissues as well as on the bone on both sides. This anesthetizes the relevant area adequately).

1. Take a stab skin incision after marking the pedicle on the skin.
2. *Entry point:* The tip of Jamshidi needle is placed on the outer border of the pedicle in AP image (10/11 o' clock or 1/ 2 o' clock) and checked on the lateral image for the trajectory and superior–inferior position as desired depending upon the fracture location **(Figure 10)**. (*Tip:* One can 'walk' the transverve process/facet to

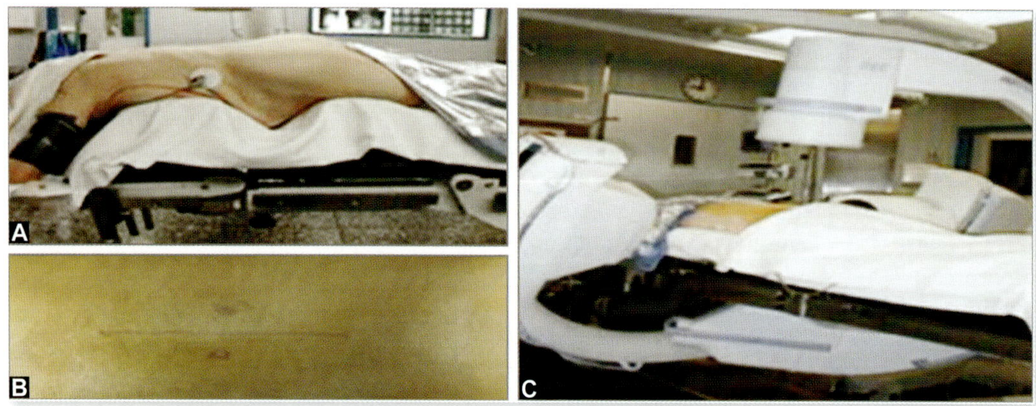

Figures 7A to C: (A) Patient positioning with horizontal bolsters; (B) Skin marking of pedicle; (c) Using two C-arms simultaneuosly to save time and radiation

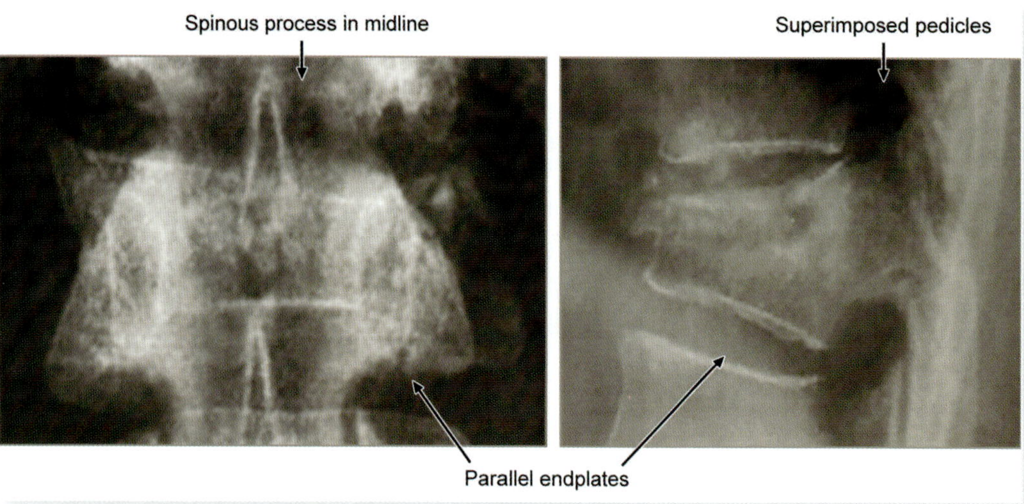

Figure 8: 'Squaring' of vertebra

reduce the number of C-arm shoots). The needle is then advanced (in the AP view) by about 15–20 mm (*Tip:* The transverse angle of the pedicle must be kept in mind) and stopped as soon as it reaches the medial border of the pedicle. At this position the needle tip should be just beyond the level of posterior cortex of the vertebral body. If in the lateral view the needle is not yet beyond the level of posterior cortex of the body, then the needle will have to be directed a bit lateral to avoid entering the epidural space and neural damage. If the needle is far beyond the posterior 1/3rd of the vertebral body, it will have to be redirected more medially to reach the midline and avoid lateral placement of the needle in the vertebral body. Once this position of the needle tip is confirmed, it can be advanced with the guidance of only lateral images. The needle tip is advanced up to junction of anterior 1/4th and posterior 3/4th of the vertebral body on the lateral image. The final position of the needle is confirmed in the AP view, where the needle tip should be near/at the midline. (*Tip:* The needle tip interpretation in the AP and the lateral view must be in relation to the shape of the vertebra. The tip of IBT should be at the junction of anterior 1/4ths and posterior 3/4th of the vertebral body).

3. Remove the trocar of the needle and insert a blunt guidewire into the vertebral body. Its position simulates the position of IBT. At this stage it is important to check the position of wire in both AP and lateral view. (*Tip:* Do not apply excess pressure on the guide wire to avoid anterior perforation).
4. After confirming guidewire position, remove the Jamshidi needle and introduce the larger working cannula (introducer) over the guide wire. The working cannula should be advanced just beyond the level of the posterior wall in lateral view, so that it is fixed there. Thereby, it reduces the chances of cement leakage . The guidewire is now removed.
5. At this stage, a biopsy can be taken if required. Most kits have biopsy system in them. The passage is smoothened with a drill, so that the balloon does not burst due to

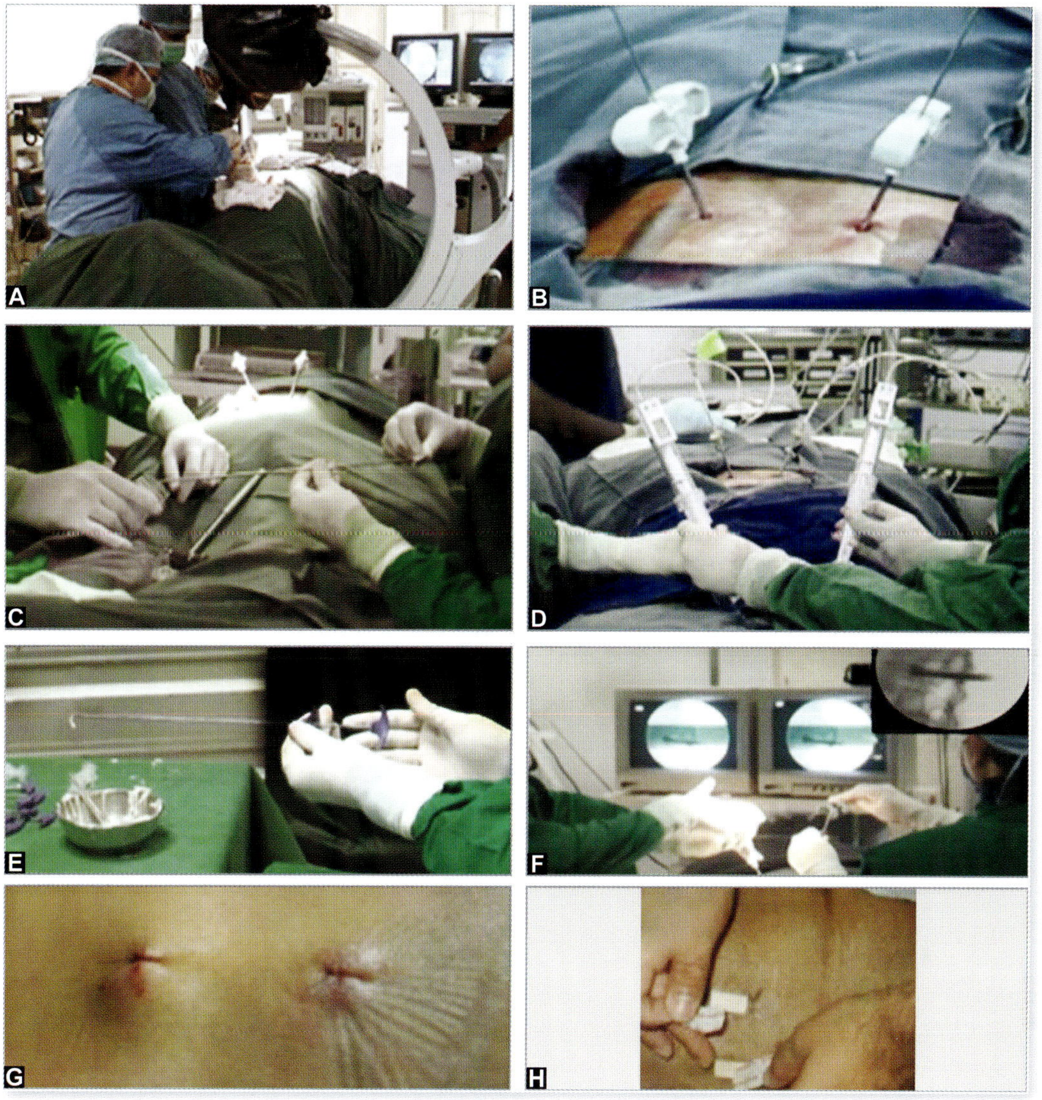

Figure 9: Stepwise procedure of kyphoplasty

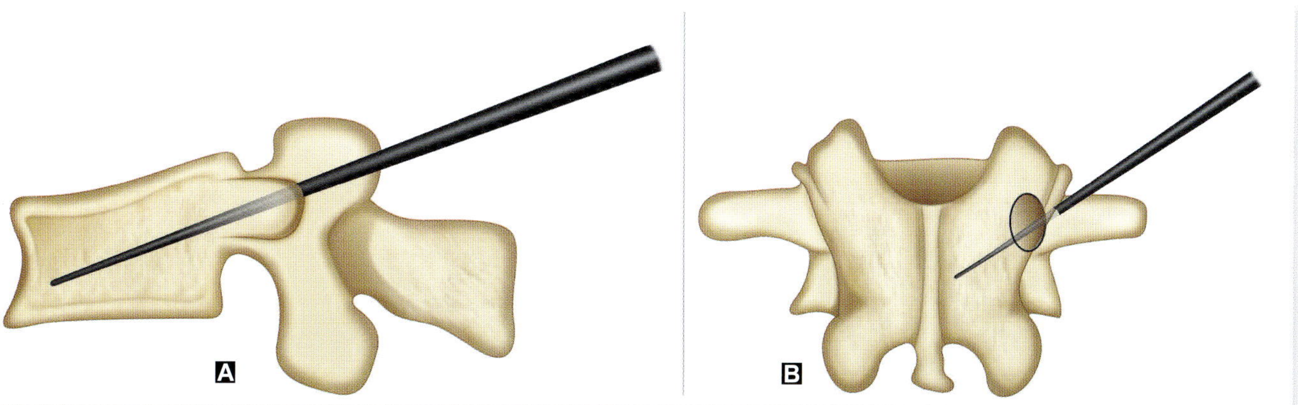

Figure 10: Diagrammatic representation of entry point in transpedicular approach

sharp body edges while inflating. The second needle is inserted in the same fashion from the opposite pedicle.

6. An appropriated size balloon is chosen according to size of the vertebra (20 mm for thoracolumbar/lumbar and 15 mm for higher thoracic). The balloon tamps and the pressure syringe system with contrast is prepared as per manufacturer guidelines. The balloons are introduced simultaneously from both sides and inflated stepwise (0.25 mL increments) with the help of pressure syringe . The pressure is seen on the inline pressure gauge. (*Tip:* In the lateral view when the balloons are inflated till about 25% volume of the vertebral body, an AP view is taken to determine the position of the balloons in relation to the lateral walls). The balloons are then further inflated till adequate body height restoration is achieved or maximum volume or pressure is reached or the balloons are seen kissing in the midline or contact with cortical walls is seen. For fresh fractures usually 150 psi is sufficient. Larger pressures up to 300 psi may be needed in older fractures. One should be careful not to break the endplate or the posterior wall which could lead to cement leakage. (*Tip:* Look out for asymmetric balloon inflation).
7. Remove both the balloons after deflating them fully, keeping the introducer in place. Mix the cement while the balloon is being deflated. The volume of the two balloons will be the approximate quantity of cement to be injected.
8. Keep cement loaded in the bone fillers. Each bone filler will accommodate about 1.5 mL of cement. It usually takes 3-5 minutes for PMMA to reach toothpaste like consistency. (*Tip:* When the cement is injected freely in air, it should not form droplets of cement but flow out like toothpaste). Also, the cement should not stick to the gloves easily.
9. Now carefully fill the bone cavity with cement from both the sides simultaneously under strict fluoroscopic control. Look out for cement leakage. 3–5 mL of cement per vertebral level is usually sufficient. (*Tip:* When injecting cement from the opposite side, the previous bone filler should not be removed to prevent backflow). In case of cement leakage outside the vertebral body, switch to the opposite side. Under no circumstances shall the cement be injected with pressure.
10. The PMMA cement takes about 10–13 minutes to cure. The introducer should be removed after the curing period with rotating movement to break the cement away from the cannula tip.
11. The skin usually does not require formal closure. Dry gauze dressing is kept for a day to soak the ooze. At the time of discharge, it is our usual practice to send the patient with a 'bandaid' dressing.

Percutaneous Unilateral Extrapedicular Kyphoplasty

In the thoracic spine central placement of the balloon is difficult due to narrow pedicles, which do not accommodate the wide introducer and the pedicle angle does not allow medial angulation. Thus in thoracic spine the extrapedicular (transcostovertebral) approach is gaining popularity. It has an added advantage of being away from the neural structures and uses single balloon.

Steps

1. In the AP view "square" the affected vertebra as mentioned above. Locate the costal angle associated with the affected vertebral body. Place a transverse stab incision immediately superior to its cranial to its cranial border. This is usually 5–10 cm lateral from the midline. The Jamshidi needle is introduced from craniolateral towards the costovertebral joint **(Figure 11)**. (*Tip:* Make contact with the neck of the rib or the transverse process).

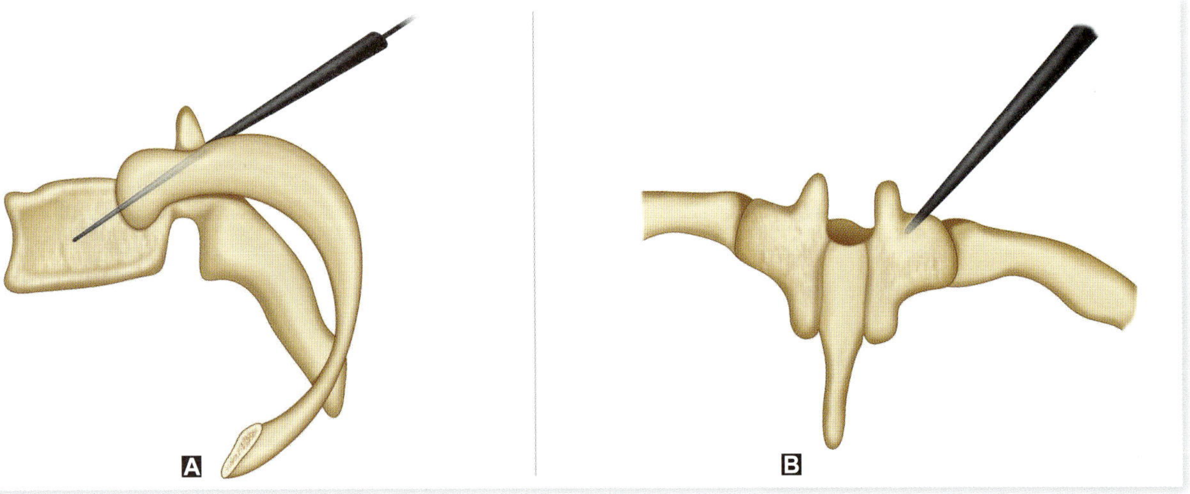

Figure 11: Diagrammatic representation of entry point in extrapedicular approach

2. With the needle tip "walk" along the neck of the rib under the transverse process and through the ligament complex of the costovertebral joint until the lateral pedicle wall is reached.
3. At this point, in the AP view the needle tip is at the craniolateral circumference (11 o'clock of the left side) of the targeted pedicle and the lateral view should show the needle tip anterior to the facet joint at the level of midpoint of the pedicle and close to the base of the pedicle (where the pedicle meets the vertebral body). If the needle posterior to the facet joint, it means that it is on the transverse process and needs repositioning.
4. Now, tap the needle with gentle blows through the lateral pedicle cortex. At this point the needle tip should be inside the pedicle ring in the AP view. Care must be taken that until the needle tip passes beyond the posterior vertebral wall in lateral view, it should not breach the medial pedicle wall. Once this is achieved, the needle tip is allowed to cross the pedicle and thereafter the midline.
5. These steps should be followed strictly to avoid spinal perforation. The rest of the steps are as described before with guide wire and working cannula.

Open Unilateral Interlaminary Kyphoplasty[4]

Done only for cases where an open neural decompression procedure has to be performed. It is best to reserve this procedure for below the conus level to avoid handling the cord.

1. After open decompression, retract the dural sac medially and expose the posterior wall of the fractured vertebra .
2. Now kyphoplasty can be performed with the working cannula placed centrally under C-arm guidance. A single balloon positioned in the centre of the vertebral body is sufficient.
3. **Tip:** Do not create additional entry sites on the posterior wall of the body which may act as paths of least resistance for the cement to flow into the canal.
4. At the end of the procedure the canal has to be checked for cement leakage

Figure 12 shows C-arm images showing each step of procedure

Tips to Minimize Radiation

1. Use intermittent fluoroscopy instead of continuous.
2. To check the needle position under C-arm during insertion hold the needle with Kocher forceps instead of hands.
3. Lead aprons/shields can be used to cover the areas outside the drapes and even to the sides of the table to minimize radiation scatter from under the table.
4. Placing the X-ray tube of C-arm on the opposite side of the surgeon can reduce the radiation by 10 times.
5. Computer-assisted navigation can be used for needle placement. This reduces radiation by up to 76%. However, the balloon inflation and cement injection should be under fluoroscopic guidance.
6. Radiation attenuation gloves may be used.

Postprocedure Protocol

Patient is mobilized in same evening. Brace usually is not advised. Patient is discharged within 24 hours after post-procedure spine and chest X-rays.

It is important emphasize the fact that treatment of osteoporosis is essentially medical management and regular follow up is essential. DEXA scan, if not done earlier is done in the same admission. (*Tip:* The authors strongly believe that the patients are most receptive to counseling in this period and this opportunity of patient education and medical management should not be missed). The patient is reviewed at one month, 3 months, 6 months and then yearly.

COMPLICATIONS

Overall kyphoplasty is a safe and effective procedure.[5] Vertebral augmentation procedures have been shown to be superior to non surgical management of OVCF with respect to pain relief and quality of life. Complications do occur in kyphoplasty, and most of them are avoidable. These are classified as related to technique and others.

Technique-related Complications

Malpositioning of Cannula (Figure 13A)

In principle, the structures surrounding the pathway of the needle are at risk due to malpositioning causing nerve damage as well as perforation of walls of vertebra. Wall perforations also act as sites of cement leakage, especially in the veterbral canal. *Tip:* Paying strict attention to needle placement on fluoroscopy can minimize these events.

Endplate Fracture and Lateral wall Fractures (Figure 13B)

Lateral wall and endplate fractures can occur during inflation of the balloon (BRC). It can damage the adjacent disk and adjacent vertebral endplate fracture. Cannula tip should be guided into the fracture zone away from these structures. It may also occur due to nonuniform expansion of balloon due to heterogenous bone structure. Careful needle placement and watchful expansion of the balloon under fluoroscopy avoids these complications. *Tip:* Another technique described is controlled segmental balloon

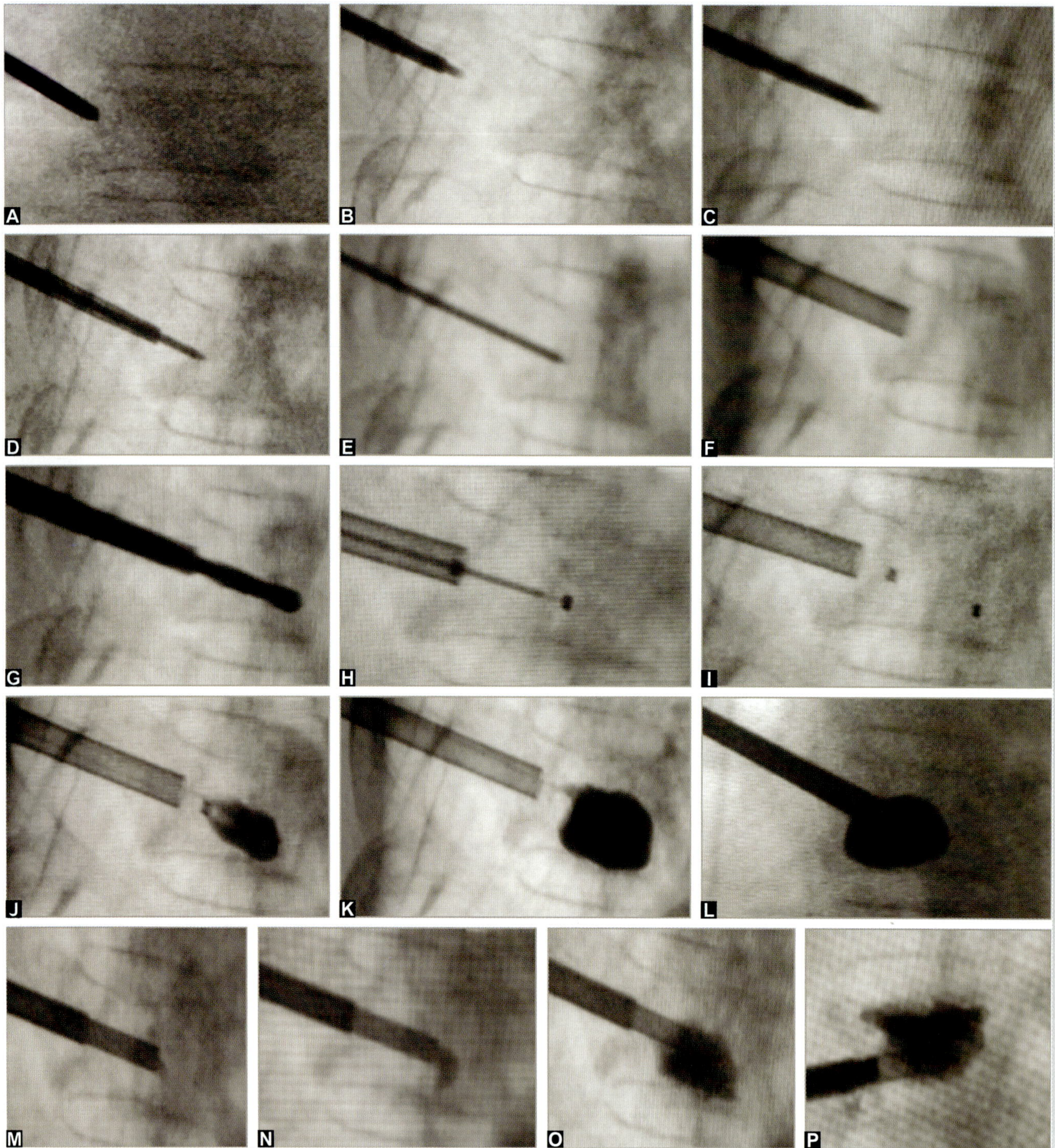

Figures 12A to P: C-arm images of kyphoplasty performed in D11 vertebra: (A) Position of needle in anteroposterior view for entry in extrapedicular approach; (B) Position of needle in lateral view for entry in extrapedicular approach; (C) Crossing pedicle; (D) Insertion of K-wire; (E) Needle removed over K-wire; (F) Working cannula inserted; (G) Drill inserted through cannula; (H) Balloon entered through cannula; (I) Stylet of balloon removed; (J) Initial inflation of balloon; (K) Final inflation of balloon in lateral view; (L) Final inflation of balloon in anteroposterior view; (M) Bone filler device inserted; (N) Cement insertion; (O) Final picture in lateral view; (p) Final picture in anteroposterior view

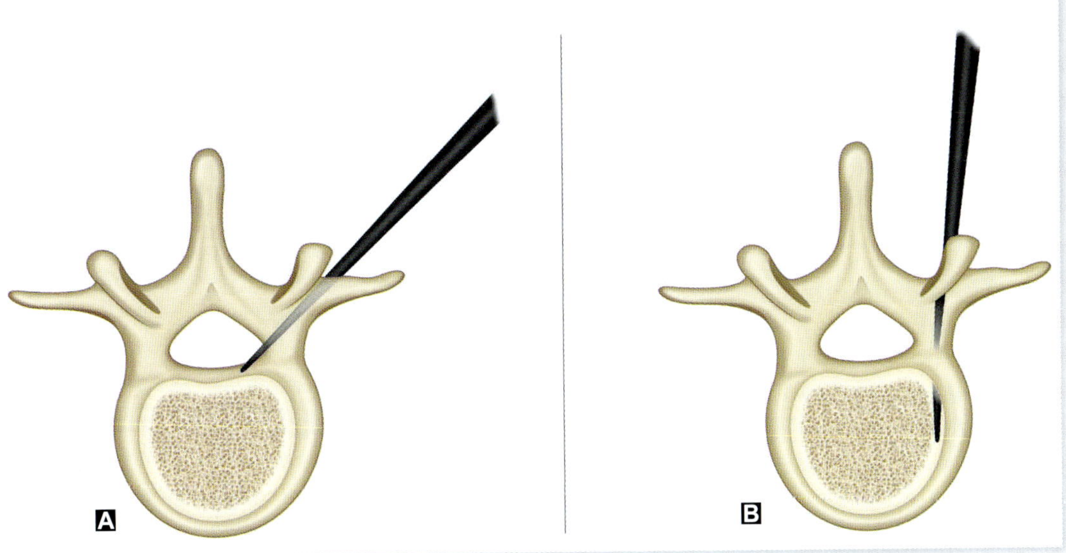

Figures 13: (A) Medial placement of cannula causes neurologic injury; (B) Lateral placement of cannula leads to wall rupture during inflation

expansion, wherein sequentially increasing lengths of the balloon is advanced outside the tip of the introducer into the fracture zone and inflated creating a uniform cavity.[6.]

Vertebral Fracture Recollapse after Balloon Deflation

Fractures with osteonecrosis are mobile and get easily reduced; however they tend to collapse after balloon deflation. *Tip:* Lordotic positioning will help maintain the vertebral height. Another technique is to inject cement from one side while the other balloon is kept inflated.[7] However, this carries a risk of balloon rupture due cement heat. The cement should never be injected under pressure in a bid to fill the collapsed cavity.

Balloon Rupture

As such balloon rupture is not a technical failure, although it can cause contrast seepage and increased procedure time. Balloon rupture can be due to sharp bony edges. It can be avoided by slowly inflating the balloon or curetting the sharp edges before inflation. Air embolism is a theoretical possibility and balloons must be purged of any trapped air before insertion and inflation.

Local Cement Leakage

The average rate of cement leakage in kyphoplasty is 18% with only 0.5% being symptomatic.[5] Cement leakage in kyphoplasty is comparatively less than in vertebroplasty (44%). Use of high viscocity cement, low injection pressure and compaction of the surrounding bone by balloon inflation sealing the defects prevents extravasation of cement. Cement leakage is classified as cortical (adjacent soft tissue, adjacent disk space), epidural (spinal canal and the neuroforamina) and anterior venous. Cement leak is most commonly asymptomatic; however, major complications and deaths have been reported. Cement leakage close to neural structures can cause radiculopathy and spinal cord compression. For mild symptoms expectant or symptomatic treatment is adequate as they usually resolve. For symptomatic cord compression, formal surgical decompression is required.

Several factors affect cement leakage. Most crucial is cement injection consistency. A toothpaste-like consistency is ideal. Undue force applied during injection will also result in cement extravasation. About 3–5 mL is adequate to stabilize the fracture and restore stiffness of the vertebral body. However, excess of cement injection leads to leakage. *Tip:* If using nonreadymade cements, then opacification with barium sulfate powder should be adequate (30%). Careful fluoroscopic monitoring during PMMA injection is imperative. On first recognition of cement leakage, injection from the same side should be interrupted or even terminated. Intraosseous venography is an option but not routinely performed.

Nontechnique-related Complications

Transient Hyperalgesia

The postulated mechanism of hyperalgesia is local inflammatory reaction to cement polymerization and exothermic reaction. It can also be because of tissue stretch during balloon inflation. It usually settles with NSAIDs.

Cardiorespiratory Effects

Transient desaturation and bradycardia during cement injection is not uncommon. It is due to monomer toxicity. Interruption of injection till the anaesthetists 'settles' the patient is advised. The balloon inflation or cement injection can displace blood and marrow fat. This can lead to symptomatic or asymptomatic pulmonary emboli. PMMA has a thrombogenic potential which may cause pulmonary artery occlusion when it reaches the pulmonary vasculature. Local venous extravasations are common and may be associated with delayed pulmonary events.[8] Routine post operative chest x rays have therefore been advised by some authors.[5] Cement bolus has also been reported to embolize into the cardiac chambers as well, requiring surgery[9] and causing pulmonary necrosis requiring pulmonary wedge resection.[10]

For symptomatic patients with peripheral/small emboli conservative treatment and follow-up is adequate. Acute symptomatic patients should receive anticoagulants. Embolectomy may be necessary for those with severe symptoms.[11]

Infection

Postoperative infection can appear locally as wound infection, or it may present as spondylodiskitis. Infections may occur early or seed even after months. A high index of suspicion is required for early detection. MRI is the investigation of choice. Early infections may settle with appropriate antibiotics. In advanced cases surgery is required and anterior surgery is usually necessary to remove the cement which now acts as a foreign body [12.]

Adjacent Fractures

There is a mixed reporting in literature about increased or decreased incidence of adjacent level fracture after vertebral augmentation. Some authors have reported that correction of deformity and subsequent sagittal alignment favors biomechanically toward lesser incidence of adjacent fractures.[5] On the other hand a meta-analysis of level I–II studies on complications of kyphoplasty found increased incidence of adjacent level fractures, which was more than historical data on adjacent level fractures in patients treated nonsurgically.[13] The results are further confounded by the fact that not all studies report antiosteoporotic treatment. Intradiskal cement leakage and positive sagittal balance are risk factor for adjacent fractures other than osteoporosis itself.

Late Collapse and Instability

The authors have noticed several cases of late onset instability;[14] classified as intravertebral and intervertebral. Intravertebral instability results when there is collapse of the vertebral body around the cement. The cement causes stress shielding of the bone around it which causes osteolysis and bone resoprtion rather than healing due to continuous micromotion. Intradiskal cement leakage leads to accelerated degeneration of the disk and later, erosion of the endplate of the adjacent vertebra leading to intervertebral instability. This is further exacerbated if there is gross kyphosis in a high demand back. Some of these patients develop bridging osteophytes which may stabilize the instability. For others, posterior instrumentation is warranted.

Mortality

The perioperative mortality is less than 1%.[13] Of note here is that these patients are frail and OVCF itself has an increased mortality rate.

Miscellaneous

Rib fractures are described because of pressure in prone position while inserting the needle.

Procedure site bleeding have also been described.[15]

ACKNOWLEDGMENTS

We acknowledge Dr Viral Shah and Dr Praveen Saxena (The Spine Clinic Team, Ahmedabad) for providing **Figures 7 and 9.**

REFERENCES

1. Dalbayrak S, Onen MR, Yilmaz M, Naderi S. Clinical and radiographic results of balloon kyphoplasty for treatment of vertebral body metastases and multiple myelomas. J Clin Neurosci. 2010;17(2):219-24.
2. Rahamimov N, Mulla H, Shani A, Freiman S. Percutaneous augmented instrumentation of unstable thoracolumbar burst fractures. Eur Spine J. 2012;21(5):850-4.
3. Fürstenberg CH, Grieser T, Wiedenhöfer B, Gerner HJ, Putz CM. The role of kyphoplasty in the management of osteogenesis imperfecta: risk or benefit? Eur Spine J. 2010;19 (Suppl) 2:S144-8.
4. Boszczyk BM, Bierschneider M, Schmid K, Grillhösl A, Robert B, Jaksche H. Microsurgical interlaminary vertebro- and kyphoplasty for severe osteoporotic fractures. J Neurosurg Spine. 2004;100(1 Suppl):32-7.
5. Papanastassiou ID, Phillips FM, Van Meirhaeghe J, Berenson JR, Andersson GB, Chung G, et al. Comparing effects of kyphoplasty, vertebroplasty, and non-surgical management in a systematic review of randomized and non-randomized controlled studies. Eur Spine J. 2012;21(9):1826-43.
6. Saliou G, Lehmann P, Vallée JN. Controlled segmental balloon kyphoplasy: a new technique for patients with heterogeneous vertebral bone density. Spine (Phila Pa 1976). 2008;33(7):E216-20.

7. Saliou G, Rutgers DR, Kocheida EM, Langman G, Meurin A, Deramond H, Lehmann P.Balloon-related complications and technical failures in kyphoplasty for vertebral fractures. AJNR Am J Neuroradiol. 2010;31(1):175-9.
8. Wardlaw D, Cummings SR, Van Meirhaeghe J, Bastian L, Tillman JB, Ranstam J, et al. Efficacy and safety of balloon kyphoplasty compared with non-surgical care for vertebral compression fracture (FREE): a randomised controlled trial. Lancet. 2009;373(9668):1016-24.
9. Dash A, Brinster DR. Open heart surgery for removal of polymethylmethacrylate after percutaneous vertebroplasty. Ann Thorac Surg. 2011;91:276-8.
10. Rothermich MA, Buchowski JM, Bumpass DB, Patterson GA. Pulmonary Cement Embolization After Vertebroplasty Requiring Pulmonary Wedge Resection. Clinical Orthopaedics and Related Research. 2014;472(5):1652-7.
11. Tozzi P, Abdelmoumene Y, Corno AF, Gersbach PA, Hoogewoud HM, von Segesser LK. Management of pulmonary embolism during acrylic vertebroplasty. Ann Thorac Surg. 2002;74:1706-8.
12. Abdelrahman H, Siam AE, Shawky A, et al. Infection after vertebroplasty or kyphoplasty. A series of nine cases and review of literature.Spine J. 2013;13(12):1809-17.
13. Bouza C, López-Cuadrado T, Almendro N, Amate JM. Safety of balloon kyphoplasty in the treatment of osteoporotic vertebral compression fractures in Europe: a meta-analysis of randomized controlled trials. Eur Spine J. 2015;24(4):715-23.
14. Nagad P, Rawall S, Kundnani V, Mohan K, Patil SS, Nene A. Postvertebroplasty instability. J Neurosurg Spine. 2012; 16(4):387-93.
15. Lee MJ, Dumonski M, Cahill P, Stanley T, Park D, Singh K. Percutaneous treatment of vertebral compression fractures: a meta-analysis of complications. Spine (Phila Pa 1976). 2009; 34(11):1228-32.

Scope of Minimally Invasive Techniques in Spinal Infections

Arvind G Kulkarni, Navin Mewara

ABSTRACT

The primary goals for treating infectious spinal conditions are to make an accurate diagnosis, isolate the causative organism, and prescribe effective antibiotic therapy on the basis of the culture reports. A positive culture is extremely important for successful treatment and prevention of further morbidity. Surgically collected samples have shown to have a greater chance of giving positive results as compared to CT guided fine needle samples. Surgical drainage and/or reconstruction with/or without fixation is usually indicated when there is no or poor response to antibiotic therapy, systemic toxicity with evidence of large collections, progressive spinal deformity or instability or neurological impairment. However, the incidence of perioperative morbidity is particularly increased in elderly patients or in those with a poor general condition. With improved instrumentation and techniques in minimally invasive spine surgery (MISS), spinal infections can be successfully treated by minimally invasive debridement followed by pharmacological treatment, without causing any destabilization to spine. Where major reconstruction and fixation procedures are deemed mandatory, various MIS techniques can be utilized to decrease the surgery-related morbidity and allow for faster rehabilitation. These procedures are associated with steep learning curve. With the advent of intraoperative navigation, the exposure to radiations can be drastically reduced.

INTRODUCTION

Infectious spinal conditions are becoming increasingly prevalent, especially in elderly or immunocompromised patients or those with medical comorbidities. This increase has been due to vast improvements in medical care and prolonged life expectancies. The standard choice of treatment in cases of mild infection is antibiotic administration and bed rest. To procure a sample of tissue for biopsy and culture many techniques have been employed. The rate of pathogen identification varies widely, from 36 to 92%.[1-6] Open transpedicular biopsy does increase the changes of isolation of organism but is associated with major surgical morbidities.[9] A CT-guided biopsy is a less invasive procedure used to obtain specimens for pathogen identification with varying results and an inherent risk of exposure to the radiations. Anterior debridement and reconstruction with or without posterior instrumentation are the traditional gold standard surgical procedures for cases that require being treated surgically. But this is associated with high rates of postoperative complications, especially in immunocompromised patients with many comorbid diseases or in the elderly.[8] Over the last few decades, spinal surgery has been modified to become minimally invasive. In degenerative spinal disorders, MISS has proven to reduce blood loss, muscular trauma, and the hospital stays.[9] However, with an increase in the experience with MISS, it is also gaining popularity for patients with spinal infections. The innovations in techniques like intraoperative navigation have helped increase the accuracy of these procedures and reduce the overall exposure to radiations.

Rationale of MISS

1. Decrease retractor associated muscle crush injury.
2. Avoid subperiosteal dissection and detachment of muscle attachments.
3. Limit surgical corridor without compromising on the field of vision.
4. Reduce bony resection thus causing less destabilization.

MIS techniques that can be employed in spinal infections can be broadly categorized as:

1. Needle based
2. Tubular retractor based
3. Endoscopic techniques and
4. Thoracoscopic techniques.

Scope of MISS in spinal infections

1. To obtain specimens for culture
2. Drainage of epidural abscess
3. Percutaneous debridement of infected diskin early stage
4. Anterior debridement and reconstruction followed by posterior MIS screw fixation.
5. Utilization of MIS direct lateral interbody fusion (DLIF/XLIF) techniques
6. All posterior MIS: Transforaminal debridement with interbody fusion and percutaneous pedicle screw fixation and
7. Integration of MIS techniques with intraoperative navigation to increases the accuracy and decrease the amount of exposure to radiation.

Scenario where MISS serves extremely useful

1. Immunocompromised individual,
2. Extremely sick and
3. Elderly or those with multiple medical comorbidities.

Advantages of using MISS technique

1. Less blood loss and lesser use of blood products,
2. Lesser hospital stay,
3. Quicker rehabilitation which is extremely important in these patients, and
4. Reduced overall cost.

VARIOUS MIS TECHNIQUES

MIS techniques for spinal infections range from percutaneous transpedicular biopsy to the use of tubular decompressions with or without percutaneous fixation and its integration with the intraoperative navigation system.

Percutaneous Transpedicular Biopsy (PTB)

Obtaining biopsy specimen from the affected vertebral body and disk space is extremely important for initiation of proper antibiotics. This can be done in various ways. An open biopsy has minimal sampling error but is a major procedure associated with increased morbidity. Paraspinal needle biopsy of vertebral lesions is also associated with its own set of complications.[10] CT-guided needle biopsies have a high incidence of false-negatives as well the risk of exposure to radiations. In cases of spinal infections, the reported accuracy of spinal biopsy varies from 36 to 92%.[5-6,11-16] Fouquet et al. obtained bacteriological diagnosis in nine (36%) of 25 patients biopsied, using a Mazabraud trocar.[11] Staatz et al. reported[11] (76%) positive cultures for 21 patients, using CT-guided, percutaneous, catheter drainage. Rankine et al. who analyzed 20 patients undergoing percutaneous spinal biopsy for a spinal infection, isolated an organism in six of 12 (50%) patients not taking antibiotics, whereas an organism was isolated in only two of eight patients taking antibiotics.[5] Y S Chooi et al.[14] showed 70% positive cultures in pyogenic spinal infection using transpedicular biopsy.

Furkan Yapici et al.[15] retrospectively evaluated 33 patients who had undergone transpedicular biopsy for vertebral body lesions. 13 of the 17 percutaneous biopsies' (76.5%) and 14 of the 16 open biopsies' (87.5%) specimens were adequate for diagnosis. The adequacy of the specimen for determining a final diagnosis was higher in open biopsy than in percutaneous transpedicular biopsy ($P > 0.05$). The limited number of patients was the most important limitation of their study. They concluded that comparative prospective studies with more cases are needed to determine the reliability and the adequacy of open and percutaneous transpedicular biopsy in the thoracolumbar spine.

Ashizwa R et al.[16] performed percutaneous transpedicular needle biopsy on 28 thoracic and lumbar vertebral bodies with a thin trocar (2.0 mm outer diameter) under fluoroscopic guidance. The accuracy rate of diagnosis with this biopsy method was 92% without significant intra- or postoperative complications. They concluded that the less invasive technique has a good potential to provide a correct preoperative diagnosis of thoracic and lumbar lesions so that more effective treatment can be determined.

Procedure

The fully awake patient is asked to lie prone on the radiolucent table. Intravenous sedation may be given. The chosen vertebral level and the pedicle to be probed are marked in the AP view. In the same view, the C-arm is manipulated along the inclination of the pedicle until an end-on or bull's eyes view of the pedicle is obtained. The entry point, of the needle, is anesthetized followed by the periosteum surrounding the pedicle and the area at the junction of superior facet. A Jamshedi needle is positioned in an end-on view of the pedicle. A stab incision is made. The needle is tapped genty with a mallet through the pedicle into the intended area of the vertebral body **(Figures 1A and B)**. The track is kept within the margins (medial, lateral, superior, and inferior) of the pedicle. The lateral view on fluoroscopy ensures the correct anterior trajectory.When the needle tip was in a satisfactory position; the needle is moved slightly in situ so that the bone sample could be collected easily. Core biopsy samples were sent for histopathological examination in a sterile container. If more tissue is required, the needle is tilted in various directions to improve tissue sampling. The procedure may be repeated on the opposite side if required. The integrity of the pedicle margins must be preserved at all times, especially the medial and inferior

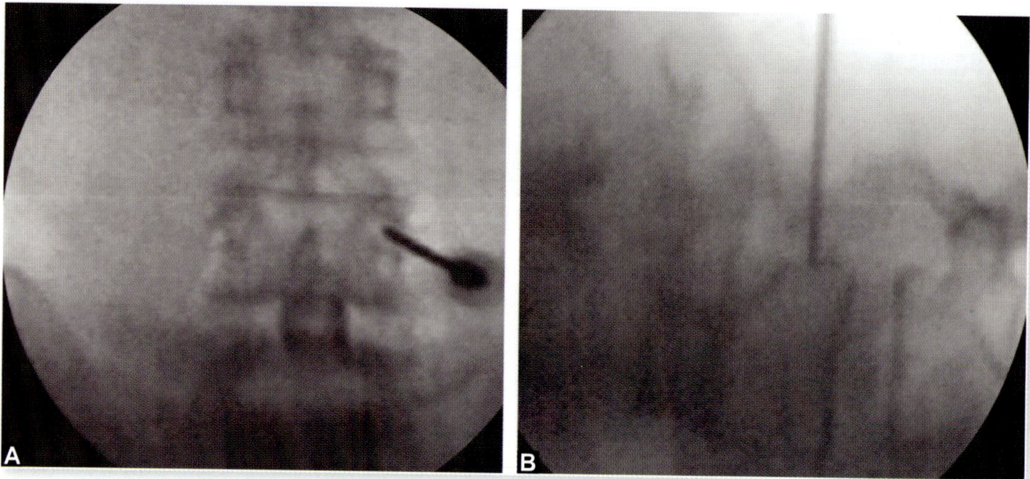

Figures 1A and B: (A) A true AP view with entry site for the Jamshedi needle; (B) Lateral view showing the needle entering the vertebral body

borders. This is to prevent the spread of hematoma, infection or tumor into the spinal canal. No drain is needed.

Advantages

Minimally invasive PTB has the following advantages[14,16,17] as compared to the other techniques:

1. It has shown to yield high cultures in both pyogenic and granulomatous conditions.
2. It can be performed under local anesthesia.
3. Fluoroscopic monitoring enables realtime positioning of the needle.
4. Serious needle related complications from percutaneous needle biopsy are uncommon.
5. More than 50% of vertebral body tissue, including the disk, can be accessed via a unilateral transpedicular approach.
6. Similar to vertebroplasty procedures thus is familiar to most and can be done quickly and safely.

Percutaneous Endoscopic Diskectomy and Drainage (PEDD)

Percutaneous endoscopic diskectomy was first employed for treating uncomplicated herniated disks in the early 1980s. Recently, numerous minimally invasive, percutaneous, endoscopic procedures for lumbar disk herniation have been developed for spinal surgery, with clinical outcomes comparable to those of conventional open surgery.[18,19] The minimal invasiveness and acceptance of the technique led the authors to apply it in treating infectious spondylitis in select cases. Obtaining a sufficient amount of material for microbiological examination directly from the infected region is possible. Additionally, eradication and irrigation of infected and necrotic tissue from a disk and even an epidural space facilitate a fenestration similar to open debridement.[20,21]

Procedure

Under local anesthesia and conscious sedation, the target site is localized with a spinal needle passed 8–10 cm away from the midline under fluoroscopic guidance. A guide-wire is inserted through the spinal needle into the central disk space and the spinal needle is withdrawn. A small stab incision (about 1 cm) is placed, a dilator and the cannulated sleeve are passed **(Figures 2A and B)**. The dilator is withdrawn and a cutting tool is used to harvest a core of impacted biopsy specimen. Percutaneous debridement using the biopsy forceps and shaver is followed by normal saline irrigation **(Figure 2C)**. Finally, a drainage tube is inserted into the debrided disk space and connected to a negative-pressure Hemovac **(Figure 2D)**. The biopsy specimen contained disk material and parts of vertebral endplates of adjacent vertebrae. Each biopsy is examined for microorganisms and examined histopathologically.

Yang et al.[1] evaluated 15 patients with infectious spondylitis who were treated by percutaneous endoscopic diskectomy and drainage (PEDD) and associated appropriate parenteral antibiotics. The patients had presented with intractable back pain requiring narcotic pain control and bed rest. The inclusion criteria were (i) early stage spondylitis (clinical, pathological and radiological); (ii) complicated spondylitis in patients of advanced age and/or with a compromising medical condition. Patients with an infection associated with epidural abscess resulting in the neurological deficit were excluded. Thirteen patients (86.7%) reported immediate relief of back pain following PEDD. The remaining two patients, who had persistent infection and severe back pain, underwent anterior debridement with accompanied autograft interbody fusion one week and two weeks after PEDD, respectively. Of these, 13 patients who had improved, two experienced recurrent intractable pain with progressive kyphotic deformity, identified radio-

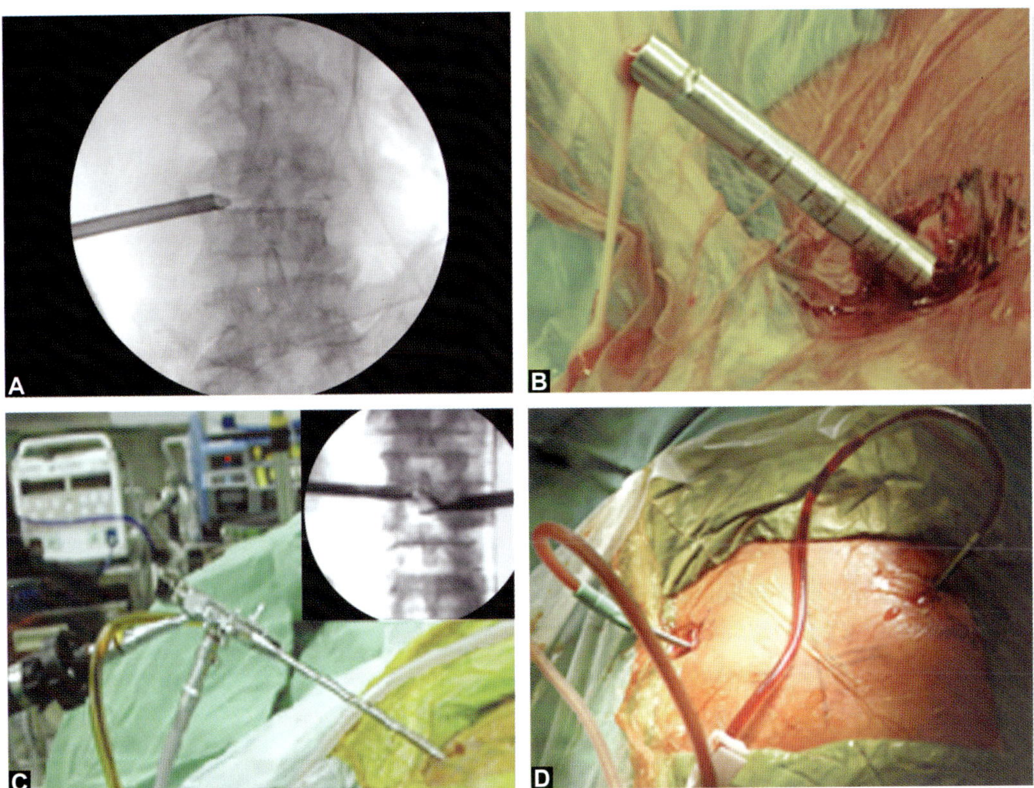

Figures 2A to D: (A and B) Cannula positioned into the disk space under fluoroscopic guidance; (C) Use of forceps and other instruments to withdraw as much infected tissue as possible; (D) After percutaneous endoscopic debridement, portal working sheaths, for continuous lavage[22]

logically, underwent surgical treatment at one month and eight months after PEDD, respectively. Causative bacteria were identified in13 (86.7%) of 15 biopsy specimens. Eleven patients responded to PEDD and were successfully treated with at least a six-week course of parenteral antibiotics therapy or full-course antimicrobial chemotherapy. However, no surgery related complications or side effects were noted during at least 12 months of follow-up. Four of 15 patients underwent anterior debridement and fusion with autograft because the pathogens or progressive infection had not been identified. Extensive osteolytic destruction of the vertebral body, with spinal instability or kyphotic deformity, was observed in these four patients. The authors concluded that PEDD is an effective alternative to spinal biopsy and should be considered prior to extensive anterior surgery for infectious spondylitis in carefully selected cases. It is especially recommended for patients with early stage spinal infection or serious medical problems.

Li-Chen Hsu et al.[22] retrospectively evaluated the clinical outcomes of bilateral portal percutaneous endoscopic debridement and lavage with a dilute povidone-iodine solution in the treatment of patients with single level lumbar pyogenic spondylitis, in 22 patients. Causative bacteria were identified in 19 (86.4%) of 22 biopsy specimens. Eighteen patients had satisfactory relief of back pain and uneventful recovery after this treatment. The success rate was 81.8% (18 of 22). Both visual analog scale and modified Mac Nab criteria scores improved significantly in successfully treated patients. No major surgical complications were noted, except for 3 patients who had residual or subsequent paresthesia in the affected lumbar segment.

Tsai-Sheng Fu et al.[23] in their study showed that PEDD is an effective alternative and should be considered prior to extensive anterior surgery for infectious spondylodiskitis, particularly in patients with early stage spinal infections or serious medical conditions

Hsin-Chuan Chen et al.[24] evaluated the safety and effectiveness of computed tomography- (CT-) assisted PEDD in the treatment of infectious spondylodiskitis of the thoracic and upper lumbar spine in 41 immuno-compromised patients. A number 5 Fr C1 angiographic catheter was placed at the affected level under CT guidance, as a guide to avoid injury to visceral organs, major vessels, and the spinal cord. Under intravenous pain control but awake, a percutaneous endoscopic guidewire was inserted directly through the angiographic catheter and advanced slowly to the infected area with the assistance of fluoroscope without penetrating the angiographic catheter wall and injuring any related structures. The angiographic catheter is now removed and sequential dilators were inserted along the endoscopic guidewire to perform PEDD. They concluded:

1. The CT-guided catheter prevents many complications normally associated with percutaneous endoscopic surgery in the thoracic and upper lumbar area.
2. This procedure has a high rate of the causative-pathogen identification and also provides good infection control and pain relief.
3. The safe and minimally invasive nature of this procedure broadens the application of operative treatment for infectious spondylodiskitis, even in the thoracic and upper lumbar level, and prevents progressive deformity when prolonged antibiotic treatment is used.
4. It is a promising and safe treatment strategy when treating patients in poor health, immunocompromised or elderly patients.
5. Neurological involvement may be the only contraindication for this procedure.

Tubular Decompression

While percutaneous endoscopic techniques are not widely used by all surgeons, surgery through a tubular retractor is a familiar technique to many spine surgeons.

Procedure

The patient is placed prone on two horizontal bolsters under general anesthesia. The level and extent of involvement are carefully evaluated on preoperative MRI studies. The entry site is then marked about one cm paramedial and a spinal needle is inserted at the disk level with the help of fluoroscopy. Skin and fascia are then incised and sequential tubular dilators (METRx, Medtronic Sofamor Danek) are used to dock an 18 mm diameter retractor tube on the inferior part of the superior lamina **(Figure 3A)**. The microscope is then brought in **(Figure 3B)**. A hemilaminectomy is completed using high-speed drilling and Kerrison rongeurs. The ligamentum is opened subsequently to release and drain the infectious material. Once spontaneous drainage ends, small angled pituitary suction tips can be connected to silastic tubing and placed down into the epidural space. Copious irrigation is performed through these tubes until all infectious material is evacuated. Drains are not placed at the completion of the procedure. Cultures are taken during the evacuation for postoperative adjustment of the patient's antibiotic regimen.

Reihsaus et al.[25] determined that laminectomy was the procedure recommended by most authors and should be performed emergently following diagnosis of spinal epidural abscess. However, laminectomy over several levels, especially in the cervicothoracic spine, and particularly in children and young adults, carries the risk of development of spinal deformity.[26-30]

Extensive SEA decompressed through conventional surgical approach requires extensive exposure and also associated with high rates of morbidity and mortality like increased blood loss, increased pain, delayed mobilization, and longer hospital stay and recovery time.[31-33] Sam Safavi-Abbasi et al.[34] described the use of minimally invasive tubular retractor system for treatment of multilevel spinal epidural abscess in 3 cases. They used tubular retractors at two or more levels for irrigation, evacuation, and drainage of multilevel SEA. Tubes were inserted at the most upper and lower levels of the SEA. A third tube may also be used in the middle of the SEA level. The patients received 4 to 6 weeks of sensitive antibiotics. Subsequent MRI after completion of therapy showed resolution of the disease process. They concluded that a minimally invasive tubular retractor system can be used safely in the thoracolumbar spine to evacuate the pus collection, avoiding multilevel laminectomies and subsequent risk of instability and extensive exposures in SEA.

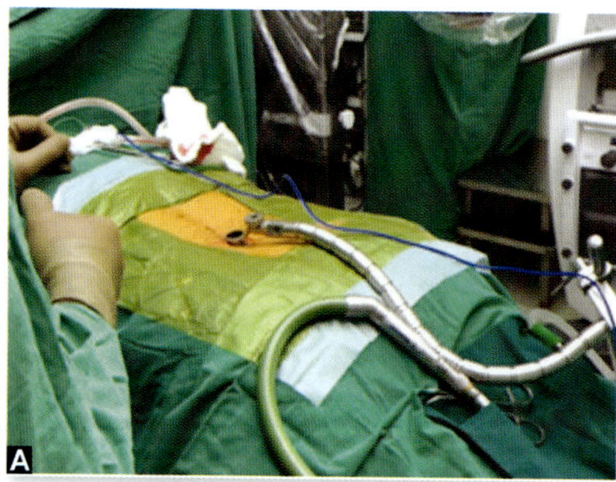

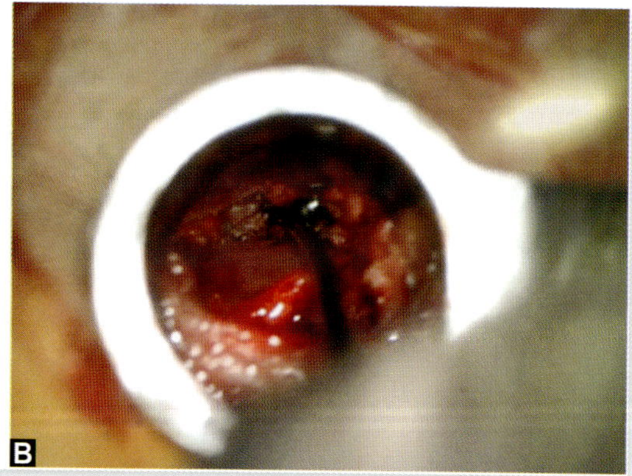

Figures 3A and B: (A) Docking of an 18 tubular retractor; (B) Microscopic view

Tubular Decompression and Interbody Fusion with Percutaneous Pedicle Screw Fixation

Posterior Transforaminal Approach

Lumbar pedicle screw fixation with transforaminal lumbar interbody fusion (TLIF) is an established, safe, and effective surgical technique in patients with infective spondylodiskitis. It provides an adequate surgical debridement and enables immediate stabilization, if necessary.[35] Nevertheless, open pedicle screw fixation with TLIF is an invasive surgical intervention that may be associated with several risks.[36] Therefore, minimally invasive techniques have been developed for degenerative diseases and have been applied in infected cases to minimize tissue damage, reduce narcotic requirements, decrease blood loss, and, therefore, potentially avoid prolonged immobilization.[37-40] This is of great interest especially in spondylodiskitis patients who frequently suffer from severe comorbidities.

Procedure

Under general anesthesia the patient is placed prone on two vertical bolsters. Two 3 cm incisions are placed approximately 4 cm paraspinal at the invovled level for passage of guidewires into the pedicles of the involved segment. The 22 mm diameter tube is docked at the ipsilateral facets over the sequential dilators. Facetectomy and hemilaminectomy are done to decompress the ipsilateral side of the spinal canal. Furthermore, the contra-lateral side of the spinal canal can also be reached if required by tilting the tube and the table toward the contralateral side. After adequate decompression, interbody fusion is performed. Ipsilateral pedicle screws are passed through the same incision and stab incisions are used for contra lateral screws. Rod is introduced with the help of a zig assembly. When using intraoperative navigation an extra-2 cm midline incision is placed at one or two level above the affected segment in order to fix the reference frame to the spinous process

Anja Tschugg et al.[41] retrospectively studied the safety and efficacy of a minimally invasive transforaminal lumbar interbody debridement and fusion plus pedicle screw fixation in lumbar spondylodiskitis and compared it to an open surgical approach. Out of 67 patients analyzed in this study,48 had undergone an open TLIF and rest underwent the same procedure through MIS technique using expandable tubular retractor. Epidural abscess detected on preoperative MRI could also be removed adequately by this surgical technique. The two groups were compared at the time of initial diagnosis, the day of admission, on the third postoperative day, before discharge, and after 3-month follow-up. Data were collected using the patients´ health records and magnetic resonance imaging (MRI). C-reactive protein (CRP), hemoglobin, and complete white cell count were analyzed routinely. Their results showed that patients who underwent MIS had significantly lower pain scores at discharge compared to patients undergoing the open surgical technique, whereas no differences could be revealed 3 months after surgery. MIS group was associated with less intraoperative blood loss and shorter hospital stay. Decision-making is predominantly based on the individual surgeon's preference and skill. The patients who were treated by the open approach were evidently sicker. Less postoperative pain before discharge was detected in the MIS group. They concluded that the open technique was effective in all varieties of spondylodiskitis inclusive in epidural abscess formation. MIS can be applied safely and effectively as well in select cases, even with an epidural abscess. Nevertheless, prospective randomized controlled clinical trials would be mandatory to develop evidence-based treatment recommendations.

Viezens L[39] retrospectively evaluated 148 patients comparing the safety and efficacy of minimally invasive and open surgery over a period of nine years. The patients were divided into two groups, 75 underwent MIS and 73 open surgery. The two groups did not differ in terms of age, body mass index, American Society of Anesthesiologists score, comorbidities, septic disease, or preoperative neurologic deficit. The two methods were associated with similar postoperative stays in the intensive care unit, overall hospital stays, complication rates, and postoperative survival. However, MIS was associated with a significantly shorter operating time, a lower perioperative need for blood products, and, as expected, and increased intraoperative fluoroscopy duration. They concluded that MIS is safe and effective for spontaneous pyogenic thoracic and lumbar spondylodiskitis.

Lateral Transpoas Lumbar Interbody Decompression and Fusion (LLIF)

The lateral retroperitoneal transpsoas approach has demonstrated utility in providing an adequate surgical corridor for interbody fusion in patients with degenerative back pain, scoliosis, spondylolisthesis, trauma, and tumor, among other indications.[42-50] Although the lateral trans-psoas approach has been effectively studied for these indications, there have been very few dedicated reports of its utility in the treatment of spinal infections.

Advantages[50-55]

1. As spondylodiskitis predominantly affects the anterior and middle columns of the lumbar spine, sparing the posterior elements, LLIF may provide an ideal treatment option because it provides a direct surgical corridor to the vertebral body without disrupting the unaffected posterior elements or traversing the neural elements and risking injury.

2. The great vessels do not have to be mobilized, as is necessary with a true anterior approach.
3. Decreased tissue trauma, blood loss, and operative time, which are further valued in the treatment of this patient population who generally present in a poor medical condition.
4. In the obese population decreases the working distance to reach the vertebral bodies, as the pannus often falls forward in the lateral position.
5. The lateral positioning is more tolerable for obese patients, as opposed to the more traditional posterior approach where they may experience decreased oxygenation and/or ventilation.

Procedure

Under general anesthesia, the patient is positioned in the standard lateral decubitus position. The level is identified under fluoroscopy. After an oblique incision, blunt dissection is used to dissect down to the level of the psoas muscle, at which point sequential dilator tubes are used to traverse the psoas. After ensuring adequate safe placement, the tubular retractor system is docked and fixed with the table mount. The disk space and vertebral bodies are then exposed and debrided extensively. Multiple cultures and specimens are sent for pathological analysis. After complete debridement and end plate preparation, interbody fusion is completed with a cage and graft. This is followed by anterior +/- posterior fixation.

Patel NB et al.[56] presented a series of 6 patients with diskitis and osteomyelitis who were surgically treated via a minimally invasive lateral transpsoas approach to the lumbar spine (DLIF/XLIF). The patients underwent debridement with a discectomy and partial or complete corpectomy, with polyetheretherketone or titanium cage placement with only two patients requiring additional posterior fixation with percutaneous pedicle screws. The postoperative CT scans demonstrated satisfactory debridement and hardware placement. All patients experienced significant pain improvement and could ambulate within a few days of surgery. The 1-year follow-up data demonstrated stable hardware with good fusion and the patients continued to have pain improvements. They concluded that due to the significant co morbidities in this patient population, a minimally invasive approach is a suitable surgical technique.

Qiyou Wang et al.[57] described the application of minimally invasive extreme lateral interbody fusion (XLIF) in combination with percutaneous pedicle screws fixation in the treatment of lumbar tuberculosis (TB) in an elderly patient. They concluded that satisfying results can be obtained with this procedure in terms of correcting spinal deformity, eradicating infection, achieving spinal decompression and obtaining functional improvement in the treatment of lumbar TB if proper surgical indications are correctly followed.

Video-assisted Thoracoscopic Surgery (VATS)

In the early 1990s, VATS techniques were applied to the treatment of spinal disease simultaneously by both Rosenthal et al. in Germany and Mack et al. in the United States.[58,59] Recently VATS have been used for management of thoracic and thoracolumbar junction pathologies, including thoracic diskherniation, fractures, tuberculosis spondylitis, idiopathic scoliosis, neuromuscular spinal deformity, congenital scoliosis, tumours.[60-79]

Advantages[62-64,66,72,74,76-79]

1. Anterior and anterolateral reconstruction can be performed to provide effective anterior load-bearing.
2. Avoids rib resection or rib retractors.
3. Excellent direct intraoperative visualization of the abnormality.
4. Treatment of multisegmental abnormality without the need for additional rib resection.
5. Avoidance of division of the diaphragm and significantly reduced injury to the chest wall.
6. Reduction of pain, better cosmetic effect, lower perioperative morbidity and an earlier return to normal activity.

Disadvantages[66-68,72-74,75,77,80]

1. Extremely steep learning curve for proper thoracoscopic surgery technique, such as, establishing proper operative orientation under the angled 2-dimensional endoscopic image and performing the operation through the smaller portals with long surgical instruments at longer distances from the target area.
2. The posterior elements, the contralateral pedicle, or contralateral transverse process cannot be exposed.
3. The costs for thoracoscopic instrumentation are high.

Complications

1. Intraoperative bleeding due to damage of the segmental vessels and intercostal vessels. It is important to identify the segmental vessels during the procedure at the midportion of the vertebral body. Although ligation of the segmental vessels is a time-consuming procedure, it eliminates catastrophic intraoperative or postoperative bleeding.
2. Transient intercostal neuralgia is the second most common complication, but it usually resolves spontaneously in one to 2 weeks.
3. Pulmonary atelectasis or pleural effusions.

4. Postoperative chylothorax is an uncommon complication, but a potentially lethal disorder).

A retrospective analysis of 38 patients with tuberculosis of dorsal and lumbar spine was done by Pankaj Kandwal et al.[81] Here, the patients were divided into two groups. Group A: 23 patients, those who had been treated with video-assisted thoracoscopic surgery (VATS) with anterior debridement and fusion (anterior/posterior) and Group B: 15 patients who had undergone posterior surgery using expanding tubular retractors and percutaneous posterior pedicle screw instrumentation. The indications of surgery in both the groups were neurological deficits not responding to antituberculous chemotherapy for 4–6 weeks or instability (anteroposterior or lateral translation; kyphosis). All the patients received antituberculous treatment (ATT) for minimum 3–4 weeks before surgery and then postoperatively for a total duration of 12 months.

Minimally invasive operative procedures in VATS group included: (1) Debridement and drainage of abscess; (2) Debridement, decompression, and reconstruction with rib graft; (3) Debridement, decompression, anterior titanium mesh cage, and posterior pedicle screw instrumentation and (4) Debridement, decompression, and anterior instrumentation. Operative procedures in group B included MISTLIF with percutaneous screws.

Good surgical decompression and interbody fusion were achieved by both the groups. Postoperative improvement in the ODI and VAS scores was significantly achieved. In VATS group the most common complication was conversion to open thoracotomy, seen in three patients. Two had prolonged (5 days) intercostal drainage tube in situ due to a persistent air leak. One patient had a superficial wound infection. In MISTLIF group, one patient reported pseudoarthrosis with screw loosening and clincoradiological evidence of persistent disease at six months of follow-up; she later improved clinically with the second line of antitubercular chemotherapy with good fusion status.

Future is Here: Intraoperative Navigation

In order to improve the identification of anatomic structure and the accuracy of pedicle screws placement, the intraoperative fluoroscopy and computed tomography-(iCT-) guided navigation has been developed and may play a significant role in MISS .

In their study, Meng-Huang Wu et al.[82] aimed to evaluate the safety and efficacy of using iCTguided navigation in simultaneous minimally invasive anterior and posterior surgery for infectious spondylitis. With the patient in lateral decubitus and the reference array fixed to the iliac crest, pedicle screws were first inserted with the aid of iCT-guided navigation. This is followed by simultaneous minimal access spinal surgery (MASS) for anterior decompression and reconstruction. The anterior spine lesions localized by

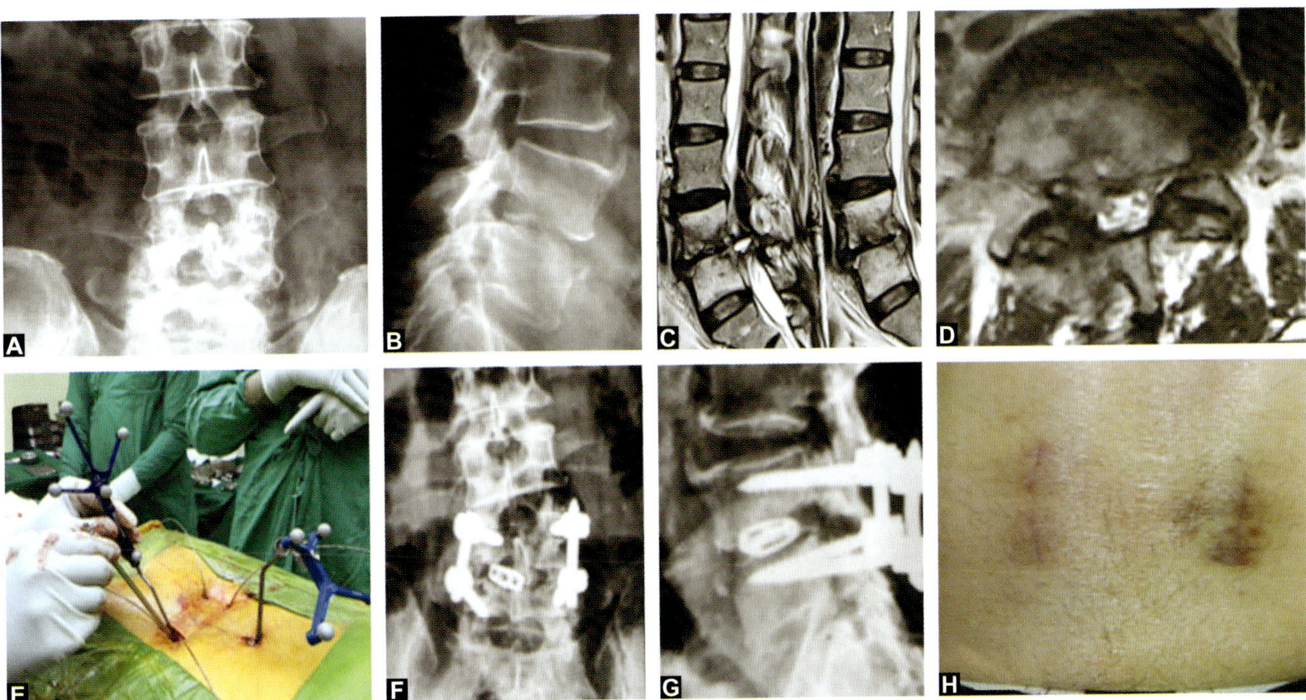

Figures 4A to H: (A to D) X-ray and MRI showing L4–L5 sponylodiskitis, in a 50-year-old male, 6 weeks postdiskectomy; (E) Introperative images showing a reference frame for the navigation at the spinous process of L2 with guidewires inserted into all four pedicles and use of a navigable probe to guide for the tubular decompression and interbody fusion; (F and G) Immediate postoperative X-rays; (H) Postoperative wound healing

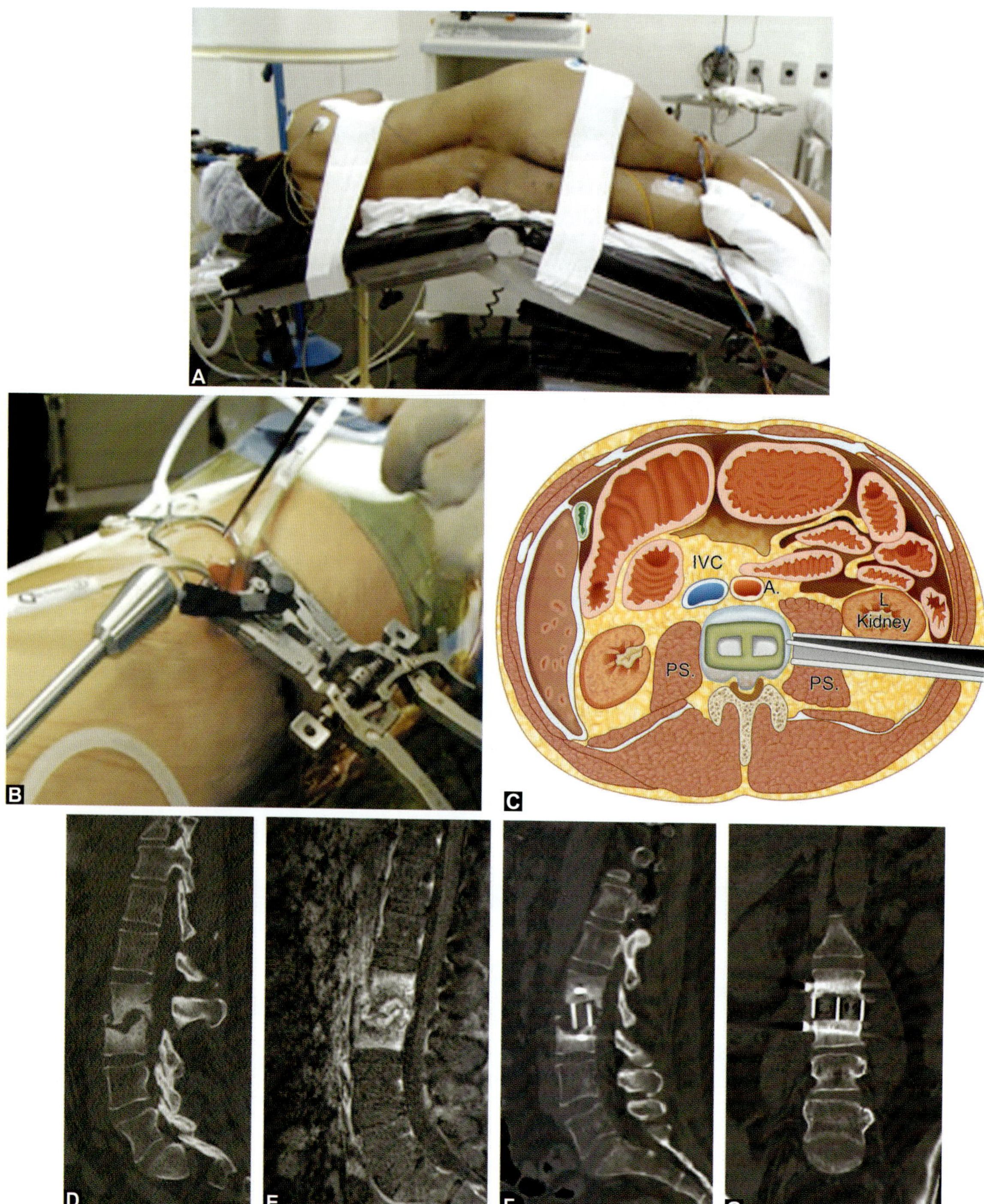

Figures 5A to G: (A) Intraoperative lateral position with a break in the table at the level of greater trochanter; (B and C) Use of tubular retractor and the trans-psoas corridor used to access the diskspace via a retroperitoneal approach; (D and E) Preoperative CT scan of the lumbar spine without contrast and T1-weighted MRI with contrast demonstrating L2–L3 spondylodiskitis; (F and G) Immediate postoperative CT scan without contrast demonstrating interval debridement with placement of a polyetheretherketone interbody graft with lateral plate and screws[56,83]

iCT-guided navigation perioperatively is targeted followed by curettage and debridement of the lesion site, obtaining tissue specimens, decompression of the epidural space, and placement of autogenous bone struts from the ilium or excised rib into the intervertebral space. Finally, the connecting rods were inserted and anchored in pedicle screw heads to achieve stabilization. Out of 54 pedicle screws employed, 53 screws were placed correctly. There was a significant improvement in terms of clinical (ODI and VAS scores); neurological (ASIA impairment scale) and radiological (Cobb's angle) parameters. They concluded that iCT-guided navigation approach can provide a good intraoperative orientation and visualization of anatomic structures and also high pedicle screw placement accuracy. The author regularly uses intraoperative navigation for the routine MISTLIF.

CONCLUSION

MIS in conjugation with intraoperative navigation is here to stay. It has proven the test of time. A transpedicular biopsy is safe and low morbid procedure that can be performed under local anesthesia with high rates of positivity. PEDD can be safely performed for early stage spinal infections without any evidence for instability with high changes of positive cultures and effective irrigation of the infected segments. Tubular decompression of the epidural abscess can be performed at multiple levels without causing instability of the involved segments. MISTLIF and LLIF can be employed in conditions demanding stabilization. VATS can be used for decompression and fixation of the affected segments but has its own set of advantages and disadvantages. MIS provides a less morbid opportunity to the already compromised individuals with the added advantages of less blood loss, lesser hospital stay and early mobilization that are essential in this group of patients. Each procedure is associated with steep learning curve and surgeon can choose any of these according to his training and the demand of the situation.

REFERENCES.

1. Yang SC, Fu TS, Chen LH, Niu CC, Lai PL, Chen WJ. Percutaneous endoscopic discectomy and drainage for infectious spondylitis. Int Orthop 2007;31:367-73.
2. Chew FS, Kline MJ. Diagnostic yield of CT-guided percutaneous aspiration procedures in suspected spontaneous infectious diskitis. Radiology. 2001;218(1):211-4.
3. Fu MJ, Chen LH, Chen WJ. Minimally invasive percutaneous endoscopic discectomy and drainage for infectious spondylodiscitis. Biomedical Journal. 2013;36(4):168-74.
4. Parker LM, McAfee PC, Fedder IL, et al. Minimally invasive surgical techniques to treat spine infections. Ortho Clin N Am 1996;27(1):183-99.
5. Rankine JJ, Barron DA, Robinson P, et al. Therapeutic impact of percutaneous spinal biopsy in spinal infection. Postgraduate Med J. 2004;80(948):607-9.
6. Staatz G, Adam GB, Keulers P, et al. Spondylodiskitic abscesses: CT-guided percutaneous catheter drainage. Radiology. 1998;208(2):363-7.
7. Kasraeian S, Allison DC, Ahlmann ER, et al. A comparison of fine-needle aspiration, core biopsy, and surgical biopsy in the diagnosis of extremity soft tissue masses. Clin Orthop Relat Res. 2010;468:2992-3002. doi: 10.1007/s11999-010-1401-x.
8. Carragee EJ. Instrumentation of the infected and unstable spine: A review of 17 cases from the thoracic and lumbar spine with pyogenic infections. J Spinal Disord. 1997;10:317-24.
9. Kulkarni AG, Bohra H, Dhruv A, Sarraf A, Bassi A, Patil VM. Minimal invasive transforaminal lumbar interbody fusion versus open transforaminal lumbar interbody fusion. Indian J Orthop. 2016;50(5):464-72.
10. Kattapuram SV, Khurana JS, Rosenthal DI. Percutaneous needle biopsy of the spine. Spine. 1992;17:561-4.
11. Fouquet B, Goupille P, Jattiot F, Cotty P, Lapierre F, Valat JP, et al. Discitis after lumbar disksurgery: Features of "aseptic" and "septic" forms. Spine. 1992;17:356-8.
12. Haaker RG, Senkal M, Kielich T, et al. Percutaneous lumbar discectomy in the treatment of lumbar discitis. Eur Spine J. 1997;6:98-101.
13. Vinicoff PG, Gutschik E, Hansen SE, et al. CT-guided spinal biopsy in spondylodiscitis. Ugeskr Laeger. 1998;160:5931-4.
14. Chooi YS, Ozlan IM Kamil, Fazir M, et al. Percutaneous Transpedicular Biopsy of the Spine. Med J Malaysia. 2007;62(1).
15. Furkan Yapici, Yunus Atici, Mehmet Bülent Balioglu, Akif Albayrak, Deniz Kargin, Yunus Emre Akman, et al. A comparison of two techniques: open and percutaneous biopsies of thoracolumbar vertebral body lesions. J Craniovertebr Junction Spine. 2015; 6(1):36-9.
16. Ashizawa R, Ohtsuka K, Kamimura M, et al. Percutaneous transpedicular biopsy of thoracic and lumbar vertebrae—method and diagnostic validity. Surg Neurol. 1999;52:545-51.
17. Dave BR, Nanda A, Anandjiwala JV. Transpedicular percutaneous biopsy of vertebral body lesions: a series of 71 cases. Spinal Cord. 2009;47:384-9. doi:10.1038/sc.2008.108; published online 23 September 2008.
18. Hermantin FU, Peters T, Quartararo L, Kambin P. A prospective, randomized study comparing the results of open discectomy with those of video-assisted arthroscopic microdiscectomy. J Bone Joint Surg Am. 1999;81:958-65.
19. Yeung AT, Tsou PM. Posterolateral endoscopic excision for lumbar diskherniation: surgical technique, outcome, and complications in 307 consecutive cases. Spine. 2002; 27:722-31.
20. Bavinzski G, Schoeggl A, Trattnig S, Standhardt H, DietrichW, Reddy M, et al. Microsurgical management of postoperative diskspace infection. Neurosurg Rev. 2003; 26:102-7.

21. Hadjipavlou AG, Mader JT, Necessary JT, et al. Hematogenous pyogenic spinal infections and their surgical management. Spine. 2000;25:1668-79.
22. Li-Chen Hsu, Tzu-Ming Tseng, Shih-Chieh Yang, Hung-Shu Chen, Cheng-Yo Yen, Yuan-Kun Tu. Bilateral Portal Percutaneous Endoscopic Debridement and Lavage for Lumbar Pyogenic Spondylitis. Orthopedics. 2015;38(10):e856-63.
23. Tsai-Sheng Fu, Lih-Hui Chen, Wen-Jer Chen. Minimally Invasive Percutaneous Endoscopic Discectomy and Drainage for Infectious Spondylodiscitis. Biomed J 2013;36:168-74.
24. Hsin-Chuan Chen, Teng-Le Huang. A Minimally Invasive Endoscopic Surgery for Infectious Spondylodiscitis of the Thoracic and Upper Lumbar Spine in Immunocompromised Patients. Bio Med Res Intern Vol. 2015; Article ID 780451. p. 8.
25. Reihsaus E, Waldbaur H, Seeling W. Spinal epidural abscess: a meta-analysis of 915 patients. Neurosurg Rev. 2000;23:175-205.
26. Aizawa T, Sato T, Ozawa H, Morozumi N, Matsumoto F, Sasaki H, et al. Sagittal alignment changes after thoracic laminectomy in adults. J Neurosurg Spine. 2008;8:510-6.
27. Fischer EG, Greene CS Jr, Winston KR. Spinal epidural absecc in children. Neurosurgery. 1981;9:257-60.
28. Lange M, Tiecks F, Schielke E, Yousry T, Haberl R, Oeckler R. Diagnosis and results of different treatment regimens in patients with spinal abscesses. Acta Neurochir (Wien). 1993;125:105-14.
29. Löhr M, Reithmeier T, Ernestus RI, et al. Spinal epidural abscess: prognostic factors and comparison of different surgical treatment strategies. Acta Neurochir (Wien). 2005;147:159-66.
30. Yasuoka S, Peterson HA, MacCarty CS. Incidence of spinal column deformity after multilevel laminectomy in children and adults. J Neurosurg. 1982;57:441-5.
31. Pradilla G, Nagahama Y, Spivak AM, et al. Spinal epidural abscess: current diagnosis and management. Curr Infect Dis Rep. 2010;12:484-91.
32. Schultz KD Jr, Comey CH, Haid RW Jr. Pyogenic spinal epidural abscess: a minimally invasive technique for multisegmental decompression. J Spinal Disord. 2001;14:546-9.
33. Tahir MZ, Hassan RU, Enam SA. Management of an extensive spinal epidural abscess from C-1 to the sacrum. Case report. J Neurosurg Spine. 2010;13:780-3.
34. Sam Safavi-Abbasi, Adrian J Maurer, Craig H Rabb. Minimally invasive treatment of multilevel spinal epidural abscess. J Neurosurg Spine. 2013;18(1):32-3.
35. Lu ML, Niu CC, Tsai TT, Fu TS, Chen LH, Chen WJ. Transforaminal lumbar interbody debridement and fusion for the treatment of infective spondylodiscitis in the lumbar spine. Eur Spine J. 2015;24:555-60.
36. Carreon LY, Puno RM, Dimar JR, et al. Perioperative complications of posterior lumbar decompression and arthrodesis in older adults. J Bone Jt Surg Am. 2003;85(11):2089-92.
37. Rieger B, Jiang H, Ruess D, Reinshagen C, Molcanyi M, Zivcak J, et al. First clinical results of minimally invasive vector lumbar interbody fusion (MIS-VLIF) in spondylodiscitis and concomitant osteoporosis: a technical note. Eur Spine J. 2016. doi:10. 1007/s00586-016-4928-z (epub 2016 Dec 27)
38. Turel MK, Kerolus M, Deutsch H. The role of minimally invasive spine surgery in the management of pyogenic spinal discitis. J Craniovertebr Junction Spine. 2017;8:39-43.
39. Viezens L, Schaefer C, Helmers R, Vettorazzi E, Schroeder M, Hansen-Algenstaedt N. Spontaneous pyogenic spondylodiscitis in the thoracic or lumbar spine: a retrospective cohort study comparing the safety and efficacy of minimally invasive and open surgery over a nine-year period. World Neurosurg. 2017. doi:10.1016/j.wneu.2017.02.129 (epub 2017 Mar 9)
40. Khan NR, Clark AJ, Lee SL, Venable GT, Rossi NB, Foley KT. Surgical outcomes for minimally invasive vs open transforaminal lumbar interbody fusion: an updated systematic review and meta-analysis. Neurosurgery. 2015;77:847-74.
41. Tschugg A, Hartmann S, Lener S, Rietzler A, Sabrina N, Thomé C. Minimally invasive spine surgery in lumbar spondylodiscitis: a retrospective single-center analysis of 67 cases. Eur Spine J. 2017. doi: 10.1007/s00586-017-5180-x. [Epub ahead of print]
42. Patel VC, Park DK, Herkowitz HN. Lateral transpsoas fusion: indications and outcomes. Sci World J. 2012;2012:893608.
43. Acosta FL, Liu J, Slimack N, et al. Changes in coronal and sagittal plane alignment following minimally invasive direct lateral interbody fusion for the treatment of degenerative lumbar disease in adults: a radiographic study. J Neurosurg Spine. 2011;15:92-6.
44. Arnold PM, Anderson KK, McGuire Jr RA. The lateral transpsoas approach to the lumbar and thoracic spine: a review. Surg Neurol Int. 2012;3:S198-215.
45. Dakwar E, Cardona RF, Smith DA, et al. Early outcomes and safety of the minimally invasive, lateral retroperitoneal transpsoas approach for adult degenerative scoliosis. Neurosurg Focus. 2010;28:E8.
46. Eck JC. Minimally invasive corpectomy and posterior stabilization for lumbar burst fracture. Spine J. 2011;11:904-8.
47. Isaacs RE, Hyde J, Goodrich JA, et al. A prospective, nonrandomized, multicenter evaluation of extreme lateral interbody fusion for the treatment of adult degenerative scoliosis: perioperative outcomes and complications. Spine (Phila Pa 1976). 2010;35:S322-30.

48. Karikari IO, Nimjee SM, Hardin CA, et al. Extreme lateral interbody fusion approach for isolated thoracic and thoracolumbar spine diseases: initial clinical experience and early outcomes. J Spinal Disord Tech. 2011;24:368-75.
49. Marchi L, Abdala N, Oliveira L, et al. Stand-alone lateral interbody fusion for the treatment of low-grade degenerative spondylolisthesis. Sci World J. 2012;2012:456346.
50. Ozgur BM, Aryan HE, Pimenta L, et al. Extreme Lateral Interbody Fusion (XLIF): a novel surgical technique for anterior lumbar interbody fusion. Spine J. 2006;6:435-43.
51. Hatzenbuehler J, Pulling TJ. Diagnosis and management of osteomyelitis. Am Fam Physician. 2011;84:1027-33.
52. Lew DP, Waldvogel FA. Osteomyelitis. Lancet. 2004;364:369-79.
53. Mann S, Schutze M, Sola S, et al. Nonspecific pyogenic spondylodiscitis: clinical manifestations, surgical treatment, and outcome in 24 patients. Neurosurg Focus. 2004;17:E3.
54. Mylona E, Samarkos M, Kakalou E, et al. Pyogenic vertebral osteomyelitis: a systematic review of clinical characteristics. Semin Arthritis Rheum. 2009;39:10-7.
55. Moller DJ, Slimack NP, Acosta Jr FL, et al. Minimally invasive lateral lumbar interbody fusion and transpsoas approach-related morbidity. Neurosurg Focus. 2011;31:E4.
56. Neal B Patel, Zachary H Dodd, Jason Voorhies, Eric M Horn. Minimally invasive lateral transpsoas approach for spinal discitis and osteomyelitis. Journal of Clinical Neuroscience. 2015; 22:1753-7.
57. Qiyou Wang, Yichun Xu, Ruiqiang Chen, Jianwen Dong, Bin Liu, Limin Rong. A novel indication for a method in the treatment of lumbar tuberculosis through minimally invasive extreme lateral interbody fusion (XLIF) in combination with percutaneous pedicle screws fixation in an elderly patient. A case report. Medicine (Baltimore). 2016; 95(48): e5303. Published online 2016 Dec 2. doi: 10.1097/MD.0000000000005303.
58. Rosenthal D, Dickman CA. Thoracoscopic microsurgical excision of herniated thoracic discs. J Neurosurg. 1998;89:224-35.
59. Mack MJ, Aronoff RJ, Acuff TE, Ryan WH. Thoracoscopic transdiaphragmatic approach for adrenal biopsy. Ann Thorac Surg. 1993;55:772-3.
60. Al-Sayyad MJ, Crawford AH, Wolf RK. Early experiences with video-assisted thoracoscopic surgery : our first 70 cases. Spine. 2004;29:1945-51.
61. Benli IT, Alanay A, Akalin S, Kis M, Acaroglu E, Ates B, et al. Comparison of anterior instrumentation systems and the results of minimum 5 years follow-up in the treatment of tuberculosis spondylitis. Kobe J Med Sci. 2004;50:167-80.
62. Connelly CS, Manges PA. Video-assisted thoracoscopic discectomy and fusion. AORN J. 1998;67:940-52.
63. Dickman CA, Rosenthal D, Karahalios DG, Paramore CG, Mican CA, Apostolides PJ, et al. Thoracic vertebrectomy and reconstruction using a microsurgical thoracoscopic approach. Neurosurgery. 1996;38:279-93.
64. Han PP, Kenny K, Dickman CA. Thoracoscopic approaches to the thoracic spine: experience with 241 surgical procedures. Neurosurgery. 2002;51(Suppl):88 95.
65. Horn EM, Henn JS, Lemole GM, Jr, Hott JS, Dickman CA. Thoracoscopic placement of dual-rod instrumentation in thoracic spinal trauma. Neurosurgery. 2004;54:1150-3.
66. Huang TJ, Hsu RW, Liu HP, Hsu KY, Liao YS, Shih HN, et al. Video-assisted thoracoscopic treatment of spinal lesions in the thoracolumbar junction. Surg Endosc. 1997;11:1189-93.
67. Huang TJ, Hsu RW, Liu HP, Liao YS, Hsu KY, Shih HN. Analysis of techniques for video-assisted thoracoscopic internal fixation of the spine. Arch Orthop Trauma Surg. 1998;117:92-5.
68. Huang TJ, Hsu RW, Liu HP, et al. Technique of video-assisted thoracoscopic surgery for the spine: new approach. World J Surg. 1997;21:358-62.
69. Huang TJ, Hsu RW, Liu HP, Shih HN, Liao YS, Hsu KY, et al. Video-assisted thoracoscopic surgery to the upper thoracic spine. Surg Endosc. 1999;13:123-6.
70. Huang TJ, Hsu RW, Sum CW, Liu HP. Complications in thoracoscopic spinal surgery: a study of 90 consecutive patients. Surg Endosc. 1999;13:346-50.
71. Ishikawa E, Matsumura A, Ishikawa S, et al. Combined minimally invasive approach using microsurgery and thoracoscopic surgery for resecting a dumbbell-type thoracic schwannoma. Minim Invasive Neurosurg. 2002;45:251-3.
72. Johnson JP, Filler AG, Mc Bride DQ. Endoscopic thoracic discectomy. Neurosurg Focus. 2000;9:E11.
73. Khoo LT, Beisse R, Potulski M. Thoracoscopic-assisted treatment of thoracic and lumbar fractures: a series of 371 consecutive cases. Neurosurgery. 2002;51(Suppl):S104-17.
74. Kim DH, Jahng TA, Balabhadra RS, et al. Thoracoscopic transdiaphragmatic approach to thoracolumbar junction fractures. Spine J. 2004;4:317-28.
75. Lonner BS, Kondrachov D, Siddiqi F, et al. Thoracoscopic spinal fusion compared with posterior spinal fusion for the treatment of thoracic adolescent idiopathic scoliosis. Surgical technique. J Bone Joint Surg Am. 2007;89(Suppl):142-56.
76. Mack MJ, Regan JJ, McAfee PC, Picetti G, Ben-Yishay A, Acuff TE. Video-assisted thoracic surgery for the anterior approach to the thoracic spine. Ann Thorac Surg. 1995;59:1100-6.
77. Niemeyer T, Freeman BJ, Grevitt MP, Webb JK. Anterior thoracoscopic surgery followed by posterior instrumentation and fusion in spinal deformity. Eur Spine J. 2000;9:499-504.

78. Son-Hing JP, Blakemore LC, Poe-Kochert C, Thompson GH. Video-assisted thoracoscopic surgery in idiopathic scoliosis: evaluation of the learning curve. Spine. 2007;32:703-7.
79. Visocchi M, Masferrer R, Sonntag VK, Dickman CA. Thoracoscopic approaches to the thoracic spine. Acta neurochirurgica. 1998;140:737-43.
80. Lonner BS, Scharf C, Antonacci D, et al. The learning curve associated with thoracoscopic spinal instrumentation. Spine. 2005;30:2835-40.
81. Kandwal P, Garg B, Upendra B, et al. Outcome of minimally invasive surgery in the management of tuberculous spondylitis. Indian J Orthop. 2012;46:159-64.
82. Meng-Huang Wu, Navneet Kumar Dubey, Ching-Yu Lee, et al. Application of Intraoperative CT-Guided Navigation in Simultaneous Minimally Invasive Anterior and Posterior Surgery for Infectious Spondylitis. Bio Med Res Intern Vol. 2017. Article ID 2302395. p. 7. doi:10.1155/2017/2302395.
83. Abhijit Pawar, Alexander Hughes, Federico Girardi, Andrew Sama, Darren Lebl, Frank Cammisa. Lateral Lumbar Interbody Fusion. Asian Spine J. 2015;9(6):978-83. PMCID: PMC4686408.

31

CHAPTER

Minimally Invasive Spine Surgery for Spinal Intradural Tumors

Alok Ranjan, Rahul Lath

ABSTRACT

Intradural tumors are commonly found in the dorsal spine with equal distribution between cervical and lumbar region. Conventional techniques of excision of tumors involved wide laminectomy and extensive soft-tissue dissection. This had resulted in instability and other tissue-related complications. The use of minimally invasive techniques in dealing with intradural tumors has revolutionized the approach toward the intradural tumors management. The advantages of minimally invasive techniques are lesser tissue trauma, shorter incision and faster rehabilitation.This chapter deals with the management of intradural tumors through minimal access.

INTRODUCTION

The incidence of spinal intradural tumors is about 3–10 per 100,000.[1,2] Nerve sheath tumors (neurofibromas and schwannomas) and meningiomas constitute 80% of all the intradural tumors. They are generally moderate in size and eccentrically placed. They are occur commonly in the dorsal spine and are proportionately distributed in cervical and lumbar spine as well. 15% of the intradural tumors are myxopapillary ependymomas, while the remaining 5% include other tumors.[1] Intramedullary spinal cord tumors constitute 15% of all intradural tumors in the adults.[3] The common intramedullary tumors are ependymomas in adults and astrocytomas in children.

The traditional surgical approach to spinal intradural pathology is midline and Involves a Standard laminectomy.[1,3] A subperiosteal paraspinal muscle dissection is followed by removal of the spinous process, interspinous ligament, ligamentum flavum and a complete laminectomy which extends to one level above and below the lesion. In case of dumbbell tumors with foraminal and extraspinal extension a facetectomy may be required. This could result in instability requiring a spinal fusion. Large series with long-term follow-up have shown surgical complication rate of 10% and delayed instability in 6% of the patients.[4] This has led to the development of minimally invasive approaches in which a hemilaminectomy with minimal removal of the facets has been suggested.[5,6]

The tubular retraction system was introduced in 1997 by Foley and Smithfor endoscopic diskectomy.[7] Following this a variety of nonexpandable and expandable tubular retractors have been developed for minimally invasive spine surgery (MIS) (**Table 1**). The nonexpandable tubes have a fixed diametre and are used for single level procedures. The expandable systems have blades which can open in the cephalocaudal directon and in the mediolateral direction increasing the exposure. The blades can be angulated from 10 to 30 degrees improving visualization in the depth. Tredway et al. in 2006 used the X-tube for removal of spinal intradural extramedullary tumors.[2] Subsequently other authors have also used the tubular systems for removal of intradural spinal tumors and other spinal pathologies.[8-14] The results of these reports are summarized in **Table 2**.

ADVANTAGES

The advantages of MIS include shorter incision, less pain due to muscle splitting, less blood loss, early ambulation, short hospital stay and early return to work.[2,11,15] Additionally, the other advantage of MIS is that the chances of postoperative instability requiring a fusion procedure are reduced.

DISADVANTAGES

The exact confirmation of level with fluoroscopy is mandatory in MISS. Exact extant of tumor location should match the fully deployed retractor system. Even with fluoroscopy wrong level surgery is possible which occasionally requires conversion to an open surgery.[9] Dural closure is difficult

Table 1

Tubular and expandable retractor systems

Retractor system	Company	Expandable	Workinglenth/Diametre	Blade angulation
Metrx tubes	Medtronic	No	16–18 mm diameter	N/A
X-tube	Medtronic	Yes	26 mm diameter	Yes
Mast quadrant	Medtronic	Yes	30–52 mm visualization	Yes
Spotlight acess	DePuy	No	18–24 mm diameter	N/A
Pipeline	DePuy	Yes	19 mm inner diametre	Yes
(Cephalocaudal 2 level expansion)				
MARS™ port	Globus	No	Variable diameter	N/A
MARS™ 3V	Globus	Yes	18–60 mm exposure	Yes
Insight access tube	Synthes	No	16–28 mm diameter	N/A
Insight access retractor	Synthes	Yes	19–50mm expansion	Yes

N/A – not applicable

Table 2

Review of the case series of MIS for intradural tumors

Author/ year	No of patients	Pathology	System	Mean blood loss (mL)	Mean OT	Mean hospital stay	Complications	GTR (%)	Follow-up	Outcome improved
Tredway et al. (2006)	6	ID-EM	X tube	56	247 minutes	57 Hours	Nil	100	11.3 months	100%
Ogden/ Fessler (2009)	1	ID-IM	X tube	NA	NA	6 days	Nil	100	6 months	NA
Manion et al. (2011)	13	ID-EM	Quadrant and X tube	155	2.5 hours	3.1 days	Wrong level 2 CSF leak 1 Pseudomenin-gocoele 1 Conversion 1	100	1–2 years	100%
Haji et al. (2011)	20 patients with 22 tumors	ID-EM, ED	Quadrant	428	210 minutes	3 days	CSF leak 1 Foot drop 1	68	6 weeks	95% (19/20)
Lu et al. (2011)	18	ID-EM, ID-IM	Pieline	153	239 minutes	4.9 days	Pseudomenin-gocoele 1	94.4	16 months	Functional improvement 100%
Dahlberg et al. (2012)	9	ID-EM	Quadrant	<200 in 9, 200-400 mL in 2	126 minutes	NA	Sensory deficit 2	100	9–38 months	78% (7/9)
Nzokou et al. (2013	13	ID-EM, ED	Spotlight	219	189 minutes	66 hours	Nil	12/13 (92)	21	92%
Gandhi et al. (2013)	26 patients 27 surger-ies	ID-EM ID-IM non tumor	Quadrant	197	213 minutes	3 days	Meningitis 1 wound break 1 redo 1	11/14 tumor 78.5	474 days	92%

Abbreviations: ID, intradural; EM, extramedullary; IM, intramedullary; ED, extradural; OT, operation time; GTR, gross total resection; NA, not available.

due to limited space and may require a patch with dural sealant if primary closure is not possible. Some authors have used special applicators for dural closure.[9] Presently MIS is limited to tumor which extends over 3 or lesser levels. It can be done for dorsal or dorsolaterally placed tumors but it would be difficult for purely ventral tumors. Recurrent tumors have scar tissue and for these the open approach is still preferred.

The complications reported with MIS procedures for intradural tumors are wrong level surgery, CSF leak with pseudomeningocoele formation, incomplete resection, new neurological deficit, meningitis and wound dehiscence.[9-12,14]

Techniqueusing the Metrx tube and Mast Quadrant System (Medtronic, Memphis, TN): The decision to do MIS for spinal intradural tumor is based on the size, location and pathology **(Table 3)**. Following induction the patient is positioned in prone position. The tumor is approached from the left or right depending upon its location. A paramedian approach is used at the involved level which is confirmed with fluoroscopy. The incision is made 1.5–2.5 cm lateral to the midline. A K-wire is used to start the procedure and confirm the level under fluoroscopic guidance. Serial dilators **(Figure 1)** are used to split the muscle following which the Mast Quadrant retractors are placed and the blades are expanded to the desired length and then angulated to maximize the exposure **(Figures 2 and 3)**. The operating microscope is brought in and a high speed drill is used for the hemilaminectomy which can be extended to one level above and below **(Figure 4)**. Dura is opened and the tumor is excised using standard microsurgical techniques **(Figure 5)**. Larger tumors may have to be decompressed with the CUSA prior to dissection and removal. Following the hemostasis, watertight dural closure is done and a dural sealant (TISSEL, Baxter) is used to reinforce the closure **(Figure 6)**. With the non-expandable tubular systems, dural closure can be a challenge and authors have used a knot pusher to assist in the closure.[2,13] Some authors have used dural substitutes for the closure while Mannion et al. have used non penetrating titanium clips for dural closure.[9,14] Following dural closure the retractor system is removed

Table 3

Relative indications and contraindications for MIS in intradural tumors

The right case for MIS intradural tumor surgery
• Tumorless than 3 spinal levels
• Benign tumors, such as schwannoma and neurofibroma
• Eccentric location of tumor
• Where spinal cord manipulation or retraction is not needed
• Lumbar region is the best location.
The wrong case for MIS intradural tumor surgery
• Large intramedullary tumor where radical surgery is the goal.
• Intradural tumor where prognosis changes if radical surgery without spilling the operative field is of immense importance, such as in myxopapillary ependymoma.
• Tumor with significant vascularity
• Ventrally located tumor in relationship to spinal cord in cervical and dorsal spine
• Where spinal cord retraction or significant manipulation is anticipated
• Recurrent tumor with presence of scar tissue.

Figure 1: Serial dilators being applied

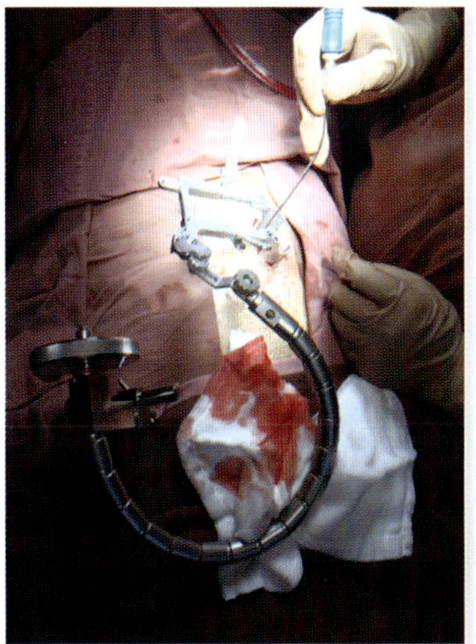

Figure 2: Mast quadrant system opened

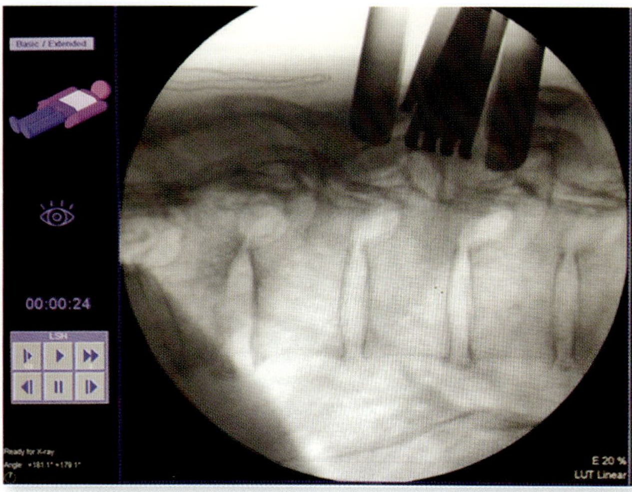

Figure 3: Retractor blades opened and level confirmed under fluoroscopy

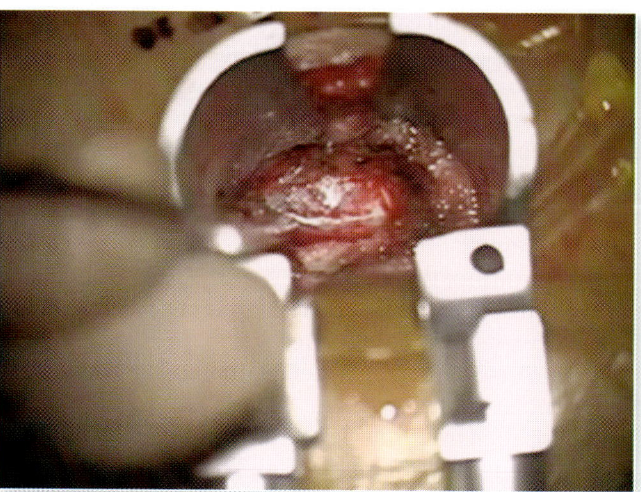

Figure 4: Hemilaminectomy done and dura exposed

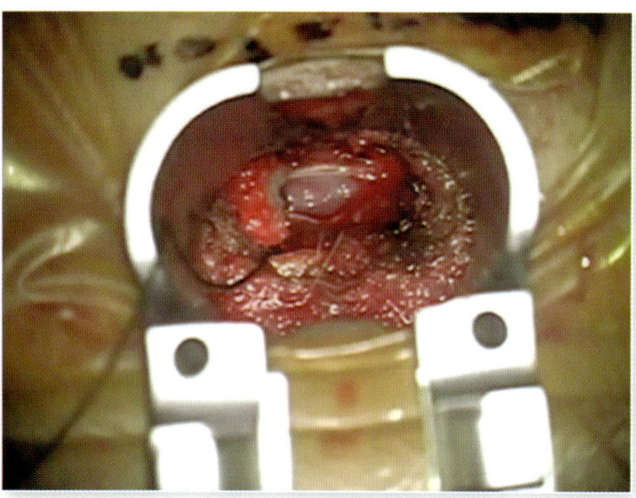

Figure 5: Dural opening

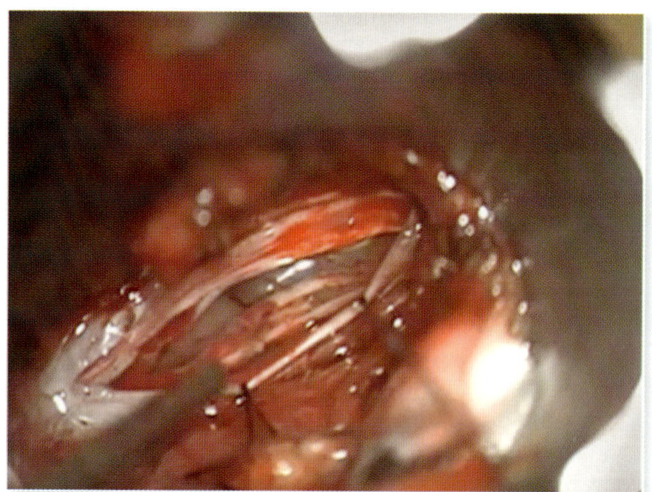

Figure 6: Dural retraction and exposure of tumor

and the muscle layers closes automatically over wound obliterating any dead space. For tumors that have foraminal and extraspinal extension, a facetectomy is done and if there is instability a fusion can be done with percutaneous pedicle screw systems like the Sextant (Medtronic, Memphis,TN).[9] The technique of dural closure and essential steps of the surgery are summarized in **Tables 4 and 5**.

FUTURE DIRECTIONS

Image-guided navigation, the O-arm and MIS robotic spine surgery are being used increasingly in the MIS procedures[15] and have also been used for spinal intradural tumors.[9]

CASE ILLUSTRATION

An illustrative case of MIS for intradural tumor is presented. A 33-years old lady presented with back pain and paresthesiain the left lower limb. MRI showed an intradural tumor at the L3 level more towards the left side **(Figure 7)**. There were no postoperative complications and the postoperative MRI showed complete excision of the tumor with the left hemilaminectomy and intact midline structures and the facet **(Figure 8)**.

Table 4

Various techniques of dural closure

1. Arachnoid can be closed using a very low current holding the two blades of the bipolar together.
2. Dura can be closed using 7/0 ethilon.
3. Dura can be approximated by using titanium clips.
4. Fibrin glue is an important addition.
5. If there is a dural defect then an appropriately sized fascia or dural substitute can be overlayed and fibrin glue applied.
6. Fascia can be obtained either from fascia lata or by extending the skin incision and harvesting from under the skin without disturbing the retractor system.

Table 5

Essential steps during surgery

1. Fluroscopic localization is the single most important surgical step in MIS surgery.
2. No part of tumor should be out of operating field and this should be determined by fluoroscopic confirmation in relationship to the MRI scan
3. Retraction system is on one side of midline and spinous process. Entry should be on the side of tumor as seen in MRI scan.
4. Adequate bone drilling, undercutting the spinous process in midline, and avoiding facetal distruction laterally has to be done prior to the dural incision.
5. Confirming that adequacy of dural exposre in relationship to tumor extent is mandatory prior to opening the dura.
6. Extradural hemostasis is done prior to opening the dura by using bone wax, bipolar coagulation and surgical technique. Once the dura is opened and CSF comes out, the extradural oozing will be more due to decompression of extradural bleeding points.
7. Dural opening should be more towards midline as dural retraction is technically easier on lateral side using hitch stiches to retract the dura by hitching to muscle. Special care to be taken during MIS tumor excision.
8. The vascular pedicle has to be completely coagulated and then cut as the nerve root retracts out of operating field and subsequent hemostasis would be difficult.
9. Retraction of spinal cord (in the thoracic and region) is to be avoided as the degree of retraction is difficult to control.

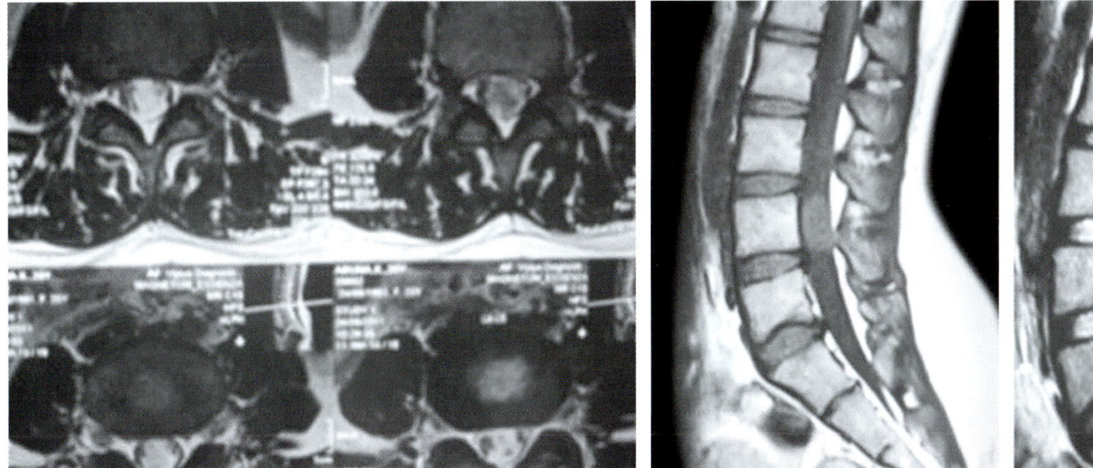

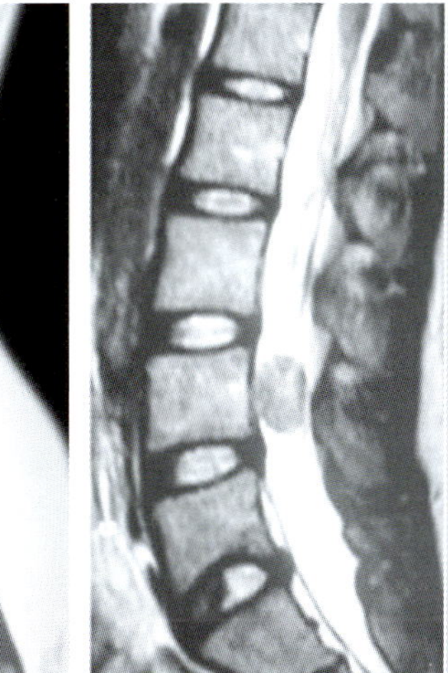

Figure 7: Preoperative axial and sagittal MRI showing an intradural tumor at L4 level

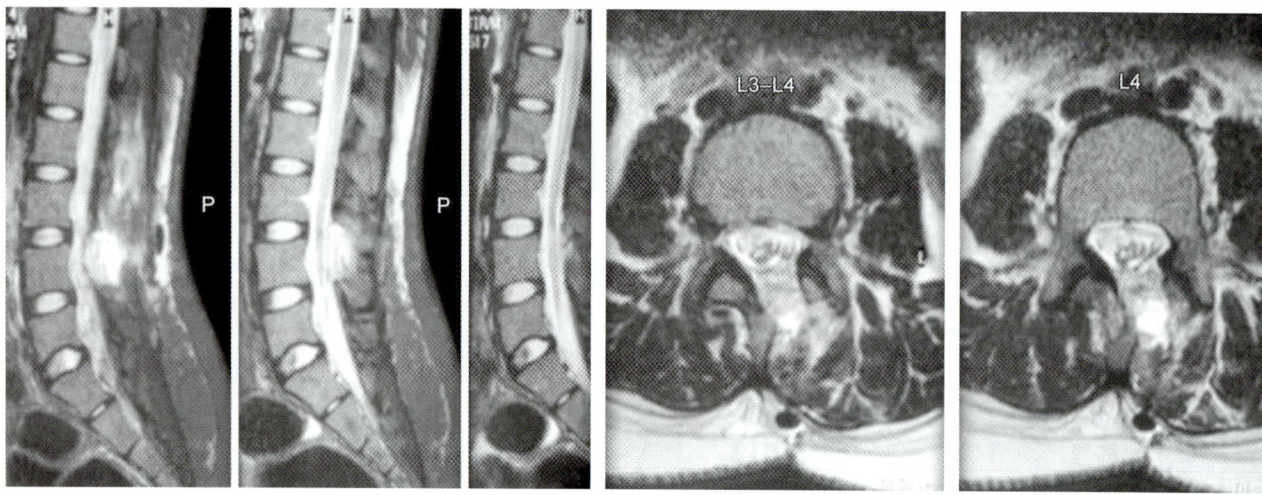

Figure 8: Postoperative axial and sagittal T2 MRI showing complete excision of tumor with a left hemilaminectomy and intact midline structures and facet joint

REFERENCES

1. Agrawal BM, Birch BD, McCormick PC, Resnick DK. Intradural Extramedullary Spinal Lesions. Chapter 102 Spine Surgery Third edition. Benzel EC. Elsevier–Saunders: Philadelphia. 2012;(2):991-8.
2. Tredway TL, Santiago P, Hrubes MR, Song JK, Christie SD, Fessler RG. Minimally invasive resection of intradural-extra-medullary spinal neoplasms. Neurosurgery. 2006;58 (1 Suppl): ONS52–ONS58.
3. McCormick P. Intradural Extramedullary Tumors. Chapter 187. In Schmidek and Sweet Operative Neurosurgical Techniques Sixth edition Volume 2. Ed:Quinones-Hinojosa A Elsevier Saunders Philadelphia. 2012. p. 2127-33.
4. Seppala MT, Haltia MJ, Sankila RJ, Jaaskelainen JE, Heiskanen O. Long-term outcome after removal of spinal schwannoma: a clinicopathological study of 187 cases. J Neurosurg. 1995;83:621-6.
5. Oktem IS, Akdemir H, Kurtsoy A, Koc RK, Menku A, Tucer B. Hemilaminectomy for the removal of spinal lesions. Spinal Cord. 2000;38:92-6.
6. Pompili A, Caroli F, Cattani F, Crecco M Giovanetti M, Raus L et al. Unilateral limited laminectomy as the approach of choice for the removal of thoracolumbar neurofibromas. Spine. 2004;29:1698-702.
7. Foley KT, Smith MM. Microendoscopic discectomy. Tech Neurosurg. 1997;3(4):301-7.
8. Ogden AT, Fessler RG. Minimally invasive resection of intramedullary ependymoma: case report. Neurosurgery. 2009;65:E1203-4.
9. Mannion RJ, Nowitzke AM, Efendy J, Wood MJ. Safety and efficacy of intraduralextramedullary spinal tumor removal us- ing a minimally invasive approach. Neurosurgery. 2011;68 (1 Suppl Operative):208-16.
10. Haji FA, Cenic A, Crevier L, Murty N, Reddy K. Minimally invasive approach for the resection of spinal neoplasm. Spine (Phila Pa 1976). 2011;36:E1018-26.
11. Lu DC, Chou D, Mummaneni PV. A comparison of mini- open and open approaches for resection of thoracolumbar intradural spinal tumors. Clinical article. J Neurosurg Spine. 2011;14:758-64.
12. Dahlberg D, Halvorsen CM, Lied B, Helseth E. Minimally invasive microsurgical resection of primary, intradural spinal tumors using a tubular retraction system. Br J Neurosurg. 2012;26(4):472-5. doi: 10.3109/02688697.2011.644823. Epub 2012 Jan 12.
13. Nzokou A, Weil AG, Shedid D. Minimally invasive removal of thoracic and lumbar spinal tumors using a nonexpandable tubular retractor. J Neurosurg Spine. 2013;19:708-15.
14. Gandhi RH, German JW. Minimally invasive approach for the treatment of intradural spinal pathology. Neurosurg Focus. 2013;35(2):E5.
15. O'Toole JE. The future of minimally invasive spine surgery. Chapter 4. Clinical Neurosurgery. 2013;60:13-9.

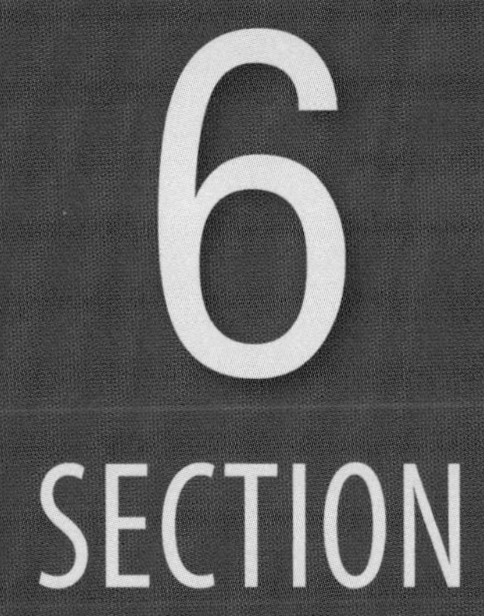

Pain Management

Section Outline

32

CHAPTER

Epidural Steroid Injection

DK Baheti

ABSTRACT

Epidural steroid injections (ESI) is here to stay as conservative treatment approach for chronic back pain as they have benefitted millions of patients suffering of back pain. There are two different ways to do EPI: one is transforaminal and another is interlaminar.

The use of fluoroscopy for ESI has added new dimension for perfection and to have maximum pain relief. ESI can be given via cervical, lumbar and caudal routes.

This chapter describes these procedures in a stepwise manner and also highlights the protocol, indications and contraindications of transforminal ESIs.

INTRODUCTION

Epidural steroid injection (ESI) are the placement of steroids into the epidural space and for many years they have benefitted millions of patients for the treatment of axial and radicular back pain.[1] they are of diagnostic and therapeutic purpose.

Earlier or even today, ESIs are done in consulting rooms with a "blind approach"; i.e. without the fluoroscopy. The author strongly believes that any interventional pain treatment procedure without fluoroscopy is unethical and dangerous to the life of patient. On top of it the blind approach has fallacies, such as it does not confirm placement of needle and drug may not reach the target, i.e. nerve root. The unexpected reaction to local anesthesia and possibility of vasovagal reactions are always there. It is unethical medicolegally too.

With the advent of fluoroscopy, the transforaminal approach the ESIs has become widespread and more effective as drug is delivered accurately to the site of pathology. Although efficacy of epidural steroids still remains controversial. Some studies reported significant improvement of symptoms.[2,3] A meta-analysis of the epidural steroid injection literature from 1996 to 1993 revealed a 14% positive treatment effect over placebo.[4,5]

HOW DOES EPIDURAL STEROID INJECTION WORK?

The basis behind the use of epidural steroid injections is that chemical mediators are released from a disk after injury to that disk. This results in the release of phospholipase A2 (PLA2) from the nucleus pulposus into the epidural space.[6] PLA2 is an enzyme found in high concentrations in disk material and is highly inflammatogenic and propagates an inflammatory cascade with the liberation of arachidonic acid with inflammatory responses via leukotrienes and prostaglandins.

The epidural steroids act by blocking PLA2 activity and can exert an anesthetic like activity by blocking nociceptive C-fiber conduction.[7] This effect is reversed when the corticosteroid is removed, suggesting a direct membrane effect. The neither glucocorticoid receptor sites have also been located on nor epinephrine and 5-hydroxytryptamine neurons within the dorsal horn substantia gelatinosa.[8]

Anatomy of Epidural Space

The epidural space lies between the osseoligamentous structures lining the vertebral canal and the dural membrane surrounding the spinal cord and the nerve roots.[9] The anterior epidural space is bordered anteriorly by the vertebral body, intervertebral disk; and posterior longitudinal ligament and posteriorly by the thecal sac. The posterior epidural space is bordered anteriorly by the thecal sac and posteriorly by the ligamentum flavum and the laminae. Each spinal nerve exists within an intervertebral foramen, bordered anteriorly by the vertebral body and the disk, posteriorly by the facet joint, and superiorly and inferiorly by the pedicles of the adjacent vertebrae.

Evaluation

Evaluation of a patient with back pain should begin with a detailed history and physical examination. Inquire about the type, intensity of pain along with radicular symptoms to the extremities, including pain, numbness, paresthesiae, or weakness. Pain may be associated with neurogenic claudication. One should also look for presence of red flags, such as footdrop, motor paralysis then it is an emergency, so refer to spine or neurosurgeon.

The physical examination may reveal paresthesiae in a dermatomal distribution, weakness in a myotomal distribution, and a positive straight-leg raise (SLR).

It is mandatory to correlate the clinical findings with the imaging study findings, such as X-rays, MRI for correct diagnosis and to decide the type of ESI to achieve maximum benefit.

The electrodiagnostic signs of radiculopathy may be helpful, but are not an absolute prerequisite to ESIs.

In some patients is necessary to perform facet block or by provocative diskography to decide source of pain before radiofrequency ablation of medial branch or to know the level of diskogenic pain.

Indications and Applications

The main clinical indications for epidural steroid injections include:

1. Disk degeneration or herniation, spinal nerve root compression.
2. Spinal nerve root inflammation.
3. Spinal stenosis.
4. Case of radiculopathy has not responded to nonsurgical conservative measures, and whose pain is likely to have an inflammatory basis.

Contraindications

Absolute Contraindications

Absolute contraindications to epidural steroid injections include:

1. Presence of **Red flags,** such as footdrop, motor paralysis.
2. Unwilling patient to consent to the procedure.
3. Evidence of an untreated infection at the site of the injection.
4. Pregnancy
5. Bleeding diathesis.

Relative Contraindications

1. Known allergy to the medications and dye
2. Concurrent use of anticoagulant medication
3. Known systemic infection
4. Immunosuppresion
5. Severe respiratory or cardiovascular compromised patient.
6. Anatomic, congenital or surgical changes preventing safe administration of medication into the epidural space.
7. If the patient has a known allergy to the medications used for the procedure, premedication may then be required depending on the severity of the allergic reaction.

Equipments

1. C-arm fluoroscope with printer.
2. Lead aprons, thyroid shield, eye cover, radiation gloves
3. Tuohy epidural needles 16 or 18 gauge with LOR syringe-for interlaminar.
4. Spinal needle, 22 or 23 gauge short bevel needle (transforaminal).
5. 25 gauge 1.5-inch needle for administration of local anesthetic.
6. Leur lock syringe 3 mL, 5 mL,10 mL and extension tubing 10/25 cm.

Medications

a. Normal saline
b. Water soluble, non-ionic radiographic contrast medium (Omnipaque).
c. Inj. Xylocard (preservative-free xylocaine) or bupivicaine (0.125%–0.5%).
d. Inj. Aurocort (preservative free corticosteroid-preferably) or triamcinolone, betamethasone 6–18 mg, Depomedrol 20–80 mg or dexamethasone.
e. Injection hylase or hyaluronidase for caudal adhesiolysis

Suggested Volume for ESIs

1. Interlaminar: 6–8 mL
2. Transforaminal:1 cc per nerve root, i.e. 10 mg of steroid with normal saline (author prefers to dilute steroid with normal saline).
4. Caudal: 5–10 mL.

Protocol[10]

The suggested protocol is as follows:

Preprocedure Check

1. Evaluation and documentation of history, symptoms, signs and investigations such as X-ray, CT scan, MRI, electromyography, nerve conduction study.
2. Explain the procedure details, side effects, complications, if any to patient and relatives.
3. Informed consent must be explained in the language in which patient and his relatives understand, before signing of informed consent form.
4. Hospital admission for few hours to few days as the case may be.
5. Investigations, such as bleeding time, clotting time, INR ratio (if patient on anticoagulants); HIV HCV and HbSAg.
6. Interventional pain treatment procedure (IPTP) should be done either in operating room or procedure room equipped with monitoring and resuscitation facilities
7. Anesthetist stand by and sedation, if necessary
8. Monitoring of blood pressure, pulse, NIBP, and SaO_2 all the time
9. Secure IV line and IV antibiotic cover
10. Aseptic precaution, such as wearing of gown, gloves, preparation of the area.
11. Lead gowns along with thyroid shield, radiation counter and radiation gloves for all procedure or operating room.
12. Keep talking to the patient while performing the procedure to allay the fear and anxiety.
13. Follow **Rule of three Ds,** i.e. Direction, Depth, and Destination. Aim for **Tunnel vision.**

APPROACHES FOR CERVICAL OR LUMBAR EPIDURAL STEROID INJECTION

1. **Interlaminar:** Approach both midline and paramedian, involves insertion of an epidural needle midway between the laminae of the adjacent vertebrae and forwarding the needle with loss of resistance or hanging drop techniques with normal saline. Avoid using air in loss of resistance syringe.
2. **Transforaminal** approach involves insertion of a 23 gauge spinal needle into the superior portion of an intervertebral foramen just inferior to the pedicle.

Cervical Epidural (Interlaminar)

Stepwise Approach

1. Anesthetist stand by with monitoring of vital signs is mandatory.
2. Patient in prone position with a pillow under the chest with the neck flexed. The arms can be placed at the patient's sides **(Figure 1)**. Prepare and drape the area.
3. Identify C7–T1 interspace under fluoroscopy by marker. The C-arm is placed in AP plane with a slight tilt cranial or caudal, to visualize the desired foramen, as wide as possible. The skin is anesthetized with 1% or 2% lidocaine or xylocard with one inch needle.

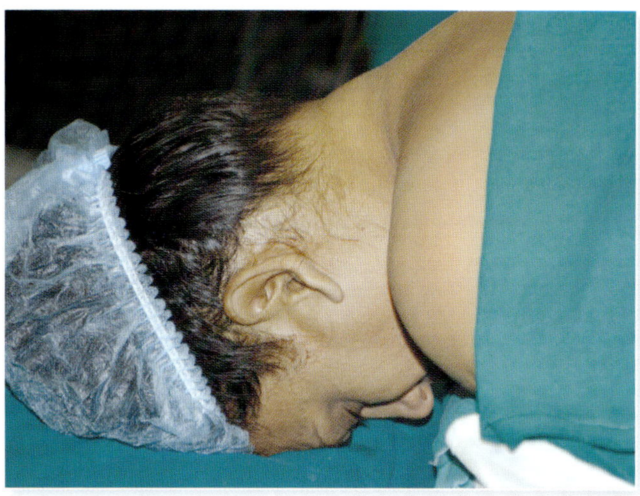

Figure 1: Position for cervical epidural

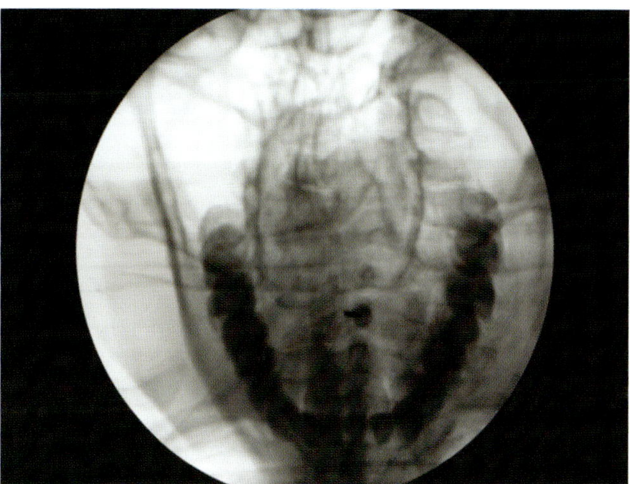

Figure 2: Cervical epidural-tunnel vision

4. Tuohy needle 18 or 20 gauge with drop of saline at the hub of needle and directed toward epidural space slowly and gently by maintaining tunnel vision **(Figure 2)**, till drop is sucked in. Now attach loss-of-resistance syringe filled with 1–2 cc of normal saline to confirm injection of saline without resistance.
5. After negative aspiration for absence of cerebrospinal fluid and blood, inject 1–2 cc of nonionic contrast. The spread of the dye should be confirmed in anteroposterior and lateral position under fluoroscopy **(Figure 3)**.
6. After confirming spread of dye, 80 mg of preservative free injection triamcinolone acetonide (Aurocort) 40 mg or dexamethasone 4–8 mg mixed with 3 cc of normal saline can be injected. Never inject local anesthetic in cervical epidural space, as it can be fatal if enters intrathecally as margin of safety in nil.

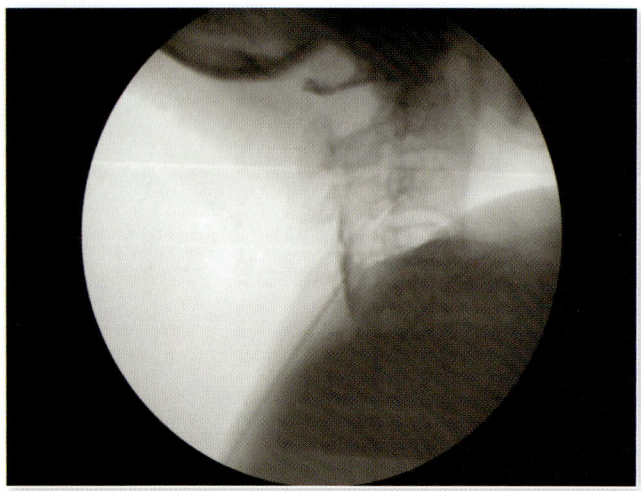
Figure 3: Cervical epidural: Spread of dye (Lateral view)

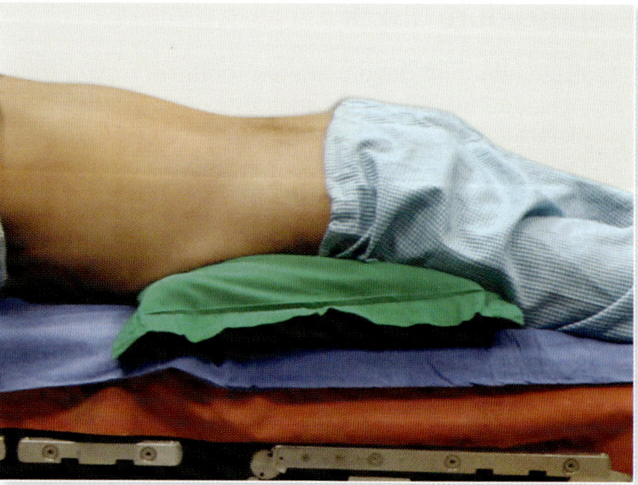
Figure 4: Position for lumbar epidural

7. Inject 1-2 mL local anesthetic in the needle track, while withdrawing of the needle to reduce postprocedure local pain.
8. The patient is then observed in recovery with monitoring of vital signs.

Transforaminal Lumbar Epidural

Step Wise Approach

1. Patient is placed prone with pillow under pelvis **(Figure 4)**.
2. After preparation, draping visualize the lumbar spine in AP position Now rotate C-arm in an oblique position about 20° to visualize typical scotty dog picture **(Figure 5).**
3. Put a skin marker on skin directly 6 o'clock position of the pedicle. Inject LA.
4. A 23 gauge 5-inch needle is then advanced under fluoroscopic guidance toward the target point, i.e. 6 o'clock position. Now push 23 gauge spinal needle into the foraman slowly maintaining tunnel vision, i.e. end on view in AP position of fluoroscope **(Figure 6)** and in lateral view. The tip of the needle should enter the neural foramen just under the pedicle **(Figure 7).**
5. Now attach 10 cc extension tubing and check for any CSF or blood by negative aspiration, and inject, 1 cc of radiopaque contrast Inj. Omnipaque under continuous fluoroscopy. Confirm the spread of dye in epidural space in AP and lateral position **(Figure 8)**.
6. Now inject steroid (Inj. Kenacort or dexamethasone). The author uses 10 mg of Aurocort (preservative free triamcenalone) per nerve root. Some pain physician uses Kenacort or dexamethasone.
7. Shift patient to recovery room for monitoring of vital signs.

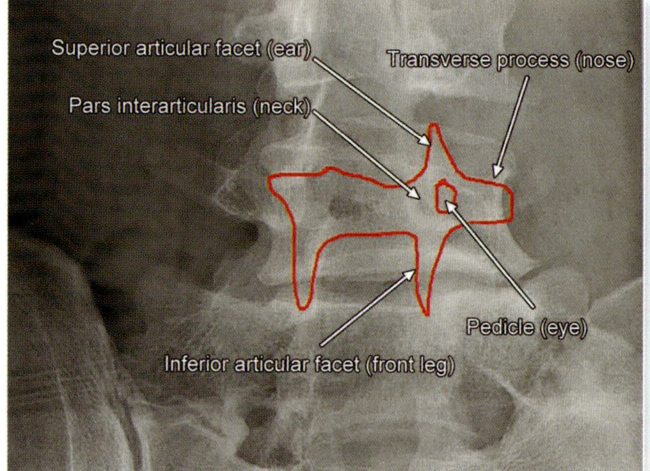

Figure 5: Scoty dog

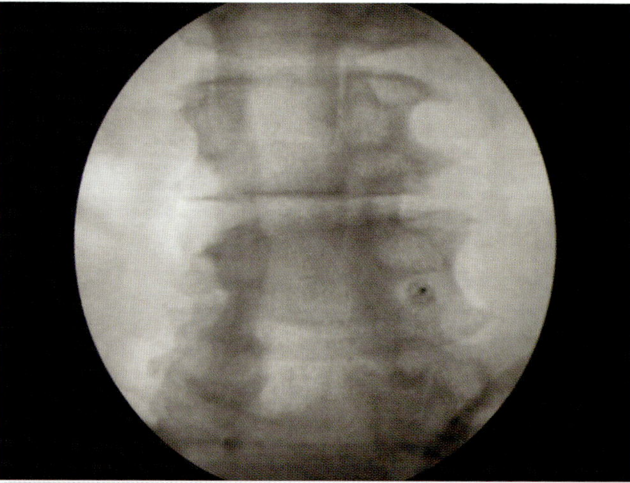
Figure 6: TFLE: Tunnel vision

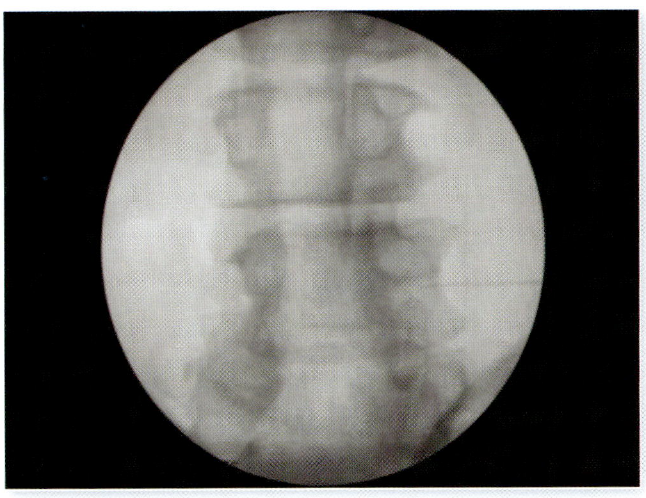

Figure 7: TFLE: Needle position: Lateral view

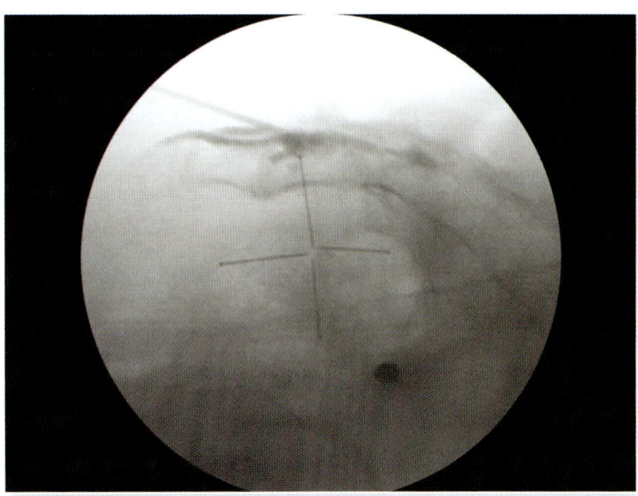

Figure 9: Caudal epidural dye spread: Lateral view

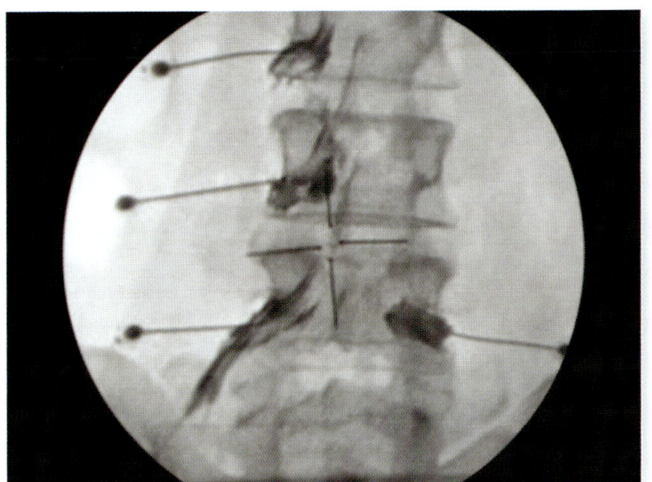

Figure 8: TFLE: Dye spread (AP view)

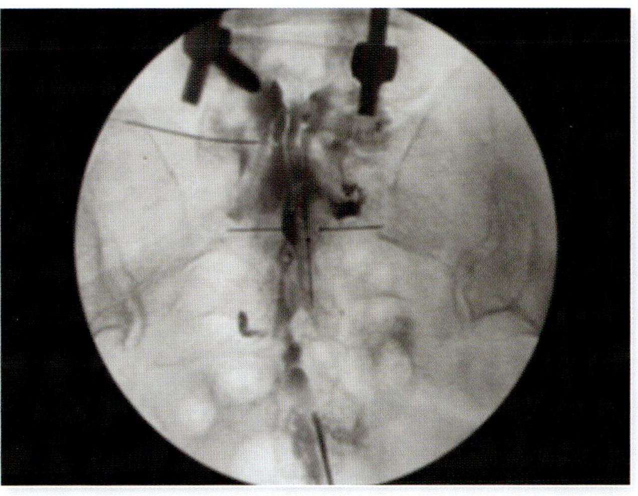

Figure 10: Caudal epidurogram (AP view)

Caudal Epidural

1. After obtaining of informed consent, patient is placed prone on the fluoroscopy table, with a pillow under the lower abdomen and toe directed inwards. Start procedure with C-arm in lateral position.
2. Palpate both posterior superior ilieac spine and confirm with marker under fluoroscopy
3. After inject local anesthesia, hold 21guage spinal or 20 gauge Tuohy needle at 90°, direct vertically downwards to hit sacrococcygeal membrane.
4. Then with 45° advanced needle in to the caudal epidural space.
5. Confirm with loss of resistance
6. After negative aspiration inject Inj. Omnipaque 3–5 cc slowly and confirm spread of dye in lateral **(Figure 9)** and anterior posterior view **(Figure 10)**.
7. Shift patient to recovery room for monitoring

POSTPROCEDURAL CARE

Following the injection the patient should be monitored for vital signs.

Observe for any skin rashes, hives shortness of breath, wheezing, increase in pain level, persistent nausea or vomiting, persistent headache which worsens upon sitting. Patient can be discharged after few hours.

POSTPROCEDURE CHECK

- Documentation in the form of print out, CD—One copy for record and one for patient.
- Postprocedure monitoring of vital signs.
- Follow-up advice must include
- Dosage and schedule of medications
- Explain about possible side effects of the drug

- Date and time of next visit
- Driving instruction to the patient if driving by himself.

COMPLICATIONS

The risks are infrequent and divided into complications of needle placement or medication side effects.

Needle-related

Pain at the injection site, nerve root injury, spinal cord injury, epidural hematoma, epidural abscess, meningitis, osteomyelitis, and postdural puncture headache.

Medication-related

1. Weakness in lower extremity secondary to motor block.
2. Cardiac arrhythmia, seizure, and hypotension.
3. Allergic reactions.

Late side effects steroid related, such as fluid retention, transient weight gain, hyperglycemia, and hypertension.

Very rarely Cushing syndrome, facial flushing, and steroid myopathy may also occur with any of the medication administered.

CONCLUSION

With the advent and use of fluoroscopy the transforaminal approach became widespread, with the thought that epidural steroids would be more effective if they were delivered more accurately to the site of pathology.

Epidural steroid injections are here to stay for the treatment of axial; radicular neck and back pain; and in post laminectomy patients due to epidural adhesions or implant related.

Author very strongly believes and advocates that these procedures should be done under fluoroscopic control and monitoring of vital signs.

REFERENCES

1. Derby R, Kine G, Saal J, Reynolds J, Goldthwaite N, White A, et al. Response to steroid and duration of radicular pain as predictors of surgical outcome. Spine. 1992; 17:S176-83.
2. Dilke TFW, Burry HC, Grahame R. Extradural corticosteroid injection in the management of lumbar nerve root compression. BMJ. 1973; 2:635-7.
3. Derby R, Bogduk N, Kine G. Precision percutaneous blocking procedures for localizing spinal pain. Part 2. The lumbar neuraxial compartment. Pain Digest. 1993; 3:175-88.
4. Bogduk N. Spine update: epidural steroids. Spine. 1995; 20:845-8.
5. Rapp SE, Haselkorn JK, Elam K, et al. Epidural steroid injection in the treatment of low back pain: A meta-analysis. Anesthesiology. 1994; 81:A923.
6. Rydevik B, Brown MD, Lundborg G. Pathoanatomy and pathophysiology of nerve root compression. Spine. 1984;9: 7-15.
7. Saal JS, Franson RC, Dobrow R, et al. High levels of inflammatory phospholipase A2 activity in lumbar disk herniations. Spine. 1990;15:674-8.
8. Johansson A, Hao J, Sjolund B. Local corticosteroid blocks transmission in normal nocioceptive C-fibers. Acta Anesthesiol Scand. 1990;34:335-8.
9. Fenton DS, Czervionke LF. Image-guided Spine Intervention. Saunders. 2003;5:99-126.
10. Baheti DK. Protocol for Interventional pain procedures: A suggested format—nterventional Pain Management-A Practical Approach. New Delhi: Jaypee Medical Publishers. 2009. pp 50-3.

33 CHAPTER

Radiofrequency Ablation of Facet Joints

Doshi Preeti P

ABSTRACT

Facetogenic pain is a common source of cervical and low back pain but often remains underdiagnosed and undertreated. Radiofrequency ablation of facet joints is a minimally invasive percutaneous technique for effective and meaningful control of pain arising from facet or zygapophyseal joints. When clinically suspected, a diagnostic block is performed to establish facet as a pain generator. If it yields a positive result, radiofrequency ablation is considered for longer-term pain relief. Radiofrequency ablation is a technique utilizing thermal energy to cause reversible and precise destruction of medial branch of dorsal ramus nerve innervating the affected facet joints. Imaging guidance is essential for precise placement of needles to improve the outcome of the procedure.

INTRODUCTION

Facet or zygapophyseal joints can be clinically important source of chronic cervical, thoracic, and lumbar spine pain. These are responsible for various functions on an ongoing basis, including weight bearing which subject them to stress and degeneration resulting in pain and disability.

Lumbar facet joints are a well-recognized source of low back pain and referred pain in the lower extremity in patients with a prevalence of 27–40% revealed by controlled diagnostic studies. In1996, Lord et al. using a diagnostic double blind placebo controlled local anesthetic blocks in patients with chronic neck pain after whiplash injury reported overall prevalence of cervical zygapophyseal joint pain as 60%. The prevalence of facetogenic pain arising from cervical and lumbar regions is much higher as compared to thoracic region due to the greater mobility of these regions resulting in enhanced wear and tear in these two regions.

A continuum of therapies including interventions ranging from simple to complex is available for managing chronic spinal pain in clinical practice. Interventions may be indicated when pain remains persistent after an adequate trial of conservative management. The most important requirement for a successful and satisfactory outcome is to establish a correct clinical diagnosis and suitable therapy goals. Interventions can have diagnostic, therapeutic and prognostic value. Diagnostic blocks may help establish or rule out a clinical diagnosis. Therapeutic interventions are used to control or eliminate pain and to facilitate rehabilitation.

Neurolysis or ablation is known since centuries to interrupt nociceptive pathways at various levels and to effectively control pain on a long-term basis. Neurolysis can be achieved by a multitude of techniques, such as either by the application of chemical, heat, cold, surgical disruption, and ionizing radiation or focused ultrasound.

Radiofrequency ablation is minimally invasive, target selective percutaneous technique that has been in clinical use for more than three decades and has demonstrated success at reducing pain for a meaningful duration ranging from 6 months to 18 months in patients with chronic facetogenic spinal pain. A hollow insulated cannula [Teflon coated along entire length with metalbare tip] is positioned as parallel and adjacent as possible to the target medial branch. A thermistor probe inserted through it and connected to a radiofrequency generator. The energy flowing from the tip of the cannula creates a heat lesion in the 80–85°C range mostly about the length of the exposed active tip and in proportion to the diameter of the probe.

Radiofrequency ablation is a refined technique based on temperature controlled destruction of the target nerve. Since the current involves use of a special equipment to produce high frequency energy of 300–500 kHz similar to one used in radio transmitters, it was aptly termed Radiofrequency current. The usual objective is to deposit enough RF power to raise the temperature of the target tissue to above 45–50°C. This is termed as "lethal temperature range "as cells exposed to such temperature for more than 20 seconds or more are known to be destroyed by heat. The term radiofrequency ablation has several synonyms such as radiofrequency thermo coagulation or radiofrequency rhizotomy or radiofrequency neurotomy. This technique is the most widely accepted technique and the most effective one in the present time. The innovation of pulsed radiofrequency has shown promise for neuropathic pain but again does not have adequate positive evidence till date to support its use. Successful use of these techniques requires specialized training and in depth knowledge of neural anatomy. RF Ablation has shown promise when used responsibly in properly selected patients and in conjunction with a multidisciplinary approach to address pain.

HISTORY AND EVOLUTION

Some important landmarks in the evolution of Radiofrequency ablation to the stage of its current practice are as follows:

1. 1920s: Harvey Cushing did a series of experiments to show utility of RF technique.
2. 1930s: Radiofrequency (RF) neurolysis was used for the first time in clinical practice for the treatment of chronic intractable pain when Kirschner using diathermy produced high current lesions of Gasserian ganglion for relief of trigeminal neuralgia.
3. 1950s: Hunsperger and Wyss proposed that instead of direct current, use of high frequency alternating current may be more appropriate.
4. 1950s: First commercially available RF generator was produced by Cosman and Arnoff based on which most of the current lesion generators have evolved.
5. 1960: Mundinger using a thermocouple for stereotactic brain surgery pioneered early neuroablative techniques with deep brain RF lesioning.
6. 1975: First application for spinal pain by Shealy who used RF probe to interrupt posterior ramus [medial branch] for facet joint pain in lumbar region. His studies appeared to demonstrate improved outcomes compared with the often poor results obtained from open neurosurgery procedure for the relief of intractable pain.
7. 1980s: MannoSluijter developed percutaneous RF technique for cervical, lumbar, thoracic and sacral discogenic pain syndromes using small diameter RF needles under local anesthesia using fluoroscopy a current could be passed through the electrode that would reliably produce the patient's concordant pain following which the appropriate RF thermal lesion could be produced.
8. 1994: Sluijter developed pulsed RF which was more of neuromodulation.

GENERAL PHYSICS AND PRINCIPLES OF RADIOFREQUENCY ABLATION

The main components of the circuit required to produce neurolysis of the target nerveare as follows **(Figure 1)**:

1. Active electrode (thermistor) which delivers the current from the generator to the tissue.
2. Ground pad (passive or dispersive electrode).
3. RF generator machine.

Radiofrequency current is a high frequency (500–1000 KHz), low energy current that can build an electromagnetic field between electrodes. This will make the free charged ions move back and forth in a radiofrequency movement in fluid media called "ionic dissipation". The friction will produce a rise of temperature that will be transmitted and sensed in the active tip of electrode which is able to measure it.

The radio frequency lesion generator **(Figure 2)** can deliver stimulation and lesioning options after satisfactory placement based on the impedance and temperature monitoring which are displayed in digital and analog formats on it. The resistance to the flow of current from target tissue called impedance is an important parameter which indicates position of the cannula tip to the operator. [1] The impedance drops to 200 Ω in case of short circuit and can be around 2000 Ω in event of a disconnection.

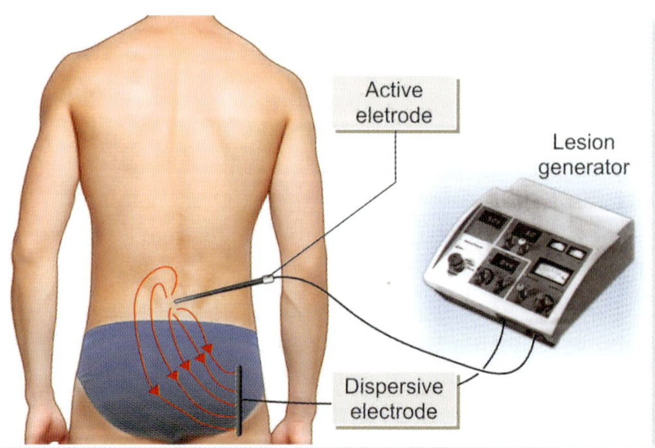

Figure 1: Basic circuit

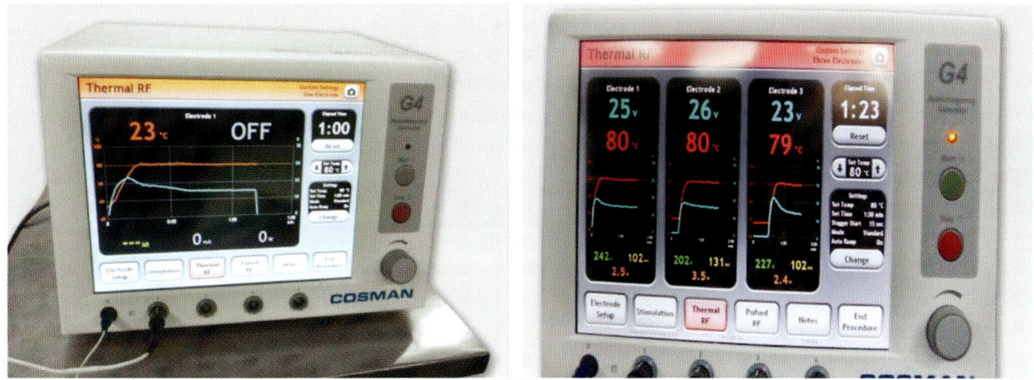

Figure 2: RF lesion generator

The active electrode must be close to the target nerve, ganglion or to plexus. The grounding pad is placed on patient's body surface to complete the circuit. The current from the thermistor heats the surrounding tissue due to the resistance which in turn heats the tip of the electrode. The temperature at the tip of the electrode is measured by a thermocouple and is displayed on the generator. The heat generated is proportional to the amount of current per unit area that flows in the region of the electrode. The thermistor itself doesnot generate heat but is heated due to local tissue warming. The ground pad has a greater surface area so as the current flows from active to the passive electrode and along the path, the current density reduces. This helps in preventing heating and tissue damage at the passive electrode. Heating of the active electrode is an important safety feature of this system, because tissue damage is related to the temperature generated. The newer electrodes have a low thermal coefficient, meaning that the electrode absorbs heat well and heats rapidly, leading to a faster response and improved safety of the system. Excessive heating causes more diffuse and permanent tissue damage. It is possible to boil tissues and these tissues may then adhere to the electrode and be avulsed when the electrode is removed.

It has also been suggested that the electric field rather than temperature induces changes in the nerve cells and has a neuromodulatory effect on pain processing mechanisms at the dorsal root ganglion, dorsal horn, and molecular levels by changing gene expression in pain-processing neurons.[2] This is of greater relevance in application of pulsed mode radiofrequency lesion as compared to the conventional mode.

Most electrodes are available in different configurations with number of sizes and lengths. Both reusable and disposable needles are available. The exposed or the uninsulated tip portion is crucial as it delivers RF energy. The four important variables of RF cannula are total length of cannula and length, sharpness (sharp/blunt) and shape [curved/straight] of active or uninsulated tip. An appropriate type of cannula is selected for the desired purpose. For example, an 18-gauge reusable electrode with a 2 mm exposed tip is suitable for radiofrequency denervation of the trigeminal nerve, whereas a 22-gauge electrode 10 cm long cannula with a 10 mm exposed tip is appropriate for lumbar facet denervation.

Lesion

The lesion generated at the tip of the cannula is usually in a shape of an inverted cone.

In vitro evidence suggests that the lesion radius is maximal at the part of the exposed electrode farthest from the tip **(Figure 3)**. The actual tip may not even be incorporated in the lesion, and this has important clinical implications. Nerves in contact with the tip may be only partially blocked, and an electrode placed tangential to the nerve generates a more effective lesion. It is crucial to create a lesion of a desired size.

The size and consistency of the lesion is determined by the following five factors:

1. Electrode tip configuration: The lesion produced is directly proportional to the distance from the active electrode tip and the cannula diameter. The thermal lesion is effective approximately 2 mm past the tip of the cannula. However, a circumferential 4–5 mm lesion is produced around the radius of the length of the cannula. The cannula should be placed parallel to the nerve for best results. Larger cannula generates bigger lesion but at the expense of more tissue trauma on insertion, unwanted neural destruction and larger reversible zone e. g. 18 G electrode generates a lesion with radius 2. 2 mm (larger size) as compared to 22 G which generates a lesion of 1.9 mm.
2. Temperature generated: The local tissue reaction is directly proportional to the temperature generated at the electrode tip. At 42-45°C temporary neural blockade

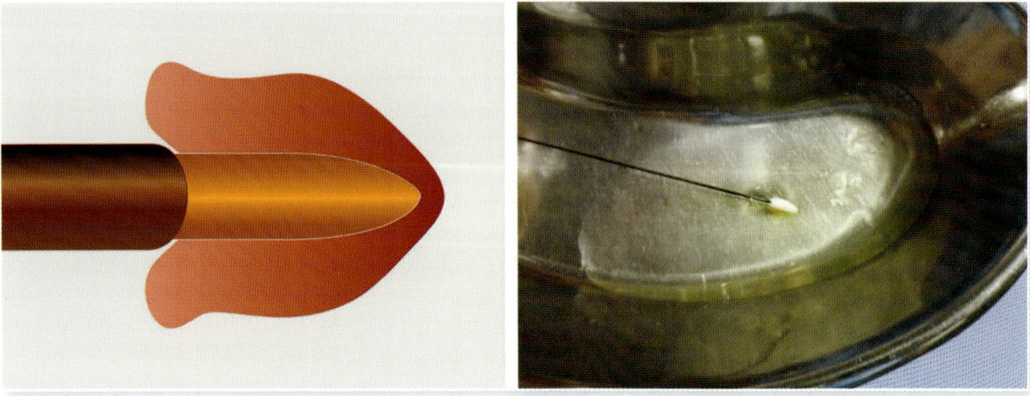

Figure 3: Shape of RF lesion at the tip

occurs. Above 45°C, irreversible tissue injury occurs. Thermo coagulation of the nerve cell with long-term loss of function begins at 60°C and loss of all nerve function at >65°C. To ensure complete denervation, the tradition RF lesioning is done at 80°C for 90–120 seconds.

3. Local tissue characteristics: Tissues of low electrical impedance, such as blood, CSF, lung tissue or any other tissue in homogeneity can cause lesions of irregular size and shape. Blood may also act as a heat sink, removing heat from the area and thereby limiting the temperature rise and reducing the lesion size.
4. Rate of thermal equilibrium: The lesion size is more uniform if there is a rapid thermal equilibrium between the tissues. Conversely, if there is slow and incomplete equilibrium, the lesion is erratic. Usually the thermal equilibrium is complete by 60 seconds.
5. Time: The lesion size initially rises exponentially with time but becomes independent of time after approximately 30–90 seconds **(Figure 4)**. Cosman and Cosman were first to determine the lesion size for a given electrode tip size and temperature. They concluded that at a tip temperature of 75°C, the lesion size would only increase by 20% beyond 30 seconds, and it did not increase much after 60 seconds. [3] The lesion is said to be 85% complete by 30 seconds, 94% complete by 60 seconds and hence duration of 60–90 seconds is considered adequate in regular use.

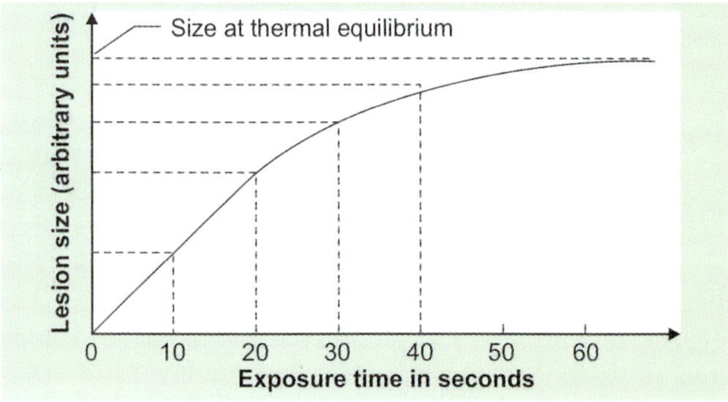

Figure 4: Graph of lesion size vs time

ADVANTAGES OF RF LESIONING OVER OTHER NEURODESTRUCTIVE TECHNIQUES

a. Minimally invasive percutaneous procedure.
b. Lesion size can be accurately controlled allowing precise lesioning without damaging important structures in the vicinity.
c. Procedure can be done under local anesthesia with or without sedation.
d. Measurement of impedance and feature for sensory and motor stimulation permits accurate placement of cannula on the desired target.
e. Lesions can be reproduced for similar degree of analgesia in case of pain recurrence in the same distribution.
f. Recovery is rapid allowing the patient to resume work or daily activity faster.
g. Minimum morbidity and mortality.

INDICATIONS

Radiofrequency ablation is useful for long-term pain control in a variety of indications for spinal pain. Facetogenic pain is the common indication for spinal pain with a success rate of about 60–70% with a meaningful duration ranging from 6–18 months. Pain originating from facet joint is common but underdiagnosed component of low back pain and neck pain. This pain is often not amenable to surgical intervention and is difficult to manage conservatively. Steroid injections generally provide pain relief for a shorter duration. RF ablation denervates one or more facet joints and provides long-term, good quality pain relief as per requirement in well-selected patients.

PATIENT SELECTION CRITERIA

A fundamental criterion for the selection of patients for lumbar medial branch blocks is that serious possible causes of spinal pain, such as infection, tumors, vascular disease, and metabolic disease have been excluded by careful history and thorough examination, laboratory tests and medical imaging if necessary.

Patients with cervical or back pain of moderate severity for a duration of more than three months, which has failed to respond to conservative management, should be examined to clinically establish facet origin pain. If the type of pain is deemed appropriate for radiofrequency ablation and all the above contraindications are ruled out, a diagnostic block should be undertaken with local anesthetic drug.

Controlled comparative blocks are ideal in selecting patients for radiofrequency ablation. Patient should be ideally subjected to two sets of diagnostic blocks performed on two separate occasions at least two weeks apart with two different local anesthetic agents. A true-positive response to comparative local anesthetic blocks is one in which the patient reports almost complete relief of pain for a shorter duration when a short-acting agent is used, and for a longer duration when a long-acting agent is used. Such a response is referred to as "concordant" in that it is concordant with the expected action of the agents used.

Before the procedure, the patient must have realistic expectations and must understand that the aim is to reduce the pain and single target lesioning may not be sufficient necessitating complementary blocks for better pain relief.

CONTRAINDICATIONS AND LIMITATIONS

Absolute

- Infection
- Coagulopathy or continued use anticoagulant drugs
- Pregnancy
- Failed diagnostic block
- Patients with significant psychological problems
- Deafferentation pain which may be aggravated by destruction of the nerve.

Relative

- Patients with pacemaker
- Pain relief lasting less than three months with previous neurotomy.

MINIMAL STANDARDS AND RECOMMENDATIONS

RF treatment is the most described minimally invasive and effective procedure preferred over more invasive and expensive treatment modalities in the multidisciplinary approach to pain management. The following recommendations are followed in practice:

- Multidisciplinary patient selection using validated selection criteria
- Prior diagnostic block/blocks in most indications
- Full explanation of the procedure and Informed consent
- Fluoroscopic or imaging guidance
- Standardized report on the intervention including impedance, voltage, temperature, time, radiographic pictures in patient record
- Standardized patient follow up with validated assessment tools
- Accurate training of physicians on the anatomy, technical aspects, hands-on experience and radiation protection

Patient Preparation

In the Wards

As like most interventions in pain management the following should be followed:

- Thorough explanation of the procedure
- Written consent with possible side effects of the intervention
- Confirm the stoppage of anti-platelet agents 3–5 days prior to the procedure
- Blood tests as necessary
- Confirm the nil by mouth status if sedation is planned
- Confirm the morning dose of antihypertensive or similar drugs in special group patients
- Intravenous access
- Intravenous antibiotic as appropriate.

In the Procedure Room

- Basic monitoring and all necessary resuscitation equipment and drugs
- RF machine is checked for the test mode: The test mode produces a 100 Ω phantom load resistor across the output so that the unit is tested before using it for the procedure
- Check availability of appropriate configuration cannula as per target nerve
- Radiation protection gears: Lead apron, thyroid shield, eyewear, gloves
- Ground pad to be applied to the patient
- Thermistor connection to be attached to the radiofrequency machine

PROCEDURES

Lumbar Facetogenic Pain

Applied Anatomy

To perform effective ablation, knowledge of anatomy of dorsal rami and medial branches which innervate each facet joint, is essential. The level of medial branch is determined depending on the affected facet joint. Forone facet in most situations two adjoining level medial branches are targeted. The medial branches of the L1–L4 dorsal rami all assume an analogous course. Each medial branch crosses the root of the transverse process of the vertebra below. Thus the L3 medial branch crosses the L4 transverse process, and the L4 medial branch crosses the L5 transverse process. Each nerve runs in the groove formed by the junction of the transverse process and the superior articular process at each level. Subsequently, each medial branch runs under the mamilloaccessory ligament as it curves medially to enter the multifidus muscle. This ligament holds the nerve in place and affords little variation in the location of the nerve as it crosses the junction of the superior articular and transverse processes.[4] It is important to note that the number of medial branches to be targeted is different from the corresponding facetjoint, e. g. L4–5 facet isinnervated by medial branches of L3 and L4 **(Figure 5)** dorsal rami which in turn are branches of corresponding segmental nerves.

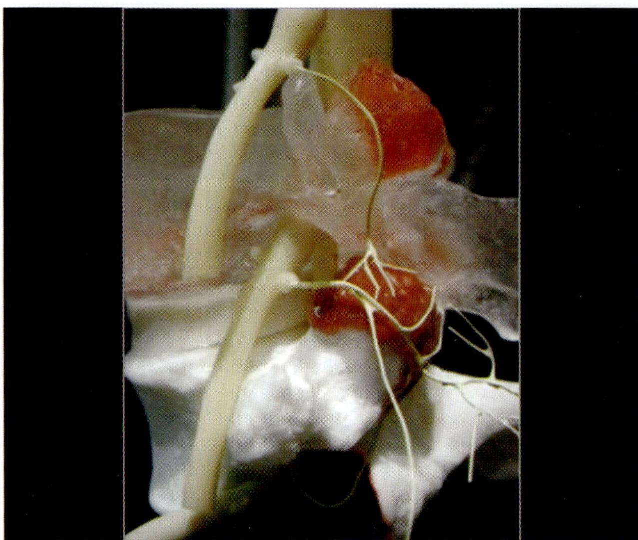

Figure 5: Medial branch anatomy

Procedure

1. After full explanation of the procedure,the patientis placed in prone position on the operating table with pillows under the hips and chest with the arms by the head-side **(Figure 6)** and all resuscitative equipment at hand in the OT.
2. After squaring the endplates, the fluoroscope or C-arm is positioned in an ipsilateral (10-25°) oblique projection to obtain a scotty dog view until the groove between the base of superior articular and medial end of the transverse process where medial branch is located is clearly visualized.
3. To denervate L4–5 and L5–S1 facet joints, entry points are marked overlying the grooves at the L4, L5 and S1 level depending on the side of desired lesion. In these grooves run the posterior primary rami of L3, L4 and L5.
4. Under due asepsis, under fluoroscopy guidance, after local anesthetic injection, RF cannula is introduced and placed at the groove as shown in **Figure 7**.
5. Biplanar fluoroscopy gives an additional confirmation of correct placement of the RF needle **(Figure 8)**.
6. The stylet of the cannula is then removed and replaced by the thermistor probe. The RF cannula has a well-insulated shaft to protect the nearby tissues from electrical burn. The tip of the cannula is bare which in contact with the desired target.
7. Check for the impedance on the RF machine (normally should be between 200 ohms and 600 ohms). The stimulation mode is now started. Sensory stimulation is done at 50 Hz up to 2 V to confirm the accuracy of electrode position. Patient should get paraesthesia in the

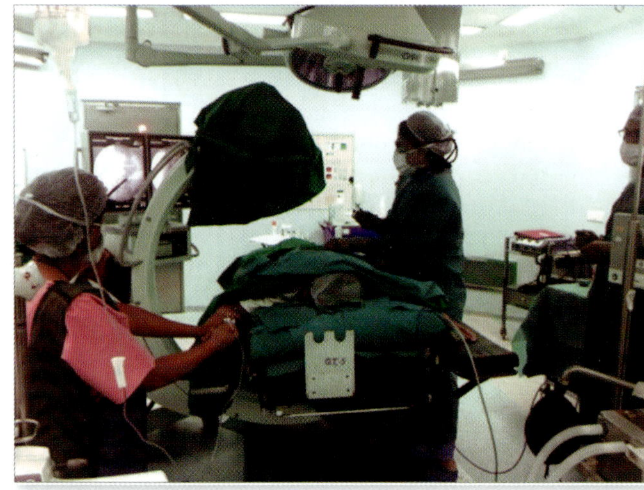

Figure 6: OT setup for RF ablation

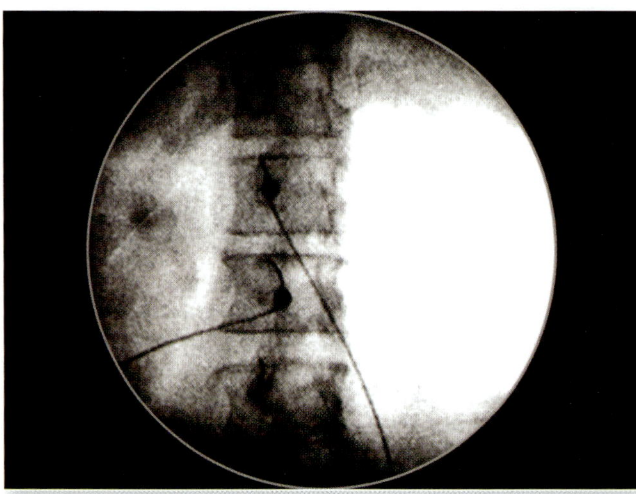

Figure 7: Oblique fluoroscopic view

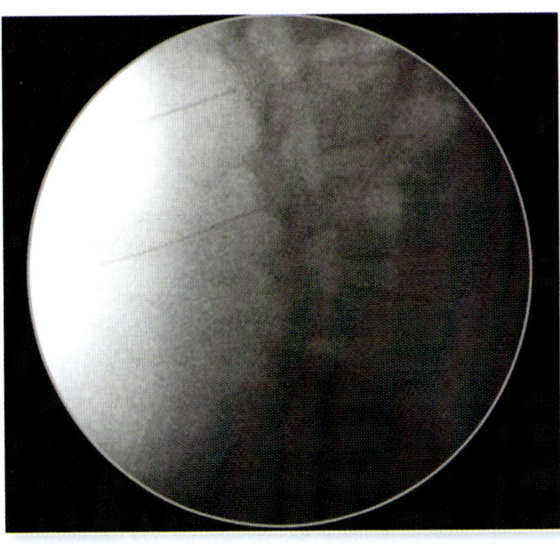
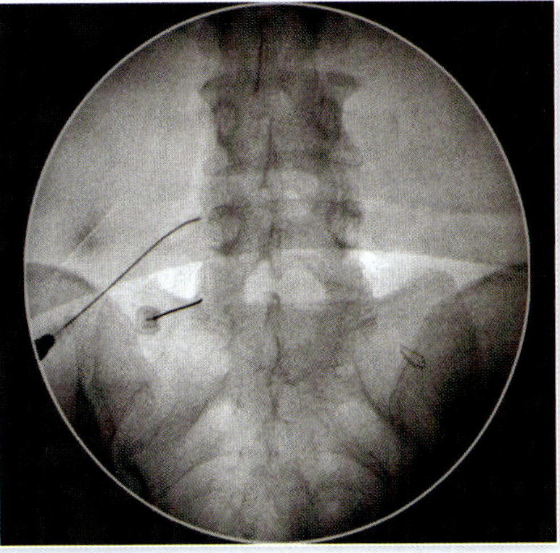

Figure 8: Lateral and AP views with needles in situ

affected area only. This can be elicited in 50–70% of the patients. This is followed by motor stimulation at 2 Hz which can be increased up to 3 V. For medial branch just a small twitch in the distribution of multifidus muscle may be noticed. No sensory or motor stimulation of adjoining segmental nerve should occur.

8. Once the position is confirmed on the desired target, 1mL of local anesthetic with or without 5 mg methyl prednisolone is injected through the cannula to decrease the discomfort during coagulation and reduce incidence of post procedure neuritis.
9. The lesion is carried out at 80°C for 90 seconds. Usually, one and sometimes two additional lesions are done after slight repositioning of the cannula to take care of anatomical variations **(Figure 9)**.

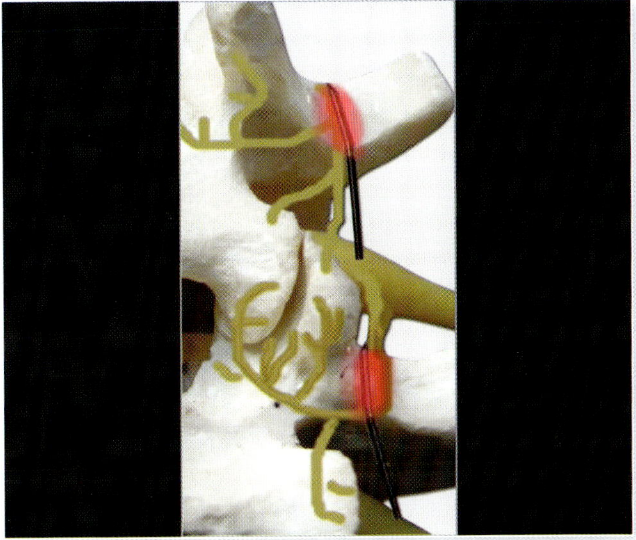

Figure 9: RF lesion

Cervical RF Ablation

Again here it is important to have thorough knowledge of anatomy before embarking on the procedure.

Anatomy

The structures innervated by the cervical medial branches include the cervical zygapophyseal joints, paramedian and deep cervical muscles, multifidus, semispinalis cervicis and interspinales.

Anatomic studies have shown that the C3-4 to C7-T1 facet joints are supplied by the medial branches of the cervical dorsal rami with each joint receiving supply from the medial branches above and below its location. In contrast, C2-3 joint is innervated by the third occipital nerve as it crosses the back of the joint. The C5 medial branch courses across the centroid of the articular pillar of C5 **(Figure 10)**. The C4 and C6 medial branches are between the centroid and the base of the SAP while the C3 and C7 branches lie on the SAP **(Figure 11)** At the C3 level, two medial branches are present: the C3 deep medial branch, which is involved in the innervation of the C3–4 zygapophyseal joint, and the C3 superficial medial branch, which is the third occipital nerve and which innervates the C2–3 zygapophyseal joint. In lateral views **(Figure 11)**, the C3 deep medial branch is usually found running across the upper half of the C3 articular pillar, but sometimes it crosses the lower half of the C2–3 zygapophyseal joint. The third occipital nerve crosses the C2–3 zygapophyseal joint, and may be located anywhere from opposite the apex of the C3 superior articular process to opposite the bottom of the C2–3 intervertebral foramen.

Procedure

The main indication for cervical radiofrequency medial branch neurotomy is long-term relief of pain following

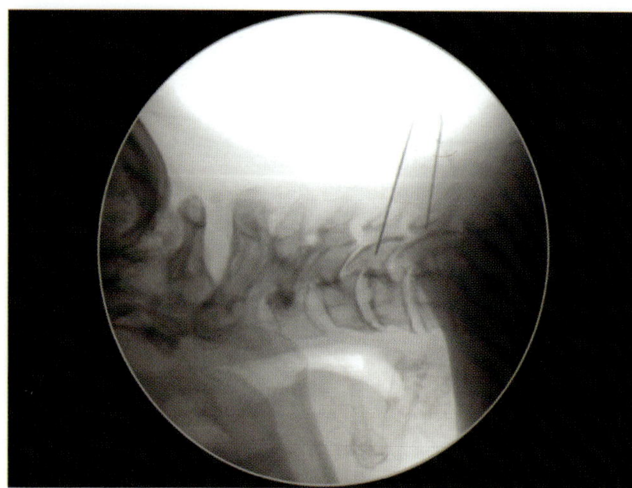

Figure 10: Lateral view with needle on centroid of C5 vertebra

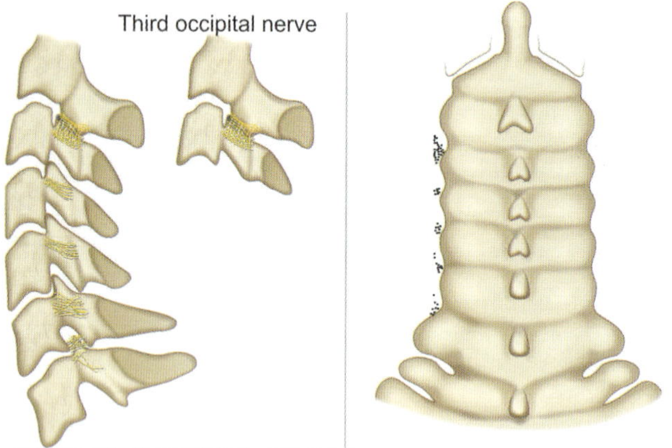

Figure 11: Cervical medial branch anatomy

controlled diagnostic blocks of the target medial branches. These blocks may be placebo-controlled blocks or comparative local anesthetic blocks.

The patient may be positioned either prone or in lateral position with the target side uppermost. The lateral position is more comfortable for the patient and poses no additional difficulty for the operator but for targeting the lower cervical levels prone position is preferred.

In cross section, the articular pillars of the cervical vertebrae are curved, and the medial branches wrap around this curve. A straight electrode, however, will place a lesion only tangential to this curve. Therefore, if a maximal length of nerve is to be coagulated, the electrode must be introduced along each of two paths; a sagittal path, to be tangential to the lateral sector of the pillar (3 o'clock or 9 o'clock); and an oblique path, 30° from sagittal, in order to be tangential to the anterolateral sector of the pillar (2 o'clock or 10 o'clock). Using a single placement will coagulate less of the length of the nerve, and is associated with lesser duration of relief. A three needle approach to each level is advocated with a 2 stage insertion. Initially the medial branch is anesthetized via a standard medial branch block and the muscles in the area are also infiltrated with local anesthetic. This marker needle is left in place to facilitate the placement of the oblique RF needle. Then the RF needles are inserted using oblique and sagittal passes. Oblique is suggested to be performed first as it is the most difficult. Target is anterior 1/3 of the SAP and on AP projection is on the convexity above the concavity of the pillar. A 30-degree oblique approach is used and the needle is inserted without any craniocaudad beam angulation. 2–3 lesions are made serially as the needle is linearly retracted after each lesion. Lesioning parameters are 80°C for 90 seconds. The sagittal pass needle is placed without any obliquity in the beam but with a declination of the fluoroscopy beam to the same angle as the zygapophyseal joints on lateral fluoroscopic views. The lateral aspect of the lateral mass at the waist of the pillar is lesioned using the same parameters.

Thoracic RF Ablation

This procedure is indicated in patients diagnosed to have facetogenic pain and who have had a positive response to controlled comparative diagnostic block. Lesion parameters are similar to lumbar region.

Patient is placed in prone position on a radiolucent table after preparation as for other regions.

Target Identification

The target level must be carefully and accurately identified under continuous AP fluoroscopic screening by counting from T1. The target landmarks are the transverse processes. Care should be taken to name the target joint and target transverse processes correctly as their segmental nerves will be different from those of the target nerves.

For the nerves from T1 to T4 and for the T9 and T10 nerves, the target point will be the dorsal surface of the transverse process, opposite the lateral end of its superior border. [5] This point is not the superior lateral corner of the transverse process, but lies slightly medial to it. Essentially, it lies at the medial end of the curve of the corner. At upper thoracic levels, the target point lies slightly more medially than at lower thoracic levels. If the transverse process is short and obscure, it may be brought into better relief by rotating the C-arm away from the side of interest. As this is done, the transverse process appears to elongate (This is referred to as "Pinocchio view", referring metaphorically to the growth of Pinocchio's nose). For the T11 and T12 nerves, the target point will be like that for lumbar medial branches, viz. at the junction of the root of the superior articular process and the root of the transverse process. This point is best seen and approached along an ipsilateral oblique view, i. e. a 'Scotty dog' view. For the nerves from T4 to T8, the eventual target point does not rest on bone, but the initial approach is like that for typical thoracic levels, and is based on first identifying the tips of the transverse processes in an AP view. However, instead of the transverse process the initial target is the dorsal surface of the rib that articulates with the transverse process. The T6 and T7 medial branches appear consistently to be suspended in the inter transverse space. The T4, T5 and T8 nerves may sometimes cross the tip of the transverse process.

Potential Postprocedural Complaints

1. Vasovagal reaction (hypotension, bradycardia, nausea).
2. Pain (injection site, radicular, corticosteroid flare).
3. Headache (corticosteroids).

Postprocedure Instructions

1. Local Icepack application for soreness due to the lesion.
2. Patient might need simple analgesics or muscle relaxants to reduce soreness at the injection site.
3. Patient should be reassured that the effect of the RF lesion takes 10–14 days to realize the pain relief.

Potential Complications of Radiofrequency Neurotomy

- Allergic reaction to drugs used (to nonionic contrast agent, local anesthetic, corticosteroid or latex causing urticaria, laryngeal edema, bronchospasm, anaphylaxis)
- Bleeding
- Cardiovascular (dysrhythmias, congestive heart failure, hypotension, bradycardia, vasovagal reaction)
- Neurologic injury (direct neural trauma, compression from hematoma or abscess, radicular or vertebral artery trauma, arterial particulate injection, seizure)
- Infection (cellulitis, osteomyelitis, epidural abscess, discitis, meningitis, arachnoiditis, sepsis)
- Urologic (urinary retention, incontinence)
- Adverse local anesthetic drug reaction due to excess dose (CNS and cardiovascular toxicity, anxiety, incoherent speech, light-headedness, perioral parethesias, blurred vision, tremors,drowsiness, seizures, cardiac arrest, excessive intrathecal or epidural local anestheticinjection resulting in spinal block or leg weakness)
- Adverse steroid reaction (facial flushing, injection site hypopigmentation, subcutaneous fat atrophy, increased appetite, fluid retention, gastritis, malaise, euphoria, insomnia,headache, immunosuppression, aseptic meningitis, arachnoiditis, congestive heart failure,increased intraocular pressures, adrenal insufficiency, steroid myopathy, mania, hyperglycemia, hypertension, epidural lipomatosis, menstrual irregularity)

OUTCOME OF RADIOFREQUENCY THERMAL ABLATION CURRENT EVIDENCE

The evidence for the efficacy of RF ablation of medial branch of facet joints has remained controversial. A 10-year prospective clinical audit of radiofrequency denervation of the lumbar facet joints by Michael Gofeld et al. report that proper patient selection and anatomically correct radiofrequency denervation of lumbar fact joints do provide long-term pain relief. The indicated level of evidence for radiofrequency neurotomy as per USPSTF criteria is from level II-2 to II-3 based on one randomized trial and 2 observational studies. Based on Guyatt et al.'s criteria, the recommendation is 1B or C strong for radiofrequency neurotomy.[6]

RF denervation of the cervical and lumbar medial branches has the most solid evidence ASIPP's analysis 7 of five systematic reviews concluded that RF treatment of the medial branch of the cervical spine utilizing the multiple lesioning technique and strict inclusion criteria requiring 100% pain relief following diagnostic blocks is strong for short- and long-term relief of cervical facet joint pain. There is insufficient evidence to support the use of RF denervation of C2–C3 for the management of cervicogenic headache.

CONCLUSION

Radiofrequency ablation features on the top in the algorithm for managing multiple chronic pain problems when conservative methods fail to relieve pain in an adequate manner on long-term basis. As in many of these patients we have no surgical option to control pain, RF ablation emerges as a useful option mainly due to its safety, efficacy and minimally invasive nature. There is enough evidence in the literature to support its use in some common indications like facetogenic cervical, lumbar or thoracic pain. Refinement in the technology withimproved generators which can perform multiple simultaneous lesions can enable time-saving to permit use in elderly patients. Also with availability of different configurations of cannulae the use of radiofrequency ablation is expanding in clinical practice with many new emerging indications. Facet RF Ablation is an effective treatment for mechanical back and neck pain due to facetogenic pathology. It should be used in conjunction with suitable exercise program which can help to minimize stress on diseased segment and improve outcome.

REFERENCES

1. Schwarzer AC, Wang S, Bogduk N, et al. Prevalence and clinical features of lumbar zygapophysial joint pain: a study in an

Australian population with chronic low back pain. Ann Rheum Dis. 1995;54:100-6.
2. Lord SM, Barnsley L, Wallis B, Bogduk N. et al. Percutaneous radiofrequency neurotomy for chronic cervical zygapophyseal joint pain. N Eng J Med. 1996;335:1721-6.
3. Cosman ER. Jr, Cosman ER Sr. Electric and thermal field effects in tissue around radiofrequency electrodes. Pain Medicine. 2005;6;6;405-24.
4. Shealy CN. Percutaneous radiofrequency denervation of spinal facets. J Neurosurgery. 1975;43:448-51.
5. Gauci CA. A Practical Manual of RF Procedures in chronic pain management; 2004.
6. Higuchi Y, Nashold B, Sluijter M et al. Exposure of the dorsal root ganglion in rats to pulsed radiofrequency currents activates dorsal horn lamina I and II neurons. Neurosurg. 2002;50: 850-6.
7. Van Zundert J, Sluijter M, VanKleef M. Thermal and Pulsed Radiofrequency; Interventional Pain Management: Image guided Procedures; Textbook by P Prithvi Raj. 2008;56-63.
8. Bogduk N, Long DM. Lumbar medical branch neurotomy: A modification of facet denervation. Spine. 1980;5:193-201.
9. Stolker RJ, Vervest ACM, Groen GJ. Percutaneous facet denervation in chronic thoracic spinal pain. Acta Neurochir (Wien). 1993;122: 82-90.
10. Sukdeb Datta, Marion Lee, Frank J Falco, et al. Systematic assessment of diagnostic accuracy and therapeutic utility of lumbar facet joint interventions. Pain Physician. 2009;12: 437-60.
11. Boswell MV, Trescot AM, Datta S, et al. Interventional techniques: evidence-based practice guidelines in the management of chronic spinal pain. Pain Physician. 2007;10:7-111.

34

CHAPTER

Failed Back Surgery Syndrome

Sandeep Diwan, Miraj

ABSTRACT

Failed back surgery syndrome is one of the debilitating diseases following spinal surgery. The pain mechanism is complex which can include nociceptive and neuropathic components. There are wide variety of causes for the back pain and equally many interventions in the management of this complex scenario.

INTRODUCTION

The term "failed back surgery syndrome (FBSS)" has an imprecise definition and includes different morbid conditions following spinal surgery that are associated with persistent pain and disability.[1-3]

FBSS is defined as persistant or recurrent back pain and leg pain after a precise technically adequate lumbar spinal surgery. There is no indication of of macroscopic pathology justifying reoperation.[4]

The complex pain incorporates both nociceptive and neuropathic components and involves the sympathetic nervous systems, occasionally.

CAUSE OF PERSISTENT PAIN

It has been substantiated that a significant corelation exists between the degree of epidural fibrosis and existing pain fact. This was confirmed through epiduroscopic examinations.[5]

The major causes for pain following spine surgery are *Chronic spinal pain without spinal surgery.*

Epidural adhesions can occur from leaking disks, without prior spinal surgery.[6]

Chronic Spinal Pain with Spinal Surgery

The chief causes of persistent pain syndromes, postspinal surgery are related to:[7-12]

- Epidural fibrosis
- Lateral and foraminal stenosis
- Progressive facet joint degeneration
- Segment instability, and
- Myofascial pain.

A fibrous connective tissue causing epidural fibrosis into a postoperative hematoma has been demonstrated (dogs postlaminectomy epidural space).[13] Fibrous tissue in the epidural space may adhere to the dura mater and nerve roots; this causes a mechanical tethering of the nerve roots or the dura. Fibrosis with neural compression can lead to increased neural sensitivity. Studies in animal models support the clinical and imaging findings with evidence of pain in the presence of epidural scarring.

Myofascial Pain

The results of different studies have supported the hypothesis that myofascial pain may contribute to failed back surgery syndrome.[14]

Natural Process

It was proved that the degenerative changes can develop regardless of the type of surgery. Thus in spite of an excellent surgical work, the progressive facetal degeneration or hypertrophy, spinal canal stenosis and foraminal stenosis contribute significantly to FBSS.[15-17]

Psychosocial Factors

There are often psychological and social factors at play that have an impact on the outcome of spinal surgery, and that is what makes this a complex condition easy to diagnose but difficult to treat.

Literature supports that psychosocial variables affect surgery outcomes, and that psychological screening can assist healthcare providers in deciding who is an appropriate candidate for spine surgery.

Several variables are identified that predict with 90.7% accuracy which acute back pain patients went on to develop chronic back pain.[18]

Most Common Cause

The two most common causes[19] by far are:
- Recurrent disk prolapse and
- Epidural fibrosis, or a combination of both.

Micromovement Theory

Failed fusion theory not demonstrable on X-ray or MRI may be the cause of persisting back pain – the "micromovement theory".[19]

MANAGEMENT

Multidisciplinary Team

Successful management of this condition requires management within the context of a multidisciplinary team as patients benefit from a range of treatment options including:
- Cognitive—behavioral,
- Pharmacological (chemical neuromodulation) injections and
- Neuromodulation approaches.[20]

Initial Assessment

Following staged assessments are done:
- A comprehensive biopsychosocial assessment.
- Assess pain severity and its impact on function and quality of life
- Assess for dorsal column function
- Assess associated deafferentation in the affected painful area
- Obtain the relevant records regarding previous treatments
- Spinal surgery, impant X-rays and recent MRI
- Pain assessment scores.

Imaging the Failed Back

A recent magnetic resonance imaging is screened for:
- Postoperative diskitis.
- Residual disk herniation
- New or lateral disk herniation
- Foraminal stenosis.

Magnetic resonance scanning is sensitive in identifying causes, such as postoperative diskitis.[21] Residual disk herniation is differentiated from epidural scarring, as this has implications for further treatment options. Exclude new or recurrent lateral disk prolapse in patient with a new onset of symptoms and signs of a radicular nature. A Gd-DTPA enhanced MRI is particularly valuable in differentiating disk and scar.

Consultation with a spine surgeon is necessary in these setting. Foraminal stenosis is one of the most common causes of persistent back pain following surgery.[22]

PHARMACOLOGICAL INTERVENTION

Case report dictates the effectiveness of gabapentin in postoperative epidural fibrosis after spinal surgery.[23] A large randomised controlled trial failed to show efficacy of pregabalin in neuropathic pain associated with radiculopathy.[24]

Strong opioids for chronic pain are being re-evaluated because the side effects from the long-term. Strong opioids cause immune suppression, endocrine suppression, reduced libido and an overall detrimental effect.[25]

Pharmacological treatment options are helpful only in a minority of patients with FBSS.[26-28]

The recent guidelines for the management of neuropathic pain suggests oral amitrityline, gabapentin and pregabalin as the first line of treatment (NICE).[29]

Spinal Intervention Techniques

Indications

Chronic intractable low back pain due either to postlumbar laminectomy syndrome or spinal stenosis with or without radicular findings of at least 6 months duration.

FBBS is a local pathology and treament modalities are directed towards the suspected area obtained from clinical —MRI examination.
- Spinal interventions, such as caudal epidural steroids,[30] transforaminal epidural steroid injection[31] and facet joint denervation[32] should be considered.

The above treatment options are a bridging treatment options until a more definative modality is decided. This allows the patient to comply with on-going exercises, reduce medication use and avoid repeat surgery.

Caudal Steroids

Fluoroscopic caudal epidural injections **(Figure 1)** are utilized for function- limiting chronic low back and lower extremity pain secondary to post surgery syndrome. A more than 50% pain relief in 56% of the participants with local anesthetic only and 61% with local anesthetic and steroids (6 mg of non-particulate betamethasone) was observed.[33]

Technique (Figure 1)

- Patient is in prone position
- The fluoroscope is adjusted to visualize the caudal epidural space.
- The part is prepped and draped.
- Local anesthesia is infiltrated at the point of needle insertion.
- A 22–23 G spinal needle is inserted.
- A pop is appreciated as the needle penetrates the sacrococcygeal ligament.
- Contrast is injected to delineate the caudal epidural space.
- The space is identified both in AP and lateral views.
- A 25 mL 0.2% bupivacaine, 40 mg (MPS) steroid and 75 mg clonidine are injected after careful aspiration.

Transforaminal Blocks

Transforaminal blocks have a major role as a stop gap treatment option. The severe radicular pain is taken care of until a more definitive treatment is implemented.

Patients with radicular pain after failed back surgery and treated with transforaminal steroids, the outcomes reported is at least 50% relief for 3 months.[34]

A Typical Patient with FBSS (Figure 2)

Annular disk bulge with focal central and left paracentral protrusion at L4–5 **(Figure 3)**. This is causing thecal sac indentation.

A left lateral recess and bilateral neural foraminal encroachment Facet arthropathy compromising the foramen.

Compression of left traversing L5 and exiting L4 nerve root **(Figure 4)**.

Technique (Figure 5)

- The patient is in prone position.
- The back is prepped and draped.
- The level of the intervention is screened and the image intensifier is positioned to gain optimal images.
- It is slight oblique towards the needle insertion. The final image is scotty dog, and the needle tip should be at 6'o clock position of the mouth of scotty dog **(Figures 6 and 7)**. (The scotty dog is not appreciated in the old patients because of the distorted anatomy secondary to degenerative changes and in osteoporosis).
- At times the patient perceives paraesthesia as the needle is close to the nerve in the perineural sheath.
- A 1 mL contrast (nonionic) delineates the nerve course (light yellow).
- The spread should be intraforaminal and epidural (dark yellow).
- The site of drug deposition in transforaminal blocks **(Figure 8)**

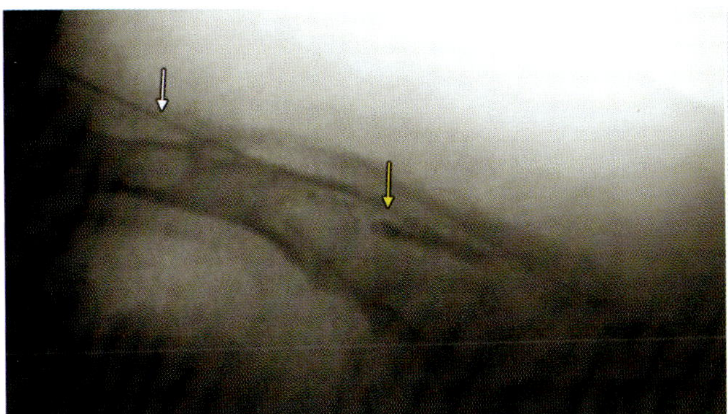

Figure 1: Caudal epidural (Sandeep Diwan 2014–15 Sancheti Hospital, Pune). Needle in the caudal epidural space. Contrast delineates the spread across the caudal space and the sacral root. The contrast reaches the level of the L5–S1 intervertebral disk

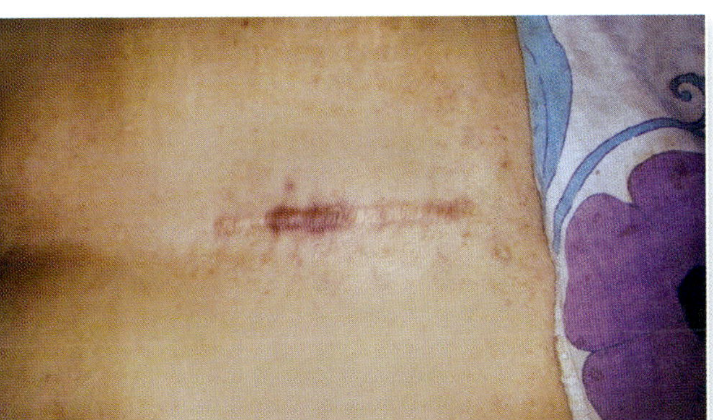

Figure 2: Postlaminectomy back scar

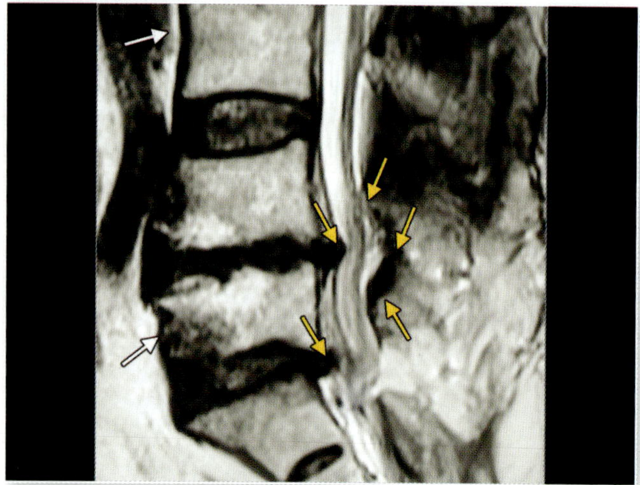

Figure 3: MRI in FBSS

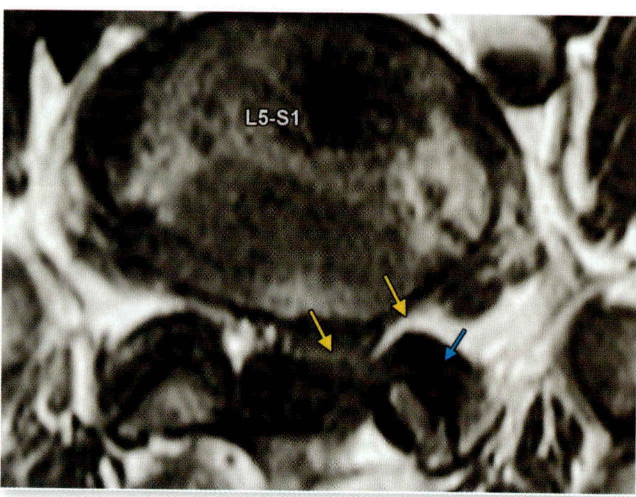

Figure 4: MRI in FBSS: Foraminal disk bulge and severe compression of left traversing S1 root

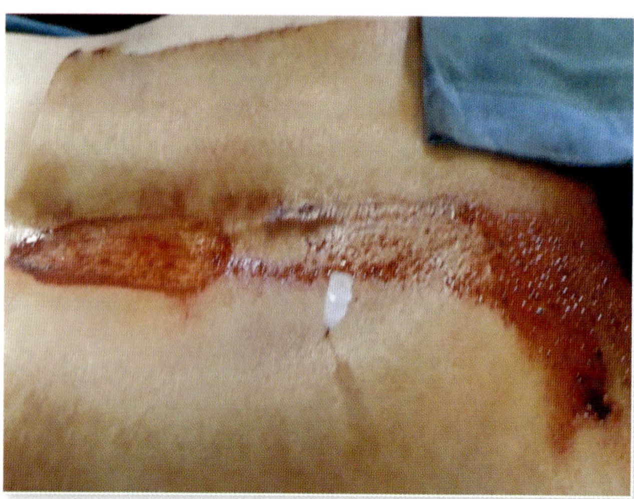

Figure 5: L5–S1 transforaminal block.Needle placed in left transforaminal area (Clinical view)

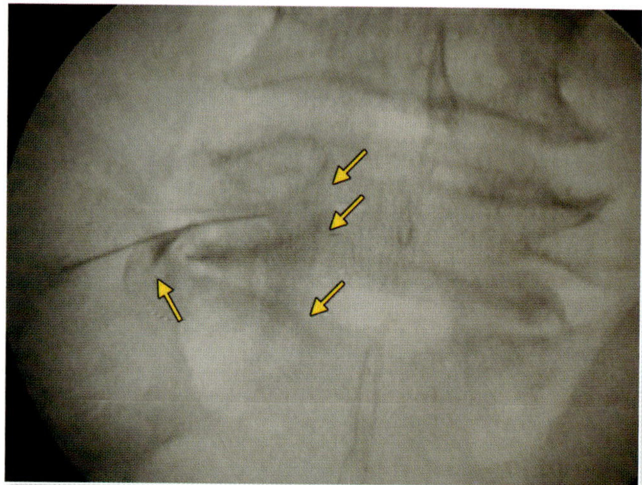

Figure 6: L5–S1 transforaminal block. Needle placed in left transforaminal area (Endoscopic view)

Caudal Steroids Versus Transforaminal Epidural Steroids

Translaminar epidural and caudal epidural steroids are dorsal approaches wherein the drug spreads ventrally by diffusion. The dorsal median septum confines the drug to ipsilateral side.[35]

A transforaminal approach allows high concentration drug to be delivered precisely to the the target area - the ventral epidural space.

A caudal epidural provided 34% pain relief in postlaminectomy syndrome.[36]

In a retrospective study, 50% of patients had 50% pain relief after transforaminal injections in postlaminectomy syndrome.[37]

In a prospective study the outcome of transforaminal was statistically significant than the caudal epidural steroids.[38]

Radiofrequency Lesioning of the Dorsal Root Ganglion

In refractory FBSS, the pulsed radiofrequency (PRF) of the dorsal root ganglion (DRG) is indicated **(Figures 9 and 10)**. The DRG modulates the pain transmission. APRF of the DRG

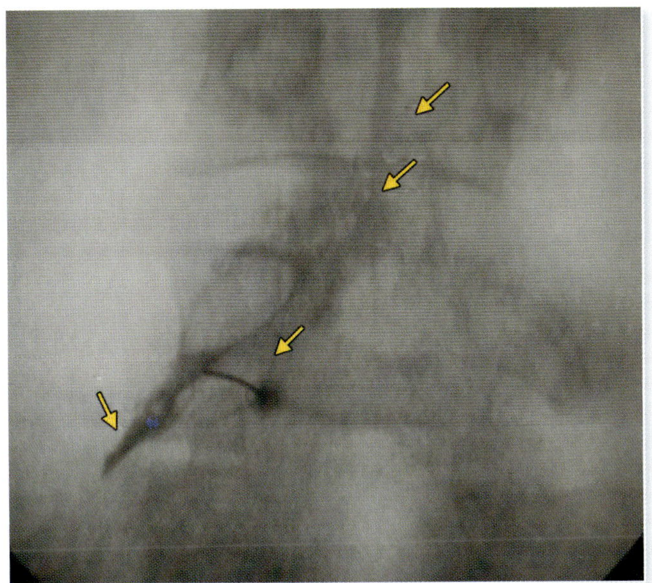

Figure 7: L5–S1 transforaminal block (right oblique). Contrast spread in the root sheath and epidural space

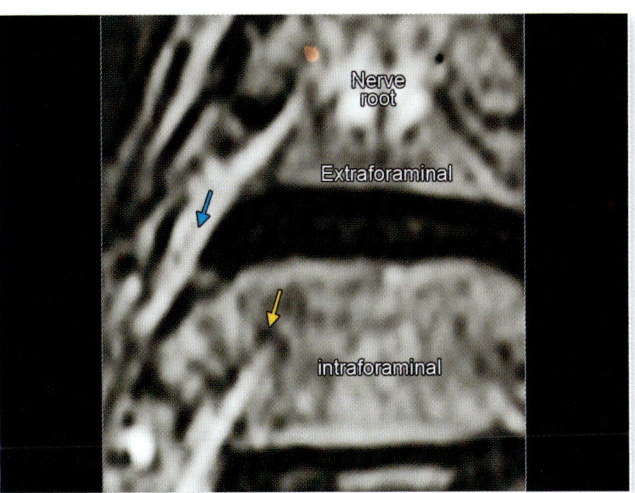

Figure 8: Intra- and extraforaminal nerve root

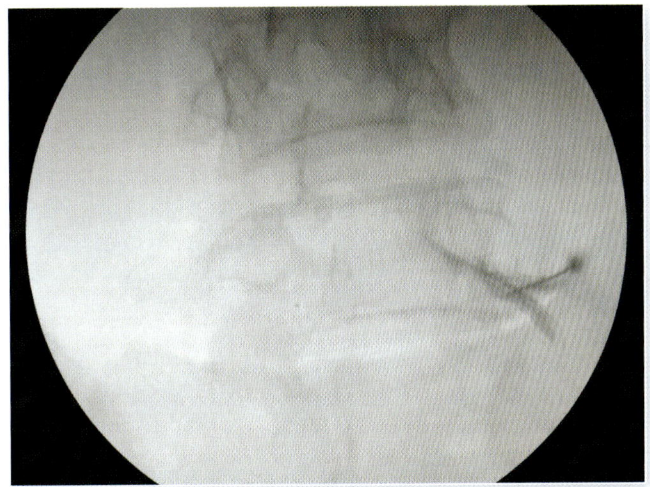

Figure 9: Radiofrequency needle at the dorsal root ganglion

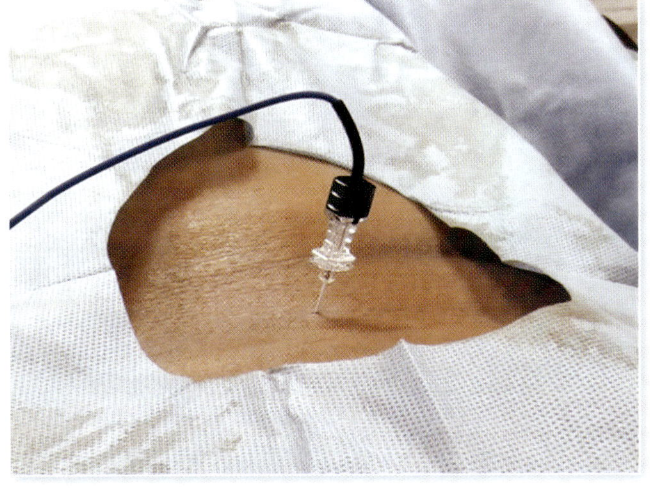

Figure 10: Pulsed RF of DRG at 42 d for 60 seconds in a process

followed by conventional RF of the lumbar median branches (LMBB) will have successful outcome.

FBSS and Spinal Hardware

Patients presenting with spinal hardware and radicular pain are the worst of FBSS to manage the persistant pain. The spinal intervention techniques are challenging due to the distorted anatomy. These patients have refractory pain to oral analgesics and patches.

A stop gap management in the form of transforaminal epidural steroids and lumbar median branch blocks are initial interventional procedures.

Patient had Severe Back and Radiating Leg Pain

The transforaminal (TFESI) and the lumbar medial branch blocks are difficult in patients with spinal hardware. The spinal anatomy is distorted and needle tips cannot be visualized under the spinal hardwares **(Figures 11 to 13)**.

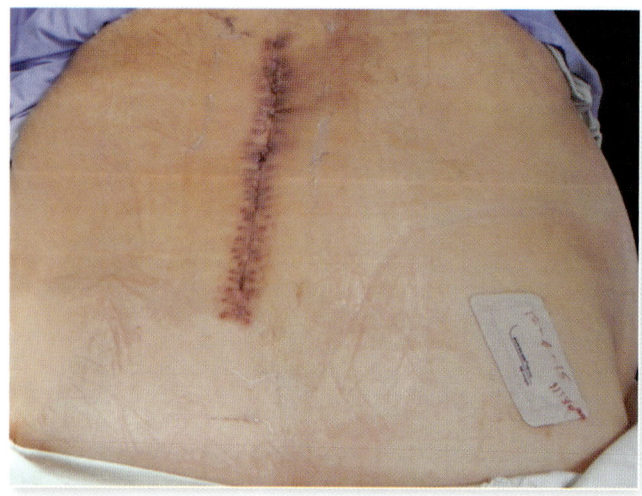

Figure 11: A patient with severe back and radicular pain on buprenorphine patch

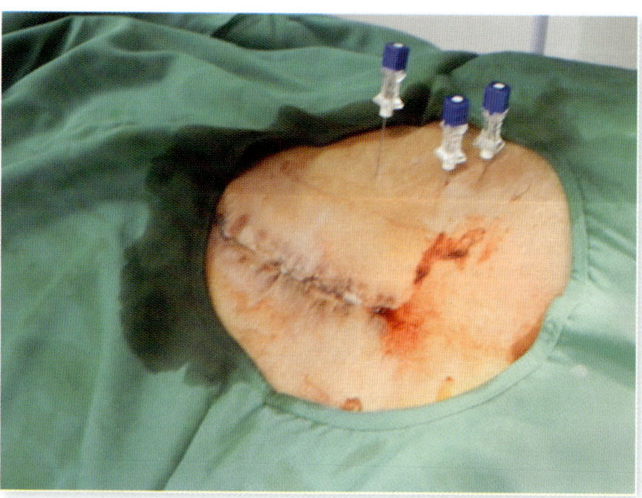

Figure 12: A multiple LMBB and TFESI in process

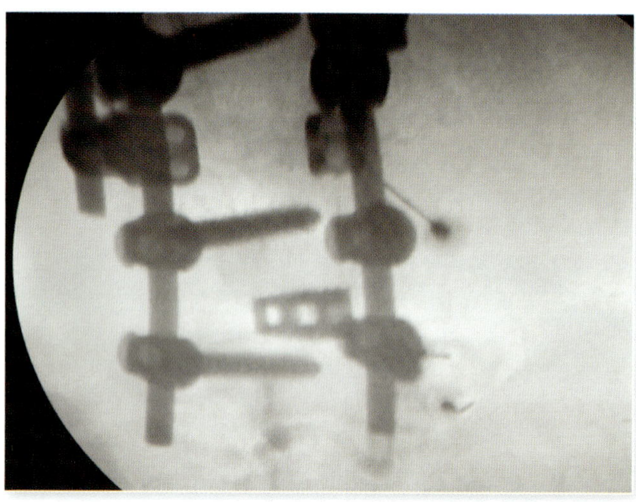

Figure 13: Needle tip imaged under fluoroscopy

PERCUTANEOUS ADHESIOLYSIS

Epidural neuroplasty (lysis of epidural adhesions) is an interventional technique that was developed at Texas Tech Health Sciences Pain Center in 1989.

Percutaneous adhesiolysis is a procedure designed to lyse epidural scarring in patients with persistent low back and leg pain due to postlumbar surgery syndrome or spinal stenosis.[39]

The most recent systematic review showed a strong (Level I or II-1 using the United States Preventive Services Task Force (USPSTF)[40] criteria for the use of adhesiolysis for post-lumbar laminectomy syndrome.

Aim and Prerequisites of the Procedure

- The adhesiolysis is performed as a one-day procedure.
- A soft-tip, wire-bound flexible catheter, steroids, local anesthetic, and hypertonic saline.
- A filling defect on fluoroscopy targets the area.
- The defect should resolve on completion of the procedure.

Technique

- Appropriate preparation with intravenous access, antibiotic administration, and appropriate sedation.
- Flurooscopic guided 18 G epidural needle is introduced into the sacral epidural space.
- A dilute nonionic contrast is injected to obtain a sacro - lumbar epidurogram.
- Identification of the filling defects is carried out by examining the contrast flow into the nerve roots
- Epidurography is confirmed and a 18 g epidural catheter is inserted to the area of filling defect or the site of pathology determined by MRI. or patient symptoms (**Figures 14 and 15**).

(A Racz catheter if avalaible is a steerable catheter and can be directed towards the site of lesion.)

Adhesiolysis

- 6 mL normal saline or 3% sodium chloride and
- 80 mg methylprednisolone.

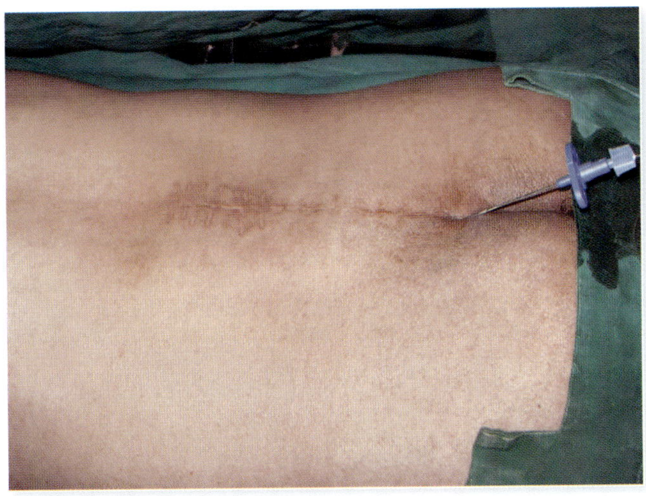

Figure 14: 18 G Tuohy in caudal epidural space

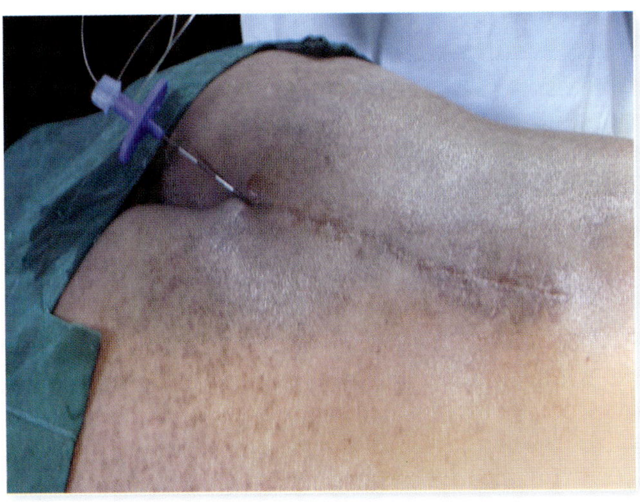

Figure 15: Epidural catheter in caudal–lumbar epidural space

Role of Hypertonic Saline

The pain conducting transmitters release from neuromuscular junctions are attenuated when exposed to hypertonic solutions.[41] Osmolar depletion of water content within the peripheral axons results in decreased nerve conduction.[42]

Clinical Effectiveness of Percutaneous Adhesiolysis

In patients with FBSS where in a prior conservative modalities of treatments, including fluoroscopically directed epidural steroid injections had failed, received epidural adhesiolysis. There was improvement is patients pain symptoms in 49% at the end of 3 months, 43% at 6 months and 49% at 12 months.[41]

This study provided evidence for the effectiveness of adhesiolysis.[41]

In a one-day adhesiolysis, as a modality of treatment for FBSS a 97% improvement was observed at the end of 6 months as compared to conservative treatment where the improvement was 46%.[43] The procedures was repeated 1–3 times. Patients in the treatment group also showed significant improvement in functional and psychological status. The study was not blinded and there was no control group.

The role of hypertonic saline in epidural adhesiolysis is validated.[43] A 60% improvement was observed at the end of 1 year with normal saline as against 72% with hypertonic saline.

It is concluded that percutaneous adhesiolysis, with or without hypertonic saline neurolysis, is a safe and effective treatment for chronic refractory low back and lower extremity pain.[43]

Postadhesiolysis

After completion of the adhesiolysis, a repeat epidurogram is carried out by additional injection of contrast. Appropriate adhesiolysis is identified by nerve root filling as well as ventral and lateral epidural filling.

Complications

The common complications of neural blockade in the lumbar spine are related to dural puncture, spinal cord compression, catheter shearing.[42]

Infection, problems related to steroids, hypertonic saline and hyaluronidase have been reported.[42]

Unintended subarachnoid or subdural puncture with injection of local anesthetic or hypertonic saline is one of the major complications of the procedure. Hypertonic saline injected into the subarachnoid space has been reported to cause cardiac arrhythmias, myelopathy, paralysis, and loss of sphincter control.[41,42]

Slow volumes of fluid injection can induce transient neurological symptoms, such as headache or hypoacusia.

Visual impairment and retinal haemorrhage after epidural fluid injection also have been reported.[44]

SPINAL ENDOSCOPY

A CT scan and MRI can be inconclusive to diagnose epidural fibrosis.

For direct visualization of the pathologic changes inside the spinal canal, "spinal endoscopy" **(Figure 16)** may be necessary to confirm the diagnosis, dissect fibrotic tissue and injecting medications. Spinal endoscopic adhesiolysis

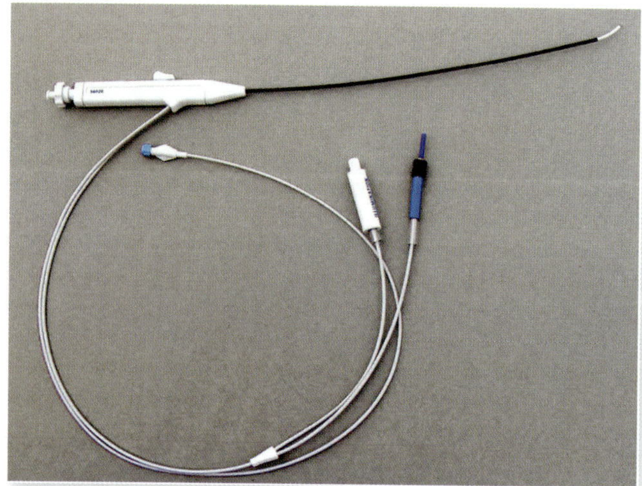
Figure 16: A spinal endoscope

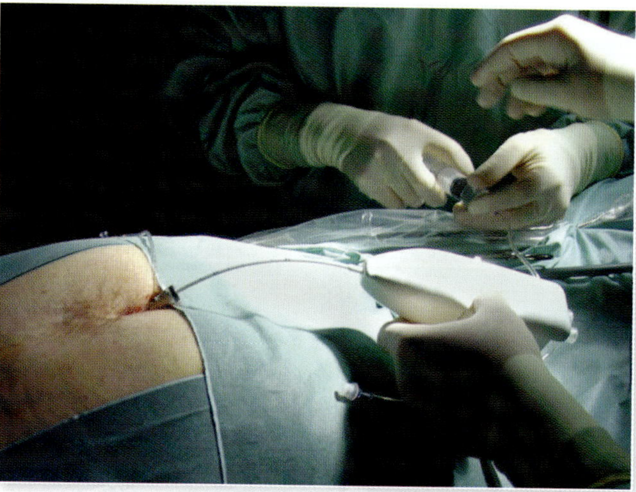
Figure 17: Epiduroscopy in process

has emerged during the 1990s after years of advances in instrumentation. Fiberoptic technology developed small flexible endoscopes with high image resolution.

Endoscopic adhesiolysis is based on the premise that the epidural space can be accessed safely by using flexible fiberoptic catheters entering via the sacral hiatus. It facilitates three-dimensional visualization of the contents of the epidural space and provides the operator with the ability to steer the catheter toward structures of interest. This procedure allows examination of a specific nerve root and its pathology and treatment by injection of a drug directly in the root, along with the ability to expand the epidural space with normal saline.

Current US Food and Drug Administration (FDA) approved indications for the use of spinal endoscopy **(Figure 17)** are as follows:

- Documentation of pathological features
- Documentation of decompression ofstructures
- Direct nerve inspection, inspection of internalfixation, and
- Delivery of therapeutic agents.

A systematic review comments that the spinal adhesions appear to be an important contributor to refractory low back and/or lumbar radicular pain especially in patients with previous (failed) lumbar spinal surgery.

Epidural[45] adhesions may compromise nerve root nutrition and contribute to persistent inflammation **(Figure 18)**. Spinal endoscopic adhesiolysis may allow improved nutrition and mobility of lumbar nerves and would allow delivery of therapeutic medications (local anesthetics and steroids) to target nerve roots **(Figure 19)**.

This systematic review of the literature of the effectiveness of spinal endoscopic adhesiolysis in managing chronic

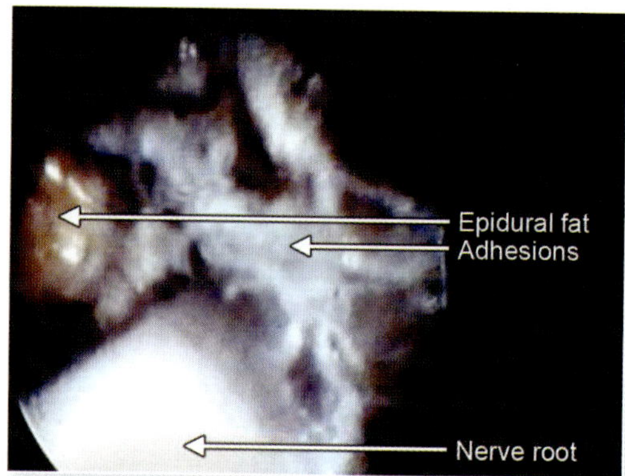

Figure 18: Structures visualized at epiduroscopy

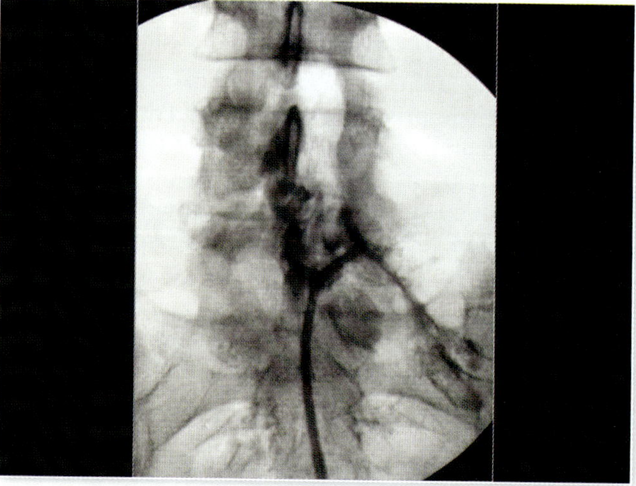
Figure 19: Postepiduroscopy epidurogram

intractable pain of post surgerysyndrome indicated evidence level II-1 or II-2 based on USPSTF criteria and one randomized trial with a recommendation of 1C/strong recommendation.[46]

Postspinal endoscopic adhesiolysis epidurogram is shown in **Figure 19**.

FBSS and the Sympathetic Nervous System

The pain in FBSS may originate from shearing compression and deformation of the dorsal root during surgery which may trigger central sensitization.[47]

The generation and maintenance of chronic pain is due to the dysfunction of autonomic nervous system.[48]

A study indicated that the skin sympathetic response (SSR) is affected in FBSS and that the dysfunction of the sympathetic nervous system may contribute to the intensity and chronicity of pain states in this group of patients.[49]

Autonomic dysfunction of the sympathetic system in FBSS may be due to several factors. The longer latency in SSR may be the result of loss of axons and preganglionic fibers. Somatic nerves are affected more which consists of non-myelinated axons.[50,51]

Injury to the somatic tissues leads to changes of excitability and neuronal activity in supraspinal and spinal centers and autonomic nervous system which is reflected in SSR.[52]

Musculoskeletal injury during surgery affects somatic tissues and autonomic nervous system.[53] This is reflected in SSR.

Chronic compression or constriction of the spinal nerves during surgery.[54] This induces the excitatory neurotransmitters like substance P, calcitonin related peptide, vasoactive intestinal peptide and

neuropeptide Y all of which play roles in allodynia and hyperalgesia.[54]

Changes in microcirculation of the tissues induced by surgery may also be responsible for dysfunction of the autonomic nervous system.[55]

Lumbar Sympathetic Block

A lumbar sympathetic block is performed to rule out the sympathetic maintained pain. Nevertheless, the improvement in microcirculation to the dorsal root ganglion will modulate the pain.

SPINAL CORD STIMULATION

A randomized controlled trial comparing repeat surgery with SCS suggested that repeat surgery has poorer results.[56]

A study[57] shows that the outcome of instrumented spinal fusion in patients with FBSS is disappointing; only 35% of the patients reported good outcome, whereas in 65% the symptoms were unchanged or worse.[57]

According to a retrospective study, the incidence of spinal instability will increase from 12% after one surgery to 50% after four or more revision surgeries.[58]

The most invasive treatment option, short of revision surgery, is spinal cord stimulation.[59] This intervention has a number of studies demonstrating its efficacy and cost-effectiveness in this population.[59] Finally, revision surgery may be used when indicated, such as with progressive neurological impairment or with issues regarding previous surgical instrumentation.[60]

Role of Neuromodulation for Failed Back Surgery Syndrome

Spinal cord stimulation (SCS) is an invasive technique that administers electrical stimulation to the dorsal columns of the spinal cord to reduce pain perception. SCS has shown to be an effective treatment for various neuropathic pain conditions.[61-67]

The SCS is less effective in

- Older patients and higher scores on the depression subscale D of the Minnesota Multiphasic Personality Inventory.[68]
- Several studies have shown SCS to be effective in treating the radicular pain after FBSS.[69,70]

A permanent implant has been shown to be effective in more than 50% of the patients with radicular pain, with an improvement in pain, function and feeling of well-being.[71]

Neuromodulation should not be considered as a last option.[70] It should be but should be offered early in the management plan.[70] Early referral and application of neuromodulation has been shown to increase its success in FBSS.[70]

The benefits of SCS are obtained when the configurations of SCS are adjusted to the patients demands.

- Configuration of active electrodes
- Stimulation frequency
- Pulse width, and
- Pulse amplitude can be

The electrical stimulation of the large-diameter fibers in the dorsal column elicits tingling sensations (paresthesia) in most patients.[72]

The perception and appreciation of this paresthesia varies to a great extent among patients and is heavily influenced by the stimulation parameters used.[73]

The frequencies of SCS that are most often used in the clinic are around 50 Hz and generally vary between 30 and 120 Hz.[74] New types of stimulation paradigms for SCS using high-frequency stimulation up to 10 kHz have been introduced.[75]

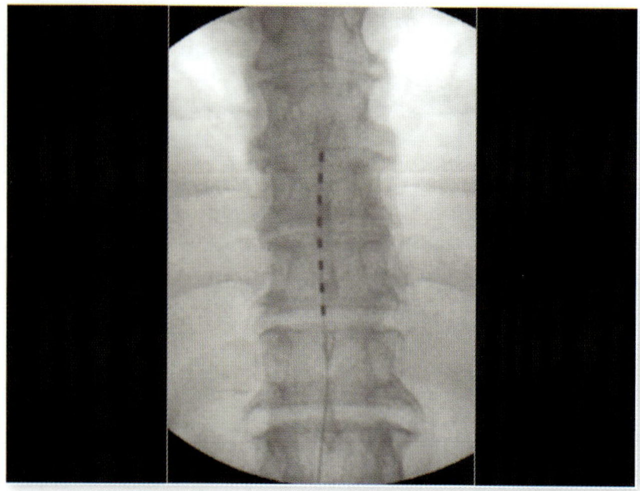

Figure 20: Epidural leads

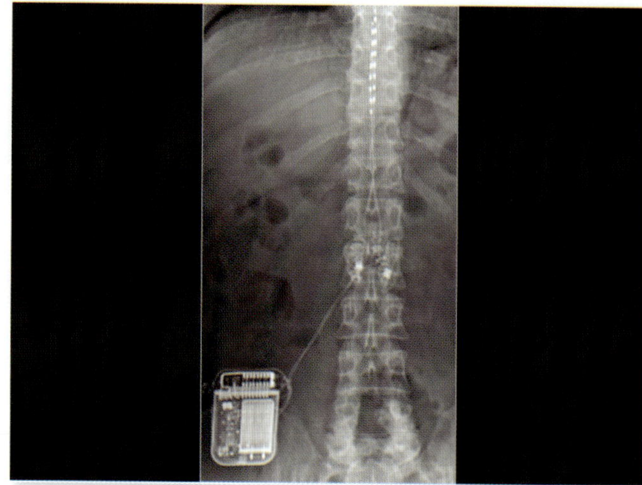

Figure 21: Spinal cord stimulator implant in situ

Neuromodulation for Failed Back Surgery Syndrome (Figures 20 and 21)

Indications

The pain is predominantly neuropathic and localised to the buttock and leg.

NICE[76] and the British Pain Society[77] have recommended trial before implantation.

There are advantages and disadvantages to a trial of SCS before proceeding to permanent implant (including false-negative or false-positive trial. The trial lead should be left in place for a week to 10 days to assess whether or not SCS is beneficial to the patient.

A 50% reduction in pain, increased function and quality of life is a successful trial.

POSTSUCCESSFUL TRIAL

The trial lead is removed, while the patient awaits implantation of the permanent lead and internal pulse generator (IPG).

There are recent trials and case reports of advanced management with neuromodulations.

High-frequency Spinal Cord Stimulation

This technique has been shown to be of particular value in patients with FBSS with a predominant lower back pain component. A frequency of about 5000–10,000 Hz is used.

There are no efficacy, cost-effectiveness or safety data from a randomised controlled trial or comparison with conventional SCS.[78]

Dorsal Root Ganglion Stimulation

A specially designed lead is placed around the dorsal root ganglion, via the epidural space.

The major advantages is possible to target dermatomes which would otherwise be difficult to target with conventional SCS (foot, groin etc).

There are minimal long-term data regarding efficacy, safety and cost-effectiveness.

Peripheral Nerve Field Stimulation[79]

A specially designed leads are approved for this use. This lead specifically targets the neuropathic back pain component of FBSS. Use of this technique, in combination with conventional SCS or alone, has been published with impressive results in case series.

The long-term efficacy is not established.

Burst Stimulation

This was introduced as a new stimulation paradigm combining features of high-frequency stimulation with conventional, tonic stimulation.[80,81]

The burst stimulation used provides pulse trains of five high-frequency pulses at 500 Hz (= 500 Hz spike frequency) occurring 40 times a second (= 40 Hz burst frequency). The pulse width is fixed at 1 msec and the amplitude is optimized for each individual patient.

Burst stimulation is indicated in chronic pain patients who are already receiving SCS treatment for at least six months.

The burst stimulation suppresses pain via the electrophysiologic gate-control mechanism before the clinical paresthesia threshold is reached.[82]

The burst stimulation causes significantly more pain reduction in patients with diabetic neuropathy and in patients with FBSS.[83] A trial period of at least two weeks of burst stimulation for every patient with a spinal cord stimulator would likely increase the efficacy of SCS therapy.[83] Further research is warranted for optimal burst stimulation parameters for patients with SCS.[83]

Intrathecal Drug Delivery System for Failed Back Surgery Syndrome

- Implanted intrathecal drug delivery systems (ITDDSs) have been used with benefit in patients with FBSS.[84-86]
- Implantation follows a trial and a careful assessment of the trial results.
- A patient with an ITDDS requires long-term regular follow-up for
  - regular pump refills,
  - to identify efficacy, side effects related to drugs delivered through the pump and neurological or endocrine issues arising as a result of this treatment.
- Intrathecal morphine, ziconotide and baclofen have approval from the US Food and Drug Administration for use in an intrathecal pump.[87]
- The use of intrathecal pumps for FBSS is questionable, but their use in palliative care is much more established.[88]

REFERENCES

1. Robaina Padrón FJ. Lumbar post-laminectomy syndrome I. Pain management using interventionist techniques.Neurocirugia (Astur). 2007;18:468-77.
2. Manchikanti L, Singh V, Cash KA, Pampati V, Datta S. A comparative effectiveness evaluation of percutaneous adhesiolysis and epidural steroid injections in managing lumbar post surgery syndrome: a randomized, equivalence controlled trial. Pain Physician. 2009;12:E355-68.
3. Rodrigues FF, Dozza DC, de Oliveira CR, de Castro RG. Failed back surgery syndrome: Casuistic and etiology. Arq Neugressionropsiquiat. 2006;64:757-61.
4. Kumar K Toth C. The role of spinal cord stimulation in chronic pain postlaminectomy. Curr Rev Pain. 1998;2:85-92.
5. Bosscher HA, Heavner JE. Incidence and severity of epidural fibrosis after back surgery: and endoscopic study. Pain Practise. 2010;(10)1;18-24.
6. Harrington JF, Messier AA, Hoffman L, Yu E, Dykhuizen M, Barker K. Physiological and behavioral evidence for focal nociception induced by epidural glutamate infusion in rats. Spine. 2005; 30:606-12.
7. Kirkaldy-Willis WH, Wedge JH, Yong-Hing K, Reilly J. Pathology and pathogenesis of lumbar spondylosis and stenosis. Spine (Phila Pa 1976). 1978;3:319-28.
8. Wenger M, Mariani L, Kalbarczyk A, Groger U. Long-term outcome of 104 patients after lumbar sequestrectomy according to Williams. Neurosurgery. 2001;49:329-35.
9. Faulhauer K, Manicke C. Fragment excision versus conventional disc removal in the microsurgical treatment of herniated lumbar disc. Acta Neurochir. 1995;133:107-11.
10. Manchikanti L, Manchukonda R, Pampati V, Damron KS, McManus CD. Prevalence of facet joint pain in chronic low back pain in postsurgical patients by controlled comparative local anesthetic blocks. Arch Phys Med Rehabil. 2007;88: 449-55.
11. Manchikanti L, Boswell MV, Singh V, Derby R, Fellows B, Falco FJ, Datta S, Smith HS, Hirsch JA. Comprehensive review of neurophysiologic basis and diagnostic interventions in managing chronic spinal pain. Pain Physician. 2009;12:E71-120.
12. Singh V, Manchikanti L, Benyamin RM, Helm S, Hirsch JA. Percutaneous lumbar laser disc decompression: A systematic review of current evidence. Pain Physician. 2009;12:573-88.
13. LaRocca H, McNab I. The laminectomy membrane: Studies in its evolution, characteristics, effects and prophylaxis in dogs. J Bone Joint Surg BR. 1974;56:545-50.
14. Zoidl G, Grifka J, Boluki D, Willburger RE, Zoidl C, Krämer J, Dermietzel R, Faustmann PM. Molecular evidence for local denervation of paraspinal muscles in failed-back surgery/ postdiscotomy syndrome. Clin Neuropathol. 2003;22:71-7.
15. Manchikanti L, Manchukonda R, Pampati V, Damron KS, McManus CD. Prevalence of facet joint pain in chronic low back pain in postsurgical patients by controlled comparative local anesthetic blocks. Arch Phys Med Rehabil. 2007;88: 449-55.
16. Dunlop RB, Adams MA, Hutton WC. Disc space narrowing and the lumbar facet joints. J Bone Joint Surg Br. 1984;66:706-10.
17. Kirkaldy-Willis WH, Farfan HF. Instability of the lumbar spine. Clin Orthop Relat Res. 1982;165:110-23.
18. Gatchel RJ, Polatin PB, and Mayer TG. The dominant role of psychosocial risk factors in the development of chronic low back pain disability. Spine. 1995;20(24):2702-9.
19. Onesti ST. Failed Back Syndrome. The Neurologist. 2004;(10)5: 259-65.
20. Chan C, Peng P. Failed back surgery syndrome. Pain Medicine. 2011;12:577-606.
21. 21.Grane P. The postoperative lumbar spine: A radiological investigation of the lumbar spine after discectomy using MR imaging and CT. Acta Radiol Suppl. 1998;414:1-23.
22. Van Goethem JW, Parizel PM, van den Hauwe L, et al. Imaging findings in patients with failed back surgery syndrome. J Belge Radiol. 1997;80(2):81-4.
23. Braverman DL, Slipman CW, Lenrow DA. Using gabapentin to treat failed back surgery syndrome caused by epidural fibrosis: A report of 2 cases. Arch Phys Med Rehab. 2001; 82(5):691-3.
24. Baron R, Freynhagen R, Tölle TR, et al. The efficacy and safety of pregabalin in the treatment of neuropathic pain associated with chronic lumbosacral radiculopathy. Pain. 2010;150(3):420-7.
25. Duthie D, Nimmo S. Adverse effects of opioid analgesic drugs. Br J Anaesth. 1987;59:61-77.

26. Turk DC, Wilson H, Cahana A. Treatment of chronic non-cancer pain. The Lancet. 2011;377(9784):2226-35.
27. Dworkin RH, O'Connor AB, Backonja M, et al. Pharmacologic management of neuropathic pain: Evidence-based recommendations. Pain. 2007;132(3):237-51.
28. Hazard RG. Failed back surgery syndrome: Surgical and nonsurgical approaches. Clinical Orthop Relat Res. 2006;443:228-32.
29. NICE. Neuropathic pain: the pharmacological management of neuropathic pain in adults in nonspecialist settings. NICE guidelines; 2010. p. 96.
30. Devulder J. Transforaminal nerve root sleeve injection with corticosteroids, hyaluronidase, and local anesthetic in the failed back surgery syndrome. J Spinal Disord. 1998;11(2):151-4.
31. Ragab A, DeShazo RD. Management of back pain in patients with previous back surgery. Am J Med. 2008;121(4):272-278.
32. Manchikanti L, Singh V, Cash KA, et al. Preliminary results of a randomized, equivalence trial of fluoroscopic caudal epidural injections in managing chronic low back pain: Part 3 – post surgery syndrome. Pain Physician. 2008;11: 817-31.
33. Management of Pain of Post Lumbar Surgery Syndrome: One-Year Results of a Randomized, Double-Blind, Active Controlled Trial of Fluoroscopic Caudal Epidural Injections Laxmaiah Manchikanti, Vijay Singh, Kimberly A. Cash, Vidyasagar Pampati, and Sukdeb Datta. Pain Physician. 2010;13:509-21.
34. Devulder J. Transforaminal nerve root sleeve injection with corticosteroids, hyaluronidase, and local anesthetic in the failed back surgery syndrome. J Spinal Disord. 1998;11:151–4.
35. O'Niell C, Derby R,Kneders L. Percise injection techniques for diagnosis and treatment for lumbar disc disease. Semin Spin Surg. 1999;11;104-18.
36. Kim SL, Sadove MA. Caudal epidural steroid in postlaminectomy syndrome: treatment for low back pain. Comprehens Ther. 1775;1;57-60.
37. Devulder J. Transforaminal nerve root sleeve injection with corticosteroids, hyaluronidase, and local anesthetic in the failed back surgery syndrome. J Spinal Disord. 1998;11:151-4.
38. JHuang. Epidural steroid for postlaminectomy syndrome: Transforaminal verses caudal. The internet journal of anesthesiology. 2006;12;1.
39. Racz GB, Heavner JE, Trescot A. Percutaneous lysis of epidural adhesions—evidence for safety and efficacy. Pain Pract. 2008;8:277-86.
40. Epter RS, Helm S 2nd, Hayek SM, Benyamin RM, Smith HS, Abdi S. Systematic review of percutaneous adhesiolysis and management of chronic low back pain in post lumbar surgery syndrome. Pain Physician. 2009;12:361-78.
41. Anderson SR, Racz GB. Heavner J. Evolution of epidural lysis of adhesions. Pain Physician. 2000;3:262-70.
42. Racz GB, Heavner JE, Trescit A. Percutaneous lysis of epidural adhesions - evidence for safety and efficacy. Pain Pract. 2008;8:277-86.
43. Laxmaiah Manchikanti, Jose J. Rivera, VidyasagarPampati, MSc, Kim S. Damron, Carla D. McManus, , Doris E. Brandon, and Sue R. Wilson, One Day Lumbar Epidural Adhesiolysis and Hypertonic Saline. Neurolysis in Treatment of Chronic Low Back Pain: A Randomized, Double-Blind Trial. Pain Physician. 2004;7:177-86.
44. Gill JB, Heavner JE. Visual Impairment following epidural fluid injections and epiduroscopy: a review. Pain Med. 2005;6:367-74.
45. Salim M Hayek MD PhD1, Standiford Helm MD2, Ramsin M Benyamin MD3, Vijay Singh MD4, David A Bryce MD5, and Howard S Smith MD6. Effectiveness of Spinal Endoscopic Adhesiolysis in Post Lumbar Surgery Syndrome: A Systematic Review. Pain Physician. 2009; 12:419-35.
46. Berg AO, Allan JD. Introducing the third U.S. Preventive Services Task Force. Am J Prev Med. 2001;20:S3-S4.
47. Rooney BA, Crown ED, Hulsebosch CE, McAdoo DJ. Preemptive-analgesia with lidocaine prevents Failed Back SurgerySyndrome. Exp Neurol. 2007;204:589-96.
48. Berker E, Dinçer N. Chronic pain and rehabilitation. Agri. 2005;17:10-6.
49. Nilay Şahihn, Lütfiye Müslümanoğlu, Ömer Karataş, Ayşegül Çakmak, Emelözcan, Ender Berker. Evaluation of sympathetic response in cases with failed back surgery syndrome. AGRI. 2009;21(1):10-5.
50. Kiylioglu N, Akyol A, Guney E, Bicerol B, Ozkul A, Erturk A. Sympathetic skin response in idiopathic and diabetic carpal tunnel syndrome. Clin Neurol Neurosurg. 2005;108:1-7.
51. Sun PC, Lin HD, Jao SH, Ku YC, Chan RC, Cheng CK. Relationship of skin temperature to sympathetic dysfunction in diabetic at-risk feet. Diabetes Res ClinPract. 2006;73:41-6.
52. Grimm DR, Cunningham BM, Burke JR. Autonomic nervous system function among individuals with acute musculoskeletal injury. J Manipulative Physiol Ther. 2005;28:44-51.
53. Nilsen KB, Sand T, Westgaard RH, Stovner LJ, White LR, Bang Leistad R, et al. Autonomic activation and pain in response to low-grade mental stress in fibromyalgia and shoulder/neck pain patients. Eur J Pain. 2007;11:743-55.
54. Son SJ, Lee KM, Jeon SM, Park ES, Park KM, Cho HJ. Activation of transcription factor c-jun in dorsal root ganglia induces VIP and NPY upregulation and contributes to the pathogenesis of neuropathic pain. ExpNeurol. 2007;204:467-72.
55. Ozgocmen S, Yoldas T, Yigiter R, Kaya A, Ardicoglu O. R-R interval variation and sympathetic skin response in fibromyalgia. Arch Med Res. 2006;37:630-4.
56. North RB, Kidd DH, Farrokhi F, et al. Spinal cord stimulation versus repeated lumbosacral spine surgery for chronic pain: A randomised controlled trial. Neurosurgery. 2005;56(1):98-107
57. Mark P Arts, Nicola I Kols, Suzanne M Onderwater and Wilco C Peul. Clinical outcome of instrumented fusion for the treatment of failed back surgery syndrome: a case series of 100 patients Acta Neurochir DOI. 10.1007/s00701-012-1380-7.
58. Hazard RG. Failed back surgery syndrome: surgical and nonsurgical approaches. Clin Orthop Relat Res. 2006;443:228-32.
59. Pain Pract. 2014 Jan;14(1):64-78. doi: 10.1111/papr.12035. Epub 2013 Feb 3.
60. Hussain A[1], Erdek M. Interventional pain management for failed back surgery syndrome. Pain pract. 2014;14(1), 64-78.

61. De Jongste MJL, Hautvast RWM, Hillege HL, Lie KI. Efficacy of spinal cord stimulation as adjuvant therapy for intractable angina pectoris:a prospective, randomized clinical study. J Am Coll Cardiol. 1994;23:1592-7.
62. Kemler MA, Barendse GAM, van Kleef M et al. Spinal cord stimulation in patients with chronic reflex sympathetic dystrophy. N Engl J Med. 2000;343:618-24.
63. Kumar K, Toth C, Nath RK. Spinal cord stimulation for chronic pain in peripheral neuropathy. Surg Neurol. 1996;46:363-9.
64. Kumar K, Taylor RS, Jacques L et al. Spinal cord stimulation versus conventional medical management for neuropathic pain: a multicentre randomised controlled trial in patients with failed back surgery syndrome. Pain. 2007;132:179-88.
65. 65. North RB, Kidd DH, Farrokhi F, Piantadosi SA. Spinal cord stimulation versus repeated lumbosacral spine surgery for chronic pain: a randomized controlled trial. Neurosurgery 2005;56:98-107.
66. Pluijms WA, Slangen R, Joosten EA et al. Electrical spinal cord stimulation in painful diabetic polyneuropathy, a systematic review on treatment efficacy and safety. Eur J Pain. 2011;15:783-8.
67. De Vos CC, Rajan V, Steenbergen W, van der Aa HE, Buschman HPJ. Effect and safety of spinal cord stimulation for treatment of chronic pain caused by diabetic neuropathy. J Diabetes Complications. 2009;23:40-5.
68. Burchiel K J, Anderson VC, Wilson BJ, et al. Prognostic factors of spinal cord stimulation for chronic back and leg pain. Neurosurgery. 1995;36(6):1101-11.
69. North RB, Kidd D, Shipley J, et al. Spinal cord stimulation versus reoperation for failed back surgery syndrome: a cost effectiveness and cost utility analysis based on a randomized, controlled trial. Neurosurgery. 2007;61:361-9.
70. Kumar K, Hunter G, Demeria D. Spinal cord stimulation in treatment of chronic benign pain: Challenges in treatment planning and present status, a 22-year experience. Neurosurgery 2006;58(3):481-96.
71. Burchiel KJ, Anderson VC, Brown FD, et al. Prospective, multicenter study of spinal cord stimulation for relief of chronic back and extremity pain. Spine. 1996;21(23):2786-94.
72. Nordin M, Nystrom B, Wallin U, Hagbarth KE. Ectopic sensory discharges and paresthesiae in patients with disorders of peripheral nerves, dorsal roots and dorsal columns. Pain 1984;20:231-45.
73. Ochoa JL, Torebjork HE. Paraesthesiae from ectopic impulse generation in human sensory nerves. Brain. 1980;103:835-53.
74. Van Buyten JP, Al-Kaisy A, Smet I, Palmisani S, Smith T. High-frequency spinal cord stimulation for the treatment of chronic back pain patients: results of a prospective multicenter European clinical study. Neuromodulation. 2012;16:59-66.
75. Tiede J, Brown L, Gekht G, Vallejo R, Yearwood T, Morgan D. Novel spinal cord stimulation parameters in patients with predominant back pain. Neuromodulation. 2013;370-5.
76. Spinal cord stimulation for chronic pain of neuropathic or ischaemic origin. NICE Technology Appraisal Guidance (2009, accessed 27 November 2012).
77. Pain Society. Spinal cord stimulation for the management of pain: Recommendations for best clinical practice, (2009, accessed 27 November 2012).
78. Met I, VanBuyten JP, Al-Kaisy A. Successful treatment of low back pain with a novel neuromodulation device. In: Proceedings of the 14th North American. Neuromodulation Society Annual Meeting, Las Vegas, Nevada, USA, 2010.
79. Verrills P[1], Mitchell B, Vivian D, Sinclair C. Peripheral nerve stimulation: a treatment for chronic low back pain and failed back surgery syndrome? Neuromodulation. 2009 Jan;12(1):68-75. doi: 10.1111/j.1525-1403.2009.00191.x.
80. De Ridder D, Vanneste S, Plazier M, van der Loo E, Menovsky T. Burst spinal cord stimulation: toward paresthesia-free pain suppression. Neurosurgery. 2010;66:986-90.
81. De Ridder D, Plazier M, Kamerling N, Menovsky T, Vanneste S. Burst spinal cord stimulation for limb and back pain. World Neurosurg. 2013;10.1016/j.wneu.2013.01.040.
82. De Ridder D, Vanneste S, Plazier M, van der Loo E, Menovsky T. Burst spinal cord stimulation: toward paresthesia-free pain suppression. Neurosurgery. 2010;66:986-90.
83. Cecile C de Vos, Marjanne J Bom, Sven Vanneste, Mathieu WPM Lenders, Dirk de Ridder. Burst Spinal Cord Stimulation Evaluated in PatientsWith Failed Back Surgery Syndrome and Painful Diabetic Neuropathy. Neuromodulation: Technology at the Neural Interface Neuromodulation 2013;(onlinelibrary.wiley.com) DOI: 10.1111/ner.12116.
84. Paice JA, Penn RD, Shott S. Intraspinal morphine for chronic pain: A retrospective multicenter study. J Pain Symptom Manage. 1996;11:71-80.
85. Winkelmuller M, Winkelmuller W. Long-term effects of continuous intrathecal opioid treatment in chronic pain of non-malignant aetiology. J Neurosurg. 1996;85:458-67.
86. Long-term experience with implanted intrathecal drug administration systems for failed back syndrome and chronic mechanical low back pain. BMC Musculoskeletal Disorders 2002;3:17.
87. Deer T, Krames ES, Hassenbusch SJ, et al. Polyanalgesic Consensus Conference 2007: Recommendations for the management of pain by intrathecal (intraspinal) drug delivery: report of an interdisciplinary expert panel. Neuromodulation: Technology at the Neural Interface. 2007;10(4):300-28.
88. Smith T, Coyne PJ. Implantable drug delivery systems (IDDS) after failure of comprehensive medical management (CMM) can palliate symptoms in the most refractory cancer pain patients. J Palliat Med. 2005;8(4):736-42.

7

SECTION

Advances in MISS

Section Outline

35

CHAPTER

Robotics in Spine Surgery: An Ideal Surgical Assistant

Pramod K Sudarshan, Aditya P Panda, Sajan K Hegde

ABSTRACT

The use of robots in the field of spine surgery has evolved over a period of time and helped in performing a safe spine surgery. The major advantages are its need for smaller incisions, accurate placement of screws, lesser postoperative morbidity and faster rehabilitation. This chapter deals with the indications, techniques, available robotic systems and complications of utilizing robots in spine surgery.

INTRODUCTION

'Robot' is derived from the Czech word 'Robota' which means forced labor. World English dictionary defines robot as a mechanical device that can be programmed to carry out instructions and perform complicated tasks done by people. The first surgical application of the robot was described in 1985 to guide a needle for brain biopsy and received FDA approval in 1999. The da Vinci robotic system has been routinely used in a number of surgical disciplines, most notably urology and gynecology, with over 200,000 procedures performed worldwide in 2012 alone.

Although robotics has been employed for longer than a decade in many surgical subspecialties, it has only recently been utilized in the area of spine surgery. A review by Bertelsen et al. showed no fewer than 18 spinal robots existed, yet only five commercially available systems and only one was approved for spinal surgery: The Renaissance system (Mazor Robotics, Inc., Caesarea, Israel) and its predecessor SpineAssist.

Our experience is with the Renaissance system and the indications, technique and complications described herewith in this chapter are in relation to the system. Other robotic systems are described in the discussion section of the chapter.

INDICATIONS AND APPLICATIONS

Robotics in spine surgery can be applied in posterior surgical approaches either as open, percutaneous or minimally invasive (MIS) techniques. Main areas of application are as follows:

- Spinal fixation – Fixation in trauma (managed by percutaneous robotic guided screws and restoring the vertebral height at fractured level), degenerative conditions (using robotic guided screws for performing transforaminal/posterior interbody fusion) and spinal deformities.
  - Pedicle screws
  - Transfacet, translaminar—facet screws
  - Sacroiliac screws
- Spinal deformities
  - Scoliosis PSF, osteotomies
- Cement augmentations
  - Kyphoplasty and vertebroplasty
- Oncological applications
  - Biopsies, tumor resections
  - Revisions.

CONTRAINDICATIONS

- There are no contraindications for robotic-guided surgery as such. General contraindications for surgery do apply.
- Though the system has been applied for cervical spine surgery and upper cervical spine fixation (C1–2 transarticular screw) has been demonstrated in cadavers, it has to be adapted to the limited surgical access to the cervical region and hence, practically remains difficult.

TECHNIQUES

Patient Positioning

Positioning of patients for robotic surgery is the same as open surgeries. Adequate clearance for image acquisition should be given.

The renaissance system has a bone-mounted miniature robot designed to guide us toward accurate placement of pedicle screws. The bone-mounting feature improves the accuracy of screw placement by ensuring that inadvertent motion during the procedure does not alter the relative position of the robot with respect to the vertebra. It only acts as a guidance tool to the surgeon where the arm takes the position based on the trajectory of the screw and the surgeon has to perform drilling and screw insertion based on the same.

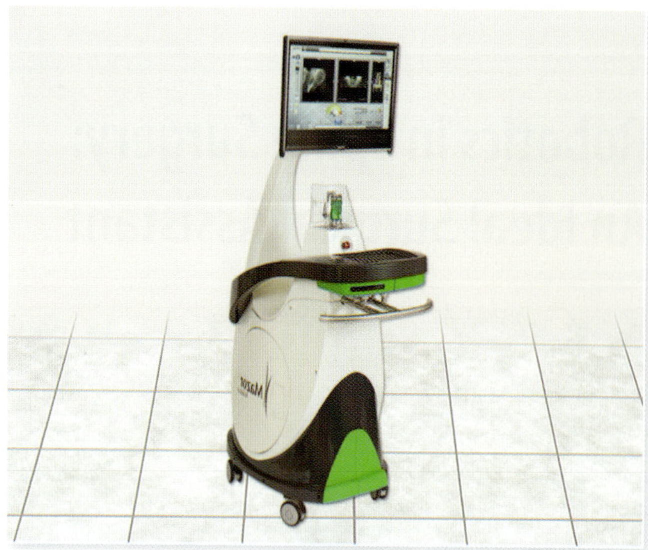

Figure 1: Computer workstation in the operation theater (Mazor Robotics, Caesarea, Israel)

Basic Steps

The robotic system works on the four basic steps:

- Plan
- Mount
- 3D Sync
- Operate

1. Preoperative planning: The computer workstation **(Figure 1)** works on a graphic 3D user interface software where all the preoperative planning is performed and real time control of the robotic motion during the procedure is handled. Patients undergo a high resolution CT scan of the spine and the protocol CD is inserted in the workstation. At our center, it is performed by a CT machine with specifications of <1 mm thickness, <0.8 mm interval and 250 FoV. On importing the CT, the segmentation of vertebra is done based on the region of interest and the approach used. Virtual placement of implants in the desired direction with appropriate width and length predicting potential collisions/complications is done. Fluoroscopy images are obtained to orient the image based on the CT setup.

2. Mounting to bony anatomy: The robotic device is handed over to the surgeon from the workstation in a sterile manner and is assembled to the plates ready for mounting. Attachment of a mounting frame (PEEK material) to the bony anatomy, usually clamped to the spinous process of the level to which targets for image registration are connected **(Figure 2)**. Other options of bed mount system or clamp and bridge mechanism can be used.

3. 3D sync: Capture of 2 fluoroscopic shots (AP and oblique) which are automatically registered to the preoperative CT images is done in the workstation. Based on the CT - fluoro-matching and accuracy, automatic segmentation of the vertebra is done and confirmed by the attending technician. Once the surgeon confirms visually regarding the accuracy of screws, operating workflow is proceeded **(Figures 3 and 4)**.

4. Operate: Once the robot is attached to the mounting frame, it moves and locks into position so that a guiding tube at the distal end of its arm is aligned with the planned screw/tool trajectory **(Figure 5)**. Drilling through the guiding tube into the pedicle either percutaneously or *via an open approach is performed under guidance and consecutively repeated for all planned implants.*

Once the guidewires are placed in all desired levels, two fluoroscopic shots (AP and lateral) to confirm the accuracy of position are taken. Cannulated screws can then be placed in the pedicles after using soft tissue dilators to provide the space for its insertion. Screws are checked for their position under image guidance and the procedure (fusion/deformity correction) is performed **(Figure 6)**.

Thereby, for the whole procedure, six images are taken—two images are taken for registration, two images for checking the guidewire position and two images for the final implant position. Radiation exposure in this system is therefore the least compared to open and other minimally invasive techniques.

POSTOPERATIVE PROTOCOL

In our experience, robotic spine surgeries have enabled faster recovery and earlier rehabilitation. Patients are mobilized out of bed and allowed to walk within 48 hours of surgery. Wound healing is significantly better with smaller incisions and minimal rate of infections in comparison to open surgeries. Analgesic use is reduced and hospital stay is minimized.

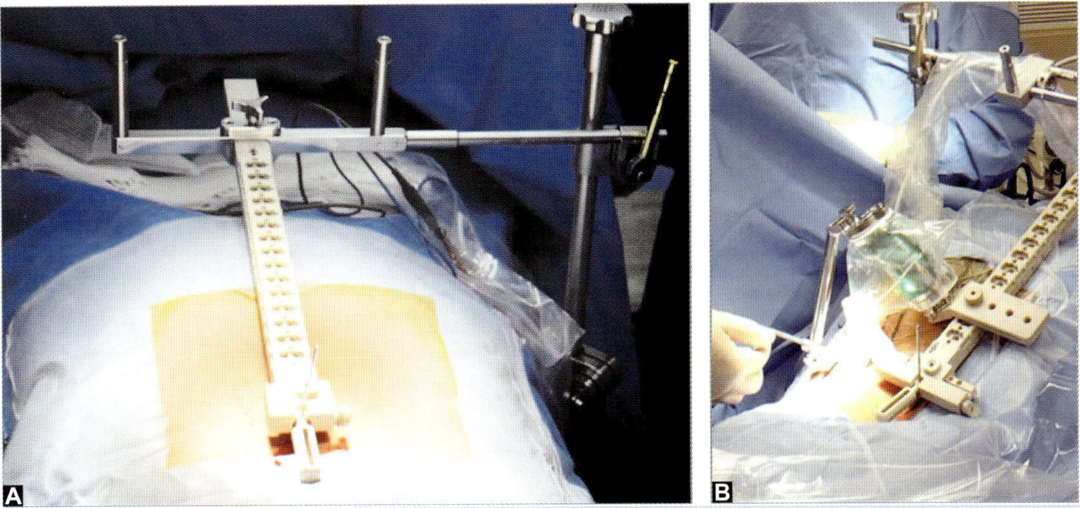

Figure 2: Bed mount system with the Hover-T attached to it guides the placement of the robot to the intended level of fixation

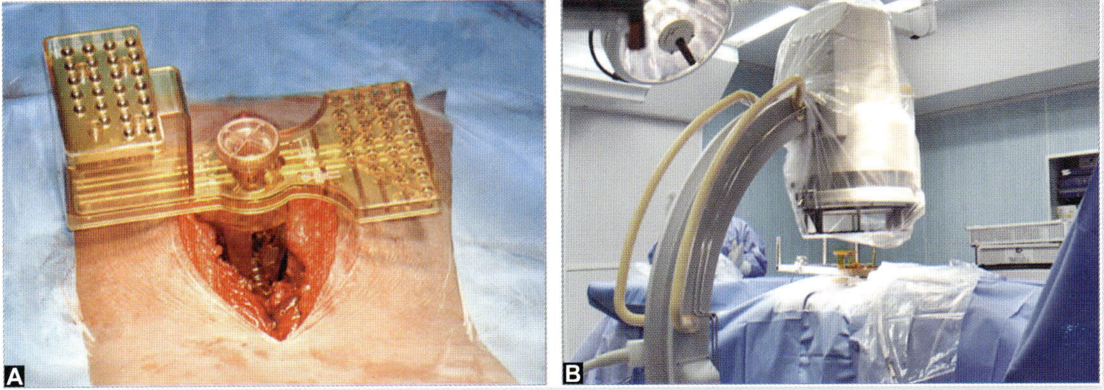

Figure 3: Placement of the image markers attached to the clamp, AP view taken to register the image in the workstation

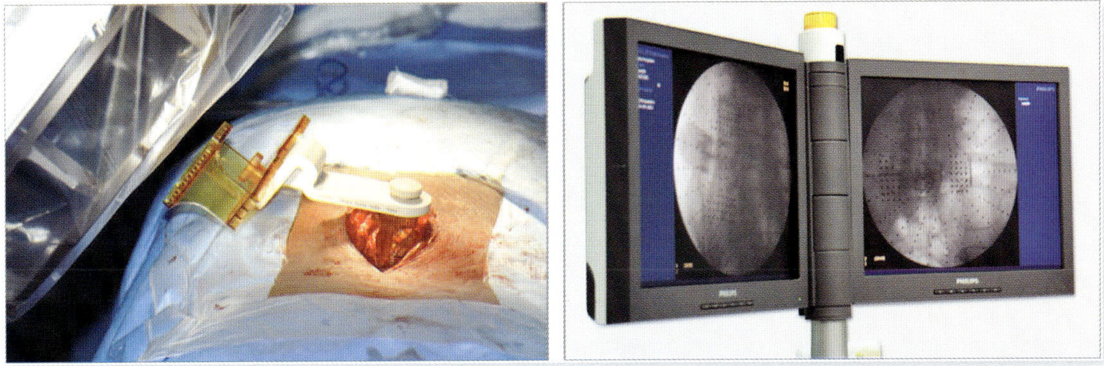

Figure 4: Use of the oblique marker extension to the clamp to obtain the oblique image, which is registered in the system

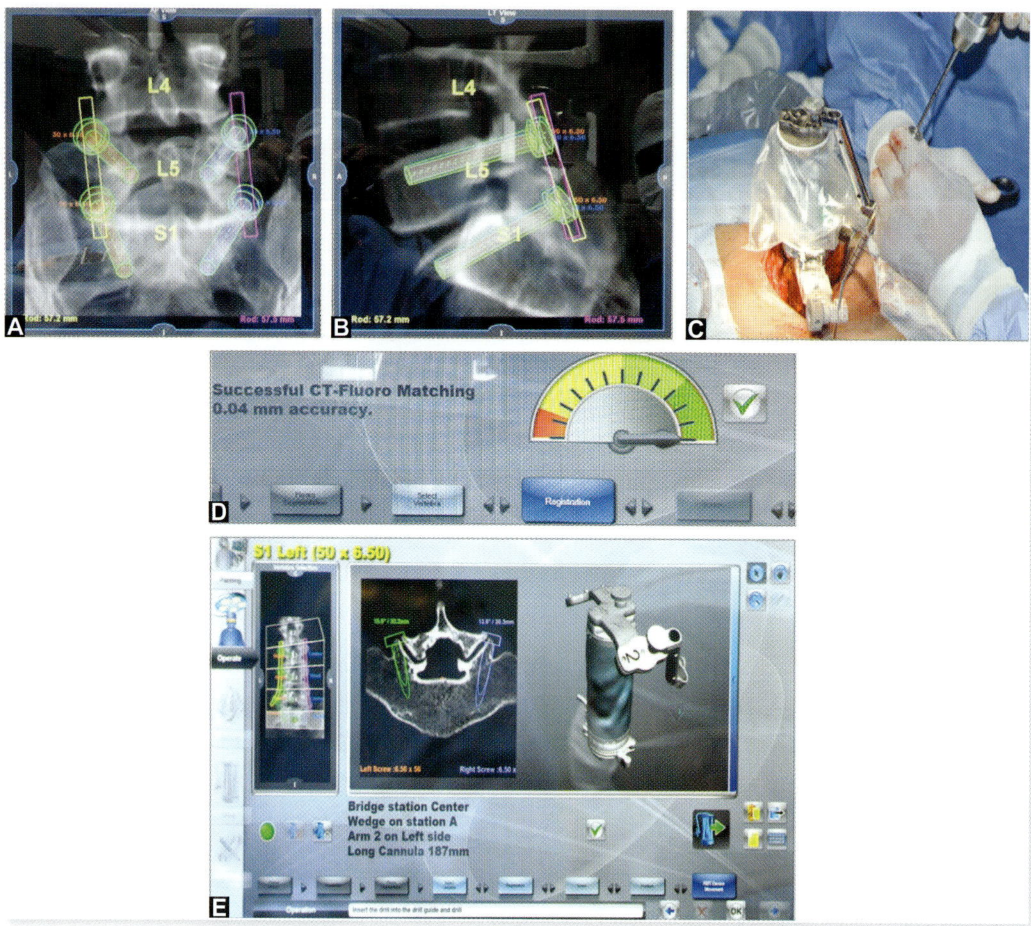

Figure 5: After checking the accuracy of the intended screw positions based on CT-fluoromatching, information about the use of wedge, the guiding arm and the length of the cannula to be used is checked in the workstation. Drilling is done through the guiding tube into the pedicle

COMPLICATIONS

We have had some occasions where screws could not be inserted due to registration failure due to technical reasons or due to error in planning. Only one patient had a skiving screw due to osteoporosis. Otherwise there have been no neurological deficits or implant-related complications specific to the robotic guided surgeries. Though the rate of infection is very minimal, it has to be considered in any surgery as a complication.

DISCUSSION

The pedicle offers the strongest point of attachment to the spine. Pedicle screws have been widely accepted as invaluable part of spinal instrumentation. Screw placement in the spine is fraught with inherent risk of injury to the nerves, spinal cord or blood vessels, as it is a free hand procedure based on the surgeon's orientation of the anatomy and guided by image intensifier, with reports of misplacement and other complications ranging from 2.5% to 40% in the literature. The disadvantage was the lack of accuracy in these machines to detect possible injury to the vital structures in complex anatomical deformities of the spine or in patients who were already operated and needed a revision surgery. In a meta-analysis performed by Kosmopoulos and Schizas, pedicle screws were assessed in a total of 16,717 pedicle screw placements according to detailed evaluation guidelines, of which 42.3% were based on postoperative CT scans, the overall weighted average of accurate lumbar and thoracic placements for the evaluated screws was only 81.9%. Thus a need for a more accurate and safe guidance device to improve the safety levels in screw placement was increasingly felt.

The recent advances in spine surgery has included minimally invasive spine surgery, also called keyhole surgery in common parlance where the entire surgery is done through one or more small incisions the sizes of

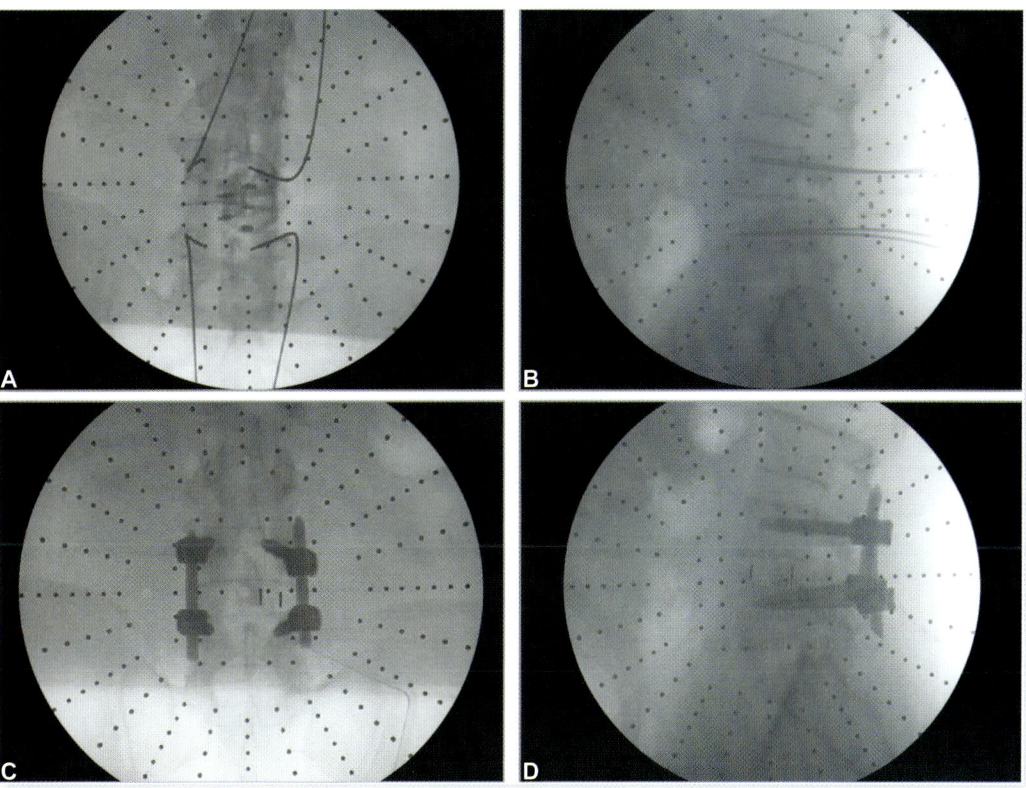

Figure 6: Once all the guidewires necessary are in place, 2 fluoroscopy images (AP/Lateral) are obtained to confirm the position. If the position is acceptable, cannulated screws are inserted over the guidewires and checked

small keyholes. This gives the patient the advantage of a faster return to work and easier rehabilitation, lesser blood loss and pain. However, more number of images has to be taken during the surgery to determine the correct level and the exactness of implant placement. This endangers the patient, surgeon and other operating room personnel to a lot of radiation hazards.

Navigation vs Robotic

The concept of a monitoring and navigating device to aid the surgeon in operating on deformed and crooked spines has been developed since the late 1990s. The early systems rely on the use of reference points on the spine, which are fed into a computer which calculated the path of a safe screw in the vertebra, based on a CT scan reconstruction of the spine. Frameless stereotaxy (also termed navigation, neuronavigation, or image guidance) has overshadowed its frame-based predecessor. The O-arm® (Medtronic, Inc., Louisville, CO, USA) is a CT scanner that permits imaging of the screws intraoperatively. In this system, a reference pin or anatomical landmark is coregistered with an acquired CT scan and is linked with a navigational software program. The reference frame is replaced by a reference-marker array, which is likewise fixed to the patient whose position is determined by either imaging studies (2D or 3D fluoroscopy). Alternatively, a pointer or laser beam is directed to surface points on the object of interest (patient's spine) and registration is then conducted by preoperative imaging study's space-coordinate system and by matching the acquired surface points to a virtual 3D model of the object of interest. Lonstein et al. report in a meta-analysis on 4,790 screws showed 0.2% neurological complications in 5.1% pedicle perforations. However, this system has its own flaws and requires the surgeon to navigate the spine, which makes the process cumbersome. Moreover it requires an alignment of surgical instrument to preplanned trajectories by hand and therefore complex hand-eye coordination and essentially remains freehand. The accuracy of such systems in large trials was suspect, Nakashima et al. in their paper on comparison of the percutaneous screw placement-precision of isocentric C-arm 3-dimensional fluoroscopy-navigated pedicle screw implantation and conventional fluoroscopy method with minimally invasive surgery reported up to 15% pedicle breach in few cases, which is highly unacceptable.

The Mazor robot renaissance spine surgery guidance system significantly improves accuracy of implant placement and reduces the radiation dosage, hospital stay, complication rate and the need for surgical revisions. It can be used for safe guidance in complex deformities and reconstructive surgeries and enables faster recovery. A retrospective, multicenter study of robotically guided spinal implant insertions published in the Spine journal 2010 showed 49% rate of less or minimally invasive procedures, which was much higher than the 5% reported in other published literature. Unlike the 2–5% rates of permanent neurologic deficits reported in the literature, SpineAssist-guided pedicle screw insertions used in this study showed reversible neurologic deficits in 0.7% (4 of 593) of the cases, none of which led to permanent neurologic deficits. Also, it reported that it required significantly shorter imaging sessions, exposing the patient and staff to approximately 50-fold less radiation when compared to non-navigated control groups.

Kim et al. in their study (2015) on monitoring of quality control of the accuracy of this robot-assisted pedicle screw fixation procedure used a cumulative summation test and concluded that the adequacy of quality control of robot-assisted pedicle screw fixation was seen even early in the application period based on the CUSUM analysis.

A 2011 European spine journal article by Kantelhardt et al. on the perioperative course and accuracy of screw positioning in conventional, open robotic-guided and percutaneous robotic-guided, pedicle screw placement using the Mazor system concluded that robot-guided pedicle screw implantation resulted in accurate placement in 94.5% compared to 91.4% in conventional screw placement. Duration of intraoperative was significantly lower in robot-guided compared to conventional procedures. Postoperative administration of new opioid analgesics, duration of postoperative hospitalization and rates of adverse events seem to be lower in percutaneous robot-guided procedures compared to open robot-guided and conventional procedures.

Barzilay et al. in 2014 published a series on robot-assisted vertebral body. Augmentation using the SpineAssist system and concluded that the use of robot guidance and pulsed fluoroscopy in vertebral body cement augmentation markedly reduces radiation exposure for surgeons and OR staff when compared with published results in similar procedures.

As far as the learning curve is concerned, Hu et al in their study concluded that the rate of successfully placed pedicle screws improved with increasing experience and the rate of the screws that were converted to manual placement decreased with increasing experience.

There are, however few disadvantages that the robotic surgery requires training to the surgeon as well as the operation theater staff personnel and it can increase the total duration of surgery. Higher cost involved in these surgeries is also an issue in developing countries.

Other Systems

The da Vinci Surgical System (Intuitive Surgical, Sunnyvale,CA) is a master-slave telemanipulator robot that received Food and Drug Administration approval for general surgery in 2000. Its advantages in general surgery and urology cases have been appreciated. However, it is not US FDA-approved for spinal procedures. The rationale for its use includes 3-dimensional imaging and improved surgical dexterity from motion scaling and tremor filtering. The decreased hospitalization time, lower morbidity, lower blood loss, and lower complication rate associated with the use of the robot are described as related to the enhanced visualization and dissection of intra-abdominal and pelvic structures in anterior lumbar surgery.

One of the clearest benefits the authors observed of performing posterior spine surgery procedures robotically using the da Vinci is the improved ergonomics for the surgeon. Apart from the dissection for the initial exposure, the surgeon may be seated for the full day of surgery at the surgeon console where height and other ergonomic adjustments can be made for optimal surgeon comfort. Ponnusamy et al. concluded that using the da Vinci system, one can perform major noninstrumented procedures **(Figures 7 and 8)** (laminotomy, laminectomy, disk incision, and dural suturing) of the posterior spine in a more ergonomic environment resulting in less "wear and tear" on the surgeon, and potentially result in fewer unintentional patient injuries. The da Vinci is designed for downscaling the surgeon's movements, assisting during tissue dissection, tumor removal, and related tasks, and does not provide any navigation information.

Robot-assisted osteosynthesis performed on10 patients by the new robot ROSA developed by Medtech was reported in the European Spine Journal in 2015. It comprises of a first floor-fixable mobile base onto which is mounted a six axes robot arm, and a second mobile base onto which is mounted a navigation camera. The robot arm supports a tool that helps guide conventional surgical instruments, and allows their accurate and stable positioning onto the target point planned by the surgeon. According to the study, with its compact floor-fixable base and rigid robotized arm, ROSA reduces the risk of secondary movement of the equipment and guarantees the reliability of the entry point and trajectory. However, it merits further studies to prove the safety and accuracy of the system.

The Miro system was developed and investigated in the German Aerospace Center. The system consisted of a lightweight robot, holding a drill guide, a control, and an optical tracking system. Kim et al developed the biplane fluoroscopy-guided robot system, which combines imaging using an O-arm with an operating system and

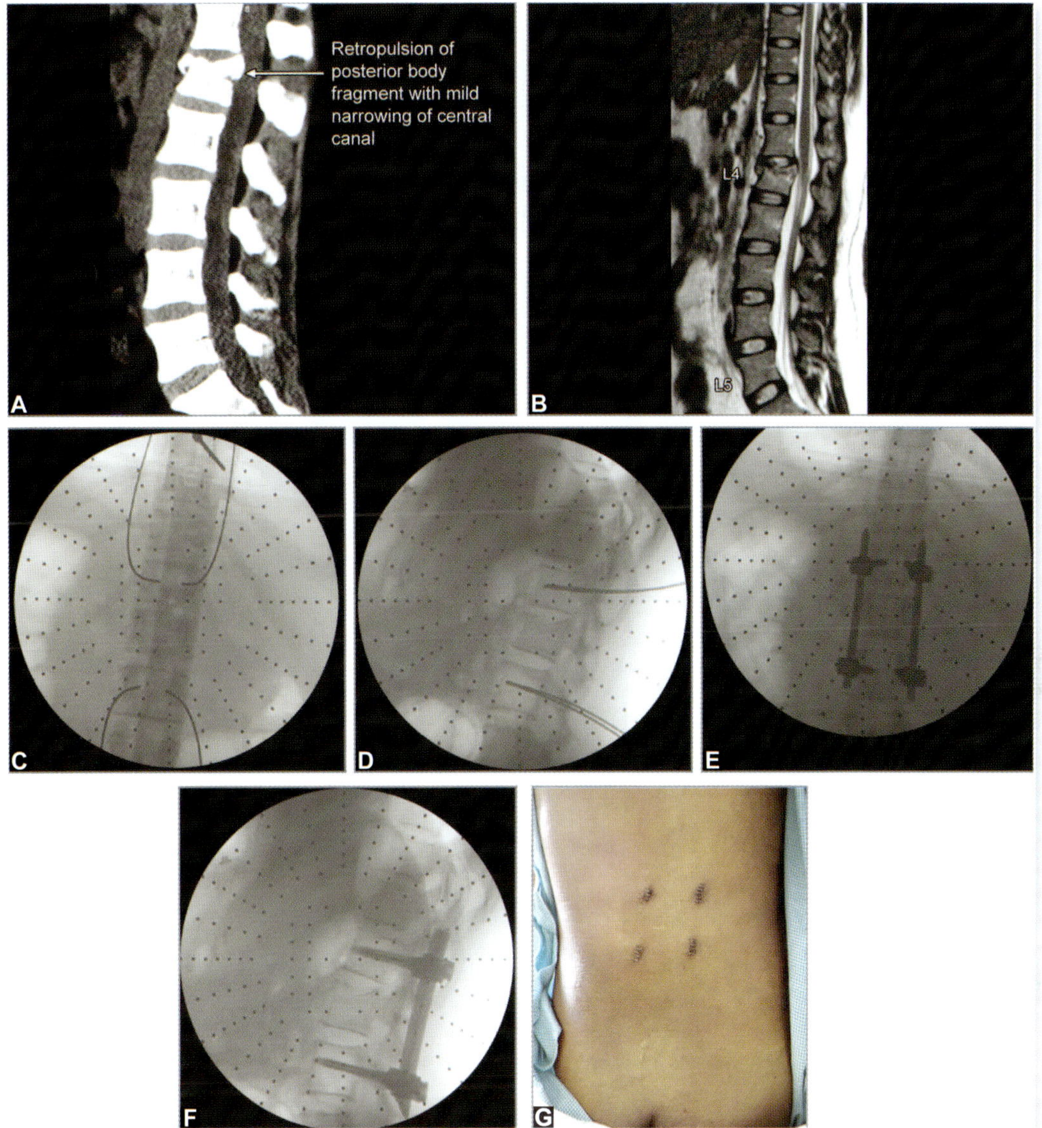

Figure 7: A 27-year-old female who sustained RTA had L1 unstable burst fracture with retropulsed fragment. Robot-guided posterior stabilization was done on the day of injury and patient was mobilized within 24 hours of injury

robot arm (Spinebot). After imaging and registration by the Spinebot, the system's software is used for planning of screw trajectories, and finally the Spinebot robot arm positions a guiding tube on the planned trajectory. The Spine Bull's-Eye Robot is a remote-controlled instrument, which places guiding wires under pedicle-axis standard-view fluoroscopy.

OUR EXPERIENCE

At our center, we have performed over 220 cases using the system over the past 2 years, including complex deformity surgeries (Some case examples attached). It includes spinal deformities in 44 patients (adolescent idiopathic scoliosis 23, neuromuscular scoliosis 9, congenital scoliosis 5, ankylosing spondylitis 1, congenital kyphosis 3, degenerative 1, post-traumatic 1, failed/revision 1), degenerative conditions (single or double level lumbar disk disease with stenosis and/or degenerative listhesis-170), dorsal stabilisation for infection/ malignancy- 11 and two vertebral body lesions biopsy. The results have been excellent with achieving over 99° accuracy in screw placement compared to standard free hand accuracy and reducing the radiation exposure to the maximum.

Robotic guidance can be especially relevant to the concave vertebral scoliotic pedicles along the apex of a large curve, where pedicles are often deformed, sometimes with a transverse pedicle width of only a millimeter.

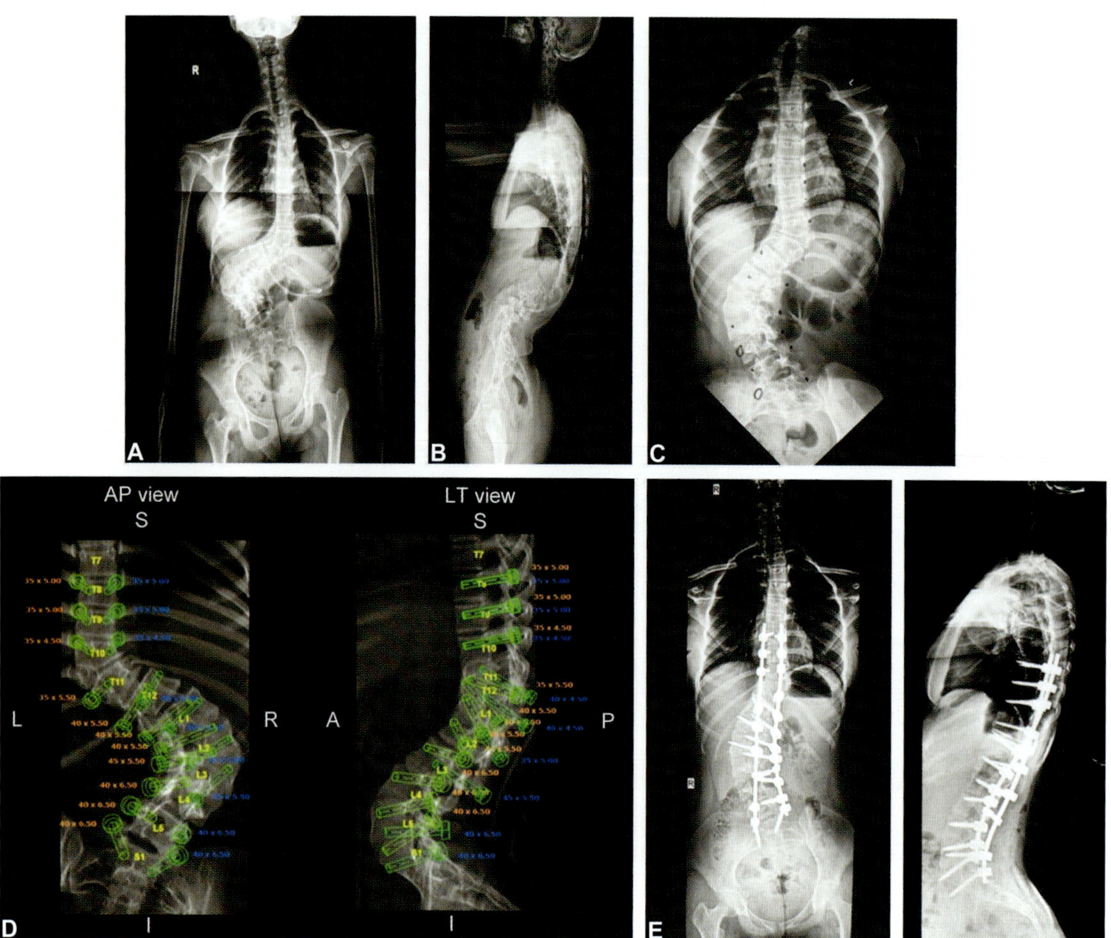

Figure 8: A 14-year-old female with adolescent idiopathic scoliosis (Lenke type V curve) with Cobb angle of 82°. Preoperative planning on the robot shows the implant position and dimensions. Accurate positioning of screws and deformity correction is seen on the postoperative X-ray

Pedicle morphometry study done at our center using the renaissance software used in robotic surgeries confirmed the high rate of hypoplastic pedicles (<4 mm) on the concave side, especially at the apex.

Our center was a part of the five-center analysis of 3,270 pedicle screws placed with robotic guidance in adolescent idiopathic scoliosis (AIS), which reported that 223 patients with AIS in five centers had a total of 3,270 pedicle screws placed using the Renaissance system with over 99% accuracy while fluoroscopy use was limited to 1.58 seconds per screw (Retrospective Analysis of Feasibility and Performance of Robotic-Guidance for Placement of Pedicle Screws in 223 Adolescents with Idiopathic Scoliosis (AIS)-presented at the SRS-IMAST 2014 in Valencia, Spain).

More so in the scenario of a very complex deformity in young adults or children where the risk of improper and dangerous surgery is high, the robot has assured us and the patient with the high safety levels it provides. Our review of all the patients operated has been excellent and we can confidently assert that the robot guided surgery has made spine surgery a safer proposition, in addition to reducing the stress on the surgeon and his team in the operation theater. The robot-guided surgery in our setup decreases the amount of radiation exposure by 10 times vis-à-vis a standard procedure. The operating room personnel too are benefitted as the radiation exposure due to an image intensifier is reduced to miniscule proportions. The surgeon and team, at the end of the day, return home with the satisfaction of having done an accurate and safe surgery.

The surgery as such is normal as a conventional surgery, but the robot finds the safest possible path. In that sense the robot does not replace the surgeon, as is the normal misconception. On the contrary, the surgeon is backed up by the foolproof planning done prior to the surgery on the robotic software.

The future of spine surgery is shaping in the direction of minimally invasive surgeries where the stress shall be on earlier return to productive activity to the patient and reduction of the hospital stay and expenses. From the surgeon's perspective too, the use of the robotic guiding systems would mean more safety levels, lesser radiation hazards and stress free situations in the operating room. As time advances, the cost hurdle will also be cleared and robotic surgery will be available for better care of all patients. Technology is ever advancing and it is the duty of the medical fraternity to keep abreast with it as the patient has the right to benefit from every such advancement.

BIBLIOGRAPHY

1. Amr Nimer Amr: Navigation and robot-aided surgery in the spine: historical review and state of the art. Dove Press Journal. 2014, september.
2. Barzilay, Schroeder, Hiller, Singer, Hasharoni, Safran, Liebergall, Itshayek, Kaplan. Robotic assisted vertebral body augmentation– a radiation reduction tool. Spine Journal. 2013.
3. Devito DP, Kaplan L, Dietl R, et al. CliniCal acCeptance and accuracy assessment of spinal implants guided with SpineAssist surgical robot: retrospective study. Spine. 2010;35(24):2109-115.
4. Hu X, Ohnmeiss D. Lieberman,I. Robotic-assisted pedicle screw placement: lessons learned from the first 102 patients. Eur Spine J 2013;22:661-6.
5. Kantelhardt SR, Martinez R, Baerwinkel S, Burger R, Giese A, Rohde V. Perioperative course and accuracy of screw positioning in conventional, open robotic-guided and percutaneous robotic-guided, pedicle screw placement. Eur Spine J. 2011;20(6):860-8.
6. Karthikeyan Ponnusamy, Samuel Chewning, Catherine Mohr, Robotic approaches to the posterior spine. Spine (Phila Pa 1976). 2009;34(19): 2104-9.
7. Kazemi N, Crew LK, Tredway TL. The future of spine surgery: New horizons in the treatment of spinal disorders. Surg Neurol Int. 2013;4:S15-21.
8. Kim et al. Monitoring the Quality of Robot-Assisted Pedicle Screw Fixation in the Lumbar Spine by Using a Cumulative Summation Test. Spine. 2015;40(2):87-94.
9. Kosmopoulos V, Schizas C. Pedicle screw placement accuracy: a metaanalysis. Spine. 2007;32:111-20.
10. Lieberman IH, Hardenbrook M, Wang J, et al. Radiation exposure using miniature robotic guidance for spinal surgery. Spine J. 2007;7:1525-35.
11. Mazor Robotics. Clinical evidence with peer reviewed publications. Available at: http://mazorrobotics.com/surgeons/clinical-evidence. Accessed May 29, 2015.
12. Russel A. Faust. Robotics in Surgery: History, Current and Future Applications; Nova Science publishers; 2007.
13. Shoham et al. Robotic assisted spinal surgery - from concept to clinical practice, Computer Aided Surgery. 2007;12(2)105-15.
14. S Kostrzewski, JM Duff, C Baur, M.Olszewski, Robotic system for cervical spine surgery. International Journal on Medical Robotics and Computer Assisted Surgery. 2011.
15. Xiaobang Hu, Isador H. Lieberman. What Is the Learning Curve for Robotic-assisted Pedicle Screw Placement in Spine Surgery? Clinical Orthopaedics and Related Research. 2014;472(6)pp 1839-44.

Lumbar Spinous Process Splitting Approach for Decompression in Lumbar Canal Stenosis

Rishi M Kanna, Ajoy P Shetty, S Rajasekaran

ABSTRACT

The use of robot has been recently introduced in field of spine surgery. It can be used in the management of wide variety of spinal pathologies. The technique has its distinct advantages of optimum accuracy and also inherent properties of minimally invasive surgery. This chapter deals with the indications, technique and complications using renaissance system.

INTRODUCTION

Lumbar canal stenosis is caused by reduction in the spinal canal dimensions due to hypertrophy of the ligamentum flavum, facet joints and or protrusion of disk into the spinal canal. In patients who present with significant claudication symptoms, surgical decompression of the stenosed spinal canal is advised. Conventional or midline micro-decompression with or without laminectomy is the standard surgical decompression technique and involves detachment of the paraspinal muscles from the spinous process and laminae and resection of the supra- and interspinous ligaments. Though the technique provides excellent results in terms of neural decompression, chronic postoperative back pain is reported in some patients, which is ascribed to intraoperative damage to paraspinal muscles and ligaments. The chronic muscle atrophy can lead to trunk extensor muscle weakness and possibly failed-back surgery syndrome.

The lumbar spinous process splitting approach (LSPS) is a recently described technique and involves exposure of the lamina by longitudinally splitting the spinous process into two halves, leaving its muscular and ligamentous attachments to the spinous process and the facet joints undisturbed. This is followed by standard microdecompression with minimal muscle dissection from the lamina. This procedure allows for better exposure of neurological structures comparable with conventional midline fenestration, while providing added advantage of minimal damage to posterior supporting structures.

INDICATIONS

- Lumbar central canal stenosis
- Central disk prolapse with stenosis.

CONTRAINDICATIONS

- Lumbar instability (>5 mm and 15°) in stress radiographs
- Revision lumbar surgery.

APPLIED ANATOMY

The muscles of the lumbar spine are made up of superficial and deep layers. The superficial layer consists of latissimus dorsi, which originates from the spinous processes and inserts into the humerus. The deep layer consists of the paraspinal muscles of the lumbar spine which are divided into two layers: the superficial portion, which contains the sacrospinalis muscles (erector spinae), and the deep short rotator muscles. The "erector spinae" is arranged into three groups namely multifidus, longissmus and iliocostalis from medial to lateral. The erector spinae is segmentally innervated and serves as the major extensor muscle of the spinal column. In standard midline exposure, the multifidus is elevated subperiosteally from the spinous process and the lamina. This may result in denervation atrophy of the muscle fibres causing weakness. In LSPSD, the muscle attachments to the bone are preserved.

TECHNIQUE

The procedure is performed under general anesthesia. The patient is placed in the prone position on a Relton Hall frame. For an L4-5 decompression, the L4 spinous process needs to be split and hence the incision is centered over this point. A posterior midline skin incision is made between the L3 and L5 spinous processes to expose the tip of L4 spinous process. After exposing the lumbodorsal fascia, the level is confirmed again by placing the needle along the wall of the spinous process till it touches the lamina. This also helps in identifying the depth of the spinous process.

The spinous process is split longitudinally in the middle using a high speed 2 mm cutting burr **(Figure 1)**. The depth is assessed by stopping 2–3 mm short of the length of the previously measured spinous process. The halves of the spinous process are divided at their base from the L4 lamina, using a curved osteotome, leaving the paraspinal muscles attached to the lateral aspect of the split spinous process **(Figure 2)**. The supra- and interspinous ligaments between L3-4 and L4-5 are also split longitudinally using a scalpel. The muscles attached to the caudal 1/3rd margin of the L4 lamina are gently dissected using an elevator. Ample working space for decompression is obtained by retracting the split spinous process laterally together with its attached paraspinal muscles using a standard microdiskectomy retractor.

The caudal margin of the L4 lamina is excised with a Kerrisons rongeur up to the attachment of the ligamentum flavum. The L4-5 ligamentum flavum is then excised in a cranial to caudal and medial to lateral manner **(Figure 3)**. "Trumpeted" under cutting preserves the lamina and pars and decreases the incidence of inadvertent iatrogenic instability. The cephalad 1/4th of the L-5 lamina is removed if required. The traversing root is then decompressed in the lateral recess and foraminal entry zone. If foraminal stenosis is observed, a foraminotomy is performed using an 1 mm Kerrisons rongeur. The end point of decompression is reached when the lateral margin of the cephalad and caudal nerve roots at the operative level are seen to be free of compression exiting freely into the foramen. After the affected nerve roots and the thecal sac are successfully decompressed, each half of the split L-4 spinous process is approximated using strong non-absorbable sutures. This is facilitated by making drill holes with a 2 mm burr in the spinous processes. Thus, a one-level posterior L4-5 decompression is accomplished by splitting the L4 spinous process and preserving the supra- and interspinous ligaments of L3-4 and L4-5, as well as the L4 spinous process, with minimal damage to the paraspinal muscles.

Routine postoperative radiographs are not required. Adequacy of decompression may be assessed by an MRI

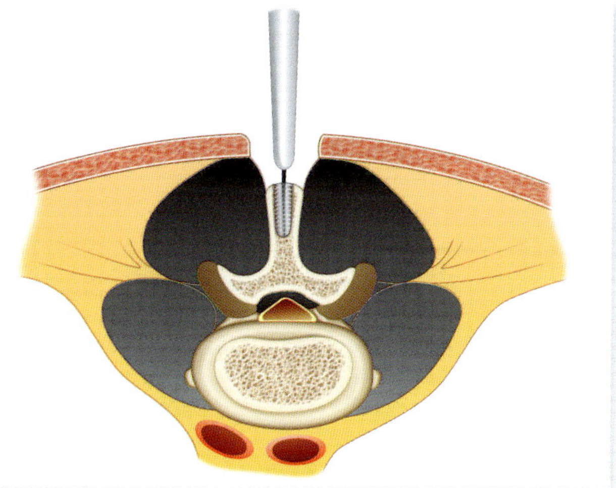

Figure 1: Technique of splitting the spinous process with a burr in the midline

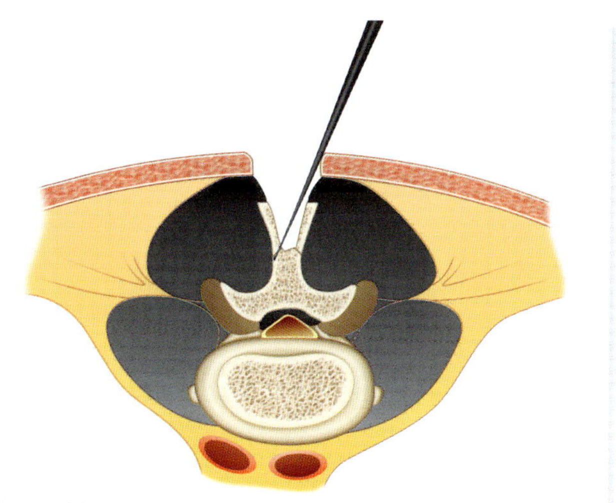

Figure 2: Separation of spinous processes along with their muscular attachments

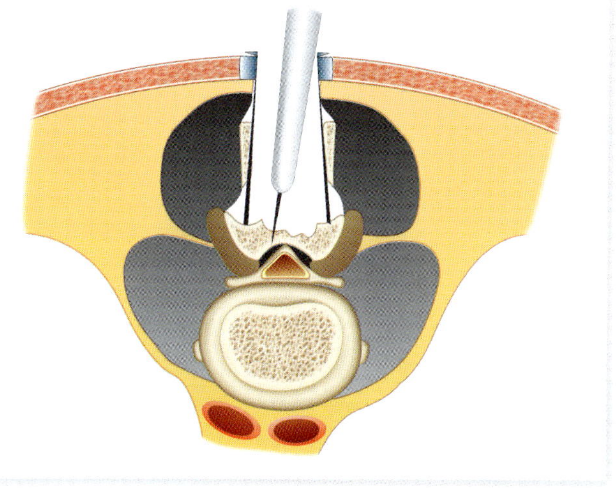

Figure 3: Split process held retracted by the MLD retractor and laminectomy being done with a burr

scan if required. The patient can be mobilised from the first postoperative day depending on the comfort levels. A lumbar sacral belt is given to support the back.

BIBLIOGRAPHY

1. Rajasekaran S, Thomas A, Kanna RM, Shetty AP. Lumbar spinous process splitting decompression provides equivalent outcomes to conventional midline decompression in degenerative lumbar canal stenosis. A Prospective, Randomised Controlled Study of 51 Patients. Spine (Phila Pa 1976). 2013;38(20):1737-43.
2. Watanabe K, Hosoya T, Shiraishi T. Spinous process splitting laminectomy preserving posterior musculoligamentous complex for lumbar spinal canal stenosis. Rinsho Seikei Geka. 2003;38:1401-8.
3. Watanabe K. Lumbar spinous process–splitting laminectomy for lumbar canal stenosis. J Neurosurg Spine. 2005;3:405-8.
4. Weiner BK, Fraser RD, Peterson M: Spinous process osteotomies to facilitate lumbar decompressive surgery. Spine. 1999;24:62-6.
5. Yong-Hing K, Kirkaldy-Willis WH: Osteotomy of the lumbar spinous process to increase surgical exposure. Clin Orthop Relat Res. 1978;134:218-20.

Computer-assisted Spine Surgery: Navigation-guided Instrumentation in Minimally Invasive Spine Surgery (Nav-MISS)

Vishal Kundnani, Tarun Dushad

ABSTRACT

Image-guided spinal instrumentation procedures in the cervical, thoracic, and lumbar spine have lower rates of screw misplacement than do those performed without image guidance. Concerns of large doses of Radiation and also growing questions on reliability of conventional fluoroscopy guided image guidance in a typical spinal procedure has led to innovation of intraoperative navigation guided instrumentation techniques.

In navigation-guided instrumentation surgical instruments are tracked in the operating room, and their positions are superimposed on to preoperatively acquired computed tomography (CT-based image guidance) or intraoperative acquired fluoroscopic images (virtual fluoroscopy). Each of these technologies has distinct advantages and limitations.

Intraoperative spinal navigation has led to advantages like enhanced precision, significantly reduced radiation exposure, particularly in minimal invasive procedures and has paved the way for newer developments for future. Navigation guidance, though infantile in current form, has been advancing rapidly in recent years, beneficially affecting a variety of surgical procedures. Future technological developments will widen its clinical application and minimize its shortcomings.

This chapter brings forth the various aspects and techniques , pitfalls, and shortcomings of navigation-guided procedures in preview of minimal invasive spine surgery.

INTRODUCTION

Percutaneous instrumentation techniques based on fluoroscopy guidance in Minimally invasive surgery (MIS), e.g. MIS-TLIF have gained popularity in recent decade with clinical outcomes comparable to or better than open conventional instrumentation techniques. Fluoroscopy Guided percutaneous instrumentation technique not only reduces immediate postoperative morbidity of extensive muscle retraction, often associated with open techniques, but also benefits with less blood loss, cosmetic Incisions, lesser postoperative pain, faster recovery, lesser infection rate and shorter hospitalization with early return to work.

Placement of percutaneous pedicle screws using conventional fluoroscopic technique has led to widening horizons and broader indications of minimal invasive spine surgery. Advancements in image-guidance technology and minimal access techniques continue to push the frontiers of minimally invasive spine surgery (MISS) further. MIS techniques carry a theoretically higher risk of misplacement with a larger learning curve in comparison with the open technique. Currently, percutaneous screw placement is most common performed using intraoperative two-dimensional (2D) fluoroscopy and the C-arm has to be repositioned throughout the procedure and repeated exposures are often needed to achieve optimal image for instrumentation resulting in greater patient and occupational radiation exposure to surgeons team compared to open techniques. The limitations associated with the use of a mobile C-arm fluoroscope include Increased surgical time, single usable real-time planar view at any given time leading to reduced precision and increasing dependence and false reliability on fluoroscope, intraoperatively. Thus procedure becomes prolonged, being more incriminatory for the patient and bearing a higher risk for infection, collateral damage due to repetitive correction and added concern of significant radiation exposure to surgical team posing cumulative radiation hazards. Moreover, recent reports indicate that cortical breaches during percutaneous pedicle screw placement can exceed in range of 15%, with neurological injury rate as high as 3–5%. Thus, utilization of methods to reduce pedicle screw misplacement and radiation exposure in MIS percutaneous instrumentation are being explored and utilized including C-arm fluoroscopy, isocentric C-arm, 3-dimensional (3D) fluoroscopy and navigation.

This led to the invention of various advanced intraoperative image guidance techniques paving way to modern-day navigation in spine surgery. The principle of navigation assisted guidance is to couple the patient images acquired by intraoperative 2D–3D fluoroscopy or CAT scans preoperatively and makes it available on a virtual platform which can be utilized in spinal instrumentation while preserving the precision accuracy without the need of radiation. A number of computed tomography (CT) and fluoroscopy-based navigation systems have been developed with demonstrated ability to increase screw accuracy, decrease radiation exposure, and reduce operative times.

This chapter deals with introduction of the indications, techniques, advantages, pitfalls, salvage, work flow and future implications of navigation-guided percutaneous instrumentation. Specific description of navigation technique in relation to MIS TLIF, commonest procedure by far is also bought forward as a example to follow.

BASICS AND CONCEPTS OF NAVIGATION

The concept of navigation is based on the notion of computer-assisted intraoperative coupling of (i) intra-operative images with (ii) patient anatomy to produce a real-time intraoperative virtual image allowing better surgical accuracy and reduced radiation exposure. This concept with advantages of better instrumentation accuracy, reduced intraoperative radiation exposure with optimized screw length and diameter in MISS is intuitive **(Table 1)**. Modern day intraoperative imaging has evolved from the use of fluoroscopy to advanced navigation systems, such as the 3D fluoroscopy, isocentric C-arm and O-arm to several CT-scan based navigation systems.

There are four fundamental steps necessary for any navigation system:

Table 1

Proposed benefits of navigation

Proposed benefits of navigation
Better instrumentation accuracy in difficult cases.
Reduces the radiation exposure significantly
Optimization of screw length and diameter.
Enables a single C-arm to provide real-time, multiplanar intraoperative guidance.

1. Transferring one or more images to a computer for subsequent processing; These images have to be acquired Intraoperatively through a wireless tracker attached to imaging modality (intraoperative fluoroscopy 2D-3D, or O-arm), or preoperatively (CT or preoperative CAT scan) and shifted to computer unit of navigation system **(Figure 1)**. This computer with a arm has an infrared camera **(Figure 1)** attached to it which sends/receives information for acquiring images from patient intraoperatively through infrared technology. Various conventional 2D imaging modalities have been utilized for intraoperative image acquisition (radiography, C-arm fluoroscopy) of patient anatomy; on other hand, newer 3D platforms, such as 3D-fluoroscopy, O arm image acquisition, cone-beam CT, and intraoperative CT/MRI are being developed for further enhancement of precise anatomical image acquisition resulting in more accurate instrumentation placement. The advantages of 2D-based systems were speed, decreased radiation exposure, and ease of use, but these systems were not as accurate as the next generation of 3D-guided navigation systems **(Table 2).**
2. Establishment of the spatial relation between the acquired images and the patient in real time. A spatial image of the patient's anatomy on the computer is created with assistance of Patient reference frame-PRF **(Figure 2)**. This PRF, with reflecting spheres or light-emitting diodes and is placed on pateint's operative surface (spinous process or iliac crest secured with percut pins), sends/receives signals from to the computer unit with optical tracking using cameras. Information about patients position to the camera utilised by the computer creating spatial image of patient in real time.

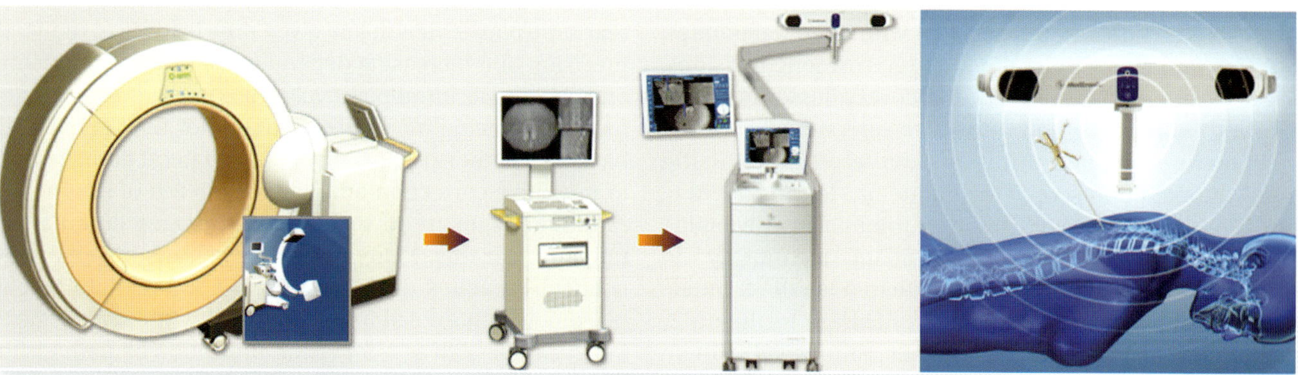

Figure 1: Images from the C-arm/O-arm console are transferred to navigation system; infrared camera of navigation system

Table 2

Different modalities of image acquisition for navigation

2D C-arm fluoroscopy	CT scan	O-arm
Avoid preoperative time and cost of obtaining especially formatted CT	Require obtaining CT scan of appropriate levels prior to surgery	Avoid need of preoperative CT scans
Image calibration process is fully automated	Manual registration process (choosing anatomical landmarks on obtained images) is time consuming and accuracy is surgeon dependent	Automatic registration process—does not need surgeon dependent registration prior to navigation
Does not provide detailed multiplanar imaging	Detailed multiplanar imaging	Detailed multiplanar imaging
Cannot compensate for causes for poor image quality like obesity, positioning of radiopaque instruments like retractors	No effect of obesity, retractors on image quality	Factors like obesity affect the image quality
Use of proper fluoroscopic techniques, such as centering the area of interest within the field of view and tangential imaging (Acquiring "true" lateral and anteroposterior views) still must be adhered to	Change in intersegmental relationships between vertebral segments during positioning for imaging and for surgery may result in inaccuracy	Images obtained in multiple planes intraoperatively—differences in anatomy due to intersegmental mobility do not affect accuracy
Fixing of reference arc is invasive which constrains the surgeon's movement and puts its own stability at risk	Fixing of reference arc is invasive which constrains the surgeon's movement and puts its own stability at risk	Reference arc fixed to the patient

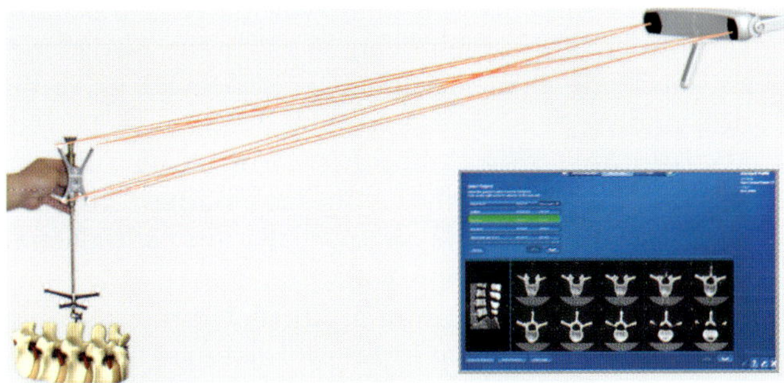

Figure 2: Recent imaging data of the patient loaded in to the software

3. "Calibration" of the acquired images (step 1) to the spatial images (step 2) sent from the PRF. This generates precision by reducing the errors of these two images of the patient acquired preoperatively by matching with the spatial image captured by PRF.
4. Superimposition or registration. This leads to registration of a "virtual surgical instrument" **(Figure 3)** onto the acquired images using measurements of the actual instrument's position, together with the information gathered in steps 1-3 to track surgical instruments and anatomy in the operative field relative to a registered

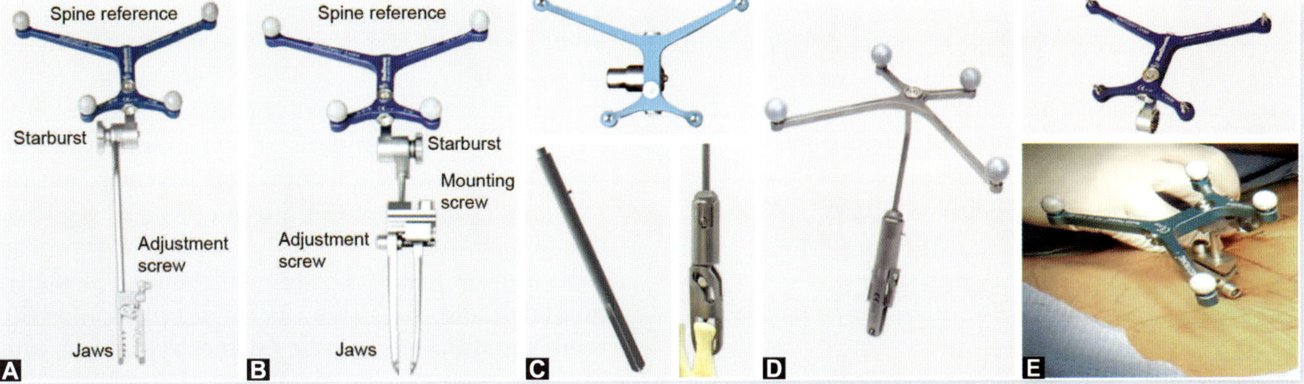

Figures 3A to E: (A) Open spine clamp and reference frame; (B) MI spine clamp and reference frame; (C) Percutaneous pin and reference frame; (D) Cervical clamp and light reference frame; (E) A patient reference frame

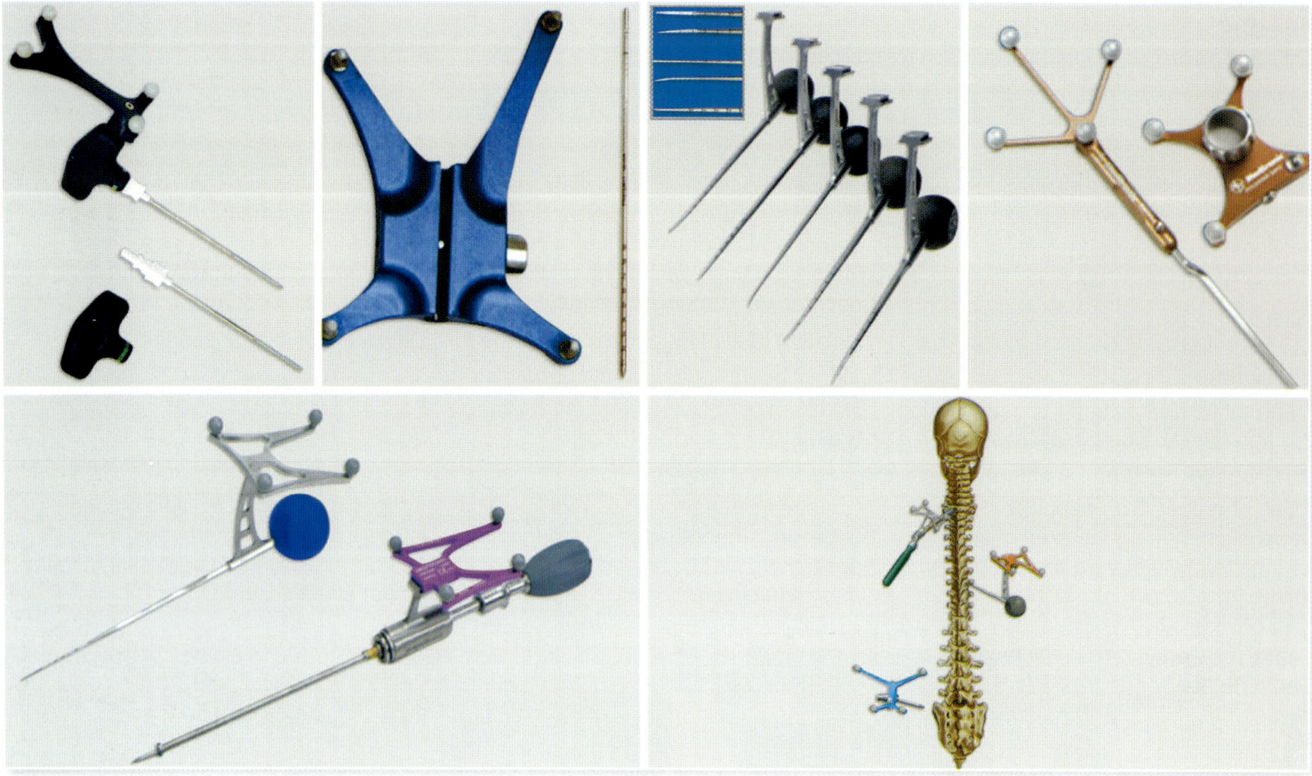

Figure 4: Surgical instruments with attached trackers or optical markers

reference point. This step helps utilize various trackers on the patients surgical position which can be visualized in real time on computer screen. Once registration has occurred, various instruments with reference markers can be appropriately localized in the surgical field, and projections in multiple planes are computed and projected for the surgeon.

When registration is completed, specialized cannulated surgical instruments can be tracked—PAK needle, passive planar, and navigable TAP **(Figure 4)** real time in relation to the reconstructed images.

Advantages with the use of this technology include the ability to image multiple levels in a single sequence, imaging accuracy in patients with prior spine surgeries at the same levels, decreased radiation exposure to the operating room (OR) staff, improved accuracy because the patient's anatomy is registered in the surgical position, and portability of the system so it can be easily transported between OTs

TECHNIQUE: NAVIGATION-GUIDED MIS PERCUTANEOUS INSTRUMENTATION IN MIS-TLIF: AUTHOR'S EXPERINECE

Steps of NAV—MISS TLIF

1. Positioning, painting, draping as in standard methods. Ensure all the equipments in place.
2. Placement of microscope, C-arm, and navigation stations so as to ensure surgeon can visualize the navigation screen clearly while navigating the screws with universal drill guide
3. Microendoscopic decompression using tubular retractors is performed using paramedian incision from symptomatic side and over the top contralateral decompression **(*see* Figure 3)**.
4. Interbody fusion—minimally-invasive microscopic transforaminal lumbar interbody fusion (TLIF) using a paramedian muscle-splitting approach with a tubular retractor. A parasagittal incision is made 3–5 cm lateral to the midline, and sequential soft tissue dilators are inserted down to the facet complex. The inferior and partial superior facetectomy is performed with Kerrison from lateral to medial to expose the posterior lateral aspect of the disk. Diskectomy is performed, and endplates are prepared followed by an interbody cage. Fluoroscopy is used to ensure satisfactory placement of the interbody cage. Then decompression of ipsilateral exiting and traversing roots are completed. The tubular retractor is angled medially, and the patient is tilted to visualize the contralateral side in cases where symptoms and magnetic resonance images showing bilateral disease. Then, decompression is done on the contralateral side where indicated **(*see* Figure 3)**.

5. Navigation-guided percutaneous instrumentation with navigable trackable percutaneous cannulated access needle–bilateral percutaneous pedicle screw-rod instrumentation is used in all cases. Screw length and size is typically predetermined from patient-specific preoperative imaging and confirmed on navigation software. Typical screw diameters were 5.5–6.5 mm at L2–L3 and 6.5–7.5 mm at L3–S1. In all cases, the screws contralateral to the planned TLIF side were placed first and the ipsilateral screws were placed after.

TECHNIQUE OF NAVIGATION-GUIDED PERCUTANEOUS INSTRUMENTATION (TABLE 3) (SEE FIGURE 7)

Conventional fluoroscopy-based navigation system combined with computer calibration unit (Medtronic Stealthstation Nav S7) and a mobile digital C-arm X-ray machine (Phillips Co.) precompatible with the navigation system is utilized commonly at authors center. The position of the navigation unit to OT table has to be kept in mind before starting **(Figure 5)**.

- The wireless tracker is attached to the Carm–IITV visible to the computer infrared camera along with all cable connections and attachments is the first step before proceeding ahead. The electro-optical camera tracks both the location of the wireless C-arm tracker and PRF and working instruments which shall be in same field of the infrared camera.
- A stab incision is placed over posterior iliac bone near PSIS for percutaneous pins to attach the PRF **(*see* Figure 2)**. A dynamic reference arc (DRA) or PRF can be attached to the spinous process of interest after mini-exposure also; however, this may lead to a separate incision. Care shall be taken to keep the patient reference frame away from surgical field and facing the infrared camera clearly. Ensure securing the PRF to prevent any movement during forthcoming steps.
- Serial fluoroscopic intraoperative 2D images of the patient on each level of interest are then obtained (True AP and true lateral) before exposure of the spine and relayed to the computer workstation for processing. Images so obtained are then transferred, acquired to the computer with digital link.
- The optical camera measures the relative position of the C-arm **(Figure 1)** and the patient at the time of image acquisition by detecting the dynamic reference arc or PRF. After calibration, computer generates a graphic

Table 3

Summary of key points in fluoroscopy-based navigation-guided MIS TLIF

Steps	*Key points*
Setup	• Position camera to maximum line of sight • Position monitor so easily visualized by surgeon • Patient positioning • Radiolucent table
Registration	• Patient's reference base placement • Firmly affix reference base to iliac crest • Acquisition of images in AP and lateral images • Register instruments
Maintaining navigational accuracy	• Check navigation accuracy on patient anatomy prior to placement of screws • Avoid changing Trendelenburg position of bed after registration • Avoid excessive banging on instruments and movements of spine • Do not adjust reference arc after registration • Always remember that the images on the screen are not in real time
Maintaining line of site	• Place reference arc between the camera and the working space for image-guided instruments • Avoid placing objects in front of reference arc
Computer surgeon interface	• Qualified OR staff interfaces and drives computer • Consider intraoperative planning function of image-guided system during screw placement • Helps to maximize screw size • Helps to guide tapping of pedicle and placement of screw down the pedicle to prevent pedicle breach
Confirming accurate instrument placement	• Perform final check with C-arm prior to leaving OR

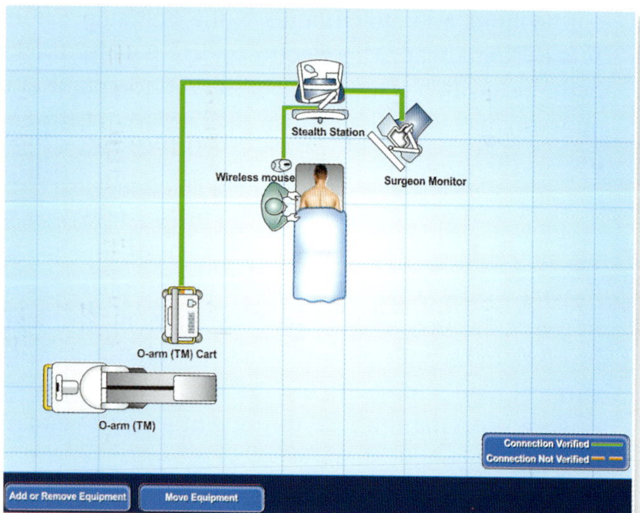

Figure 5: Completeness of circuit is denoted by a green connection on screen

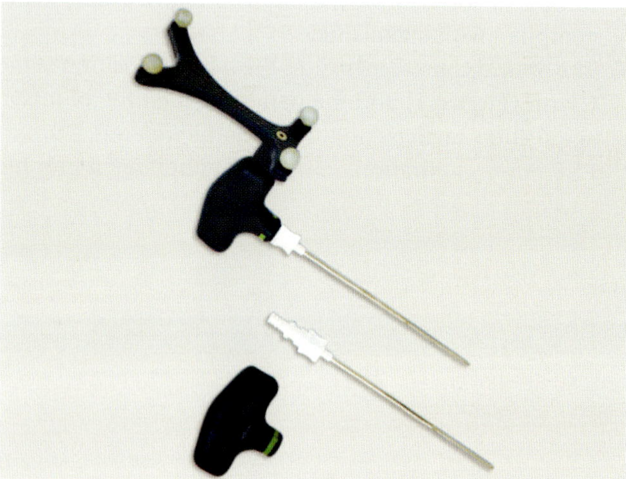

Figure 6: Cannulated percutaneous navigable access PAK needle

overlay to show the relative position of instrument with respect to fluoroscopic images. Once the system is calibrated with spatial and fluoroscopic information from at least one projection (an automated process), the computer constructs a model of the saved fluoroscopic images that permits the superimposition of a tracked surgical instrument. The real time, multiplanar position of the instrument is displayed on the workstation monitor in reference to the previously acquired fluoroscopic images.

- No surgeon-derived registration step is necessary in intraoperative image acquisition technique but is important additional step in preoperative image acquisition.
- Navigable PAK needle **(Figure 6)**: Cannulated needle universal drill guide or SureTrack navigating system and other instruments are registered and used for preparing the track for pedicle screws in the pedicle. The ideal skin incision location and each pedicle entry point and trajectory was determined and incision is given guided by navigation pointer of PAK needle. With these navigable PAK needles and inputs from monitor entry point on superolateral corner of pedicle eye is taken and pedicle cannulated with the cannulated needle guides **(Figure 7)**. Pedicles are cannulated bilaterally on both sides using a navigated cannulated PAK needle and guidewires are passed in all four pilot holes.
- The pedicles are cannulated and trocar removed **(Figure 7)** and guidewires inserted in pilot holes reaching up to half of the pedicle length. Authors recommend taking a shoot at this point to check position of guidewires as guidewires are nontrackable.
- Pedicles are tapped with navigated instrument **(Figure 7)** and pedicle screws of appropriate length and diameter **(Figure 7)**) are placed on both sides and fixed with rods. Guidewires are kept under check all the times from getting withdrawn/pulled out or being pushed forward with advancing movement of the tap.
- After having all the screws placed in all pilot holes authors recommend to check a final shoot **(Figure 7)** so as to ascertain the tulips of all screws being placed at same level so as to allow smooth rod placement process
- Rod length is then measured and rod inserted to connect the screw on both the sides completing the process.

Closure with absorbable sutures is done after a final check X-ray.

UTILIZATION OF NAVIGATION TECHNOLOGY IN MINIMALLY INVASIVE SPINE SURGERY

Benefit of navigation-guided percutaneous instrumentation can be extended to almost all percutaneous instrumentation surgeries that require intraoperative fluoroscopic control or guidance. The efficacy of navigation-guided percutaneous instrumentation has been evaluated in complex deformities, intraoperative osteotomy planning, cervical spine instrumentation and high thoracic instrumentation.

Authors have evaluated and cited benefits of navigation technology in odontoid fractures and anterior cervical fixation surgeries and have demonstrated enhanced precision and accuracy of implants with the added advantage of reduced radiation, faster surgical time and reduced requirement of biplanar fluoroscopy needed in these procedures. Posterior high cervical instrumentation can be safely performed in minimal invasive manner using navigation technology. Transarticular fixation with frameless stereotactic guidance have shown enhanced precision using navigation-guided intraoperative assistance. Percutaneous minimal invasive subaxial cervical pedicle and lateral mass fixation have also been evaluated in vivo and in vitro studies and have shown to be efficacious and safe.

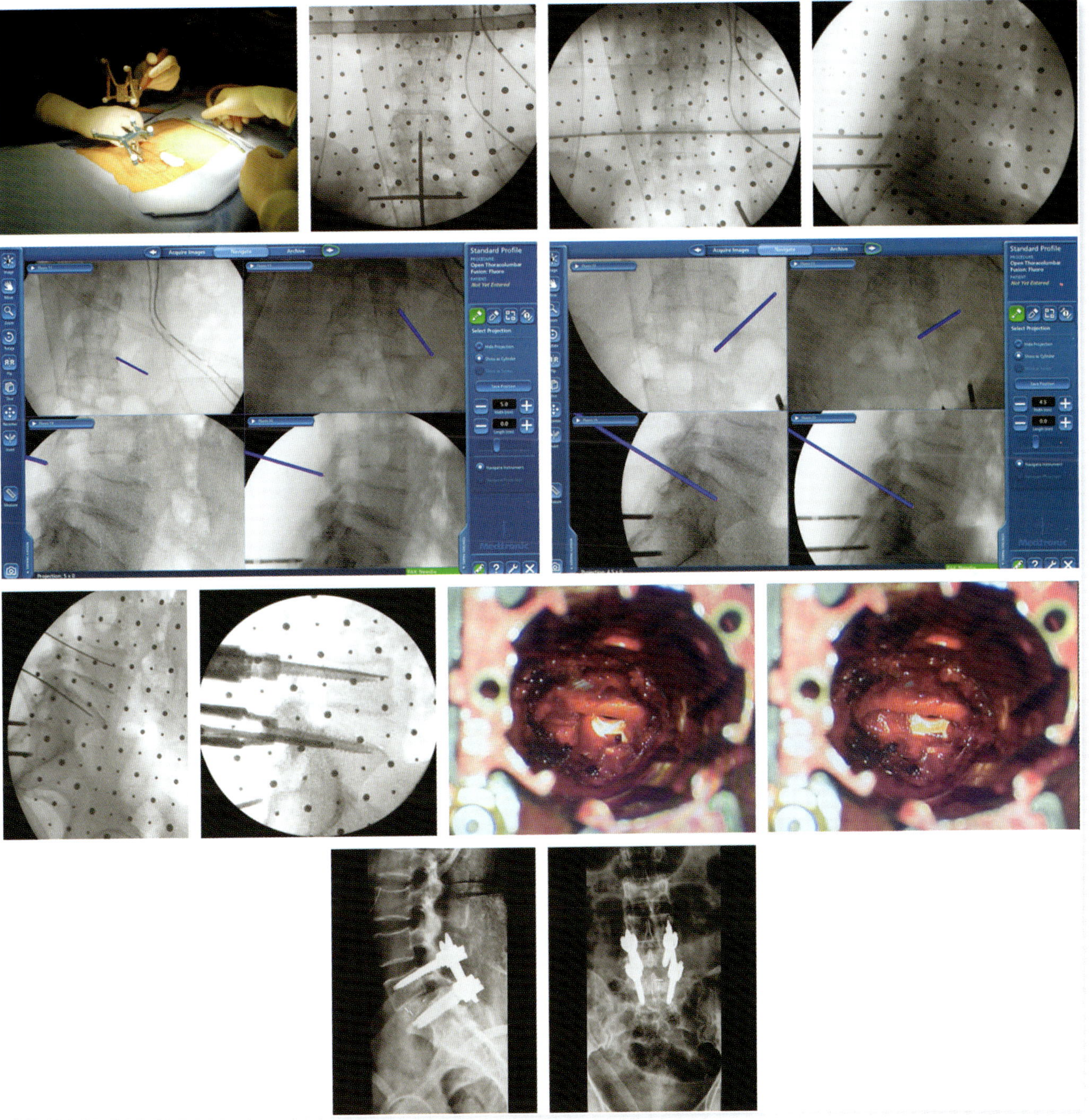

Figure 7: Steps of Nav MIS TLIF

High thoracic spinal instrumentation, particularly in deformed spine and complex deformities are of special mention and navigation assistance have shown to be of promising benefits in early studies .

Virtually every spinal instrumentation technique can be dealt within navigation-guided percutaneous manner without too much dependence on fluoroscopic control intraoperative with absolute precision.

DISCUSSION

Percutaneous placement of pedicle screws is becoming routine in spine surgery with the advent and maturity of minimally invasive techniques. The reported benefits of minimally invasive techniques compared with open procedures include reductions in blood loss, length of hospital stay, infection rates, postoperative pain, and time to return to work. Placement of percutaneous pedicle screws using the conventional fluoroscopic technique with anteroposterior and lateral images is not only time consuming but also has shown to have high rates of pedicle screw misplacement, and also exposes the patient and surgical team to considerable radiation posing significant radiation-related health hazards. Adding navigation guidance with conventional fluoroscopy in MIS instrumentation may offer several advantages. In addition to reducing occupational radiation exposure significantly, computer-assisted surgery (CAS) may be ideally suited to also address the anatomic challenges associated with percutaneous pedicle screw placement. Compared to conventional techniques, clinical reports on pedicle screw placement in the thoracic and lumbar spine using conventional three-dimensional CAS have shown a significant reduction in the misplacement rates of pedicle screws.

Accuracy of Screw Placement in Navigated vs Non-navigated surgery

MIS percutaneous instrumentation is technically more demanding with a steep learning curve. Due to loss of visual landmarks and reduced tactile feedback, percutaneous techniques mandate the use of intraoperative imaging, most commonly C-arm fluoroscopy. Recent reports indicate that cortical breaches during percutaneous pedicle screw placement can exceed 15%, 5–8 with neurological injury as high as 15%. Navigation technique have shown to significantly reduce misplacement of screws in MIS-TLIF. According to a recent meta-analysis, average pedicle screw placement accuracy was 92.1% in navigated and 87.3% in non-navigated cases. Although many clinical studies report a low incidence of neurological injury associated with misplaced screws, there is evidence that small cortical breaches can impact the biomechanical strength of a construct. George et al. demonstrated the importance of cortical containment of pedicle screws in their findings that the pull-out strength of pedicle screws with a cortical breach was 11% less than that of screws contained wholly within the pedicle. Similarly, Acikbas et al. observed that patients with malpositioned screws had reductions in early correction, increased long-term loss of correction, and greater nonunion rates. In a recent study, Waschke et al. examined the influence of CT-based navigation in 4,500 screws and demonstrated greater placement accuracy in the computer-navigated group. Verma et al found 93.3% of the computer-navigated screws and 84.7% of the conventionally inserted screws were accurately placed ($p < 0.00001$). Kosmopoulos and Schizas reported an in vivo median placement accuracy of 95.1% with and 90.3% without computer navigation, although half of the studies did not report on how placement accuracy was determined. Ravi B et al. reported no breach or acceptable breach (<2 mm) in 96.3% of cases in navigation guided MIS-TLIF. In study by Benson P Yang et al. 3% and 7.2% breach were seen with and without navigation respectively. Wei Tian et al. found that the accuracy of pedicle screw placement was 93.33% with navigation-guided MIS-TLIF. Ringel et al. reported 13% of >2 mm pedicle breach rate with the conventional fluoroscopic technique of pedicle screw placement. We, in our institutional study, found 96.67% of the pedicle screws in the navigated group were accurately placed compared to 91.67% in the non-navigated group. None of the breaches was critical and did not cause any neurological deficit or required revision.

Despite this enhanced technical accuracy, a significant clinical benefit for the patient has not so far been documented; although there is a non-statistically significant tendency toward a reduced incidence of neurological deficits by navigated pedicle screw implantation in comparison with non-navigated procedures.

Radiation in Conventional MISS and Navigation-guided Surgery

Apart from an increased accuracy, a speculated second advantage of image guidance is the reduced intraoperative radiation exposure. Although the radiation exposure of the patient remains a mostly singular event, the occupational daily radiation exposure of the dedicated spinal surgeon can lead to high cumulative lifetime doses. Fluoroscopy times of several minutes can be accumulated during MIS-TLIF or other percutaneous spine procedures. This seems to increase the risk of certain types of cancer for exposed surgeons. There is growing concerns about non-malignant health hazard also of cumulative radiation exposure including, cataract, dermatitis, skin issues dryness, etc. associated with this technique.

Long-term repeated exposure to this degree of ionizing radiation, regardless of the use of it is of great occupational health importance that, as reported by Rampersaud et al. Fluoroscopy-assisted pedicle screw implantation is associated with a 10–12 times greater radiation exposure to the spinal surgeon than in nonspinal orthopedic procedures. Ul Haque et al. estimated that surgeons were exposed to a radiation dose that exceeded the maximum recommended dose for nonclassified workers using fluoroscopy. This is of paramount importance as long-term effects of a chronic low-grade exposure are still unclear.

So far, some in vitro studies have suggested that the use of spinal navigation may significantly reduce radiation exposure in the operating room when compared with the conventional fluoroscopy guidance. In a phantom study,

Slomczykowski et al. compared the intraoperative dose of fluoroscopically-guided percutaneous pedicle screws to CT-based computer-assisted surgery and found that the intraoperative dose was reduced by the use of computer guidance instead of fluoroscopy. Although the CT dose can be significantly reduced by optimization of CT imaging, the patient dose remains higher when using a CT-based approach. In a study on 4 cadavers, Kim et al. compared surgeon exposure in a cadaveric study and fluoroscopy time without dosimetry in a patient series using conventional fluoroscopy and 2D fluoroscopy-based navigation. During surgery, fluoroscopic time was significantly reduced by navigation, whereas operating time showed no significant differences. A comparison of the radiation exposure by the use of different navigation concepts—2D fluoroscopy-based, 3D fluoroscopy-based, CT-based—versus conventional fluoroscopic guidance by Gebhard et. al. on 38 patients assessed the radiation dose by dosimeters on the radiation source, the detector, and the patient. They reported reduced radiation doses from conventional fluoroscopy to 2D fluoroscopy-based to CT-based to 3D fluoroscopy-based navigation in the operating room. Smith et al. compared radiation dose to the surgeon during pedicle screw insertion with 3D fluoroscopy- based navigation and with conventional fluoroscopic guidance using protective gear in a cadaveric study with no measurable radiation exposure in most cases of navigation assistance.

Fluoroscopy vs CT-based vs O-arm-based Navigation

Despite many advantages, it must be stated that virtual fluoroscopy is a two-dimensional (2D) navigational system with low reliability in MIS instruementation. It does not provide the detailed multiplanar imaging generated by 3D systems and, consequently, has different clinical utility. A virtual fluoroscopy system cannot compensate for causes of poor image quality, such as obesity, bowel contrast after trauma assessment, or the inadvertent positioning of radiopaque structures (e.g. retractors or patient-positioning devices). Errors in the clinical interpretation of 2D images and the extrapolation of 2D information to 3D anatomy are still dependent on the expertize of the spine surgeon. Furthermore, other disadvantages remain inherent in the nature of fluoroscopy. Clinical misinterpretation of a low quality, poorly-oriented image cannot be compensated for by any navigational system. These downsides of virtual fluoroscopy-based systems can be overcome by CT-based imaging obtained preoperatively providing 3D anatomical view for navigation. The use of proper fluoroscopic techniques, such as centering the area of interest within the field of view and tangential imaging (acquiring "true" lateral and anteroposterior views) still must be adhered to. Tian et al. examined different navigation methods and found 90.76% accurate screw placement in the CT-based group versus 85.48% in the 2D-based group.

Although preoperative CT-based image guidance is a highly effective method of intraoperative navigation, there are some notable disadvantages to the technology. The systems require a preoperative scan to be performed using a specific protocol. This can add cost and time to the preoperative workup, particularly if the patient has already had a diagnostically adequate. The registration process appears relatively straightforward in experienced hands, but there is a significant learning curve involved with properly selecting the anatomic landmarks and matching them to the image anatomy. Lastly, since the CT images are obtained before surgery with the patient in one position and the surgery is commonly performed in a different position, intersegmental relationships between adjacent vertebral levels can differ. This is particularly true in cases of spinal instability. At the very least, potential changes in intersegmental vertebral relationships mandate the use of a separate registration process for each vertebral level to be navigated.

Three-dimensional C-arm fluoroscopy (3D fluoroscopy) is a significant advancement in the rapidly developing field of image guidance and potentially represents the future of intraoperative spinal navigation. Unlike a standard fluoroscope, an isocentric C-arm is able to automatically rotate around the patient while maintaining the relevant spinal anatomy in its center. With the addition of specialized software, such a C-arm can effectively function as a computed tomography scanner. The automated image acquisition takes approximately 2 minutes. This process is somewhat analogous to virtual fluoroscopy, except that the images are identical to those provided by CT-based systems. The advantages of this innovative technology are many. The isocentric C-arm provides three-dimensional reconstructed images of the patient on the operating table. Therefore, the risk of navigation inaccuracy due to intervertebral alignment differences between the preoperative CT data set and the intraoperative position is eliminated. Since the system can display three adjacent lumbar vertebrae, separate registration solutions are unnecessary. The need for a preoperative CT scan with a specific image-guided protocol (and its cost in money and time) is eliminated. The surgeon-driven registration process is completely obviated, as navigation can commence immediately after the images have been transferred to the workstation. Lastly, a postoperative scan can be performed in the operating room to ensure accurate implant placement and/or to evaluate the thoroughness of a decompressive procedure.

2D vs 3D Navigation Systems

The desire for real-time detailed intraoperative imaging in 3D for complex revision or MIS surgery has led to the development of devices, such as the O-arm. Scattered radiation from traditional CT scans and intraoperative fluoroscopy has become a concern to the patient and health care provider. It is yet to be determined whether intraoperative 3D imaging has a preferential risk/ benefit profile compared with traditional methods of instrumentation in non-deformed thoracolumbar spine surgery. A meta-analysis of in vivo pedicle screw insertions suggested that there was a 9.2% malposition rate in CT based navigation compared with a 14.5% rate among 2D fluoroscopy. Breach rates were similar with the use of the C-arm and O-arm. The efficiency between the 2 systems was comparable, with the O-arm taking more time to set up and position but less time for instrumentation. There has been little evidence comparing the required operative time between O-arm and C-arm. In one of the earlier studies evaluating the accuracy of 2D imaging, Vaccaro et al. observed a 41% (37 of 90) pedicle wall violation after bilateral instrumentation of 5 cadavers from T4–T12. Nevertheless, with the use of an O-arm, malposition pedicle screws could be redirected before extubation. On the contrary, correction of malpositioned pedicle screws placed with C-arm guidance would require a confirmatory postoperative CT and additional surgery. Well-designed studies with consistent and clinically relevant results are needed to show a definitive advantage in using the O-arm for accurate pedicle screw placement.

In considering radiation exposure, each modality had its own safety profile. Surgeons were exposed to more radiation when using the C-arm, whereas the O-arm gave higher doses of radiation to the cadaveric specimens.

Surgical Time and Radiation Time

The navigation system set-up time, acquisition of images, their registration and learning curve of surgeon and staff for navigation may add in total surgical time. In the study by Ravi B et al., fluoroscopy time for screw placement was less than 20 seconds per case. Overall surgical time and radiation exposure time comes down with every case as you step up the ladder of learning curve. Study by Jimmy Villard et al. also shows that 3D fluoroscopy-based spinal navigation used for lumbar fusion significantly reduces the surgeon's radiation exposure time by up to 9.96 times (1884.8 cGy·cm (non-navigated) versus 887 cGy·cm (navigated)). Kim et al. in a same sort of cadaveric study found that fluoroscopic time was significantly reduced by navigation.

Clinical Outcomes with Navigation-guided Surgery vs Non-navigated Surgeries

Studies comparing the clinical outcome did not report any significant difference in intraoperative blood loss, postoperative outcome, fusion status. In the study by Benson P Yang estimated blood loss in interbody fusion surgeries with blood loss in 71.6% patients was <200 cc without any significant difference in navigated versus non-navigated group. In our study with MIS TLIF with percutaneous instrumentation, there was 128.89 ± 21.389 mL and 124.77 ± 27.15 mL (p value = 0.30) blood loss in navigated and non-navigated group respectively without any statistical difference. Tian W demonstrated significant improvement in postoperative VAS and ODI of all patients in his study of comparing navigation-guided MIS-TLIF with open TLIF. In our study also, clinical parameters (VAS, ODI) were significantly improved in both the groups without any significant difference in clinical parameters. This demonstrates that in spite of limited exposure, decompression can be done adequately in patients with MIS-TLIF. Tian W demonstrated solid fusion in 96.67% cases after 2 years follow-up with navigation-guided MIS-TLIF. Kim et al. reported in 72 patients treated with single level MIS-TLIF with 2-year fusion rate of 97%. Anand et al. reported solid fusion rate in 99% patients treated with MIS-TLIF. Seng C reported 77.5% fusion rates at 6-month follow- up with 97.3% fusion at final follow with MIS-TLIF which is close to our results.

Cost-effectiveness

Various studies have shown that spinal navigation can be used without increasing OR time, and possibly with even shorter times compared with conventional surgery. Costa et al. evaluated the cost-effectiveness of intraoperative spinal navigation with preoperative planned navigation systems. In their study of hospital costs in patients with spondylolisthesis, they concluded that the two technologies were similar in cost. Despite these data, there may be a trend to suggest a cost advantage of using image-guided navigation in high-volume centers that specialize in more complex cases and perform more than 150 cases a year.

Our Clinical Experience with Navigation-guided MIS-TLIF

In our institute, we conducted a study to compare the clinic-radiological outcome of navigated versus non-navigated MIS-TLIF in which we found that cumulative radiation dose was significantly higher in non-navigated conventional fluoroscopy-based percutaneous instrumentation MIS-TLIF group. Navigated group had 1.68 ± 0.419 mGy, 0.470 ± 0.122 Gy·cm, 46.50 ± 11.89 sec radiation dose, dose area product and radiation time respectively in comparison of 10.97 ± 2.38 mGy, 2.928 ± 0.870 Gy-cm, 119.08 ± 29.784 sec in non-navigated group as measured with digital C-arm computer assessment. Dose area product is most closely related to effective dose of radiation. It was 6.23 times higher in non-navigated group. This demonstrates that navigation can surely reduce long-term radiation exposure and aid in reducing overall radiation exposure to patient. Preacquired fluoroscopic images are used for navigation, so the surgical team can stand at a safe distance during "live" fluoroscopy, minimizing or eliminating the need for wearing lead shielding. The accuracy of screw placement was better in navigated group with 3% perforation rate out of 64 screws compared to 9% with non-navigated instrumentation MIS TLIF group. In both groups, the perforation was group 1 or group 2 with no critical breach in any series. None of the groups had any neurological complication or required revision of implant stating no added clinical benefits to the patient of navigation technology. The surgical time in our experience also improves with time and there is a definite learning involved. Clinical parameters including pain scores, disability indices and fusion rates improved in both navigated and non-navigated groups with no statistical difference in both the groups. Navigation definitely enhances the accuracy of screw placement by percutaneous methods in MIS TLIF procedure with significant reduction in radiation doses to the surgical team.

Limitations (Table 4)

Many surgeons have been hesitant to embrace navigation technology, because of early experience with tedious matched-pair point registration of numerous anatomical landmarks, excessive operative set-up times, and prolonged screw placement times. Some navigation platforms mandate the attachment of a reference arc through a separate incision. With newer generation systems, more recent reports describe image registration and set-up times between 14 and 18 minutes. Results from the current study demonstrated a relatively short set-up time of approximately 5 minutes by ancillary staff as well as reductions in screw placement time. A learning curve can be expected with the adoption of any new technology. The fact that current image guidance techniques have a learning curve that can result in surgeon frustration and longer operating room times, especially early in the surgeon's IGS experience. Also, although navigation-guided surgery is more accurate than conventional navigational techniques, it is not perfect. Failure to appreciate these limitations can result in a surgical misadventure. Navigation technology is best thought of as a supplement to, not a replacement for, the spine surgeon's experience and judgment.

Table 4

Proposed limitations of navigation in MI instrumentation

- Inability to track realtime location of guidewires which needs sequential fluoroscopic images to prevent advancement
- Questionable use in interbody cage placement or decompression
- Navigation with 2D fluoroscopy does not provide multi-planar detailed imaging
- Fixing of reference arc is invasive which constrains the surgeon's movement and puts its own stability at risk
- Navigation with 2D fluoroscopy cannot compensate for causes for poor image quality like obesity
- Prior CT obtaining (time and cost) in CT-based navigation
- Change in intersegmental relationships between vertebral segments during positioning for imaging and for surgery may result in inaccuracy in CT-based navigation
- Steep learning curve
- Current devices only image a limited number of segments; thus, for longer constructs, additional spins may be required

Future of Navigation

Use of novel surgical robotic system called BFRS, i.e. biplanar fluoroscopy, surgical planning and robotic-assist in percutaneous spinal procedures.

Use of electromagnetic technology (iMRI) for image guidance to avoid radiation exposure, to bypass requirement of direct line of sight between tracker and probe, to image larger area for longer construct.

Use of Wifi devices to transmit signals between patient frame and tracker and camera unit through internet technology for navigation; further reducing the need of radiation in intraoperative navigation and complex wiring or networking reducing the need of manpower training.

Work on new procedures like navigation-guided percutaneous lumbosacral interbody fusion (NPLSIF) to accurately establish a corridor in bone, which might open new possibilities for lumbosacral interbody fusion: if a corridor can be accurately established in the ilium and sacral ala, then it is possible to perform diskectomy and bone grafting through this corridor. In addition, employing navigation eliminates the need for exposure, so that the procedure can be performed percutaneously.

Further refinements in imaging technology, including fusion to MRI and use of multimodality techniques including endoscopy for craniocervical junction pathologies, will continue to push the limits of MISS with the goal of improving the long-term radiation safety profile of these surgical adjuncts

CONCLUSION

Use of navigation in spine surgery has improved the safety of spinal instrumentation. Improvement in navigation technology will continue to expand its applications in spine surgery. This technology, however, should not substitute for a thorough knowledge of spinal anatomy and traditional methods of instrumentation. Navigation in MIS-TLIF have added advantage of improved precision, better accuracy in intraosseous placement with significantly reduced radiation exposure in surgery in comparison of conventional fluoroscopic-guided MIS-TLIF, but there are further growth in this field is anticipated to track guidewires and aid in interbody cage placement. Certainly, there are drawbacks to and limitations of image-guided spinal surgery. Ongoing advances in this field address these limitations and appear quite promising.

BIBLIOGRAPHY

1. Esses SI, Barton LS, Vadim D. Complications associated with the technique of pedicle screw fi xation: a selected survey of ABS members. Spine. 1993;18: 2231-9.
2. Gebhard FT , Kraus MD , Schneider E , et al. Does computer-assisted spine surgery reduce intraopera- tive radiation doses? Spine (Phila Pa 1976). 2006;31:2024-7.
3. Hernanz-Schulman M, Emmons M, Price R. Fluoroscopy clinical practice: controlling dose and study quality. In: Frush DP, Huda H, eds. Categorical course syllabus in diagnostic radiology physics: from in- visible to visible—the science and practice of x-ray imaging and radiation dose optimization. Oak Brook, IL: Radiological Society of North America. 2006:133-9.
4. International Commission on Radiological Protection. Recommendations of the International Commission on Radiological Protection. Ann ICRP. 1990;21.
5. Kim CW, Lee YP , Taylor W , et al. Use of navigation-assisted fl uoroscopy to decrease radiation expo- sure during minimally invasive spine surgery . Spine J. 2008;8:58.
6. Kosmopoulos V, Schizas C. Pedicle screw placement accuracy: a metaanalysis. Spine. 2007;32:E111-20.
7. Lonstein JE, Denis F, Perra JH, et al. Complications associated with pedicle screws. J Bone Joint Surg Am. 1999;81:1519-28.
8. Mirza SK, Wiggins GC, Kuntz C, et al. Accuracy of thoracic vertebral body screw placement using standard fluoroscopy, fluoroscopic image guidance, and computed tomographic image guidance: a ca- daver study. Spine. 2003;28:402-13.
9. Rampersaud YR, Foley KT, Shen AC, et al. Radiation exposure to the spine surgeon during fluoroscopi- cally assisted pedicle screw insertion. Spine. 2000;25:2637-45.
10. Ravi B, Zahrai A, Rampersaud R. Clinical accuracy of computer-assisted two-dimensional fluoroscopy for the percutaneous placement of lumbosacral pedicle screws. Spine. 2011;36:84-91.
11. Ringel F, Stoffel M, Stüer C, et al. Minimally invasive transmuscular pedicle screw fixation of the tho- racic and lumbar spine. Neurosurgery. 2006;59(4 suppl 2):361-7.
12. Slomczykowski M , Roberto M , Schneeberger P, et al. Radiation dose for pedicle screw insertion. Fluoroscopic method versus computer-assisted surgery. Spine (Phila Pa 1976). 1999;24: 975-82.
13. Smith H, Welsch MD , Sasso RC, et al. Comparison of radiation exposure in lumbar pedicle screw placement with fluoroscopy vs. computer-assisted image guidance with intraoperative three dimensional imaging . J Spinal Cord Med. 2008;31:532-7.
14. Tian NF, Xu HZ. Image-guided pedicle screw insertion accuracy: a meta-analysis. Int Ortho. 2009;33:895-903.
15. Tian W, Xu YF, Liu B, et al. Computer-Assisted Minimally Invasive Transforaminal Lumbar Interbody Fusion May Be Better than Open Surgery for Treating Degenerative Lumbar Disease. Clin Spine Surg. 2016.
16. Villard J, Ryang YM, Demetriades AK, et al. Radiation exposure to the surgeon and the patient during posterior lumbar spinal instrumentation: a prospective randomized comparison of navigated versus non- navigated freehand techniques. Spine. 2014;39(13):1004-9.
17. Yang BP, Wahl MM, Idler CS. Percutaneous lumbar pedicle screw placement aided by computer assisted fluoroscopy-based navigation: perioperative results of a prospective, comparative, multicenter study. Spine. 2012;37(24):2055-60.

37

CHAPTER

Navigation in Minimally Invasive Spine Surgery

Benjamin Mayo, Junyoung Ahn, Benjamin Kuhns, William Long, Dustin Massel, Krishna Modi, Kern Singh

ABSTRACT

Minimally invasive spine surgeries (MIS) have distinct advantages over the conventional open procedures, the lesser tissue trauma, smaller incisions and faster rehabilitation associated with MIS. Navigation in minimally invasive surgeries has further helped to perform a safe spine surgery. Navigation can be used to deal with wide variety of spinal pathologies in all areas of the spine. This chapter deals with the techniques, indications, complications of navigation-guided minimal invasive spine surgeries.

INTRODUCTION

Several studies have demonstrated lower operative blood loss, postoperative pain, and length of hospital stay following minimally invasive spine surgery (MISS) as compared to traditional open approaches. [1,2] With advancements in surgical techniques, there has been a growing interest in improving methods for multi-planar visualization of unexposed spinal anatomy. As such, the evolution of three-dimensional (3D) intraoperative image-guidance (navigation) has paralleled the advances in MISS.[3-5] There are multiple navigation technologies currently in use, each with their own advantages and disadvantages. The purpose of this chapter is to discuss the history, evidence, and limitations of the various navigation technologies used in MISS.

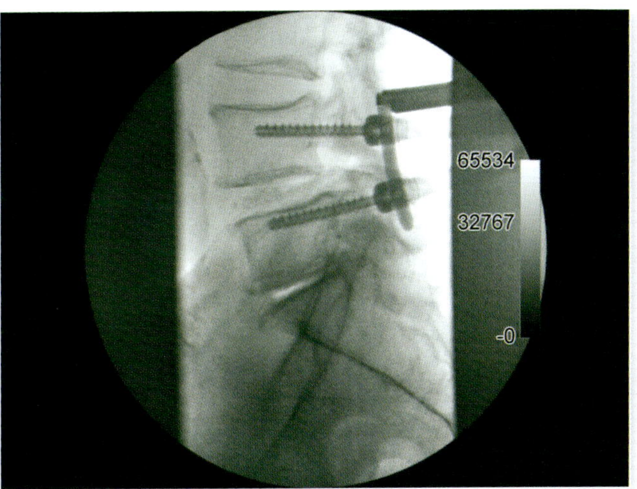

Figure 1: Intraoperative lateral C-arm fluoroscopic image of minimally invasive transforaminal lumbar interbody fusion

HISTORY, EVOLUTION AND EQUIPMENT

Prior to navigation, intraoperative image guidance relied on serial intraoperative radiographs or C-arm fluoroscopy **(Figure 1)**. Serial radiography has become less commonly used due to the time commitment for the processing of images. This delay is exaggerated if the images are of poor quality, a factor not uncommon in obese patients or in deformity surgery. Fluoroscopy can provide instant intraoperative imaging and is currently the most commonly used modality. However, the occupational radiation exposure is a concern.[6,7] Secondary drawbacks include bulky presence, technician dependence, and potential risk to the sterile field. Both methods only provide static images in one plane.

Intraoperative navigation of the spine evolved from technology used initially for intracranial stereotaxy. Specific external landmarks on the patient's body were recorded and projected onto intraoperative images. This image projection is referred to as referencing and is accomplished by a sensor attached on the patient or the "dynamic reference array". Registration is required to accurately depict the patients anatomy onto formatted images.[8] However, initial attempts at navigation were unsuccessful due to indirect and inaccurate registration of the spinal anatomy using superficial skin sensors.[9,10]

Common current image guidance equipment (hardware and software) utilizes specialized preoperative CT scans, 3D fluoroscopy, or intraoperative cone-beam CT. Preoperative CT-based image guidance uses a specific scan protocol and computer program. Images from a scanned area are transferred to a workstation to create 3D images of the patient specific anatomy **(Figure 2)**. During surgery, a probe is used to indicate specific landmarks on the dorsal bony anatomy of the spine. These selected points will register with images projected on the workstation from the preoperative scan.

Disadvantages center around the specific preoperative protocol required. Registration of anatomical landmarks can add time, expense, and redundancy to the preoperative work-up. Inaccuracies in referencing can also occur, as the segmental relationship between vertebrae may be different from preoperative scans to intraoperative position.

APPLICATION IN SPINE SURGERY

Traditional methods of lumbar pedicle instrumentation can result in misplacement rates as high as 30%.[11-13] For techniques, such as percutaneous pedicle screw placement, it is essential to optimize accuracy to avoid neurologic or vascular complications while allowing maximum pedicle fill.[14-16] Previous studies have demonstrated the increased accuracy of pedicle screw placement utilizing navigation. A meta-analysis by Shin et al. demonstrated that the risk of pedicle perforation may be significantly decreased by utilizing computer-assisted navigationwithout increasing the operative time.[17] Verma et al. performed a meta-analysis to assess the impact of computer-assisted navigation for pedicle screw placement on postoperative functional outcomes.[18] While the authors reported that navigation may be associated with a decreased risk of pedicle screw misplacement they were not able to determine any benefits in regards to clinical outcomes.

Cervical Spine

Screw placement in the cervical spine can be challenging due to the neural and vascular (vertebral arteries) elements associated with smaller bony corridors used for instrumentation, especially in the upper cervical spine **(Figure 3)**. Vertebral artery injury during upper cervical screw placement can be as high as 4.1% while pedicle screw misplacement can vary upto 12.5–18%.[16,19-22] In a cadaveric study, Holly et al. demonstrated that navigation may increase the accuracy of percutaneous posterior cervical screw placement.[23] Navigation was used in the cadaveric study for C1–2 transarticular screws, C3–6 lateral masses, or C7 pedicles screws. The majority of the screws (41/42; 97.6%) screws were accurately placed with only 1 C7 pedicle screw demonstrating a grade 1 breach.[24] In other smaller series, navigation has been successfully used for the accurate placement of occipital-condyle junction and C2 intralaminar instrumentation.[24,25]

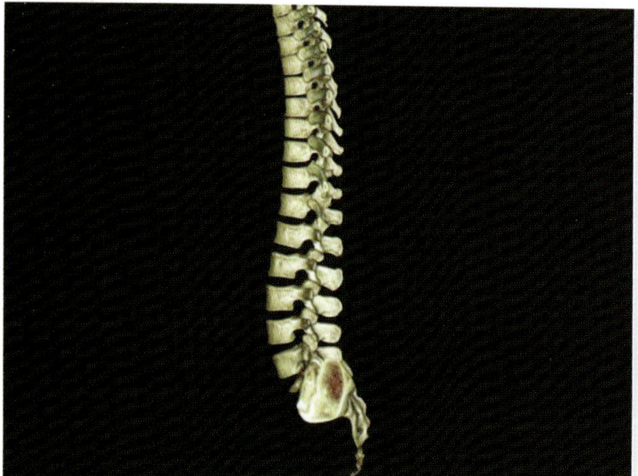

Figure 2: 3D image of the spine created by the BodyTom imaging device. 3D full spine scan

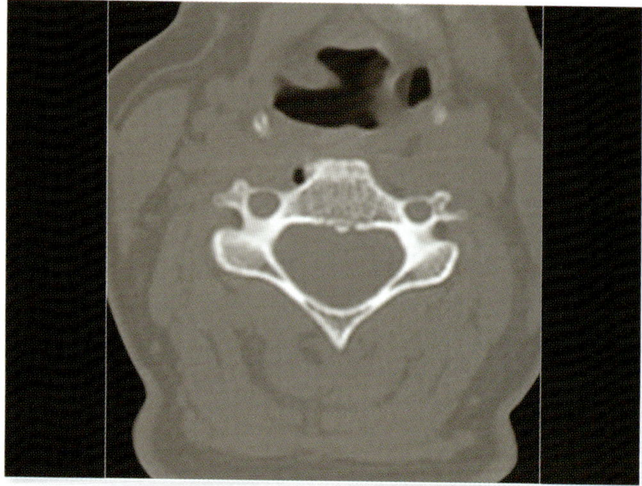

Figure 3: Axial image of cervical spine produced by BodyTom (Will label intended screw path, vertebral artery locations, and parts of vertebra)

Thoracic Spine

The variability of pedicle anatomy, the proximity of vital neurovascular structures and organs, and the poor visualization of fluoroscopic images can make instrumentation of the thoracic spine challenging as well. Studies exploring the benefits of navigation for instrumentation in the thoracic spine have focused on either small series of either cadaveric or open procedures. Traditional free hand pedicle screw misplacement in the thoracic spine has been reported as high as 55%.[26] Earlier studies of navigation in the thoracic spine reported pedicle breaches from 4.5–8.5%.[27,28] However, Allam et al. recently demonstrated 99% accuracy with navigation-based instrumentation of the thoracic spine as compared to an 89% rate for free hand techniques.[29]

Evidence regarding navigation in MISS of the thoracic spine has been more limited. In a cadaveric series, Holly et al. demonstrated a 94. 7% accuracy rate with screw placement in the thoracic pedicles.[30] The 5 recorded pedicle breaches were due to a mismatch between screws size (average 6 mm) and the pedicle width (average 4. 6 mm).

Lumbar Spine

The size, structure, and biomechanical forces make the thoracolumbar, lumbar, and lumbosacral junction susceptible to multiple pathologies. Kosmopoulos et al. pooled a collection of previous studies and estimated a median misplacement rate of 21% in lumbar pedicle screws placement when not using navigation.[31] In a combined cadaveric and clinical study, Kim et al. investigated the utility of navigation in the setting of a minimally invasive transforaminal lumbar interbody fusion (MIS TLIF).[32] The authors demonstrated that both (i) operating room time and (ii) fluoroscopy time may be decreased utilizing intraoperative navigation.

Deformity/Revision Surgery

Navigation platforms may be increasingly utilized for more complex procedures where the anatomy is altered or obscured, such as for deformity or revision surgery. Luther et al. demonstrated that navigation was more likely to be used in complex procedures ($p < 0.001$).[33] Larson et al. demonstrated an increase in pedicle screw placement accuracy (93.7% to 99.3%) in the pediatric deformity population when navigation systems were employed.[34] Scheufler et al. compared fluoroscopy to intraoperative CT navigation in patients undergoing multilevel MISS for degenerative scoliosis.[35] A total of 415 screws in 30 patients were assessed. Navigation was faster (by 35 minutes), more accurate (no misplaced screws), and safer (no radiation to surgeon).

Revision surgery can present substantial technical challenges due to alterations in the spinal anatomy.[36,37] A recent analysis of 742 total pedicle screws (313 primary, 429 revision) by Hsieh et al. demonstrated comparable efficacy rates of screw placement at 94.2% for primary and 91.6% for revision surgeries.[38] In a case report of patient undergoing revision surgery for refractory adult scoliosis, Metz and Burch suggested that computer-assisted navigation may improve the safety and efficacy of these procedures.[39] Similarly, Lim et al. reported on computer-assisted pedicle screw placement in patients who had previously undergone lumbar fusion procedures.[40] The authors concluded that navigation may be valuable in these cases as normal anatomical landmarks may be missing due to prior surgery. The utility of intraoperative navigation is intuitive for patients with complex anatomy yet the evidence is still in its infancy.

LIMITATIONS

Despite studies demonstrating the improved accuracy of pedicle screw placement, there are limitations associated with navigation, such as increased operative time and increased radiation exposure to the patient.[8] A worldwide survey of spine surgeons by Hartl et al. demonstrated that while surgeons can appreciate the clinical value of intraoperative navigation, the high cost of the equipment (in comparison to traditional 2D) and the learning curve associated with using the equipment may compel surgeons to operate without navigation.[41] This concern was supported by Bai et al. who reported that the learning curve for computer-assisted navigation may increase both operative time and the rate of screw perforation.[42] In addition, heralded benefits in improved accuracy have not necessarily been associated with improved clinical (i.e. neurological) and or functional outcomes for spine surgery patients.[18,43,44] The increase in operative time can be attributed to the time for registration of landmarks with imaging (preoperative or postoperative).[45] Intuitively, time allotted for navigation registration may increase significantly when multiple levels are involved (which may require additional registration steps).[46] This increase in time may expose spine surgeons to high doses of radiation during MISS procedures.[47] Other limitations include the segments available for visualization, upfront costs to newer technology, and lack of clinical implications. However, many of the limitations inherent within image-guided navigation systems may be alleviated by 3D intraoperative CT-guided systems.[34,48,49]

CURRENT NAVIGATION MODALITIES

Though each navigation device has its own unique benefits and limitations, each operate under the same general principle. After exposure of the patient's spinal anatomy, intraoperative CT creates a frame of referenceon the patient. Scans of the relevant anatomyare then sent to the navigation platform, and a 3D image is created for use in intraoperative registration.[35] This automated registration is beneficial for eliminating the error from poor point or surface matching, as well as its ability to recalibrate to changes in patient anatomy mid-procedure.[8,50] MISS relies on imaging to accurately characterize the surgical anatomy in the setting of limited access to landmarks and direct visualization. Without the need for anatomic registration, exposure of dorsal spinal anatomy is minimized rendering this technology ideal for MISS navigation.

Isocentric 3D C-arm

Isocentric 3D C-arm is a mobile intraoperative CT device that rotates over a 190-degree arc, keeping the distance between the target region and the imaging tube constant **(Figure 4)**. This 3D fluoroscopy device utilizes a specialized computer program and an advanced automated C-arm to acquire and synthesize multiplanar views of the spinal anatomy, typically 3–5 segments in length.[51] When coupled with navigation software, real time tracking of surgical instruments on the generated 3D images is possible **(Figure 5)**.

The benefits of 3D fluoroscopy include accurate and timely 3D reconstructed images with similar resolution to conventional CT images, without the costs or radiation exposure of preoperative CT scans. Hott et al. demonstrated similar image quality compared to postoperative CT scans, thus allowing the use of intraoperative, post-procedural images in place of a postoperative CT scan to reduce overall radiation exposure.[51] An added benefit is the reduced radiation exposure for both surgeon and patient. Smith et al. demonstrated reduced radiation exposure for surgeons when compared to conventional C-arm fluoroscopy.[43] In a prospective study of minimally invasive kyphoplasty procedures, Villavicencio et al. demonstrated an 86% reduction in radiation time, while having a minimal effect on operating time when compared to standard fluoroscopy.[52]

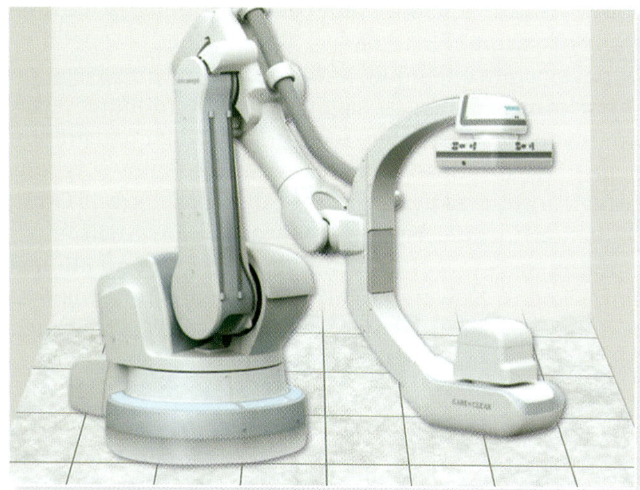

Figure 4: Isocentric 3D C-arm machine

Though reduction in radiation exposure is a critical benefit, arguably the most important advantage is the improvement in pedicle screw placement accuracy and decreased complication rates when using iso-C3D compared to conventional fluoroscopy.[53] Multiple cadaver studies have demonstrated improved pedicle screw positioning with navigation.[5,22,30] A retrospective study by Nakashima et al. showed an 8% reduction in malposition rate when using iso-C3D compared to traditional hand placement.[54]

Though there are many benefits of isocentric 3D C-arm over conventional fluoroscopy, it is not without limitations. Having only 190° of rotation limits the number of spinal levels that can be captured with each scan. This makes it a less than ideal technique for extensiveprocedures that require multiple scans to capture the full extent of the operation, as each scan interrupts the surgical procedure and increases radiation, albeit less than conventional fluoroscopy.

O-Arm

O-arm is an intraoperative cone-beam CT system that acquires images over a full 360° arc **(Figure 6)**, When compared to iso-C3D, it is capable of capturing more images, at a higher resolution, in a shorter period of time, thus decreasing the amount of interruption[55] **(Figure 7)**. Importantly, the O-arm improves on the ease and accuracy of registration as the scan can be performed following the exposure of the dorsal bony anatomy of the spine.

O-arm provides many of the same benefits as isocentric C-arm, such as decreased radiation exposure compared to conventional fluoroscopy. Tabaraee et al. demonstrated that intraoperative cone-beamed CT (O-arm) could completely avoid occupational radiation exposure to surgeon and staff as compared to C-arm.[56] Nelson et al. reported that O-arm radiation exposure to the patient was equivalent to 38 C-arm and 1.5 X-ray exposures and that the scatter radiation to the surgeon and assistant was greatest with the C-arm.[57] The use of O-arm also reduces the frequency of screw misplacement. A study by Van De Kelft et al. demonstrated a misplacement rate of 2.5%, however, with the use of navigation, all misplaced screws were detected and revised before the end of the procedure.[58]

While O-arm does have benefits over conventional fluoroscopy, such as better placement rates, it is with longer preparation times and screw placement times. However, a

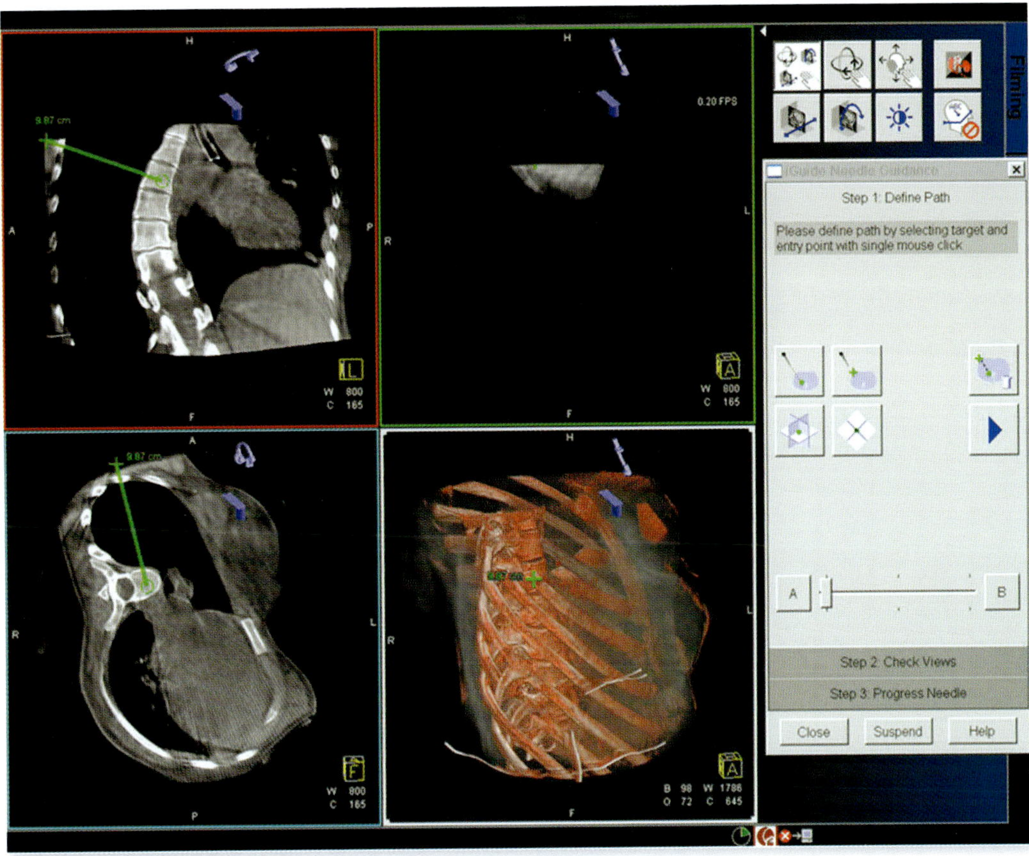

Figure 5: Intraoperative navigation screen produced by iso-C 3D

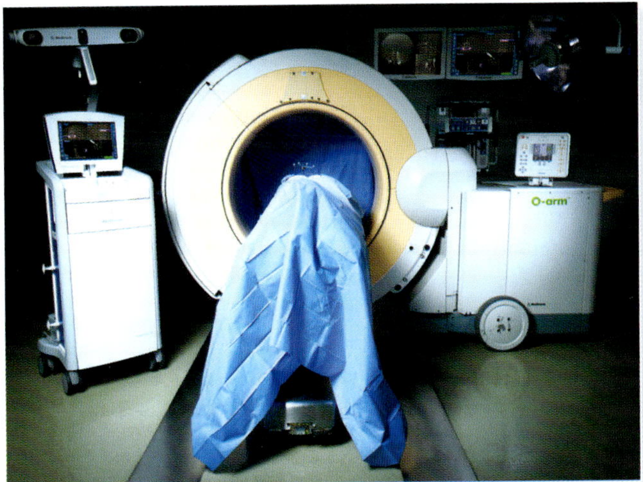

Figure 6: Example intraoperative arrangement of O-arm and Stealth navigation station

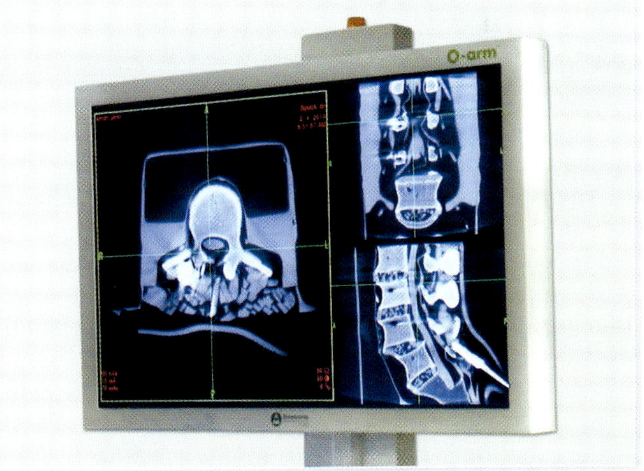

Figure 7: Intraoperative O-arm images of the lumbar spine displayed on the Stealth station

recent cadaveric study demonstrated that the operative time for pedicle screw placement was no different whether the O-arm 3D image-guided navigation or traditional C-arm fluoroscopy was used.[56] The main disadvantage is the upfront cost of the specialized equipment and the logistics of maintaining sterility during the scan (draping).

BodyTom

The BodyTom® is a portable, battery powered, full body CT scanner that was released in 2011 **(Figure 8)**. The portability of the BodyTom® allows it to be utilized in a wide range of clinical applications including cranial, spinal, head

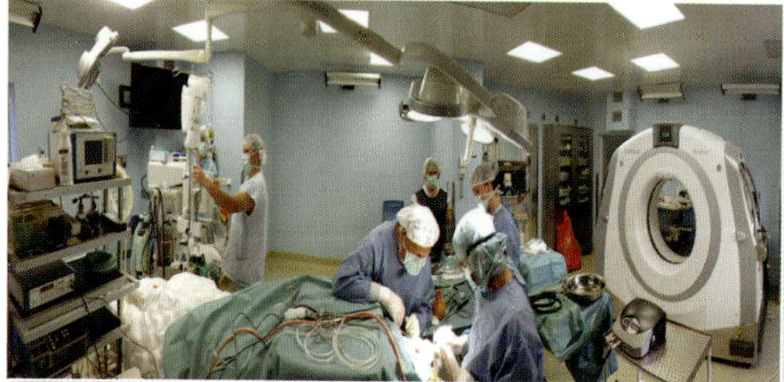

Figure 8: BodyTom machine in the operating room

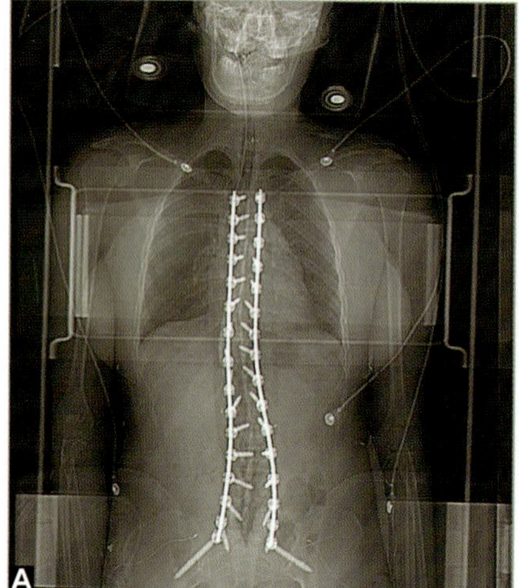

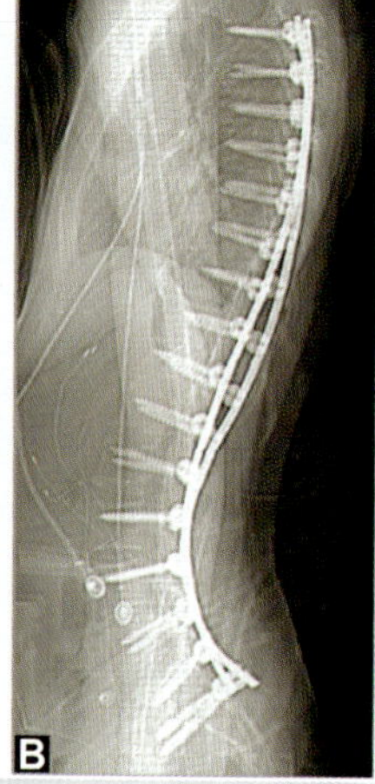

Figure 9: (A) AP; (B) Lateral images produced by the BodyTom of the full spine after scoliosis correction

and neck, trauma, and orthopedic cases.[59] It is capable of producing three-dimensional images of both bone and soft tissues, and in one pass is able to provide an image along the entire length of the spine from C1 to S5.[59] **(Figure 9)**

The BodyTom® offers surgeons several intraoperative advantages, especially during minimally invasive spine surgery.[60] Straightforward integration of images with standard surgical navigation systems allows for immediate intraoperative use and real time confirmation of instrumentation on 3D images.[60,61] This combination increases the accuracy of hardware placement and allows surgeons to double-check the hardware location before ending the procedure. As a result, the need for revision surgery due to inappropriate hardware placement should decrease.[62] The ability to image soft tissues also allows surgeons to detect complications that may have resulted throughout the procedure and subsequently correct them before leaving the operating room.[61] Additional advantages of the BodyTom® include built in internal lead shielding that prevents unnecessary radiological exposure to both the patient and operating room staff. Since the BodyTom® is still considered a new development in CT imaging, few studies have been conducted to evaluate all of its advantages and disadvantages.

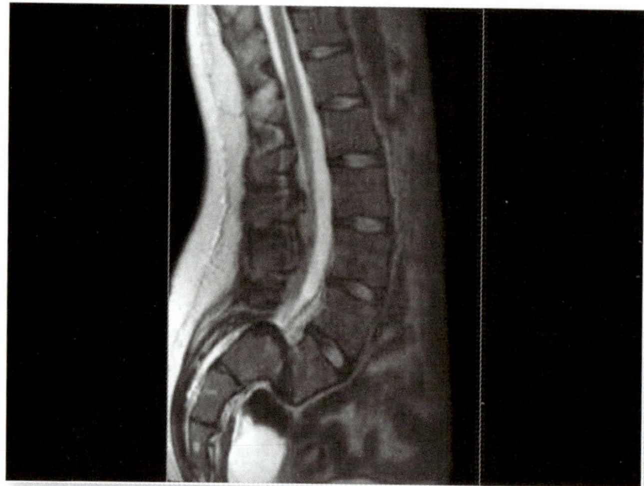

Figure 10: Lateral lumbar spine MRI depicting relevant soft tissue around the spine (Will label relevant soft tissue)

Magnetic Resonance Imaging

Intraoperative MRI is a newer technology that is well studied in brain and tumor surgery. Despite it is excellent ability to visualize soft tissue without radiation, it is not yet widely used in spinal surgery.[63] Intraoperative MRI also maintains the ability to register patient anatomy for navigation purposes through combined low field intraoperative MRI with high field preoperative MRI[63] **(Figure 10)**. One of the few studies done was by Choi et al. who prospectively investigated the use of intraoperative MRI in lumbar diskectomy surgery. The authors reported that MRI may play an important role in identifying instrument entry point on the skin and the optimal trajectory to the disk space to avoid vascular and neurologic structures. Additionally, the author found it was able to identify inadequate decompression, potentially reducing the rate of reoperations.[64]

Despite the potential benefits to intraoperative MRI, its use is complicated by many factors, most notably the relative lack of nonmagnetic surgical instruments. Additionally, the large size and immobile circular design are not easily compatible with use in the operating room.

FUTURE OF NAVIGATION

The future of navigation technology will focus on improving efficiency and accuracy of registration without delaying operative time. Additional benefits that could draw interest include reduced radiation exposure and overall cost-effectiveness. Potential future navigation technology may include intraoperative MRI, robotic systems, or electromagnetic navigation.

SUMMARY

Navigation technology in MISS may potentially improve identification of unexposed anatomy and accuracy instrumentation placement while reducing occupational radiation to the surgeon. However, the learning curve and potentially increased operative time associated with the utilization of these systems pose significant limitations. Additionally, newer technology should address radiation exposure to the patient and operating room staff. Ultimately, navigation technology should act not as a replacement, but as a supplement to surgeon judgment and experience.

REFERENCES

1. Banczerowski P, Czigléczki G, Papp Z, et al. Minimally invasive spine surgery: systematic review. Neurosurg Rev. 2014;38:11-26.
2. Spetzger U, Schilling AV, Winkler G, et al. The past, present and future of minimally invasive spine surgery: A review and speculative outlook. Minim Invasive Ther Allied Technol. 2013;22:227-41.
3. Mason A, Paulsen R, Babuska JM, et al. The accuracy of pedicle screw placement using intraoperative image guidance systems. Journal of neurosurgery. Spine. 2014;20:196-203.
4. Oppenheimer JH, DeCastro I, McDonnell DE. Minimally invasive spine technology and minimally invasive spine surgery: a historical review. Neurosurgical Focus. 2009;27.
5. Tian N-F, Huang Q-S, Zhou P, et al. Pedicle screw insertion accuracy with different assisted methods: a systematic review and meta-analysis of comparative studies. European Spine Journal: Official Publication of the European Spine Society, the European Spinal Deformity Society, and the European Section of the Cervical Spine Research Society. 2011;20:846-59.
6. Rampersaud YR, Foley KT, Shen AC, et al. Radiation exposure to the spine surgeon during fluoroscopically assisted pedicle screw insertion. Spine. 2000;25:2637-45.
7. Sanders R, Koval KJ, DiPasquale T, et al. Exposure of the orthopaedic surgeon to radiation. The Journal of Bone and Joint Surgery. American volume. 1993;75:326-30.
8. Rahmathulla G, Nottmeier EW, Pirris SM, et al. Intraoperative image-guided spinal navigation: technical pitfalls and their avoidance. Neurosurgical Focus. 2014;36.
9. Brodwater BK, Roberts DW, Nakajima T, et al. Extracranial application of the frameless stereotactic operating microscope: experience with lumbar spine. Neurosurgery. 1993;32:209-13; discussion 13.
10. Roessler K, Ungersboeck K, Dietrich W, et al. Frameless stereotactic guided neurosurgery: clinical experience with an infrared based pointer device navigation system. Acta neurochirurgica. 1997;139:551-9.
11. Castro WH, Halm H, Jerosch J, et al. Accuracy of pedicle screw placement in lumbar vertebrae. Spine. 1996;21:1320-4.
12. Laine T, Lund T, Ylikoski M, et al. Accuracy of pedicle screw insertion with and without computer assistance: a randomised controlled clinical study in 100 consecutive patients. European spine journal : official publication of the European Spine Society, the European Spinal Deformity Society, and the European Section of the Cervical Spine Research Society. 2000;9:235-40.
13. Schulze CJ, Munzinger E, Weber U. Clinical relevance of accuracy of pedicle screw placement. A computed tomographic-supported analysis. Spine. 1998;23:2215-20; discussion 20-1.
14. Davne SH, Myers DL. Complications of lumbar spinal fusion with transpedicular instrumentation. Spine. 1992;17:S184-S9.
15. Esses SI, Sachs BL, Dreyzin V. Complications Associated with the Technique of Pedicle Screw Fixation A Selected Survey of ABS Members. Spine. 1993;18:2231-9.
16. Neo M, Sakamoto T, Fujibayashi S, et al. The clinical risk of vertebral artery injury from cervical pedicle screws inserted in degenerative vertebrae. Spine. 2005;30:2800-5.
17. Shin BJ, James AR, Njoku IU, et al. Pedicle screw navigation: a systematic review and meta-analysis of perforation risk for computer-navigated versus freehand insertion. Journal of Neurosurgery. Spine. 2012;17:113-22.
18. Verma R, Krishan S, Haendlmayer K, et al. Functional outcome of computer-assisted spinal pedicle screw placement: a systematic review and meta-analysis of 23 studies including 5,992 pedicle screws. European Spine Journal. 2010;19:370-5.
19. Madawi AA, Casey ATH, Solanki GA, et al. Radiological and anatomical evaluation of the atlantoaxial transarticular screw fixation technique. Journal of Neurosurgery. 1997;86:961-8.
20. Neo M, Fujibayashi S, Miyata M, et al. Vertebral artery injury during cervical spine surgery: a survey of more than 5600 operations. Spine. 2008;33:779-85.
21. Grob D, Jeanneret B, Aebi M, et al. Atlanto-axial fusion with transarticular screw fixation. The Journal of Bone and Joint Surgery. British volume. 1991;73:972-6.
22. Wang MY. Cervical crossing laminar screws: early clinical results and complications. Neurosurgery. 2007;61:311-5; discussion. 5-6.
23. Holly LT, Foley KT. Percutaneous placement of posterior cervical screws using three-dimensional fluoroscopy. Spine. 2006;31:536-40.
24. Wolinsky JP, Sciubba DM, Suk I, et al. Endoscopic image-guided odontoidectomy for decompression of basilar invagination via a standard anterior cervical approach. Technical note. Journal of Neurosurgery. Spine. 2007;6:184-91.
25. Nottmeier EW, Foy AB. Placement of C2 laminar screws using three-dimensional fluoroscopy-based image guidance. European spine journal : official publication of the European Spine Society, the European Spinal Deformity Society, and the European Section of the Cervical Spine Research Society. 2008;17:610-5.
26. Gelalis ID, Paschos NK, Pakos EE, et al. Accuracy of pedicle screw placement: a systematic review of prospective in vivo studies comparing free hand, fluoroscopy guidance and navigation techniques. European spine journal : official publication of the European Spine Society, the European Spinal Deformity Society, and the European Section of the Cervical Spine Research Society. 2012;21:247-55.

27. Han W, Gao ZL, Wang JC, et al. Pedicle screw placement in the thoracic spine: a comparison study of computer-assisted navigation and conventional techniques. Orthopedics. 2010;33.
28. Youkilis AS, Quint DJ, McGillicuddy JE, et al. Stereotactic navigation for placement of pedicle screws in the thoracic spine. Neurosurgery. 2001;48:771-8; discussion 8-9.
29. Allam Y, Silbermann J, Riese F, et al. Computer tomography assessment of pedicle screw placement in thoracic spine: comparison between free hand and a generic 3D-based navigation techniques. European spine journal : official publication of the European Spine Society, the European Spinal Deformity Society, and the European Section of the Cervical Spine Research Society. 2013;22:648-53.
30. Holly LT, Foley KT. Three-dimensional fluoroscopy-guided percutaneous thoracolumbar pedicle screw placement. Technical note. Journal of neurosurgery. 2003;99:324-9.
31. Kosmopoulos V, Schizas C. Pedicle screw placement accuracy: a meta-analysis. Spine. 2007;32:E111-20.
32. Kim CW, Lee Y-P, Taylor W, et al. Use of navigation-assisted fluoroscopy to decrease radiation exposure during minimally invasive spine surgery. The Spine Journal: Official Journal of the North American Spine Society. 2008;8:584-90.
33. Luther N, Iorgulescu JB, Geannette C, et al. Comparison of Navigated Versus Non-Navigated Pedicle Screw Placement in 260 Patients and 1434 Screws: Screw Accuracy, Screw Size, and the Complexity of Surgery. Journal of spinal disorders & techniques. 2013.
34. Larson AN, Polly DW, Guidera KJ, et al. The accuracy of navigation and 3D image-guided placement for the placement of pedicle screws in congenital spine deformity. J Pediatr Orthop. 2012;32:e23-9.
35. Scheufler KM, Franke J, Eckardt A, et al. Accuracy of image-guided pedicle screw placement using intraoperative computed tomography-based navigation with automated referencing. Part II: thoracolumbar spine. Neurosurgery. 2011;69:1307-16.
36. Eichholz KM, Ryken TC. Complications of revision spinal surgery. Neurosurgical Focus. 2003;15.
37. Rihn JA, Harrod C, Albert TJ. Revision cervical spine surgery. Orthop. Clin. North Am. 2012;43:123-36, ix-x.
38. Hsieh JC, Drazin D, Firempong AO, et al. Accuracy of intraoperative computed tomography image-guided surgery in placing pedicle and pelvic screws for primary versus revision spine surgery. Neurosurgical Focus. 2014;36.
39. Metz LN, Burch S. Computer-assisted surgical planning and image-guided surgical navigation in refractory adult scoliosis surgery: case report and review of the literature. Spine. 2008;33:E287-92.
40. Lim MR, Girardi FP, Yoon SC, et al. Accuracy of computerized frameless stereotactic image-guided pedicle screw placement into previously fused lumbar spines. Spine. 2005;30:1793-8.
41. Hartl R, Lam KS, Wang J, et al. Worldwide survey on the use of navigation in spine surgery. World neurosurgery. 2013;79:162-72.
42. Bai Y-S, Zhang Y, Chen Z-Q, et al. Learning curve of computer-assisted navigation system in spine surgery. Chin. Med. J. 2010;123:2989-94.
43. Smith HE, Welsch MD, Sasso RC, et al. Comparison of radiation exposure in lumbar pedicle screw placement with fluoroscopy vs computer-assisted image guidance with intraoperative three-dimensional imaging. The journal of spinal cord medicine. 2008;31:532-7.
44. Villard J, Ryang YM, Demetriades AK, et al. Radiation exposure to the surgeon and the patient during posterior lumbar spinal instrumentation: a prospective randomized comparison of navigated versus non-navigated freehand techniques. Spine. 2014;39:1004-9.
45. Qureshi S, Lu Y, McAnany S, et al. Three-dimensional Intraoperative Imaging Modalities in Orthopaedic Surgery: A Narrative Review. J Am Acad Orthop Surg. 2014;22:800-9.
46. Lee TC, Yang LC, Liliang PC, et al. Single versus separate registration for computer-assisted lumbar pedicle screw placement. Spine. 2004;29:1585-9.
47. Theocharopoulos N, Perisinakis K, Damilakis J, et al. Occupational exposure from common fluoroscopic projections used in orthopaedic surgery. The Journal of Bone & Joint Surgery. 2003;85:1698-703.
48. Uhl E, Zausinger S, Morhard D, et al. Intraoperative computed tomography with integrated navigation system in a multidisciplinary operating suite. Neurosurgery. 2009;64:231-9; discussion 9-40.
49. Zausinger S, Scheder B, Uhl E, et al. Intraoperative computed tomography with integrated navigation system in spinal stabilizations. Spine. 2009;34:2919-26.
50. O-arm Surgical Imaging System]. Available at: http://www.medtronic. com/for-healthcare-professionals/products-therapies/neurological/surgical-navigation-and-imaging/o-arm-surgical-imaging-system/index. htm.
51. Hott JS, Papadopoulos SM, Theodore N, et al. Intraoperative Iso-C C-arm navigation in cervical spinal surgery: review of the first 52 cases. Spine. 2004;29:2856-60.
52. Villavicencio AT, Burneikiene S, Bulsara KR, et al. Utility of computerized isocentric fluoroscopy for minimally invasive spinal surgical techniques. Journal of Spinal Disorders & Techniques. 2005;18:369-75.
53. Ishikawa Y, Kanemura T, Yoshida G, et al. Clinical accuracy of three-dimensional fluoroscopy-based computer-assisted cervical pedicle screw placement: a retrospective comparative study of conventional versus computer-assisted cervical pedicle screw placement: Clinical article. Journal of Neurosurgery: Spine. 2010;13:606-11.
54. Nakashima H, Sato K, Ando T, et al. Comparison of the percutaneous screw placement precision of isocentric C-arm 3-dimensional fluoroscopy-navigated pedicle screw implantation and conventional fluoroscopy method with minimally invasive surgery. Journal of spinal disorders & Techniques. 2009;22:468-72.

55. Kim JM CK. Intraoperative imaging techniques in spine surgery. Semin Spine Surg. 2007;19:78-86.
56. Tabaraee E, Gibson AG, Karahalios DG, et al. Intraoperative cone beam-computed tomography with navigation (O-ARM) versus conventional fluoroscopy (C-ARM): a cadaveric study comparing accuracy, efficiency, and safety for spinal instrumentation. Spine. 2013;38:1953-8.
57. Nelson EM, Monazzam SM, Kim KD, et al. Intraoperative fluoroscopy, portable X-ray, and CT: patient and operating room personnel radiation exposure in spinal surgery. The spine journal: Official Journal of the North American Spine Society. 2014;14:2985-91.
58. Van de Kelft E, Costa F, Van der Planken D, et al. A prospective multicenter registry on the accuracy of pedicle screw placement in the thoracic, lumbar, and sacral levels with the use of the O-arm imaging system and Stealth Station Navigation. Spine. 2012;37:E1580-7.
59. BodyTom Portable Full Body Multi-Slice CT Scanner Brochure by Neurologica]. Available at: http://cdn2. hubspot. net/hub/384045/file-844471628-pdf/docs/BodyTom_Brochure.pdf?t=1437494038040.
60. Stryker and NeuroLogica Partner to Provide Surgical Navigation with the BodyTom® Portable CT Scanner. Available at: http://www. prnewswire. com/news-releases/stryker-and-neurologica-partner-to-provide-surgical-navigation-with-the-bodytom-portable-ct-scanner-238886231. html.
61. BodyTom by Neurologica]. Available at: http://www.neurologica.com/products/bodytom.
62. St. Luke's Medical Center Utilizes NeuroLogica's BodyTom® Portable Full-Body CT Scanner with Intraoperative Navigation for Complex Neurological Procedures]. Available at: http://www. businesswire. com/news/home/20131119006295/en/St. -Luke%E2%80%99s-Medical-Center-Utilizes-NeuroLogica%E2%80%99s-BodyTom%C2%AE - . Va-l0uhViko.
63. Jolesz FA. Future perspectives for intraoperative MRI. Neurosurg Clin N Am. 2005;16:201-13.
64. Choi G, Modi HN, Prada N, et al. Clinical results of XMR-assisted percutaneous transforaminal endoscopic lumbar diskectomy. J Orthop Surg Res. 2013;8:14.

38

CHAPTER

Minimally Invasive Atlantoaxial Fusion

Umesh Srikantha

ABSTRACT

Minimally invasive techniques are being increasingly used to treat disorders of the cervical spine. It reduces the postoperative neck discomfort subsequent to extensive muscle dissection associated atlantoaxial fusion procedures. The chapter describes the indications, cautions to be exercised of the technique to be employed in a minimally invasive atlantoaxial fusion procedure.

INDICATIONS

- Reducible atlantoaxial instability
- Undisplaced or minimally displaced traumatic fractures of the odontoid.

Displaced fractures that reduce partially or completely with preoperative or intraoperative traction can also be suitable candidates.

CONTRAINDICATIONS/CAUTION

- Complex craniovertebral junction abnormalities that require bilateral simultaneous joint manipulation or added decompression in the form of foramen magnum decompression or C1 arch excision
- Displaced traumatic fractures of odontoid that do not reduce on traction and hence requiring major intraoperative manipulation for reduction
- Poor neurological grade
- Cases requiring extension of construct to occiput.

Since minimally invasive atlantoaxial fusion is still in its phase of evolution, many of the above contraindications could become relative once more experience is gained in the field and specific instrumentation to aid in minimal access surgery at the CVJ is available.

RATIONALE AND APPLIED ANATOMY

Conventional C1 lateral mass screw and C2 pedicle screw placement requires midline exposure from occiput to C3-C4 to enable sufficient lateral retraction of the posterior neck muscles and visualize the described entry points for screw placement. This extensive muscular dissection causes disruption of the posterior musculoligamentous tension band resulting in impaired postoperative neck muscle function and may be responsible for persistent neck discomfort.[1-5]

Minimally invasive muscle splitting approaches, introduced for the lumbar spine, have the potential to significantly reduce muscle injury and preserve the posterior tension band.[6,7] Their superiority in minimizing blood loss, reducing the duration of hospital stay, enabling earlier return to work and improving functional outcomes as compared to conventional procedures has been shown in several studies.[8,9] Recently, several reports of extension of this technique to the cervical spine have appeared in the literature and have shown promising outcomes.[5,10-12]

Application of minimally invasive techniques to perform an atlantoaxial fusion seems reasonable as the steps of atlantoaxial joint manipulation, C1 lateral mass and C2 pedicle/pars screw placement are all done from a lateral to medial trajectory and do not require exposure of midline structures. Of importance, this preserves muscular attachments of C2 spinous process which act as stabilizers of craniocervical junction, thus preventing postoperative loss of lordosis.[4] This can be compared to transforaminal lumbar interbody fusion (TLIF), where a minimally invasive approach has shown considerable advantages over a conventional midline approach.[9,13,14] The only muscle band that needs to be transected in a minimally invasive atlantoaxial fusion procedure is the inferior oblique due to its anatomical position where it runs horizontally between the C1 posterior arch and C2 lamina. Since its function is to stabilize and aid in rotatory movements at the atlantoaxial segment, the impact of transecting this muscle is unlikely to affect outcome when an atlantoaxial fusion is being done.

Of course, needless to say, one should be thorough with the knowledge of anatomy and its variations in the region before attempting a minimally invasive atlantoaxial fusion. Practising the technique initially on cadavers, as done by the author, can help orient to the anatomy and technical difficulties associated with the procedure.

SURGICAL TECHNIQUE

After induction, intubation and firmly securing the ET tube, the patient is positioned prone on bolsters with head stabilized on a horseshoe stand and skeletal skull traction in place. A lateral fluoroscopy image of the atlantoaxial complex is done to check proper positioning, and to ensure that the atlantoaxial complex is in a reduced position while operating on cases with mobile atlantoaxial instability. The weight on the skeletal traction is limited to around 2–3 kg. While operating on cases with an odontoid fracture, gentle manipulation on the skeletal traction to reduce the fracture can be attempted. It is advisable to do such manipulation under neuromonitoring with MEP and SSEP. The following paragraph describes the technique used for a minimally invasive atlantoaxial fusion. The reader can refer elsewhere for a detailed description of the technique for inserting C1 lateral mass and C2 pedicle/ pars screws.

In the saggital plane, the C1–C2 joint and the entry points for C1 lateral mass screw and C2 pedicle/pars screw roughly corresponds to a plane about 2–2.5 cm from the midline. Hence, a vertical incision around 2.5 cm off the midline on either side, and directly above the C2 spinous process can be used to create a transmuscular tract to reach the desired area. Since the skin over the posterior part of the neck can be quite stretchable, the length of the incision need not be more than 2–2.5 cm. Once the skin and fascial incisions are made **(Figure 1A)**, blunt soft tissue dissection can be done with artery forceps or finger to palpate the inferior facet of C2. Smallest dilator should then be introduced through the dissected plane and docked on the highest point on the C2 facet **(Figure 1B)**. No effort should be made at this point to palpate the posterior arch of C1 and care should be taken not to dip the smallest dilator towards the C1–C2 joint or medially into the gap between C1 posterior arch and C2 lamina. It is preferable not to use K-wire for this step in order to avoid inadvertent neurovascular injury. Sequential dilatation is then done **(Figure 1C)** to finally place a 22 mm expandable tubular retractor overlying the C2 lateral mass **(Figure 1D)**. The retractor is then angulated superiorly and the blades expanded so as to cover the area between posterior arch of C1 and C2 lateral mass, between the superior and inferior blades of the retractor. The inferior oblique muscle, which runs transversely in the C1–C2 interlaminar space **(Figure 3A)**, is transected using cautery to expose the C1 posterior arch, posterior atlantoaxial membrane and C2 pars. The posterior atlantoaxial membrane can be divided using sharp dissection to expose the underlying venous plexus **(Figure 3B)**. Further dissection is done in between the C1 and C2 lateral masses to identify and expose the exiting C2 nerve root, C1–C2 joint space and entry points for C1 lateral mass and C2 pedicle screws **(Figures 3C to E)**. Any bleeding at this stage can be controlled with a judicious combination of gelfoam and bipolar electrocautery. Transecting the C2 ganglion gives a wide and unhindered view of the C1–C2 joint complex, but is not always required. While using a C1–C2 joint spacer [trimmed wooden block was used as joint spacer in cadavers **(Figure 2C)**], the C2 nerve root can be sacrificed if necessary; joint space distracted with a blunt penfield **(Figure 2A)**, the endplates drilled using a high speed burr, and graft can be placed within the joint space **(Figures 3F and G)**. The C1 lateral mass and C2 pedicle/pars screws can then be placed with standard technique and instruments **(Figure 2B)** **(Figures 1E and F)**. The retractor needs to be angulated more superiorly to obtain the required trajectory for C2 pedicle/ pars screw. Connecting rod can be placed directly under vision **(Figure 3H)**. For an added fusion option, a split rib graft anchored with a miniscrew, can also be placed medial to the screw-rod construct (overlying the drilled cortical surfaces of C1 posterior arch and C2 lamina) **(Figure 3I)**. Similar steps need to be repeated on the other side.

COMPLICATIONS AND AVOIDANCE

The associated complications are primarily similar to the ones encountered in a conventional atlantoaxial fusion, detailed discussion of which is beyond the scope of this chapter. However, a few additional problems can be encountered in relation to establishing minimal access to this region. Too medial an incision can give a more perpendicular visualization of the C1–C2 joint but can limit medial angulation necessary for placing C2 pedicle screws, thus increasing the chances of vertebral foraminal encroachment by the screw. Too lateral an incision can increase the depth of the working channel and also can cause the retractor to land on the lateral aspect of C2 pars, close to the vertebral foramen, thus increasing the chances of profuse venous bleeding from the vertebral venous plexus during muscle dissection, apart from putting the vertebral artery itself at risk. Hence, an ideal incision should be located around 2.5 cm lateral to the midline. Adequate care should also be taken to direct the muscle dissection track towards the centre of C2 inferior facet and not to sway too medially or laterally. Too medial a track puts the dilator

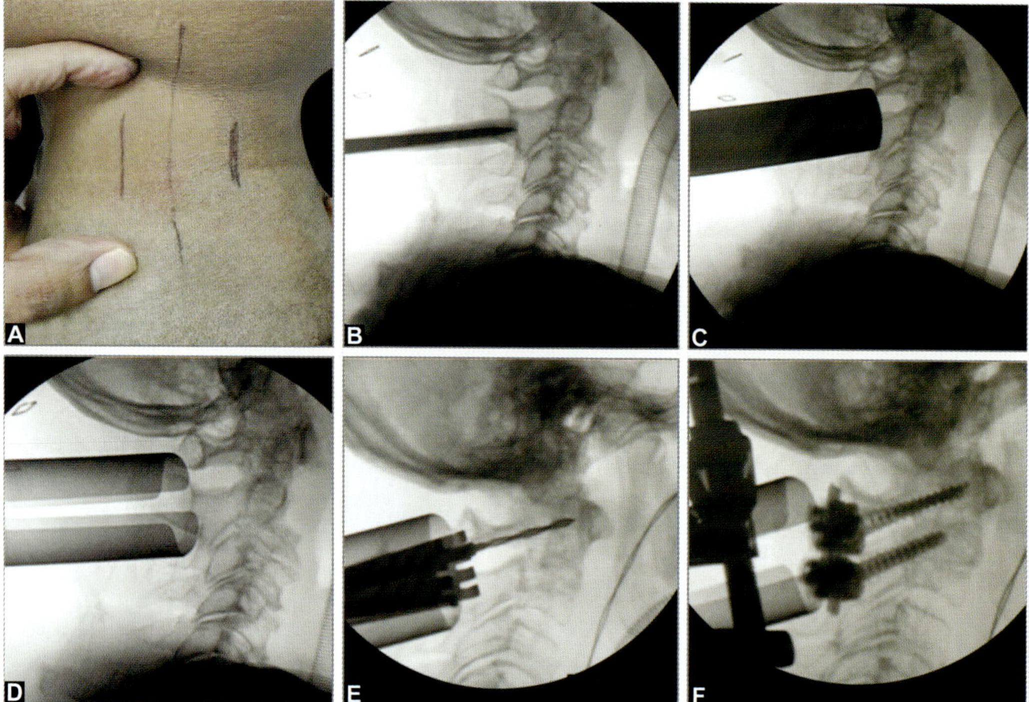

Figures 1A to F: (A) Image showing the skin marking and stretch ability of the skin in the cervical region allowing for a smaller incision; (B to E) Intraoperative fluoroscopy images: (B) Initial docking over C2 facet; (C) After sequential dilatation; (D) Placement of an expandable retractor; (E) C1 lateral mass drill hole being prepared; (F) Final construct

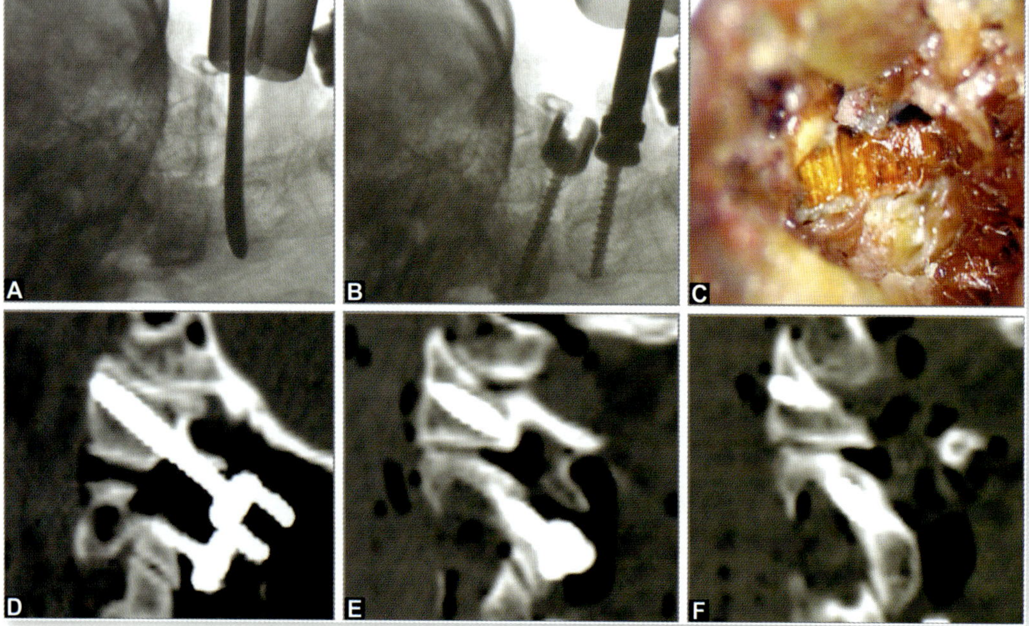

Figures 2A to F: (A) Lateral fluoroscopy image from a cadaver showing a penfield dissector within the C1–C2 joint space; (B) Final construct after placing C1 and C2 screws; (C) A fashioned wooden block has been positioned as a joint spacer; (D to F) Post-procedural CT scans in the cadaver showing the position of C1 and C2 screws

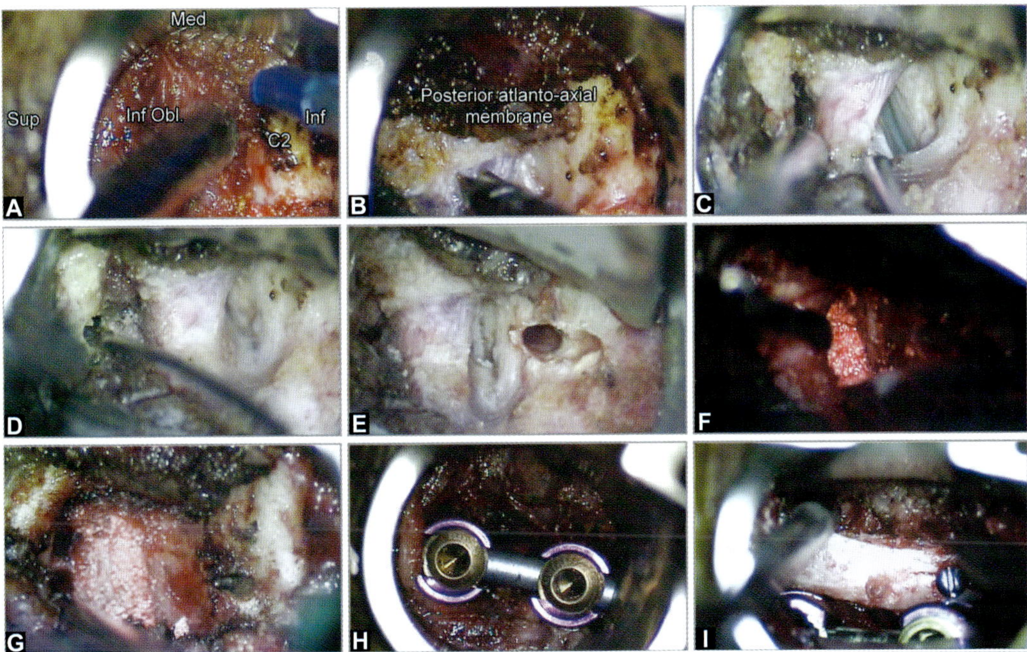

Figures 3A to I: Illustrative intraoperative images at sequential steps during the surgery. The orientation in each image is similar to that of image A that has been labeled. (A) Initial view after docking the tube. The inferior oblique muscle band can be seen running across in the C1–C2 interspace; (B) The inferior oblique muscle has been divided to expose the lateral part of the posterior atlantoaxial membrane, which is being divided. The underlying venous plexus can be visualised; (C) After dissecting around the venous plexus, the C2 nerve root has been retracted upwards to visualize the C1–C2 joint space; (D and E) Drill holes have been prepared for placing C1 and C2 screws respectively; (F) Graft has been packed within the C1–C2 joint after decorticating the articular surfaces. In this case C2 root has been retracted upwards; (G) Image from another case where C2 root has been transected to place graft inside the C1–C2 joint; (H) Final view after placing the screws and interconnecting rod; (I) A fashioned split rib graft has been placed between C1 and C2 medial to the Screw-rod construct and secured with a miniscrew.

Abbreviations: Sup, superior; Inf, inferior; Med, medial; Inf obl, inferior oblique

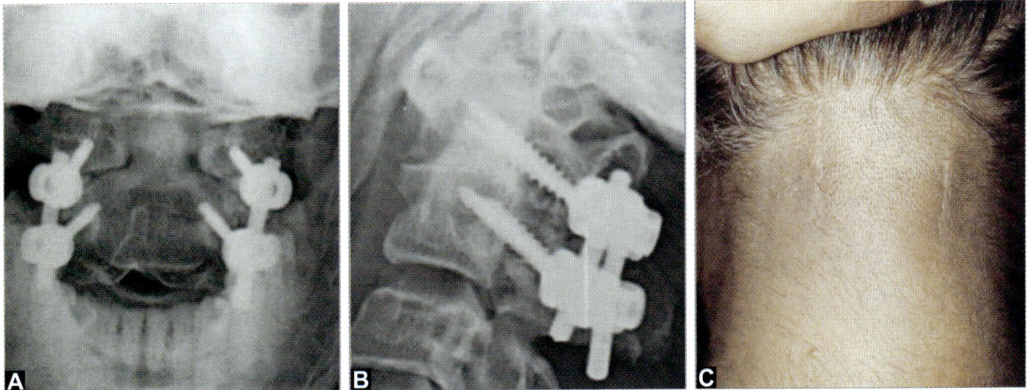

Figures 4A to C: (A) Postoperative anteroposterior; (B) Lateral radiographs showing position of screws; (C) Appearance of wound at follow-up

at risk of slipping between the laminae of C1 and C2 and potentially causing neural injury and too lateral a track can again place the vertebral artery at risk where it exits from foramen transversarium of C2 **(Figures 4A to C)**.

LITERATURE REVIEW AND DISCUSSION

Though minimally invasive techniques were initially popularized for the lumbar spine, it is being increasingly

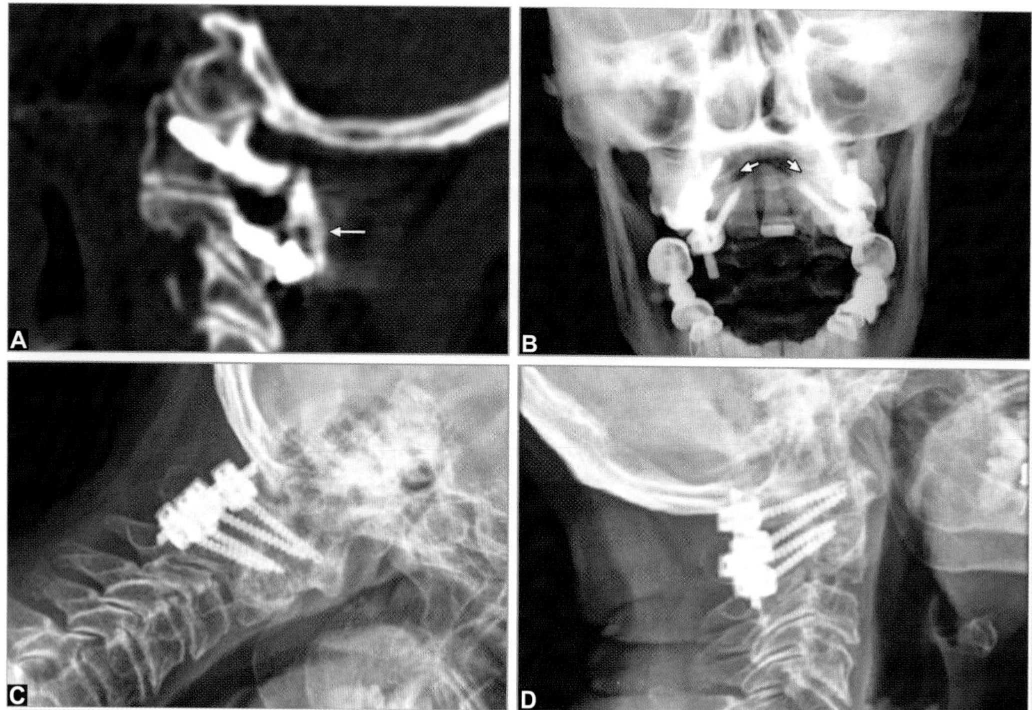

Figures 5A to D: Followup imaging in illustrative cases showing (A) Fused rib graft in a CT scan image (arrow) and (B) Fusion mass within C1–C2 joint space on an AP fluoroscopy image (arrow); (C) Flexion and (D) Extension lateral radiographs in a representative case showing no mobility

applied in the cervical spine as well. Reports of common cervical procedures like laminoforaminotomy,[15,16] lateral mass fusion[5,17] **(Figures 5A and D)** and stenosis decompression[12,18] being treated with minimally invasive techniques can be encountered in the literature.

Over the last decade, scattered reports of minimally invasive atlantoaxial fusion can be found in the literature[1-4] Using 12 fresh frozen cadavers, Bodon et al.[4] described the muscle splitting approach to the atlantoaxial joint in detail and were able to reach and identify the entry points for C1 lateral mass and C2 pars screw in all the cadavers bilaterally, though they inserted C1 lateral mass and C2 screws in only 4 cadavers. Joseffer et al.[2] initially reported one case of os odotoideum successfully treated with a minimally invasive technique using an expandable tubular retractor and later Holly et al.[1] from the same group, described the technique being used to treat 5 cases of odontoid fracture with good results in all cases. Taghva et al.[3] performed the procedure initially on 4 fresh frozen cadavers and subsequently on 2 clinical cases of odontoid fracture and described that the correct entry point for getting a lateral trajectory for placing screws was 3.5 cm lateral to midline. The author followed a similar protocol in doing a cadaveric study on 4 fresh frozen cadavers prior to applying the technique on a select cohort of 7 cases, but found that an incision 2.5 cm lateral to the midline is more beneficial as it gives a more direct view of the C1–C2 joint, prevents lateral placement of the tubular retractor and also provides sufficient lateral angulation for placement of the screws.

As has been shown in figures, in addition to placing C1 and C2 screws, minimal access to the C1–C2 region does not limit routine methods used to achieve fusion. Intra-articular drilling, graft/spacer placement, overlay interlaminar rib graft placement can all be done in minimal access as well. These steps were adequately backed by the cadaver study done prior to the clinical series. With the availability of all the above steps, achieving fusion rates similar to conventional techniques should be possible even with minimally invasive techniques.

Application of minimally invasive techniques for atlanto-axial fusion has now crossed the boundary of technical feasibility. Despite minimally invasive approach being increasingly applied for treating diseases of the cervical spine and convincing rationale and theoretical evidence of its benefit over conventional approach, one can observe a striking paucity of randomised studies comparing the two. A few studies comparing outcome between the approaches in cervical laminoforaminotomy have shown a marginal benefit for minimally invasive approach over conventional approach,[15,16] which is more than one can say about a similar procedure in the lumbar spine, i.e. microlumbar discectomy.[19,20] So, we can expect that more invasive techniques in the cervical spine like atlantoaxial fusion; cervical stenosis decompression or lateral mass fusion might reveal more convincing benefit for a minimally invasive over a conventional approach.

To summarize, minimally invasive atlantoaxial fusion can be done safely and effectively in selected cases, though the technique is not being routinely employed in clinical practice. Further studies with larger case numbers and direct comparison with conventional techniques is necessary to demonstrate the clinical benefit associated with minimally invasive approaches to this complex region.

REFERENCES

1. Holly LT, Isaacs RE, Frempong-Boadu AK. Minimally Invasive Atlantoaxial Fusion. Neurosurgery. 2010;66:A193-7. doi:10.1227/01.NEU.0000366107.69895.74.
2. Joseffer SS, Post N, Cooper PR, Frempong-Boadu AK. Minimally Invasive Atlantoaxial Fixation with a Polyaxial Screw-rod Construct: Technical Case Report. Neurosurgery. 2006;58:ONS–E375. doi:10.1227/01.NEU.0000208955.12461.C7.
3. Taghva A, Attenello FJ, Zada G, Khalessi AA, Hsieh PC. Minimally Invasive Posterior Atlantoaxial Fusion: A Cadaveric and Clinical Feasibility Study. World Neurosurg. 2013;80:414-21. doi:10.1016/j.wneu.2012.01.054.
4. Bodon G, Patonay L, Baksa G, Olerud C. Applied anatomy of a minimally invasive muscle-splitting approach to posterior C1–C2 fusion: an anatomical feasibility study. Surg Radiol Anat. 2014;36:1063–9. doi:10.1007/s00276-014-1274-x.
5. Fong S, Duplessis S. Minimally invasive lateral mass plating in the treatment of posterior cervical trauma: surgical technique. J Spinal Dis Tech. 2005;18:224-8.
6. Rahman M, Summers L, Richter B, Mimran R, Jacob R. Comparison of Techniques for Decompressive Lumbar Laminectomy: the Minimally Invasive versus the "Classic" Open Approach. Minim Invasive Neurosurg. 2008;51:100-5. doi:10.1055/s-2007-1022542.
7. Kim CW. Scientific basis of minimally invasive spine surgery: prevention of multifidus muscle injury during posterior lumbar surgery. Spine. 2010;35:S281–6. doi:10.1097/BRS.0b013n e3182022d32.
8. Fan S, Hu Z, Zhao F, Zhao X, Huang Y, Fang X. Multifidus muscle changes and clinical effects of one-level posterior lumbar interbody fusion: minimally invasive procedure versus conventional open approach. Eur Spine J. 2009;19:316–24. doi:10.1007/s00586-009-1191-6.
9. Tian N-F, Wu Y-S, Zhang X-L, Xu H-Z, Chi Y-L, Mao F-M. Minimally invasive versus open transforaminal lumbar interbody fusion: a meta-analysis based on the current evidence. Eur Spine J. 2013;22:1741–9. doi:10.1007/s00586-013-2747-z.
10. Minimally Invasive Approaches to the Cervical Spine. 2012;43:137–47. doi:10.1016/j.ocl.2011.08.007.
11. Wang MY, Levi ADO. Minimally Invasive Lateral Mass Screw Fixation in the Cervical Spine: Initial Clinical Experience with Long-term Follow-up. Neurosurgery. 2006;58:907–12. doi:10.1227/01.NEU.0000209929.38213.72.
12. Santiago P, Fessler RG. Minimally invasive surgery for the management of cervical spondylosis. Neurosurgery. 2007;60:S1–160???S1–165. doi:10.1227/01.NEU.0000215349.40925.88.
13. Parker SL, Lerner J, McGirt MJ. Effect of Minimally Invasive Technique on Return to Work and Narcotic Use Following Transforaminal Lumbar Inter-body Fusion. Professional Case Management. 2012;17:229–35. doi:10.1097/NCM.0b013 e3182529c05.
14. Minimally Invasive Transforaminal Lumbar Interbody Fusion (MI-TLIF). 2014;25:279–304. doi:10.1016/j.nec.2013.12.007.
15. Winder MJ, Thomas KC. Minimally invasive versus open approach for cervical laminoforaminotomy. Can J Neurol Sci. 2011;38:262–7. doi:10.1017/S0317167100011446.
16. Clark JG, Abdullah KG, Steinmetz MP, Benzel EC, Mroz TE. Minimally Invasive versus Open Cervical Foraminotomy: A Systematic Review. Global Spine J. 2011;1:9–14. doi:10.1055/s-0031-1296050.
17. Wang MY, Levi ADO. Minimally invasive lateral mass screw fixation in the cervical spine: initial clinical experience with long-term follow-up. Neurosurgery. 2006;58:907–12–discussion907–12. doi:10.1227/01.NEU.0000209929.38213.72.
18. Song JK, Christie SD. Minimally invasive cervical stenosis decompression. Neurosurg Clin N Am. 2006;17:423–8. doi:10.1016/j.nec.2006.06.008.
19. Arts M, Brand R, van der Kallen B, Lycklama à Nijeholt G, Peul W. Does minimally invasive lumbar disc surgery result in less muscle injury than conventional surgery? A randomized controlled trial. Eur Spine J. 2010;20:51–7. doi:10.1007/s00586-010-1482-y.
20. Jacobs WCH, Arts MP, van Tulder MW, Rubinstein SM, van Middelkoop M, Ostelo RW, et al. Surgical techniques for sciatica due to herniated disc, a systematic review. Eur Spine J. 2012;21:2232–51. doi:10.1007/s00586-012-2422-9.

39
CHAPTER

Minimally Invasive Surgery in Tuberculosis of Spine

Nitin Garg

ABSTRACT

Tuberculosis (TB) of the spine is one of the most common forms of skeletal tuberculosis. The conventional surgical management includes wide laminectomy and extensive resection of the granulation tissue. The untoward complications of these techniques are instability and need for longer fusion procedures. Minimally invasive approaches are increasingly being used in the management of TB spine. This chapter deals with the uses, indications and technique of using minimally invasive procedures in tuberculosis spine.

INTRODUCTION

Tuberculosis of spine, a paucibacillary disease, is one of the common forms of skeletal tuberculosis.[1] The management goals are to eradicate infection, prevent or treat neurological deficits, and correct and avoid spinal deformity progression. Current surgical methods include anterior debridement, decompression, fusion followed by ventral or posterior instrumentation and/or posterior decompression and fixation.[2-7] Conventional surgical approaches to the ventral aspect of dorsal spine include thoracotomy with extrapleural or transpleural access, lateral extracavitary and costotransversectomy and retroperitoneal approaches for the lumbar spine.[6-10] These are extensive approaches with associated morbidity.[11] Many of these patients are in poor general condition and may not tolerate these procedures.

Minimally invasive approaches are increasingly being used in managing various spinal disorders, such as degenerative spine, trauma and tumors.[9,10,14-17] Tuberculosis of spine is another indication for using MIS methods effectively.

We present our experience of using MIS approaches for managing tuberculosis of the dorsal and lumbar spine.

MANAGEMENT

The protocol used for managing patients with tuberculosis of the spine is the "middle path regimen" described by Tuli.[18] All patients with peridiskal involvement, preserved vertebral body height and no neurological deficits are managed with ambulatory antitubercular therapy (ATT) with an external orthosis and radiographic follow up. Surgery is considered in those with:

1. Persistent severe disabling back pain or radicular pain,
2. Neurological deficits
3. Progressive deformity, and
4. Clinical and radiographic progression of disease despite ATT.

INDICATION

The basic aims of surgery, conventional or MIS, of debridement, neural decompression and avoiding deformity progression remain the same. The morbidity however, is significantly less in MIS approaches with similar outcomes as conventional methods.

The general indications for the MIS approach are similar to those described above for surgery. The specific situations where MIS methods can be considered are:

1. Disease involving thoracic spine below D6 level
2. The lumbar spine
3. Minimum pedicle diameters of 4.5 mm, and
4. Expertise.

Vertebral level of the disease is the most important factor in deciding between conventional and MIS approaches, in addition to the limitations in the available instrumentation and surgeon experience.

LIMITATION

1. Disease affecting the craniovertebral junction, cervical spine, cervicothoracic junction and upper dorsal spine are treated using conventional approaches. Based on our experience, D6 has been chosen as a probable cut off level. The scapula acts as a hindrance for mini-open thoracotomy at these levels.
2. In addition, there is hardware limitation. The percutaneous transpedicular screw systems have 4.5 mm diameter screws as the smallest available size. Most of the pedicles in the Indian population have pedicles smaller than 4.5 mm above this level.[19]
3. In some patients, MIS approaches are not feasible due to the nature of the disease. Patients with predominantly posterior column involvement, an en-plaque epidural granulation with dorsal cord compression underwent conventional laminectomy.
4. Surgical expertise is also important criteria to decide between the conventional and MIS methods.

The description in this chapter has evolved over a period of time. Starting with most basic approaches, more complex MIS procedures were performed. A thorough radiological analysis of the X-rays, MRI and CT scans is required before considering MIS methods. In addition, dedicated equipment for minimal access spine surgery is essential. Routine anatomical landmarks are not visible, and image guidance is the key to successful outcomes. It would be better to proceed with conventional approaches in case of nonavailability of any of these rather than have suboptimal outcomes with MIS approaches. Some of the methods like DLIF are entirely new access methods and require observation and cadaveric training.

In our experience, of the 110 patients of spinal tuberculosis managed surgically from 2008 to 2016, 56 underwent conventional procedures for the following reasons: level of the disease (n = 42), nature of the disease (n = 7) and hardware limitation (n = 7). 25 out of the 42 patients had involvement of craniovertebral junction, cervical spine, and cervithoracic junction, operated by anterior cervical approach. The remaining 17 patients with upper thoracic involvement had conventional exposure due to difficulty and our inexperience in using mini-open retractors for the exposure of the upper thoracic spine and insertion of percutaneous screws at this level. Seven patients had en-plaque type of tuberculosis with epidural granulation situated dorsally without much vertebral body destruction. They underwent hemilaminectomy or laminectomy. Seven patients had hardware limitations: they were in the early part of our series when the longitude system was not available to avoid using the lordotic precontoured rods of the Sextant (Medtronics, Inc. MN, USA) in the thoracic spine. 57 patients underwent different minimally invasive procedures depending upon the level of the disease and the extent of vertebral body destruction.

SURGICAL APPROACHES

The minimally invasive approaches vary depending upon the level of the disease, the extent of vertebral body destruction, the instrumentation and surgical expertise. There are two major aims of surgery:

1. Neural decompression
2. Fixation/stabilization.

While fixation has been achieved in all of our patients using percutaneous transpedicular screw system, decompression can be achieved using either conventional methods or MIS methods.[20] In the initial part of our series, conventional approaches with lesser morbidity (like dorsolateral thoracotomy and extrapleural approach rather than ventrolateral thoracotomy and transpelural approach) were used for accessing the relevant portions of the spine for decompression and fusion. These were then supplemented with percutaneous fixation in the same sitting. As the experience in using MIS methods increased and as newer and better access channels and instrumentation were available, these could be performed by mini-open methods (like mini-open thoracotomy or DLIF). **Flowchart 1** summarizes these methods.

The most important criteria to decide between the posterior and hybrid approach is the extent of vertebral body destruction. In patients with relatively preserved vertebral body height (<25% collapse), posterior only approaches suffice. In these patients, there is no need for ventral column reconstruction and both aims of decompression and fixation can be achieved posteriorly. Patients with significant collapse require ventral column reconstruction followed by fixation.

Before we discuss the specific surgical approaches, it is important understand the basic equipment required.

Specific Requirements for Performing MIS Approaches?

MIS methods require a dedicated equipment and instrumentation. These can be divided into two broader groups:

1. Access channels.
2. Percutaneous fixation hardware.

Access channels: Tubular access channels have provided a significant advantage in spinal surgeries. They provide direct access to the area of interest, keep the muscles retracted, allow for contralateral and multilevel exposure and reduce the approach related morbidity by smaller incisions and limited muscle dissection. In our experience, we have used the METRx™ X-tube (Medtronics Inc, MN, USA) for posterior only approach. These are cylindrical tubes, of varying diameters. The tubes are of two types—fixed diameter and expandable. Expandable retractors provide wider access at the depth with similar incision sizes over the

Flowchart 1: Minimally invasive surgical approaches

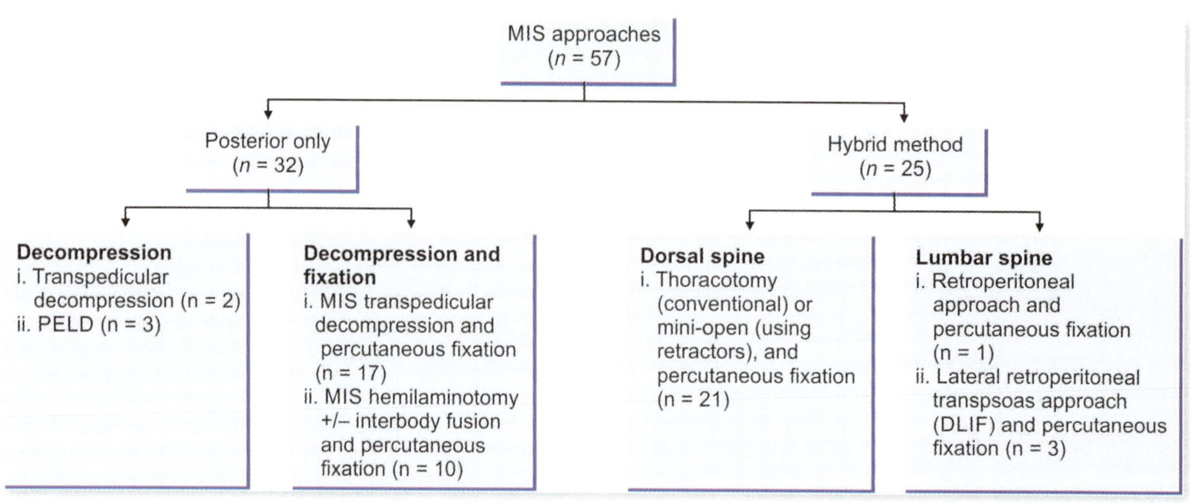

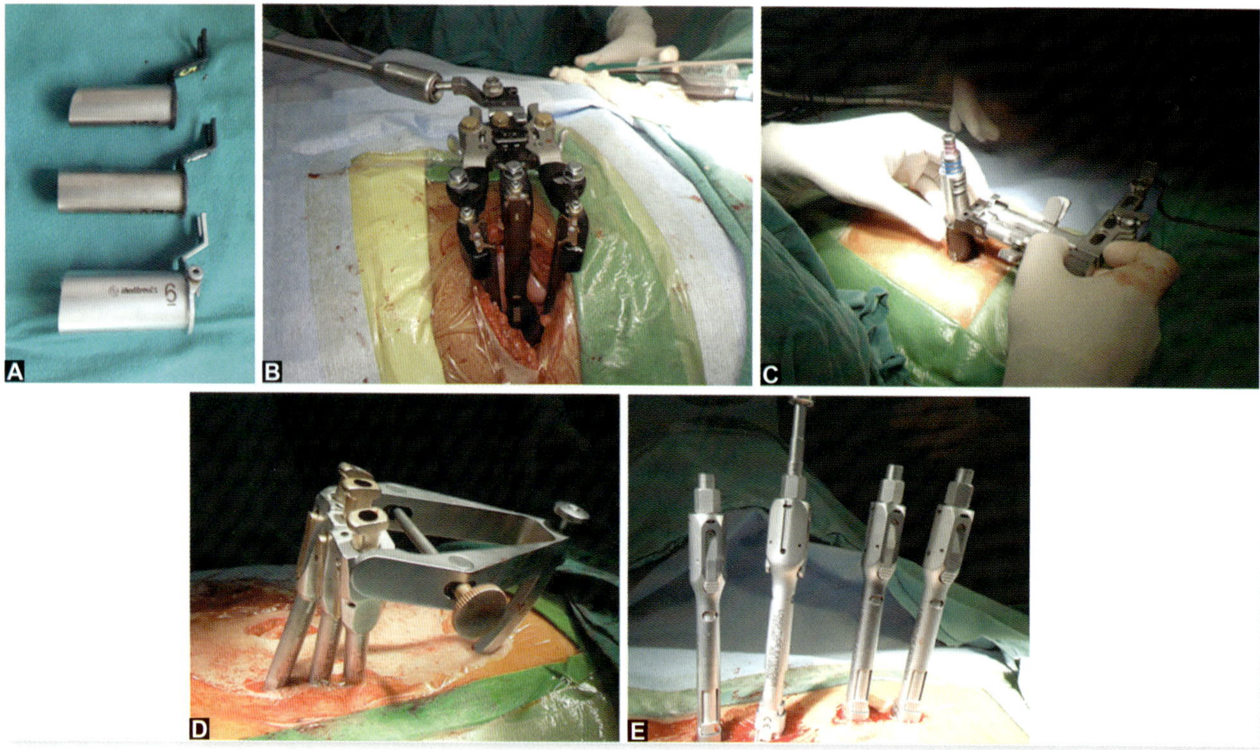

Figures 1A to E: Instrumentation. (A) Tubular ports; (B) Longer retractor system; (C) DLIF system; (D) Percutaneous system with precontoured rods; (E) Percutaneous system with free hand technique rod insertion

skin. The length of these tubes varies from 4-7 cm. These lengths are adequate to access most of the dorsal and lumbar spine posteriorly. This can be used for MIS transpedicular decompression (dorsal spine), MIS hemilaminotomy and TLIF (lumbar spine) **(Figures 1A to E).**

For lateral approaches to the thoracic and lumbar spine, longer retractors are required. In addition, there is need to retract additional structures as lung and intraperitoneal organs. These newer retractors systems (like Quadrant™, DLIF™ Medtronics Inc,; Mars™ 3V, Globus Medical Inc.,PA, USA) have longer blades, multiple blades (3-4) for craniocaudal and mediolateral retraction. In some of these systems, each blade can be replaced and manipulated individually allowing the surgeon more flexibility and avoids the need to manipulate the entire assembly **(Figures 1A to E)**. These newer systems can be used for mini-open thoracotomy and DLIF approaches. With the availability of these newer systems, the lateral exposures to the ventral aspect of thoracic and lumbar spine can be achieved by minimally invasive methods.

Percutaneous fixation systems: With percutaneous transpedicular systems, fixation can be done using minimally invasive methods. There are various systems available including the Indian systems with more reasonable costs. The difference in the systems is in the screw sheaths and manner of inserting rods. One should use a system which one is familiar with.

SURGICAL METHODS

The surgical methods can be divided into two main groups: the "Posterior-only" group and "the Hybrid" group.

Posterior-only Approach

Posterior Transpedicular Decompression Only

Method (Figures 2 to 4): Patient is positioned prone. Relevant levels are marked with C-arm. The side of the access is on the predominant epidural collection/granulation tissue. The pedicle for access is of the inferior involved vertebral body. Paramedian incision is marked under C-arm guidance. The incision can be vertical, horizontal or oblique centered on the relevant pedicle. The lumbodorsal fascia is incised, muscle split and the facet-lamina complex is exposed. At this point, the entry point and trajectory of the pedicle is marked with C-arm. The pedicle is drilled gradually enlarging it while proceeding towards the vertebral body. Once in the vertebral body, the color changes and diploic bone is visualized. C-arm in the lateral view is taken intermittently

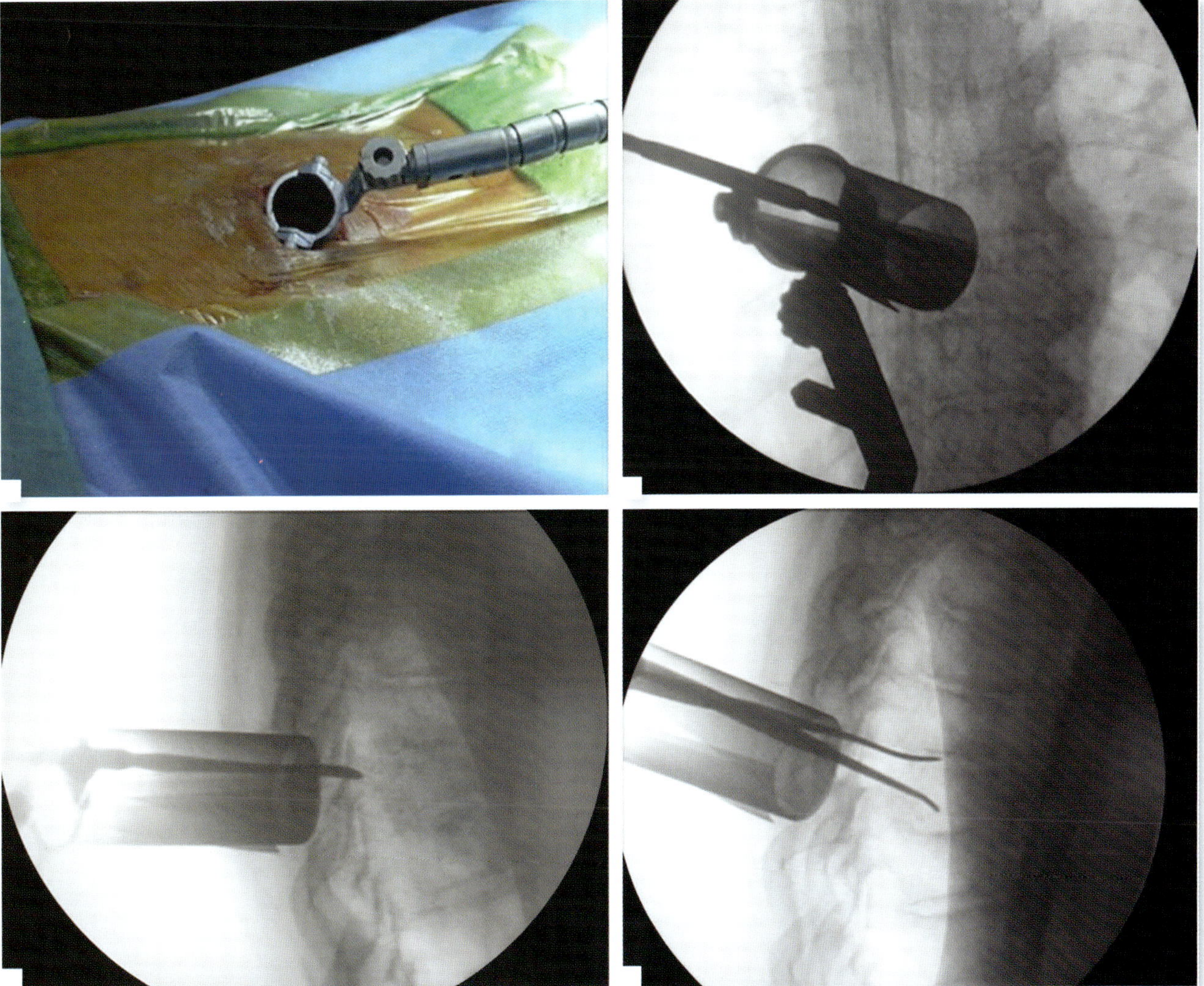

Figures 2A to D: MIS transpedicular decompression. (A) X-tube in position with medial angulation; (B) Intraoperative C-arm AP image; (C) Intraoperative lateral view; (D) Craniocaudal extent of decompression

to be sure about the trajectory **(Figures 2A to D)**. The medial and inferior wall of the pedicle is kept intact till the end to avoid early exposure of the thecal sac medially and root inferiorly. The trajectory is more towards the disc space superiorly. Once the body is reached, pus is evacuated. The pus is generally under pressure and drains spontaneously. MRI should be viewed to see the exact extent of the pus and to make sure that these are adequately evacuated **(Figures 3A to E)**. In those with granulation tissue, this is removed piecemeal using 1mm pituitary microforceps. Sequestered bone fragments are pushed ventrally using a downward curettes and then removed. 90° angled downcurette is a very useful instrument. It can be passed under the thecal sac up to the opposite side **(Figures 4A to F)**. More effective medial decompression can be achieved by endoscope assistance. In some patients especially in those with granulation tissue, 30 or 45° endoscope (4.0 mm diameter) can be passed to visualize the ventral aspect of the thecal sac for further decompression under vision **(Figures 4A to F)**. Thorough wash is given, hemostasis achieved and wound closed in layers.

Indications

1. Level: D6 to D12 vertebrae.
2. Preserved vertebral body height (<25% collapse).
3. Neurological deficits (myelopathy / severe radiculopathy).
4. Pedicle diameter <4.5 mm (instrumentation limitation of percutaneous screws).

Contraindications

i. Significant collapse.
ii. Pedicle size adequate for fixation.

MIS Transpedicular Decompression followed by Percutaneous Transpedicular Fixation

Method (Figures 5A to E): This is the preferred method in majority with dorsal tuberculosis with preserved body height but significant focal epidural cord compression with neurological deficits. The aim is to decompress the cord and achieve fixation simultaneously. The decompression is similar as described previously. This is then supplemented by percutaneous transpedicular fixation. The vertebrae fixed

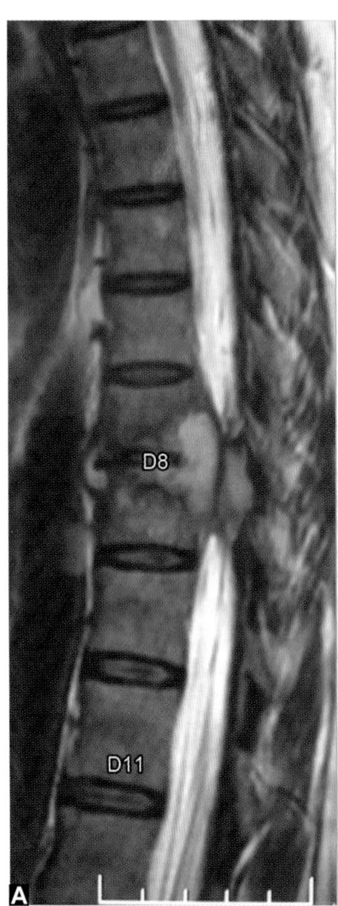

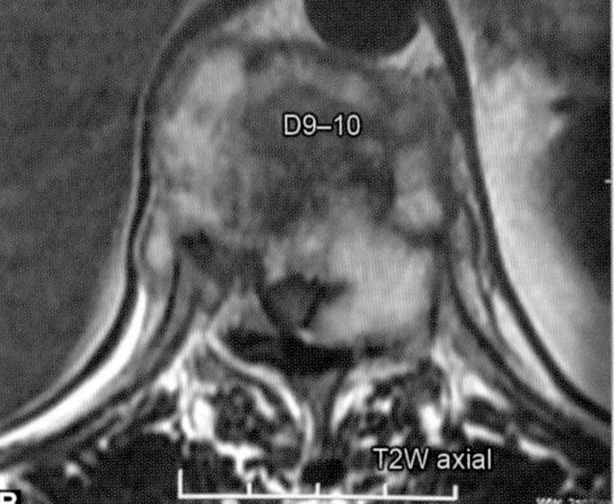

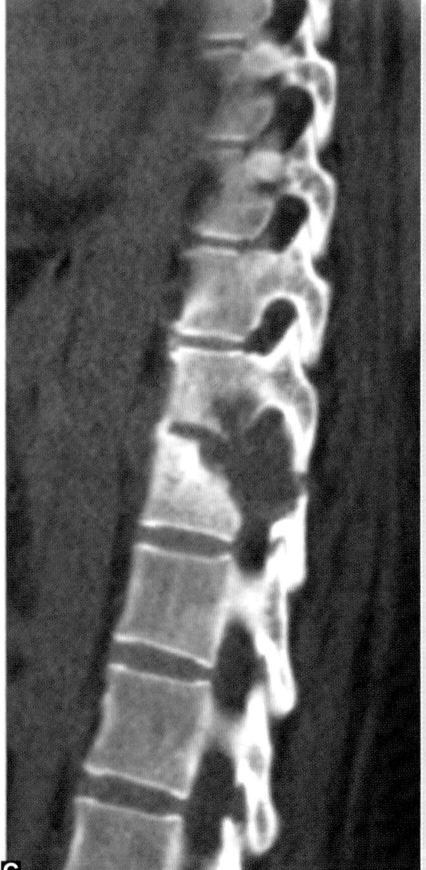

Figures 3A to C

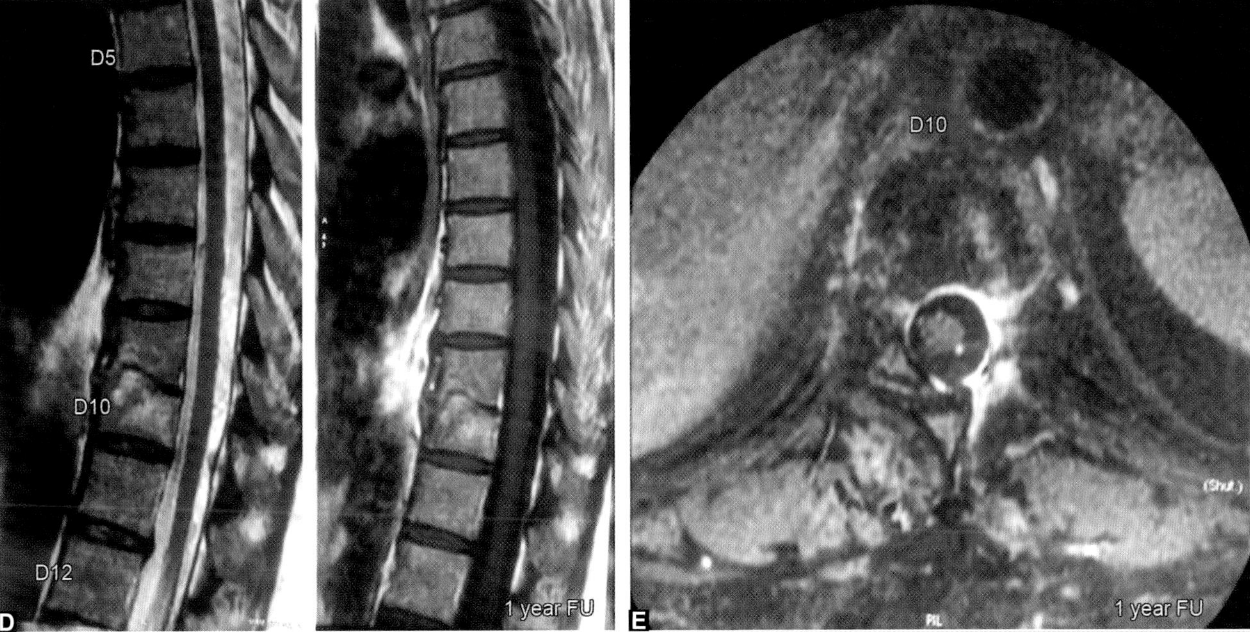

Figures 3A to E: MIS transpedicular decompression. (A) D8–9 tuberculosis; (B) Pus predominantly on the left; (C) CT scan with limited bony destruction and preserved height; (D) 1 year follow-up MRI. Vertebral body height is preserved with deformity; (E) Axial image with adequate canal and cord decompression

are adjacent to the involved vertebral bodies. In patients with the involved vertebral body of relatively preserved bony architecture (as seen on CT scan), an additional screw can be inserted in this vertebrae. The details of transpedicular screw insertion are described elsewhere in detail. In elderly patients with osteoporotic spine, the fixation can be done two levels above and below the involved vertebrae.

Indications

i. D6 to D12 vertberae.
ii. Vertebral body height preserved (<25%).
iii. Pedicle >4.5 mm diameter.
iv. Elderly patients/patients with significant comorbidities for thoracotomy.

Contraindications

i. Significant collapse (requires ventral column reconstruction).
ii. Pedicle <4.5 mm in diameter (Instrumentation limitation).

Percutaneous Endoscopic Lumbar Decompression

Method (Figures 6A and B): The approach has been described elsewhere in detail. The side of approach is based on the predominant site of symptomatology and collection. The endoscope with working channel is inserted under C-arm guidance and once the space is reached, decompression is done. Pus, granulation and sequestered bone fragment is removed piecemeal. Thorough wash is given.

Indications

i. Level - L2–3 to L4–5.
ii. Vertebral body height preserved.
iii. Radiculopathy.
iv. Predominant pus or hyperintense tissue on T2W images.
v. Tissue diagnosis.

Contraindications

i. Neurological deficit (direct decompression preferred)
ii. Significant collapse.
iii. Significant instability pain (fixation preferred)
iv. L5–1 and L1–2 are relative contraindications depending upon the rib and iliac crest angulation.

MIS Hemilaminotomy +/- fusion and Percutaneous Fixation

Method (Figures 7A to D): This approach is similar to microscopic discectomy. A hemilaminotomy is done on the predominantly affected side. The interlaminar space is widened, medial facet drilled, ligamentum flavum excised. The thecal sac and the stretched nerve root are exposed. The root is retracted to expose the PLL which is intact in almost all the patients. The PLL is bulging due to the pressure from the underlying pus or granulation tissue. The PLL is cut and decompression done. This could be done on one side or both the sides depending upon the symptomology. Following decompression, interbody fusion (TLIF or PLIF) using bone graft or cage filled with bone autograft is done. In patients

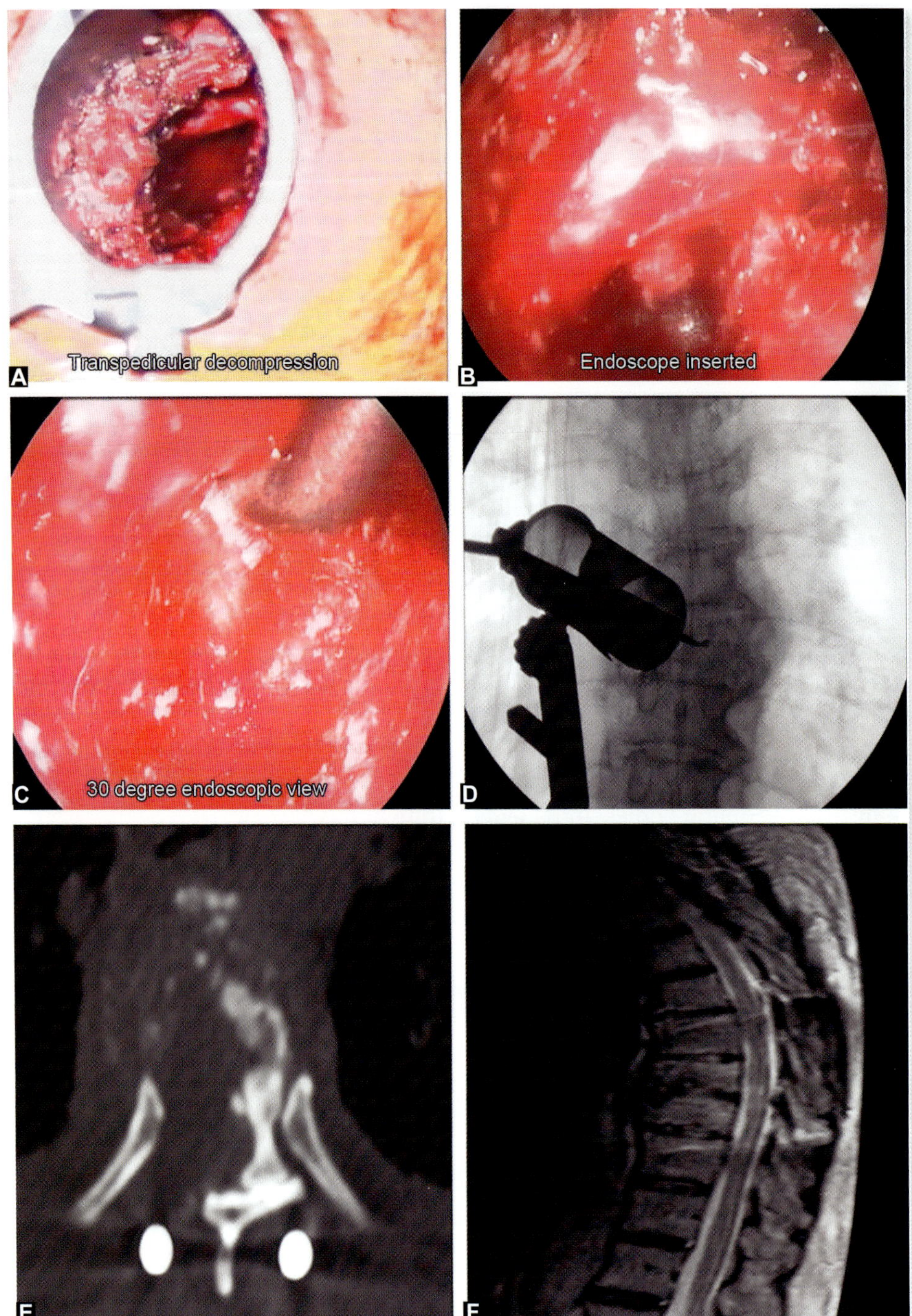

Figures 4A to F: Intraoperative images for transpedicular decompression. (A) X-tube with decompressed lateral thecal sac; (B) Endoscope being inserted; (C) Downcurettes decompressing the ventral thecal sac under endoscope vision; (D) Intraoperative C-arm image – contralateral canal decompression; (E) Postoperative axial CT showing the extent of decompression; (F) Follow-up MRI at 1 year

with more extensive disk space destruction, interbody fusion with larger grafts may not be feasible due to lumbar roots. Preoperative CT scan delineates the extent of disk space destruction and the height of graft required. It is difficult to put grafts bigger than 1.4 cm in height due to the lumbar roots. With expandable TLIF cages, interbody fusion may be possible in these subgroup of patients. Once decompression is done, bone chips are placed in the decompressed space (in case graft cannot be inserted due to size limitation). Stand-alone fixation can also be done in these subgroups in whom interbody fusion is not possible. It is important to inform the patients regarding the need for another surgery to remove

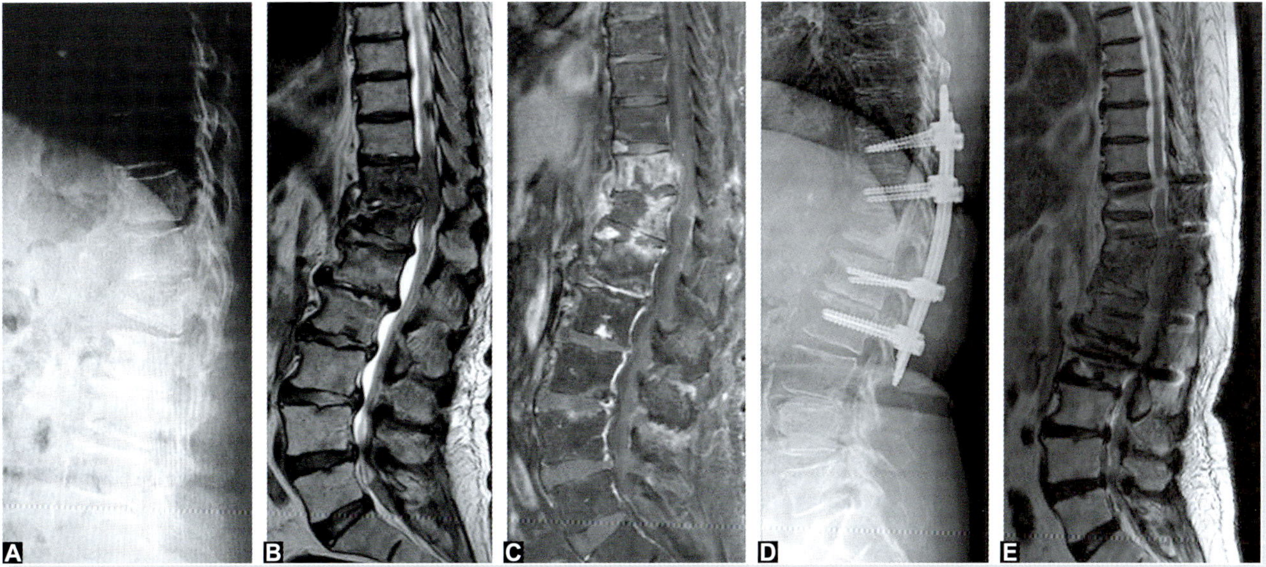

Figures 5A to E: MIS transpedicular decompression and percutaneous fixation. (A) Preoperative X-ray; (B) T2W sagittal MRI; (C) T1W sag with contrast; (D) 1 year follow-up X-ray; (E) FU MRI with complete resolution of tuberculosis

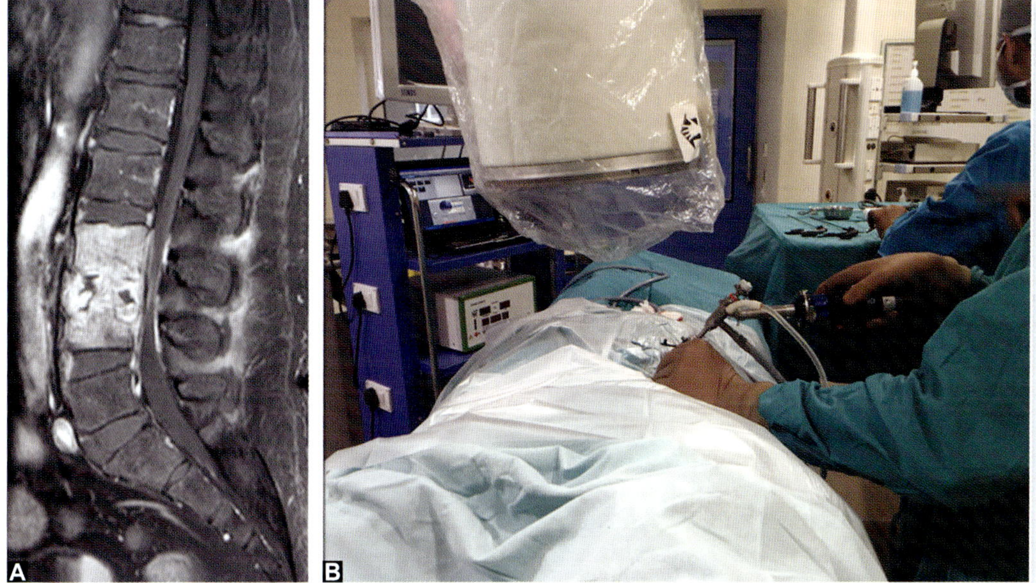

Figures 6A and B: Percutaneous transpediclar endoscopic decompression. (A) Preoperative MRI L3–4 diskitis; (B) Intraoperative image

the implants once the disease is cured. While this approach was done in our early group of patients, DLIF is done now in such cases where interbody fusion is not feasible.

Indications

1. Level L2–L5.
2. Preserved vertebral body height.
3. Neurological deficits/radiculopathy.

Contraindications

1. Significant destruction with focal kyphosis.
2. >2 vertberal body involvement.
3. Extensive disk space destruction (>14 mm)

Hybrid Approach

This is a two-step surgery done in the same sitting. The first step is ventral approach, decompression and ventral

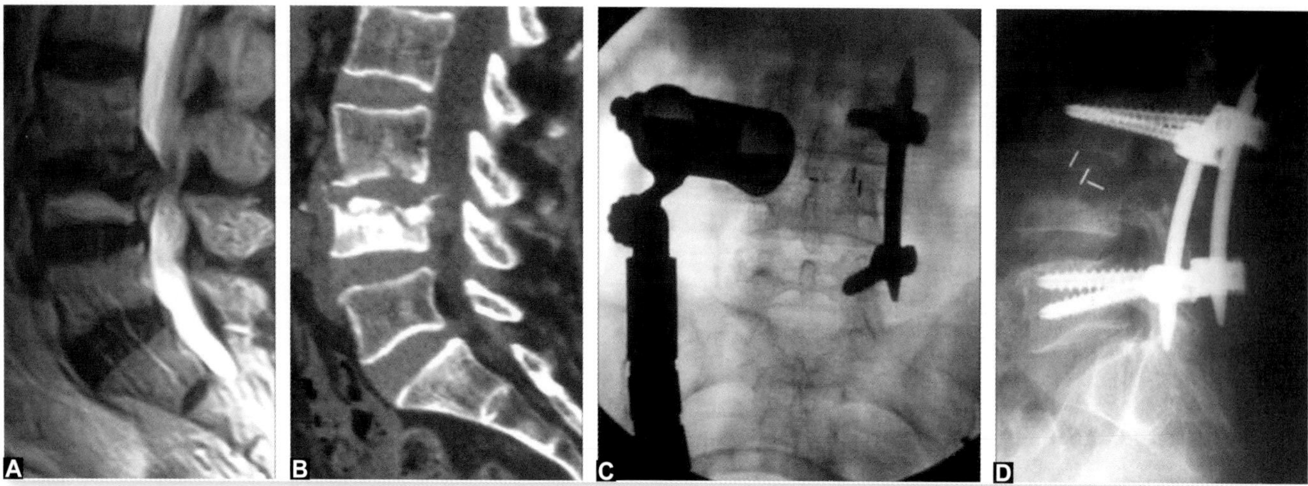

Figures 7A to D: MIS TLIF. (A) Preoperative T2W sagittal with epidural tissue and thecal sac compression; (B) Preoperative CT scan; (C) Intraoperative C-arm image with X-tube for decompression and TLIF; (D) Postoperative X-rays

column reconstruction in the lateral position. The patient is then turned prone and fixation done by percutaneous transpedicular screws.

Thoracotomy (Conventional or mini-open) and Percutaneous Fixation

Method (Figures 8A to J): Thoracotomy is done for accessing the ventral aspect of the thoracic spine. This can be a ventrolateral thoracotomy and transpelural approach or a dorsolateral and extrapleural approach. Following decompression, fusion can be performed with iliac crest or rib autograft or cages filled with bone autograft.. Mini-thoracotomy reduces morbidity. Newer long bladed retractors are used effectively for mini-thoracotomy. Patient is positioned in lateral position. The incision is marked using C-arm. Precise marking of the incision with respect to the level is important due to the limited nature of the exposure. The incision on either side of the mid-axillary line. The rib counting is not so relevant as the marking is done directly based on C-arm guidance. This is, however, a transpleural approach. Some of the retractor systems have a third blade which provides lung retraction. Once the retractors are in place, C-arm is taken to confirm the level of pathology. Internal decompression is done to remove pus, granulation tissue and sequestered necrotic bone fragments. Decompression is continued till the healthy bony margins are reached. Posteriorly, dura is decompressed till the sac is lax and pulsatile. Hemostasis is achieved. Interbody fusion is done with autologous iliac crest bone graft or cage filled with bone autograft. After confirming the positioning of the graft, thorough wash is given, retractors removed and wound is closed in layers. The patient is then turned prone and percutaneous fixation done incorporating the healthy segments on either side of the diseased segments.

Indication

1. D6 to D12 vertebrae
2. Significant body collapse.
3. Kyphotic deformity.
4. Neurological deficit (with ventral pus / granulation tissue causing cord compression).
5. 1–2 segments involved.

Contraindication

1. Involvement of L1 vertebrae (This is relative contra-indication for using retractor systems. Requires mobilization of diaphragm. Conventional extrapleural-extraperitoneal approach is better).
2. Poor respiratory reserve (extrapleural approach is better).

Retroperitoneal Approach, Decompression and Percutaneous Fixation

Method: The patient is placed in lateral position. The side depends upon the clinical and radiologically more affected site. The kidney break of the operating table is opened up to increase the space between the ribs and the iliac crest. An access surgeon for this approach is better for those not accustomed to this approach. The vertebral body is exposed, level confirmed. This is a more ventral approach with respect to the psoas muscle and the lumbar plexus is more posterior thereby eliminating risk of the injury. Direct thecal sac decompression can be achieved with this. Following decompression, interbody fusion is done with bone graft or cage filled with autograft under C-arm guidance. Wound is closed in layers; patient is turned prone; and fixation is done by percutaneous transpedicular screws.

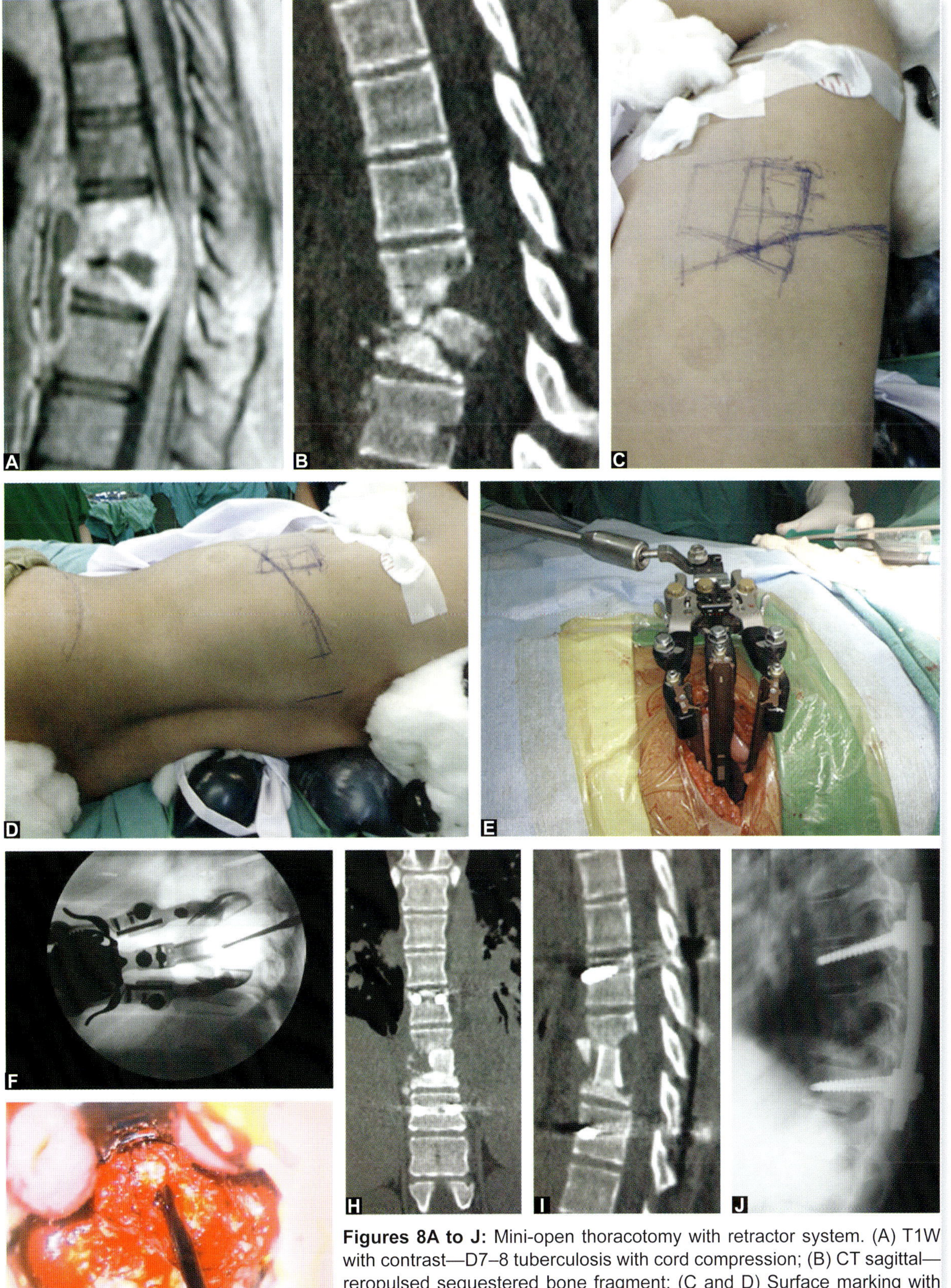

Figures 8A to J: Mini-open thoracotomy with retractor system. (A) T1W with contrast—D7–8 tuberculosis with cord compression; (B) CT sagittal—reropulsed sequestered bone fragment; (C and D) Surface marking with C-arm guidance; (E) Retractor in position; (F) Intraoperative C-arm image with localization; (G) Intraoperative image with bone grafting; (H and I) Postoperative CT with graft in situ; (J) 4 years follow-up X-ray

Indications

1. L2–L4 body involvement
2. Significant kyphotic deformity/collapse.
3. 1–2 vertebral body affected.

Contraindications

1. Preserved vertebral body height.

Minimally Invasive Retroperitoneal Lateral Trans-psoas (Direct Lateral Lumbar Interbody Fusion (DLIF) Followed by Percutaneous Fixation

Method (Figures 9 to 11): This is a more recent approach.[23] It has been used predominantly for degenerative scoliosis with canal stenosis. It provides indirect decompression with interbody fusion. The patient is positioned laterally. It is important to confirm the adequacy of the lateral position using a lateral C-arm image to be sure that the iliac crest and the lowest rib does not interfere the relevant level of the lumbosacral spine. Skin incision is marked with C-arm guidance. The incision is along the mid-axillary line. The mid-point of the vertical extent of the incision is at the relevant disc space. The incision is about 2.5–3 cm in length. After incision the skin, the abdominal muscles are split in the direction of the muscles sequentially till the preperitoneal space is reached. Monopolar cautery should be avoided to avoid injury to the iliohypogastric muscles which increases the possibility of hernia later on. Once preperitoneal space is exposed, blunt finger dissection is done to widen the retroperitoneal space. The finger is first passed inferiorly to feel for the iliac bone and then gently swiped superiorly. Posteriorly, the transverse process tip acts as a good anatomical landmark. The psoas muscle is medial to this and the belly of the psoas is felt. The smallest tubular dilator is passed using the finger as a guide. Appropriate position of the dilators confirmed with C-arm. Four zones have been described by Uribe[21] and effort is made to keep the dilator in zones 2 and 3. Once docked, electromyography (EMG) recording can be done from the relevant muscles to rule out the proximity of the lumbar plexus root to avoid

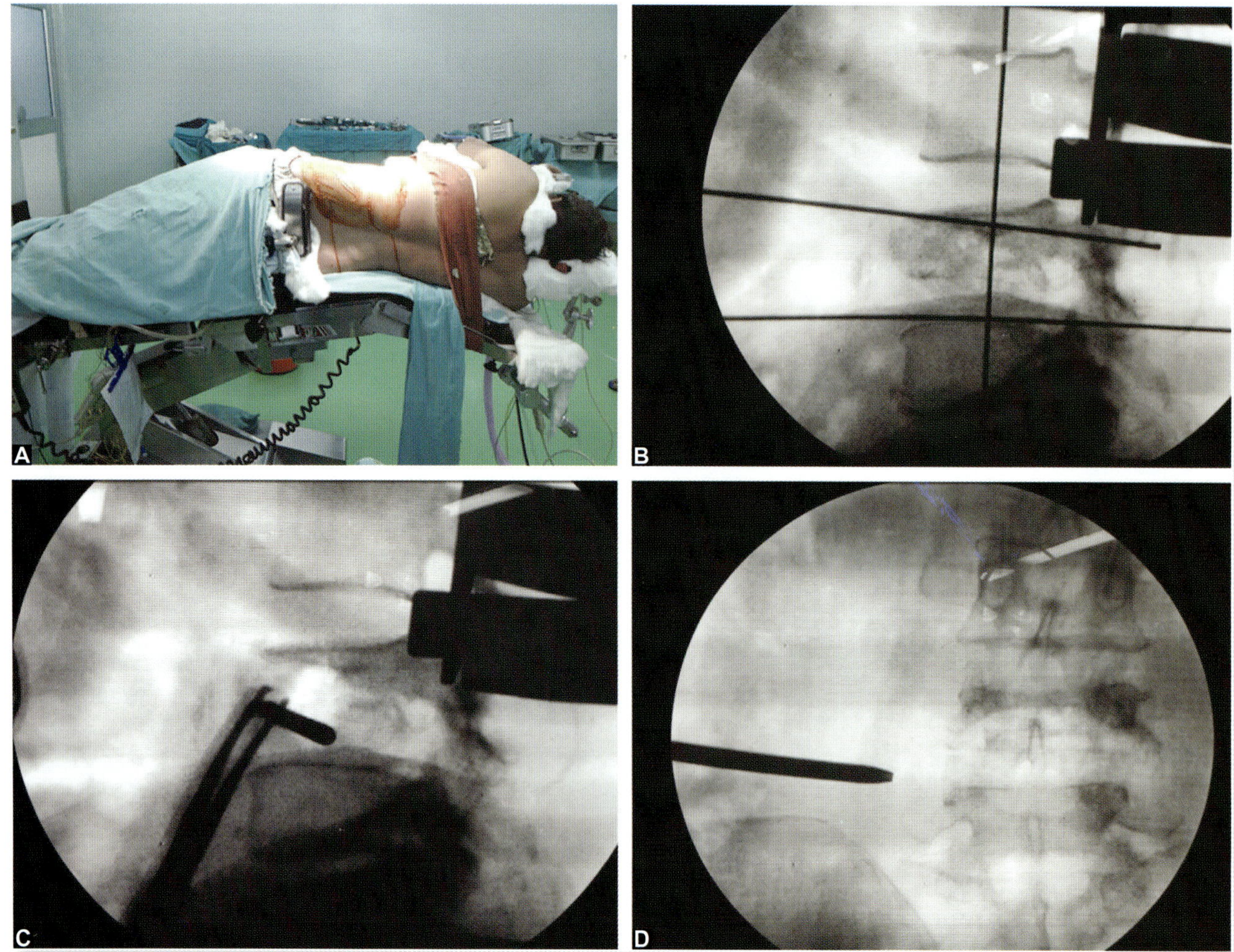

Figures 9A to D

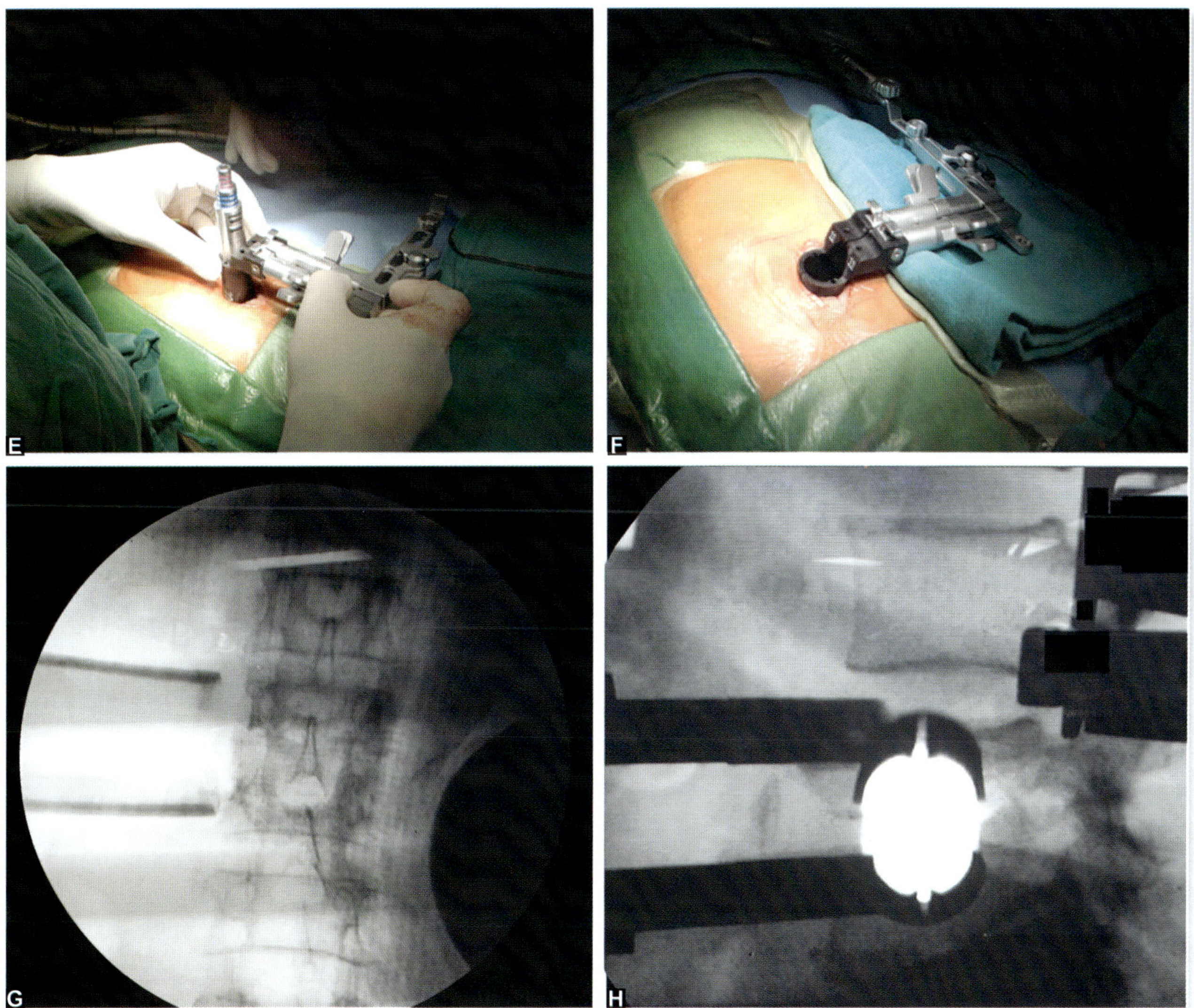

Figures 9A to H: Direct lumbar interbody fusion. (A) Position in lateral decubitus; (B) Surface marking under C-arm; (C and D) Lateral and AP view after placing first dilator; (E) Inserting the retractor over the dilators; (F) Retractor in place; (G and H) AP and lateral C-arm image with retractor docked

injury. However, this is not an essential modality and this procedure can also be done under direct vision. Sequential dilators are passed with intermittent C-arm views to be sure about the trajectory. The psoas is dissected along the direction of its fibres as the dilators are inserted. At L2 level, the genitofemoral nerve is visualized and preserved. These retractor blades are passed over the dilators. These are long (90–170 mm) and radiolucent. The lateral aspect of the vertebrae and disc space is exposed. Pus, granulation tissue and necrotic sequestered bone are decompressed. Thorough wash is given. Interbody-fusion is done with autologous iliac crest bone graft or expandable cages filled with bone graft. The retractors are gradually removed. While withdrawing the retractors slowly, any oozing from the psoas muscle is observed and controlled. Uncontrolled ooze in the psoas causes significant postoperative psoas muscle spasm. The abdominal fascia is sutured and wound closed. Patient is then turned prone and fixation done with percutaneous transpedicular screws.

Indications

1. L2–L5 disease segments.
2. Significant deformity.
3. 1–2 segments involved.

Contraindication

1. L1–2/L5–S1 disk space involved.
2. L5 body with high riding iliac crest.
3. Neurological deficits (direct decompression required, posterior approach is better).
4. Previous abdominal surgery.

It is important to understand the limitations of each of these methods. The basic aim of decompression and fixation

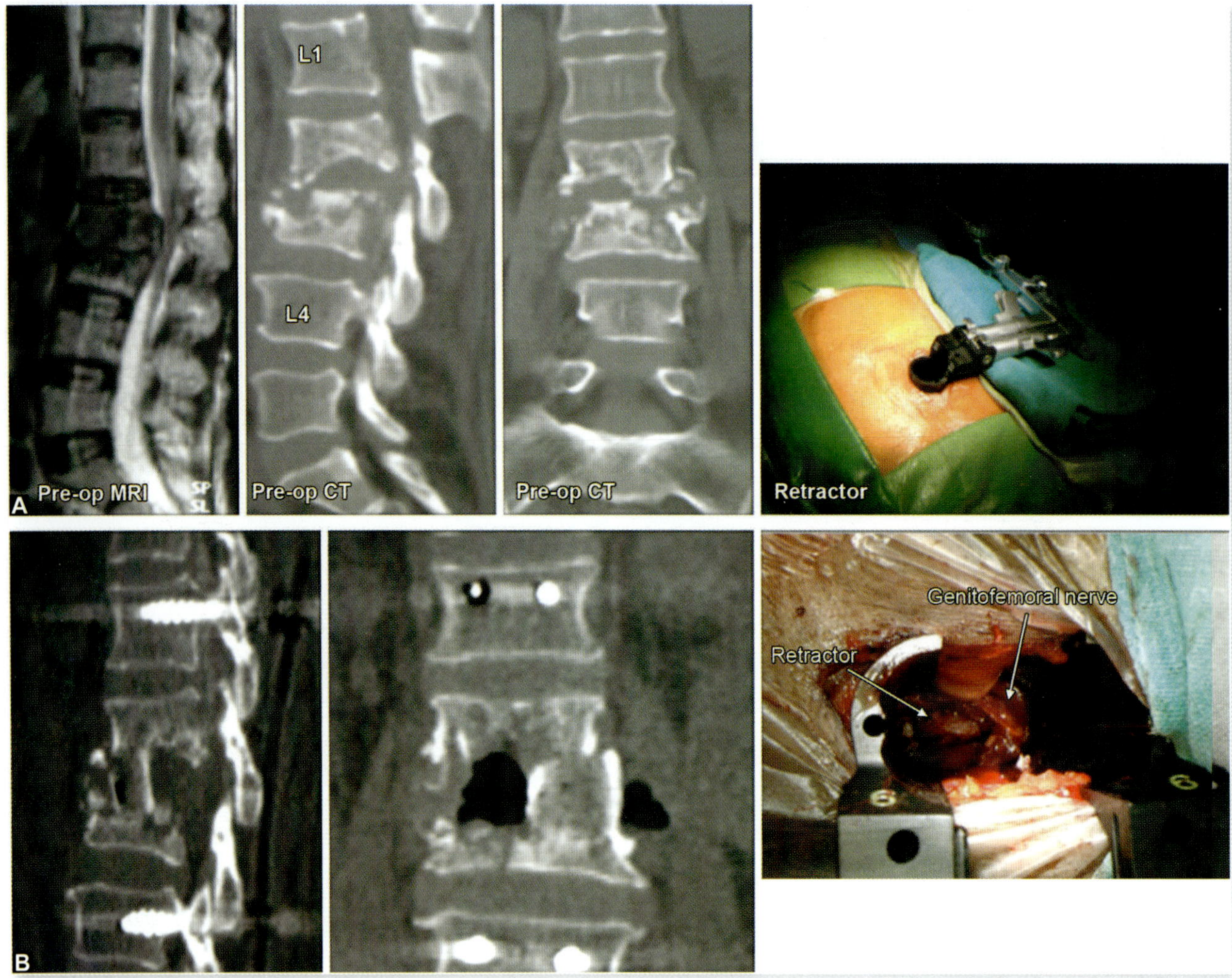

Figures 10A and B: L2–3 DLIF. DLIF, fusion followed by L1–4 fixation with percutaneous transpedicular screws

still remains the same whether one does a conventional of MIS approach surgery.

In the subsequent portion, few relevant issues shall be discussed point-wise. These specifically deal with concerns about the outcomes of MIS methods.

Other Minimally Invasive Methods and Differences with the Described Method

Video-assisted thoracoscopic surgery (VATS)—VATS has been used for ventral column decompression, debridement and biopsy[3,11,22] or in combination with percutaneous transpedicular fixation.[24,25] However, there are some limitations to this technique.[11,24] It requires additional equipment, a separate set of dedicated long instruments, steep learning curve, a two-dimensional view, hemodynamic alterations due to collapse of the lung, pleural adhesions limiting this approach and significant pulmonary complications.[11] Mini-thoracotomy, on the other hand overcomes all these limitations in addition to being familiar to the spine surgeons because the anatomical landmarks are similar to the conventional approaches. Combined with percutaneous transpedicular fixation, this hybrid MIS method helps achieve all the aims of conventional approaches using MIS principles.

Nucleotome based percutaneous aspiration[26,27], endoscopic suction and drainage[28], open transpedicular decompression[29] and transforaminal methods[23,24] have also been described for infective spondylodiskitis. These have been used predominantly for evacuation of the pus and their utility is limited in those with thicker pus or granulation tissue.[30]

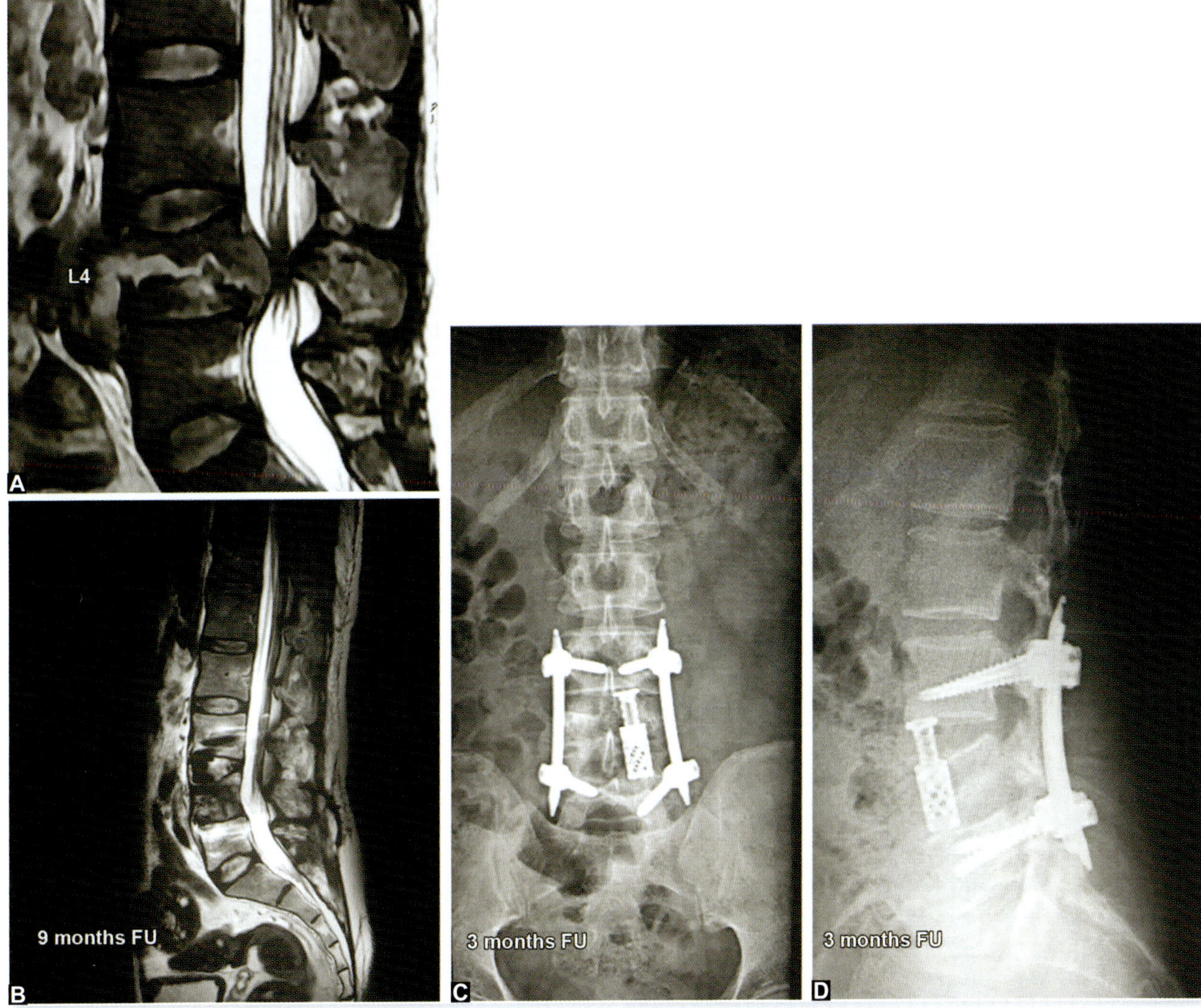

Figures 11A to D: L4 Pott's spine: DLIF + percutaneous transpedicular screws

Benefit of Posterior Only MIS Transpedicular Decompression

There are a subgroup of patients who have a focal peridiscal involvement with significant epidural pus and granulation tissue causing cord compression and neurological deficits. Conventional approaches in these patients with relatively preserved body heights may be considered an overtreatment. Keeping them on ATT medications without offering surgery may result in poor neurologic outcomes,[8] delayed or incomplete neurological recovery, and progression of deformity, causing significant pain and delayed neurological deterioration.[32,33] In these patients, MIS transpedicular decompression helps relieve cord compression, fastens neurologic recovery with minimal tissue damage. An attempt is always made to fix the adjacent healthy segments by percutaneous fixation methods. However, in the midthoracic levels, pedicle size is always a limitation for percutaneous fixation. In such patients, with preserved vertebral body height, a simple decompression suffices to relieve the compression. They are kept on external orthosis and ambulatory ATT. There is no significant deformity progression.[20]

Is Adequate Decompression Achieved by MIS Methods?

The neurological outcome is not influenced by the approach -conventional or MIS. Good neurologic recovery is achieved using either conventional[5,10] or MIS methods.[3,20,24,35] All our patients had good neurological recovery at last follow up. Thus, the misconception that wider bony decompression leads to better neurologic outcome is not appropriate. By achieving similar outcomes in various studies using MIS methods, compared to historical controls with lesser morbidity, these approaches should be used more often.

However, they require proper planning and more extensive analysis of the imaging to plan the appropriate approach.

Are MIS Methods Effective in Correction and Avoiding Deformity Progression?

Spinal deformity is a dreaded complication of tuberculosis. This is associated with significant disability and pain. Maximal deformity progression occurs during the active healing phase. Once healing occurs, deformity does not progress significantly.[2,33]

In those treated nonoperatively, there is an increase in the kyphosis by 6–15°.[29,36] In the posterior only group treated by transpedicular decompression and fixation without fusion, reasonable deformity correction can be achieved. On a long-term basis, after the disease heals, this correction is maintained and there is no significant correction loss. Importantly, this is similar in both conventional and MIS methods[4,10,20,25] So, how does internal fixation work? Internal fixation acts as an internal splint to avoid deformity progression till the healing occurs. Patients treated by posterior only approach, have predominant disc space involvement with preserved body height. Fixation allows for spontaneous fusion to occur across this diseased disc space without deformity progression.[37-39]

In our own experience,[20] mean pre-operative Cobbs' angle was 13.3 +/-4.3° in the thoracic spine. Immediately, post-operatively, these angles improved to 10.8 +/-2.8°, representing a mean correction of 2.5° (18.9%) following surgery. At a mean follow up of 30 months, there was a loss of only 2°. This is much better than the non-operative group[29,40] and similar to those seen in conventional surgeries.[4,10,25,37,39,41] In none of them, were the postoperative angles more than preoperative values. In those with only decompression without fixation, these values were 11.5° preoperatively, 12.5° postoperatively and 14.5° at last follow up.

In the hybrid group, the mean preoperative kyphosis was 19.8°, with a 4° correction achieved postoperatively and a 1.6° loss of correction at last follow up. Thus, comparative results of deformity correction can be achieved with MIS methods.

Are Complications Less with MIS Approaches?

The aims of MIS approaches are similar to conventional methods, i.e. debridement, adequate neural decompression, deformity correction and avoiding progression and early mobilization but with lesser morbidity. In our experience, a 9% incidence of complications included a dural tear and a malposition of screw but no significant approach related morbidity.[20] This is much less than 24–31% reported in conventional methods.[6,10,11] Even MIS methods as VATS have a significant risk of pulmonary complications.[3,11,24]

Do the Implants Need to Be Removed in Nonfusion Methods?

Implant removal remains controversial in those who undergo fixation without fusion, as it requires second surgery and general anaesthesia. Studies on patients with various pathologies as spinal fractures treated by percutaneous trasnpedicular fixation[12,13] infective spondylodiscitis[4] did not require implant removal. In our experience of patients with tuberculosis, there was no implant fatigue with mean follow up of 30 months (maximum, 59 months) and none of our patients have required their implants to be removed.[20]

CONCLUSION

Tuberculosis of spine is another indication for using MIS methods with good outcomes. These can be posterior only or combined ventral and dorsal approaches in the same sitting. All the aims of debridement, canal decompression, avoiding deformity progression, deformity correction and pain relief can be achieved using MIS methods. A thorough knowledge of the available instrumentation and limitations of each of these approaches is essential to use them optimally.

REFERENCES

1. Moon MS. Tuberculosis of the spine: controversies and a new challenge. Spine (Phila Pa 1976). 1997;22:1791-7.
2. Jain AK, Dhammi IK, Jain S, Mishra P. Kyphosis in spinal tuberculosis-prevention and correction. Indian J Orthop. 2010;44(2):127-36.
3. Jayaswal A, Upendra B, Ahmed A, Chowdhury B, Kumar A. Video assisted thoracoscopic anterior surgery for tuberculous spondylitis. Clin Orthop Relat Res. 2007;460:100-7.
4. Lee BH, Lee HM, Kim TH, Kim HS, Moon ES, Park JO, Chong HS, Moon SH. Transpedicular curettage and drainage of infective lumbar spondylodiscitis: technique and clinical results. Clin Orthop Surg. 2012;4:200-8.
5. Rasouli MR, Mirkoohi M, Vaccaro AR, Yarandi KK, Movaghar VR. Spinal tuberculosis: Diagnosis and management. Asian Spine J. 2012;6(4):294-308.
6. Sharkawi MM, Said GK. Instrumented circumferential fusion for tuberculosis of the dorso-lumbar spine. A single or double stage procedure? Int Orthop. 2012;36:315-24.
7. Soundararaj GD. Simultaneous anterior decompression and posterior instrumentation of the tuberculous spine using anterolateral extrapleural approach. J Bone Joint Surg Br. 2009;91(5):702-3.
8. Jain AK. Treatment of tuberculosis of the spine with neurological complications. Clin Orthop Relat Res. 2002;398:75-84.
9. Okada Y, Miyamoto H, Uno K, Sumi M. Clinical and radiological outcome of surgery for pyogenic and tuberculous spondylitis: comparisons of surgical technique and disease type. J Neurosurg Spine. 2009;11(5):620-7.

10. Pu X, Zhou Q, He Q, Dai F, Xu J, Zhang Z, Branko K. A posterior versus anterior surgical approach in combination with debridement, interbody autografting and instrumentation for thoracic and lumbar tuberculosis. Int Orthop. 2012;36:307-13.
11. Lu G, Wang B, Li J, Liu W, Cheng I. Anterior debridement and reconstruction via thoracoscopy assisted mini-open approach for the treatment of thoracic spinal tuberculosis: minimum 5 year follow up. Eur Spine J. 2012;21:463-9.
12. Court C, Vincent C. Percutaneous fixation of thoracolumbar fractures: current concepts. Ortho Traum: Surg Res. 2012;98:900-9.
13. De Iure F, Cappuccio M, Paderni S, Bosco G, Amendola L. Minimally invasive percutaneous fixation of thoracic and lumbar spine fractures. Min Inv Surg. 2012;1-6.
14. McLain RF. Spinal cord decompression: an endoscopically assisted approach for metastatic tumors. Spinal Cord. 2001;39:482-7.
15. Palmisani M, Gasbarrini A, Brodano GB, De Iure F, Cappuccio M, Boriani L, Amendola L, Boriani S. Minimally invasive percutaneous fixation in the treatment of thoracic and lumbar spine fractures. Eur Spine J. 2009;18(Suppl 1):S71-74.
16. Smith JS, Ogden AT, Fessler RG. Minimally invasive posterior thoracic fusion. Neurosurg Focus. 2008;25:E1-E9.
17. St Clair SF, McLain RF. Posterolateral spinal cord decompression in patients with metastasis: an endoscope assisted approach. Surg Technol Int. 2006;15:257-63.
18. Tuli SM. Tuberculosis of the spine: a historical review. Clin Orthop Relat Res. 2007;460:29-38.
19. Pai BS, Gangadhara, Nirmal S, et al. Morphometric analysis of the thoracic pedicle: an anatomico-radiologic study. Neurol India. 2010;58(2):253-8.
20. Garg N, Vohra R. Minimally invasive surgical approaches in the management of tuberculosis of the dorsal and lumbar spine. Clin Orthop Rel Res. 2014;472:1855-67.
21. Uribe JS, Arredoudo N, Dakwar E, et al. Defining the safe working zones using minimally invasive lateral retroperitoneal transpsoas approach: an anatomical study. J Neurosurg Spine 2010;13(2):260-6.
22. Kapoor SK, Kapoor S, Agarwal M, et al. Thoracoscopic decompression in Pott's spine and its long term follow up. Int Orthop. 2012;36:331-7.
23. Garg N. Minimally invasive lateral trans-psoas approach for tuberculosis of the lumbar spine. Ind J Neurosurg. 2014;3(1): 38-40.
24. Kandwal P, Garg B, Upendra BN, Chowdhury B, Jayaswal A. Outcome of minimally invasive surgery in the management of tuberculous spondylitis. Indian J Orthop. 2012;46(2):159-64.
25. Ringel F, Stoffel M, Stuer C, Meyer B. Minimally invasive transmuscular pedicle screw fixation of the thoracic and lumbar spine. Neurosurgery. 2006;59(4 suppl):361-7.
26. Hanaoka N, Kawasaki Y, Sakai T, Nakamura T, Nanamori K, Nakamura E, Uchida K, Yamada H. Percutaneous drainage and continuous irrigation in patients with severe pyogenic spondylitis, abscess formation and marked bone destruction. J Neurosurg Spine. 2006;4:374-9.
27. Yu MY, Siu C, Wing PC, Schweigel IF, Jetha N. Percutaneous suction aspiration for osteomyelitis: report of two cases. Spine (Phila Pa 1976). 1991;16:198-202.
28. Ito M, Sudo H, Abumi K, Kotani Y, Takahata M, Fujita M, Minami A. Minimally invasive surgical treatment for tuberculous spondylodiscitis. Minim Invasive Neurosurg. 2009;52:250-3.
29. Chacko AG, Moorthy RK, Chandy MJ. The trans-pedicular approach in the management of thoracic spine tuberculosis: a short term follow up study. Spine (Phila Pa 1976). 2004;29:E363-567.
30. Kandwal P, Vijayaraghavan G, Jayaswal A. Management of tuberculous infection of the spine. Asian Spine J 2016;10(4): 792-800.
31. Jain AK. Tuberculosis of the spine: a fresh look at an old disease. J Bone Joint Surg Br. 2010;92:905-13.
32. Tuli SM. Severe kyphotic deformity in tuberculosis of the spine. Int Orthop. 1995;19:327-31.
33. Upadhyay SS, Saji MJ, Sell P, Sell B, Yau AC. Longitudinal changes in spinal deformity after anterior spinal surgery for tuberculosis of the spine in adults; a comparative analysis between radical and debridement surgery. Spine (Phila Pa 1976). 1994;19:542-9.
34. Wang LJ, Zhang HQ, Tang MX, Gao QL, Zhou ZH, Yin XH. Comparison of Three Surgical Approaches for Thoracic Spinal Tuberculosis in Adult: Minimum 5-Year Follow-Up. Spine (Phila Pa 1976) 2016 (Epub ahead of print).
35. Sudprasert W, Choovongkomol K, Piyapromdee U, Leownorasate M. Impact on neurological recovery of transforaminal debridement and interbody fusion versus transpedicular decompression in combination with pedicle screw instrumentation for treating thoracic and lumbar spinal tuberculosis. Asian Spine J 2016;10(3):543-52.
36. Medical Research Council. A 15 year assessment of controlled trials of the management of tuberculosis of the spine in Korea and Hong Kong. J Bone Joint Surg (Br). 1998;80:456-62.
37. Yang H, Song F, Zhang L, Li N, Zhang X, Wang Y. Management of spine tuberculosis with chemotherapy and percutaneous pedicle screws in adjacent vertebrae: a retrospective study of 34 cases. Spine (Phila Pa 1976) 2016: (Epub ahead of print).
38. Zhang P, Peng W, Wang X, Luo C, Xu Z, Zeng H, et al. Minimum 5-year follow-up outcomes for single-stage transpedicular debridement, posterior instrumentation and fusion in the management of thoracic and thoracolumbar spinal tuberculosis in adults. Br J Neurosurg 2016;30(6):666-71.
39. Shen X, Huang X, Xiao S, Liu H, Zhang Y, Xiang T, et al. Surgical treatment of selected patients with multilevel contiguous thoracolumbar spinal tuberculosis by only posterior instrumentation without any bone fusion. *Int J Clin Exp Med* 2015;8(10):18611-9.
40. Medical Research Council. A 15 year assessment of controlled trials of the management of tuberculosis of the spine in Lorea and Hong Kong. J Bone Joint Surg Br. 1998;80:456-62.
41. Lee SH, Sung JK, Park YM. Single-stage transpedicular decompression and posterior instrumentation in treatment of thoracic and thoracolumbar spinal tuberculosis: A retrospective case series. J Spinal Disord Tech. 2006;19:595-602.

40

CHAPTER

Percutaneous Pedicle Screw Instrumentation

Neeraj Gupta

ABSTRACT

The invention of pedicle screws has revolutionized in the management of stabilization of spine for varied etiologies. It gives three-coloumn fixation and thus gives study constructs as compared to earlier instrumentation.The percutaneous pedicle screw insertion is the novel method of insertion and has distinct advantages over open techniques. This chapter deals with the techniques, and tips and tricks of percutaneous pedicle screw insertion.

INTRODUCTION

Pedicle screw instrumentation is a good and well accepted technique for spine instrumentation. It provides a rigid construct and gives more stability and fusion in spinal pathologies. The safety of the open techniques of pedicle screw fixation is well documented in the literature. Due to the advantages of percutaneous fixation of pedicle screws their demand is increased amongst the spine surgeons. Magerl[1] introduced percutaneous pedicle screw placement for fixation of spine in spinal fractures and osteomyelitis in 1977. Mathews and Long[2] first described percutaneous lumbar pedicle fixation with plates as longitudinal connectors.

OPEN VERSUS PERCUTANEOUS PEDICLE SCREW FIXATION

Disadvantages of Traditional Open Approach

- Extensive midline exposure
- Excessive lateral retraction of soft tissues to visualize pedicle screw entry point—increased incidence of denervation and muscle atrophy.
- Prolonged post op pain and more morbidity
- More blood loss
- Increased chances of wound infection.

Advantages of Percutaneous Pedicle Screws

- Minimal surgical incision length
- Muscle dilating approach—Less soft tissue trauma
- Less blood loss
- Shorter hospital stay
- Less anesthetic complications—so, can be useful in patients with poor general condition.
- Less postoperative pain, less morbidity

Indications

- Spinal trauma
- Degenerative disk disease
- Spondylolisthesis
- Osteoporotic fractures
- Infections.

Limitations

Patients with rotational deformities that obscure the anatomy of the pedicles on fluproscopy are not the best candidates for this procedure

PREOPERATIVE PLANNING

Physical Examination

- Evaluate spine contour—Look for any abnormal spine contour-scoliosis, etc.
- Body habitus—obesity
- Detailed neurological examination

Imaging

- Good quality X-rays of spine, both anteroposterior and lateral views
- CT can be done to look for exact diameter and angles of pedicles. It is usually done when the anatomy is obscure on plain X-rays, in osteoporosis or some deformity.

SURGICAL TECHNIQUE

Operating Room Requirements

- Radiolucent OT table
- Good quality fluoroscopy (C-arm) which can visualize pedicles in both AP and lateral planes.

Lumbar Spine Relevant Anatomy

In upper lumbar spine pedicles are oval, with height greater than transverse diameter. In lower lumbar spine pedicles are larger and more round, with relatively equal transverse and vertical diameters

- Medial angulation of pedicles increases from approximately 10° at L1 to 30° at L5. The mean sagittal angulation of pedicle increases from 2° caudal at L1 to 5° at L5.

Surgical Steps

- Patient is positioned in prone position. Area of interest is properly painted and draped.
- Pedicles should be localised under C-arm in both AP and lateral view. In AP view pedicle should be round like a bull's eye, spinous process should be in midline,and endplates should be sharp without any overlapping. In lateral view, pedicles and body should be visible without any overlapping of superior and inferior borders.
- Under C-arm guidance, by keeping long guidewire on the skin surface, midline of spine, lateral and superior margins of the pedicles are marked with sterile pen. This gives the rough idea of the postion of pedicles and reduces radiation exposure while locating the pedicles.
- Skin knife blade is kept at the intersection of lines which are along the superior and inferior borders of pedicle. Position is confirmed under C-arm. Tip of the blade is aimed at 3'o clock position on the outer margin of round pedicle.
- A 1 cm vertical incision is made through the skin and dorsal fascia. A cannulated spinal needle (Jamshidi) is placed through this stab incision and slowly directed towards the entry point of the pedicle. In obese patients the skin incision is slightly lateral.
- The starting point for both open and percutaneous pedicle screws in the lumbar spine is close to the junction of tranverse process and facet complex.
- Needle should be docked on the bone at the outer margin of the pedicle at 3'o clock position **(Figures 1A and B)**. Position should be confirmed on lateral view. At this position, needle should be at the outer wall of pedicle in midline. Cephalad and caudal angulation can be adjusted for appropriate trajectory in pedicle.

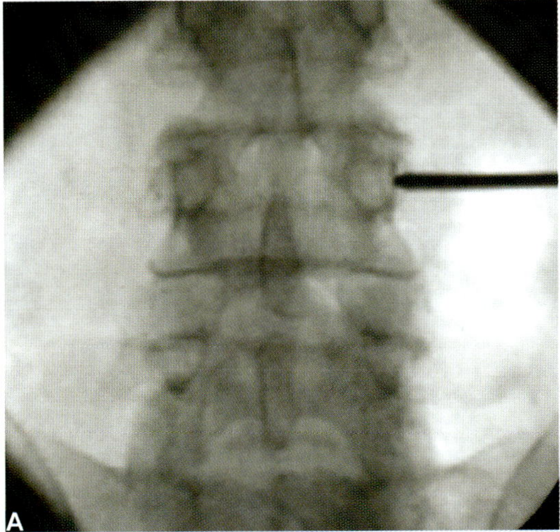

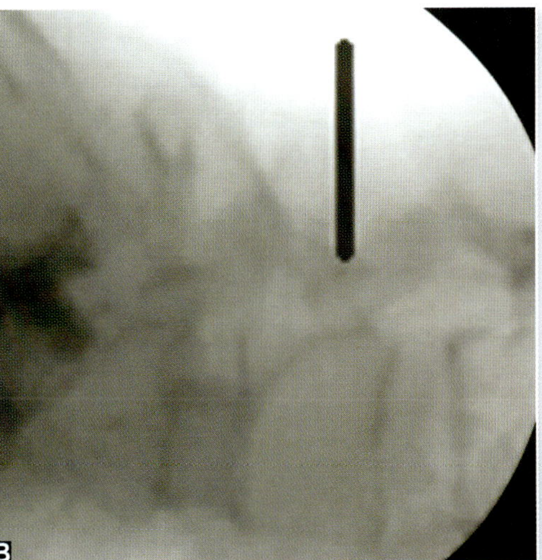

Figures 1A and B: Jamshidi needle at 3'o clock position in true AP view. Bull's eye view of pedicle is seen, spinous process in midline, without any overlapping of endplates. In lateral view, there is no overlapping of pedicle walls, and needle is placed at pedicle entry point at appropriate cephalocaudal angulation

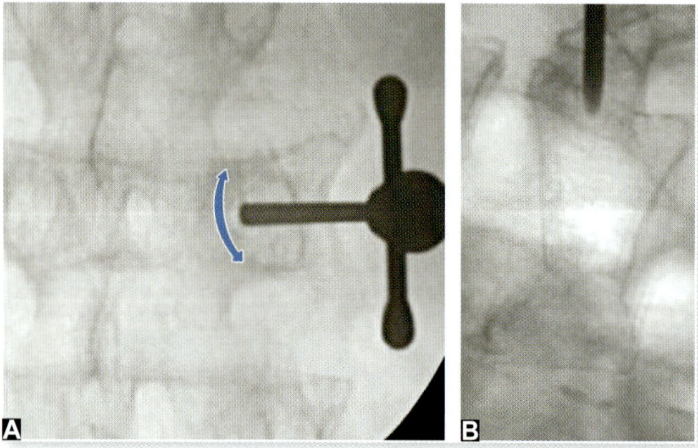

Figures 2A and B: (A) Jamshidi needle reaches inner wall of pedicle at 3–4'o clock position in AP view; (B) In lateral view, the needle just enters the vertebral body

- Needle should be advanced under C-arm guidance to avoid interlaminar placement or too medial entry.
- Using gentle twisting motion, the needle is advanced. As the needle advances and enters cancellous bone, the resistance decreases. Sudden changes in resistance should be checked in C-arm, in both AP and lateral views
- Once the needle reaches the inner wall of pedicle in AP view at 3-4'o clock position, lateral view should be checked in C-arm **(Figures 2A and B)**.Ideally, at this position the needle should have just entered the vertebral body. If at this position, the needle is too much into the body, it means that our trajectory is too much medial and needs readjustment. And, if at this position our needle has not entered the vertebral body, it means our trajectory is too much lateral and needs more medial angulation.
- Once this appropriate position is achieved, the needle is advanced into the vertebral body,1-2 cm beyond the posterior wall of vertebra under lateral view.
- Now, a K-wire or a blunt guide wire is inserted into the vertebral body through cannulated needle.
- K-wire should just exit the tip of needle on C-arm in lateral view.
- K-wire should be placed with care and should not be forced down too deeply, as it may pierce the anterior cortex and cause both great vessel or visceral injury.
- K-wire is advanced with guarded force to reach the middle of the vertebral body. Position of wire is confirmed **(Figures 3A and B)**.
- Jamshidi needle is now removed, and wire is kept in place in vertebral body. Care should be taken while removing the needle to prevent inadvertent removal of K-wire **(Figure 4)**.
- Series of dilators are placed over the wire to dilate the posterior musculature and soft tissues, for screw placement **(Figures 5 and 6)**.
- The final dilator is left in place, and tapping is done using cannulated tap over the K-wire. While tapping, position of guidewire should be checked repeatedly to prevent inadvertent advancement of K-wire, anterior to vertebral body. Tapping is usually done with a tap 0.5 mm smaller than the anticipated screw diameter **(Figure 7)**.
- Now, the cannulated pedicle screw of appropriate size is loaded on the handle and put across the K-wire in vertebral body. Again while advancing the screw, the position should be confirmed under C-arm and inadvertent advancement of K-wire should be avoided **(Figure 8)**.
- Screw heads are attached to long tabs which help in alignment of screw heads and connecting rod placement.
- Once the screw is inside the vertebral body. K-wire is removed, and screw is advanced to appropriate depths.
- Similarly screws are placed at other levels too **(Figure 9)**.
- Once the screws are placed, the tabs attached to the screw heads are brought in line using a tab aligner.
- Connecting rod, either straight or lordotic is connected to the handle. Length of rod is measured approximately by measuring the distance between the tabs. Accurate measurement can be done by putting K wires into the cannulated pedicle screw heads and then measuring the distance between them using callipers **(Figure 10)**.

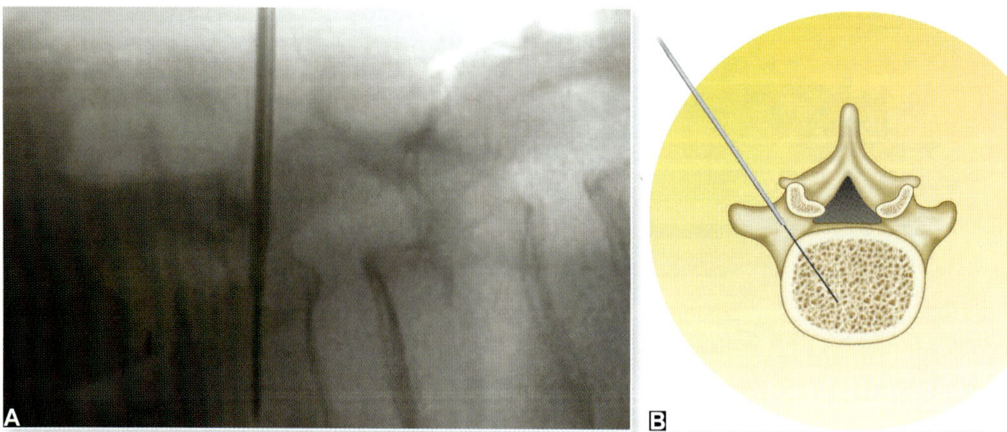

Figures 3A an B: Long wire/guidewire/K-wire inserted through the Jamshidi needle into the vertebral body

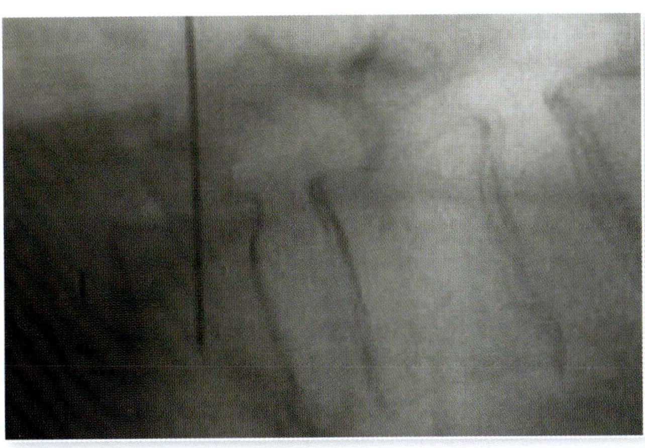

Figure 4: Jamshidi needle removed and wire left in place

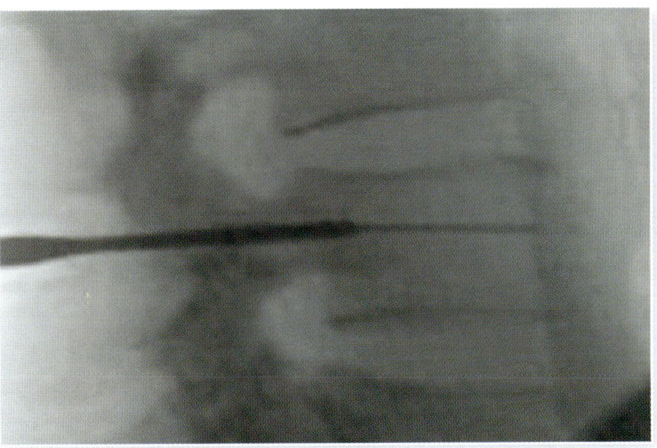

Figure 7: Tapping of pedicle with wire still inside the body

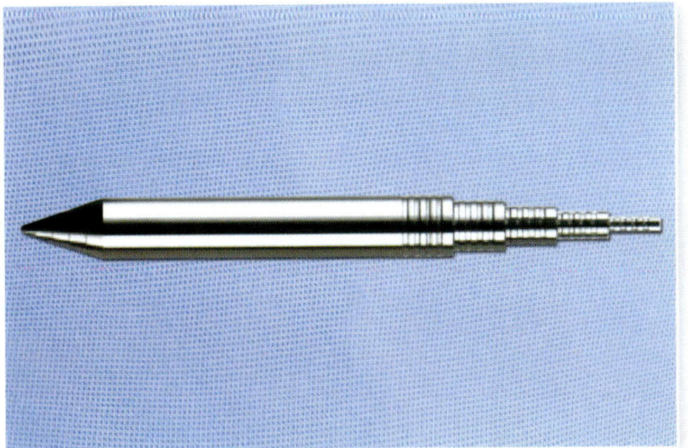

Figure 5: Serial dilators

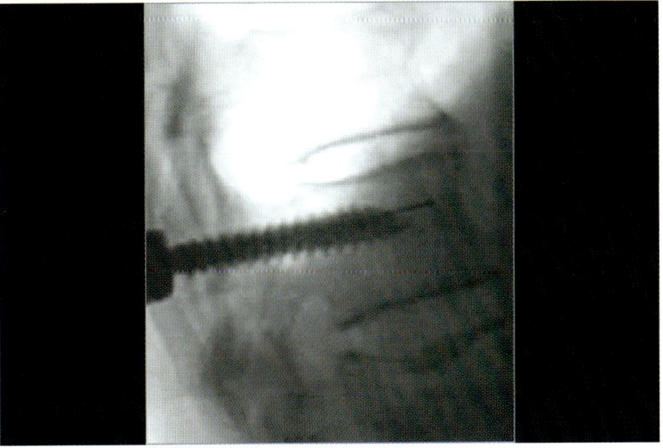

Figure 8: Pedicle screw loaded over the guidewire, and inserted in vertebral body

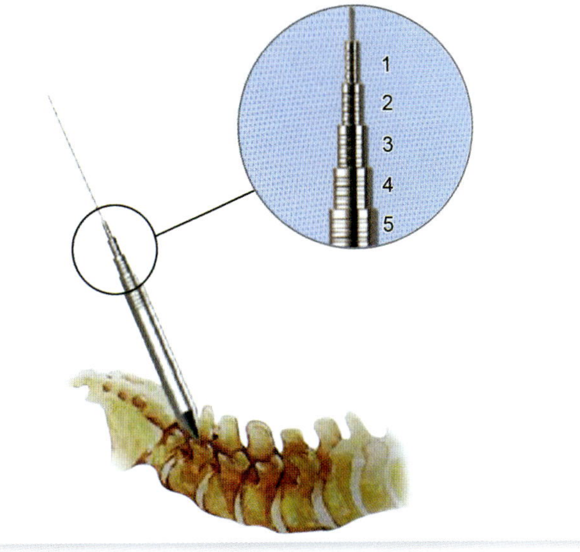

Figure 6: Serial dilators placed over the guidewire

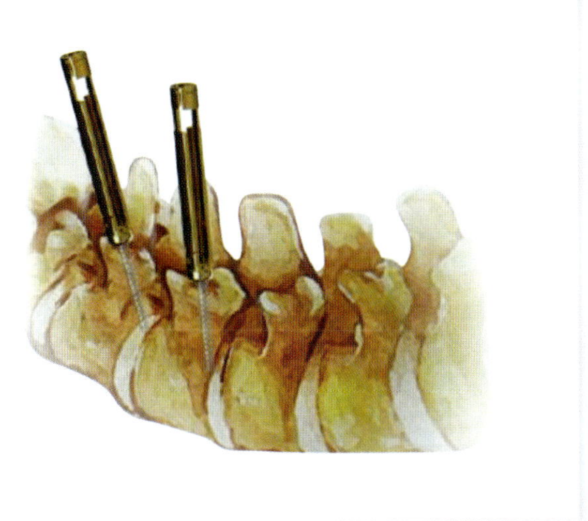

Figure 9: Screws fixed at other levels with tabs attached to the screws

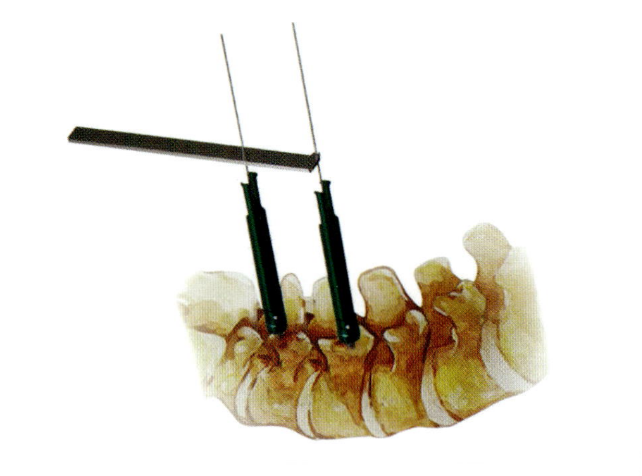

Figure 10: Measuring the distance between the wires using callipers

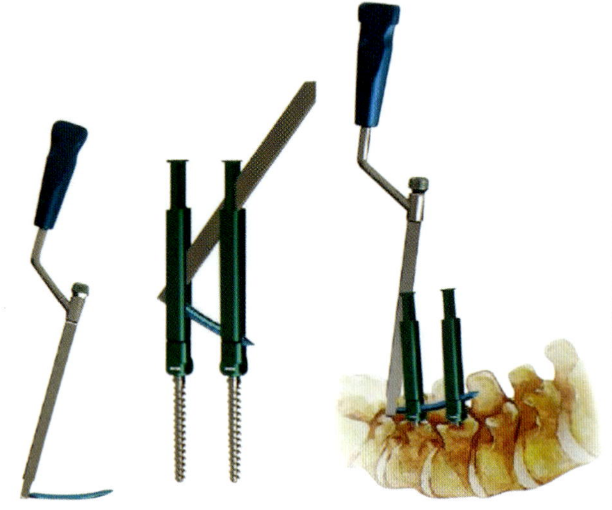

Figure 11: Rod of appropriate size is attached to rod inserter, and rod is introduced

- Rod can be inserted from both cephalad or caudad side by extending the incision of pedicle screw entry by 1-2 cm, from the side from which rod is entered(Jayon instrumentation). In some other instrumentation, there is a separate entry and skin incision for rod entry **(Figure 11)**.
- Once the rod is placed,its position is confirmed under C-arm, and adjustment is made. Rod feelers are used to check the presence of rod in each screw head.
- Now, once the rod is placed satisfactorily, the locking caps are placed in screw heads through the tabs attached and final tightening is done using the torque device attached to the screw tabs **(Figure 12)**.
- Distraction, compression and reduction can be achieved by using instrumentation attached to screw heads.

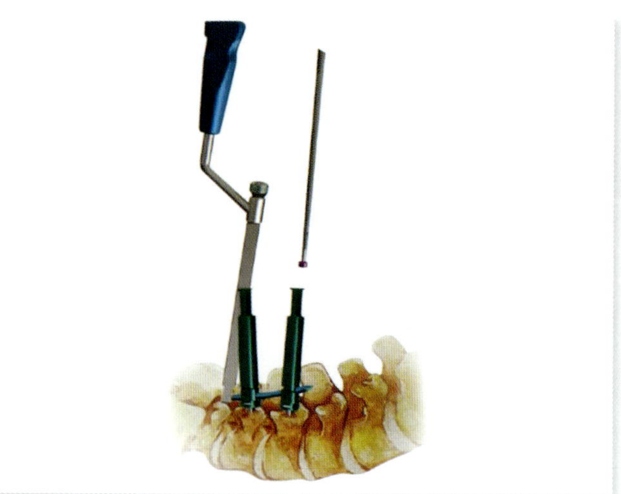

Figure 12: Locking caps being placed in screw heads with rod inserter still attached

- Tabs are now disconnected from screw heads with a device.
- Similar procedure is performed on the opposite side for pedicle screw insertion and rod fixation.

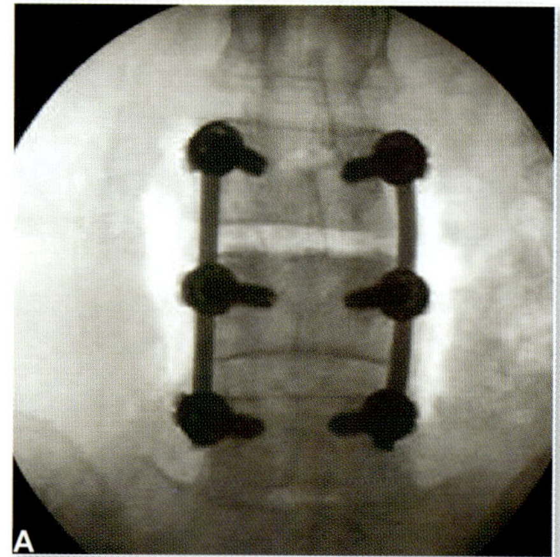

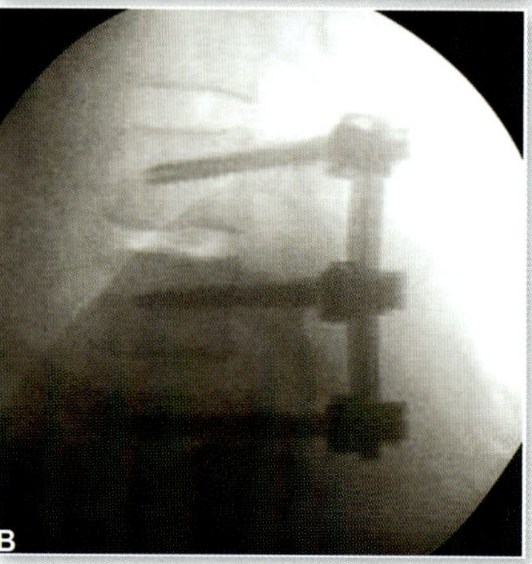

Figures 13A and B: Final image in C-arm

- Position of screws and rods are confirmed under C arm before final closure **(Figures 13A and B)**.
- Closure of deep fascia is done using Vicryl sutures after hemostasis. Skin can be closed with either Silk, nylon or skin staples.

Postoperative Protocol

- Early mobilization is encouraged depending on pain control.
- No role of braces if the fixation is adequate.

Percutaneous Pedicle Screw Fixation in Dorsal Spine

- Pedicles are small in size. Cannulation of small pedicles involve careful evaluation of preoperative CT scan and AP radiograph to ensure that pedicle can be cannulated. The pedicles must have a width of at least 3–4 mm so that Jamshidi needle can be navigated down the pedicle. Hence, percutaneous pedicle screw fixation is done safely from D8–D12 levels
- The presence of the spinal cord (vs.the cauda equina) in the thoracic spine makes the procedure a riskier one than that in the lower lumbar region, where misplacement into the spinal canal is better tolerated
- The proximity of the great vessels to the thoracic spine also increases the risk for life-threatening complications from poor screw placement.

41

CHAPTER

Tubular Retractors in Thoracic and Lumbar Spine

G Balamurali, Vignesh Pushparaj

ABSTRACT

Microscopic-assisted tubular retactor system has wide indications in dealing with the pathologies of different areas of spine. The Minimally invasive nature of these retractors helps in lesser tissue trauma, optimum visualization of intended structures, less pain and early rehabilitation. The retractors can be used in dorsal and lumbar spine as well. This chapter deals with the technique, indications and contraindications of the tubular retractors.

INTRODUCTION

This Chapter describes about the tubular retractors in the cervical spine and has detailed information regarding the tubular retractor systems, classification, advantage and disadvantages. In this chapter we will discuss regarding tubular retractor system in the thoracic and lumbar spine. The fact that tubular retractor systems have several advantages over conventional MIS techniques is well noted in the literature.[1] It offers direct visualization of the operative field, anatomical familiarity to spine surgeons, and minimizing tissue trauma. In addition to reduced blood loss, shorter operative time, reduced postoperative pain, earlier discharge, rapid return to normal activities, and other reported advantages of minimally invasive surgery, a decreased complication rate associated with these surgeries has also been noted, particularly with respect to wound infections.[2] The musculature in the lumbar spine is very strong and tubular retractor system splits the muscle instead of cutting it; hence, it has a huge added advantage of minimizing postoperative back pain by reducing muscle damage.[3] Attention to the technique and orientation, understanding of the anatomy and proper selection of patients will minimize complications and improve outcomes.

APPLIED ANATOMY OF THE THORACOLUMBAR SPINE

In thoracolumbar region. There is transition from one type of vertebral body to another. Thoracic vertebrae are smaller than the lumbar vertebrae. To fully appreciate the approach, one must understand the anatomy **(Figures 1 and 2)**. All the muscle groups are often detached as a single mass during the approach. The bony structures revealed during this approach include the spinous processes, laminae, and transverse processes. The facet joint capsules are also visualized.

INDICATION

The tubular retractors systems were first commercial available for the first time in 1997. This was used for lumbar diskectomy initially and then the system has been made available much wider.

Thoracic spine

1. Thoracic disk/ossified ligamentum flavum
2. Approach to intradural procedures (tumors)
3. Thoracic vertebrectomy (tumor, infection).

Lumbar spine

1. Microlumbar diskectomy/microendoscopic diskectomy
2. Lumbar decompression (single/multilevel)
3. Transforaminal lumbar interbody fusion/posterolateral lumbar interbody fusion
4. Approach to intradural procedures (tumors, tethered cord).

Instruments Required

- Intraoperative fluoroscopy
- Microscope

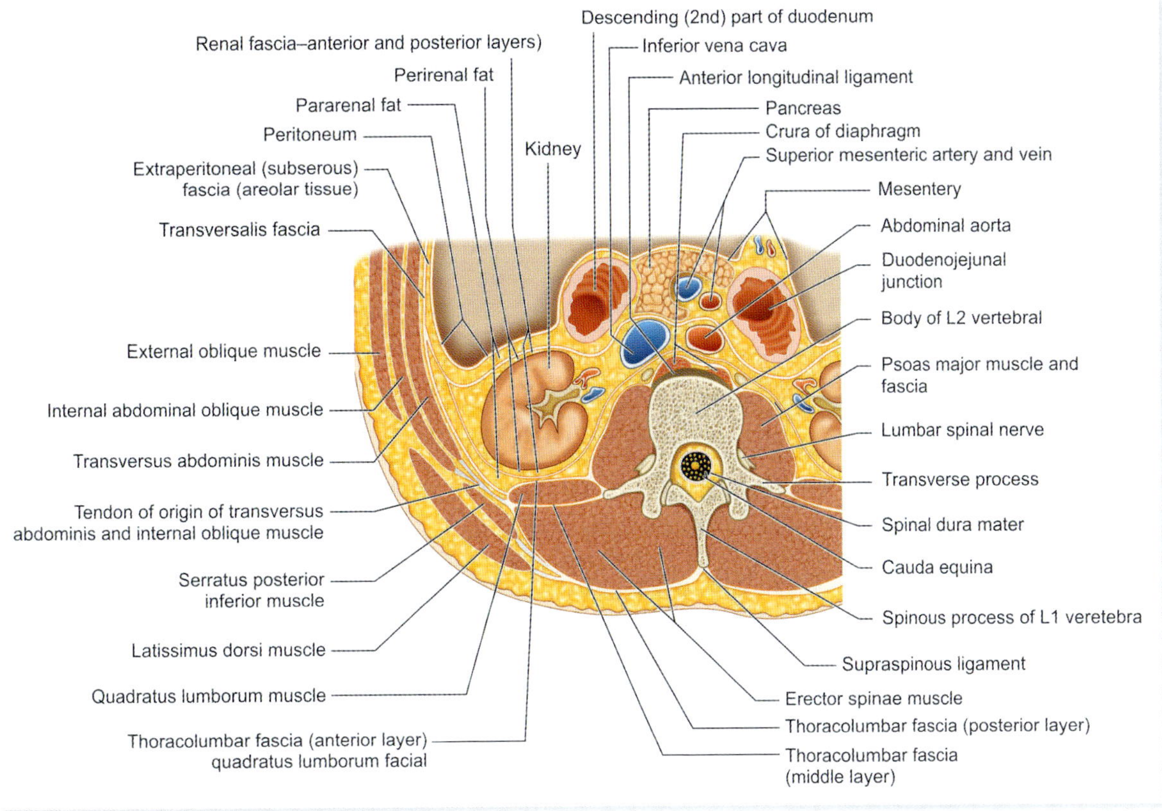

Figure 1: Axial view demonstrating posterior exposure of the thoracic spine

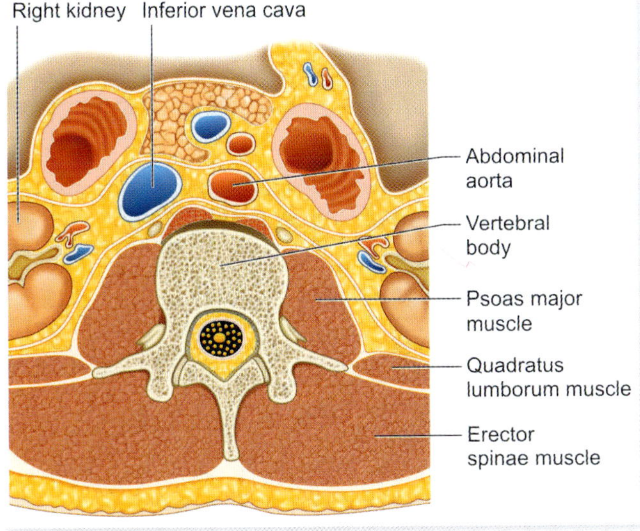

Figure 2: Axial view demonstrating posterior exposure of the lumbar spine

- Sequential dilators
- Tubular retractors with mounted retractor arm
- Microscopic instruments:
- Bayonetted high speed burr.
- Long Kerrison punches
- Pituitary roungers
- Bayonet curettes
- Bayonet suction
- Microinstruments.

TUBULAR RETRACTION

A tubular retractor system procedure is initiated by inserting a spinal needle into the paraspinal musculature at the appropriate distance off the midline toward the bony anatomy **(Figure 3)**. A K-wire can be directly used instead of a spinal needle. The placement is confirmed using lateral fluoroscopy. The docking points described in **Table 1** will vary depending on several factors like size of the patient, deformity, anatomical variation and pathology type. The measurement from midline is only an approximate guide and AP fluoroscopy can be performed if there is any doubt.

GUIDEWIRE INSERTION

After removing the spinal needle, skin and the fascia is incised. The incision length should match the diameter of the respective tubular retractor. For example, if a 14 mm

Table 1
Applied anatomy for tubular retractor docking

Procedure	*Landmark docking Point*	*Distance from midline*
Diskectomy, laminectomy, stenosis	Inferior aspect of the superior lamina	1–1.5 cm
Posterior lumbar interbody fusion (PLIF)	Medial aspect of the facet	2–2.5 cm
Pedicle screws	Transverse process/ facet junction	3–3.5 cm
Translumbar interbody fusion (TLIF)	Lateral aspect of the facet	4–4.5 cm
Far lateral disk	Junction of TP and pars of superior vertebra	4–4.5 cm

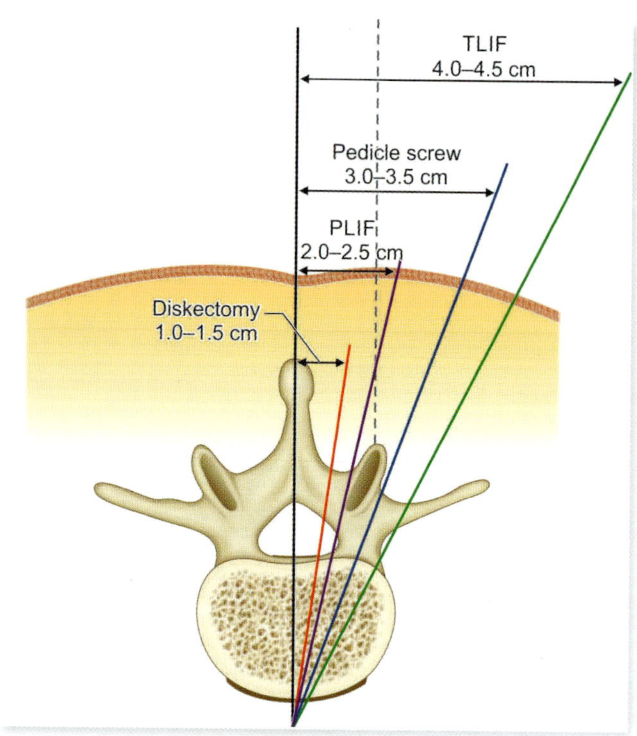

Figure 3: Guidewire insertion and specific distances from midline

tubular retractor is used, a 15-16 mm incision should be made on the skin. Incise the fascia to make tissue dilation easier. The guidewire is placed through the incision and directed toward the anatomy under lateral fluoroscopy. The guidewire is advanced through the lumbodorsal fascia. Great care must be taken to avoid penetration of the ligamentum flavum and dura with possible nerve injury or spinal fluid leak. Avoid using the sharp end; the guidewire must rest on a bony anatomy firmly at all times.

First Dilator Insertion

Soft tissue dilator is inserted in a twisting motion after removing the guidewire and advancing the dilator down the bony anatomy **(Figure 4A)**. Using the dilator, anatomy is palpated in both coronal and sagittal planes. This maneuver confirms an appropriate approach laterally and helps expedite soft tissue removal **(Figure 4B)**.

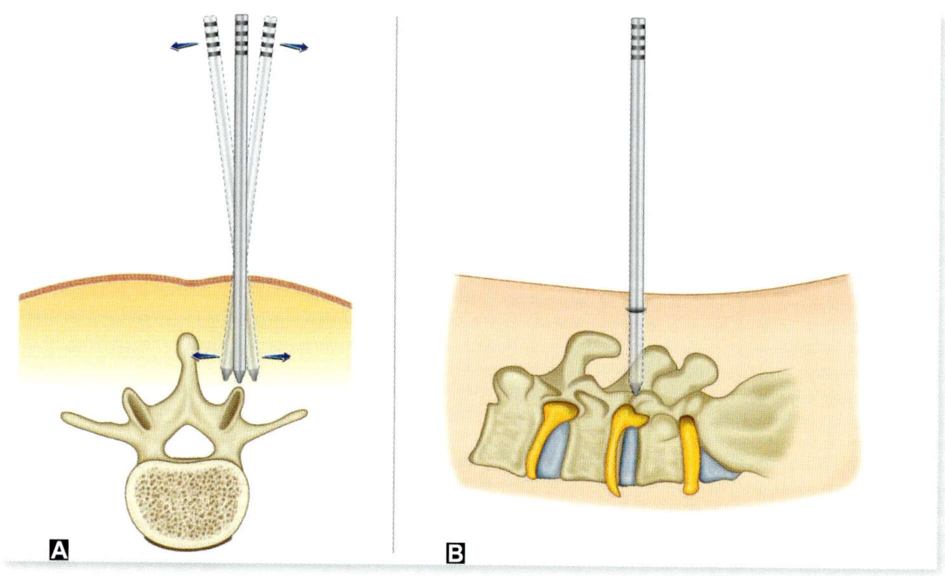

Figures 4A and B: First dilator insertion

Sequential Dilatation and Tubular Retractor Insertion

The next series of dilators are sequentially placed over each other **(Figure 5)**. Only use the number of dilators required to the preferred tubular retractor diameter. The depth markings on the dilators are noted to indicate the tubular retractor length appropriate to patient. The size of tube should be predetermined based on the pathology.

The appropriate tubular retractor is placed over the sequential dilators and seated firmly on the bony anatomy. The flexible arm is attached to the bed rail and the tubular retractor.

The flexible arm is secured and the sequential dilators are removed, establishing a tubular operative corridor. Fixed tubes or expandable tubes can be used.

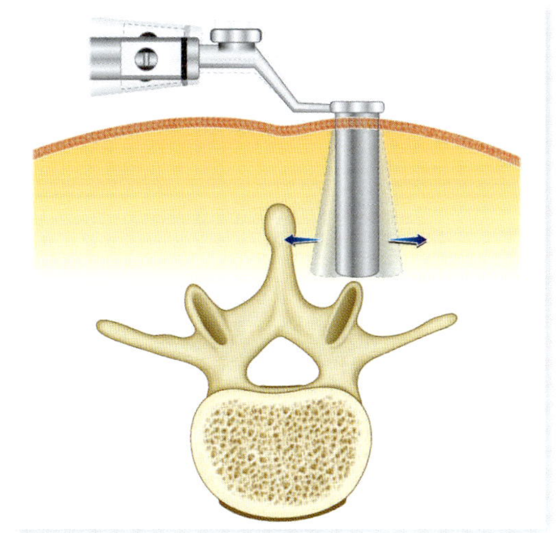

Figure 6: Repositioning the tubular retractor (wanding)

Repositioning the Tubular Retractor

An X -ray is taken at this stage to check the position of the tube in relation to the pathology. If repositioning of the tubular retractor is necessary, the retractor can be moved or angled over the pathology by the process known as wanding **(Figure 6)**. Insert the matching dilator into the tube. While downward pressure is placed on the tubular retractor, the flexible arm is unlocked, allowing the tubular retractor to be pivoted over the desired location.

Procedures in Thoracic and Lumbar Spine

Lumbar Diskectomy

The space needed for laminectomy, diskectomy and decompression is between 15 mm and 20 mm. Therefore, most surgeries for herniation of the intervertebral disk are carried out successfully with 18–20 mm cylindrical tube. In general, a tube with a maximum diameter of 20 mm and a length of 40–50 mm is used for diskectomy.[4]

Laminotomy is done with high speed drill or a Kerrison punches can be used instead. The herniated nucleus pulposus is removed as in conventional surgery. The tube position generally does not need to be altered for microdiskectomy but if it is combined with over the top decompression, tube can be angled more medially **(Figure 7)**.[5]

Direct/Indirect Decompression of the Lumbar Stenosis

Foraminal stenosis is approached in the same way as for diskectomy. For central canal stenosis, either sides or one side can be accessed with, tilting the tube **(Fig. 8)**, and then

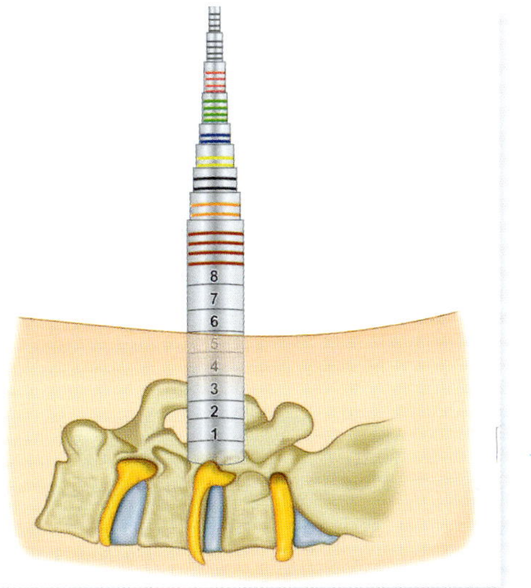

Figure 5: Sequential dilatation and tubular retractor insertion

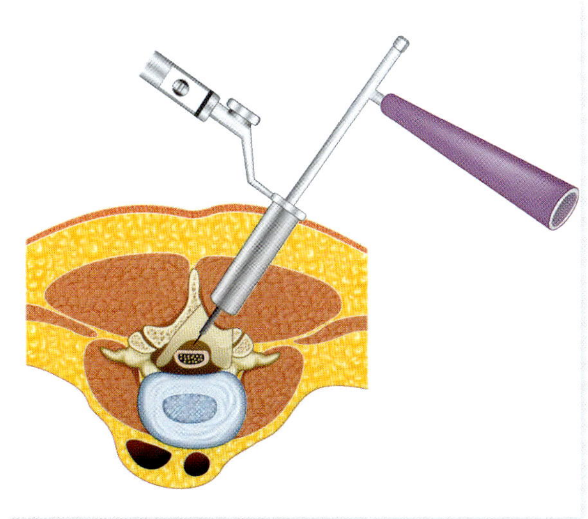

Figure 7: Tubular retractor position for lumbar diskectomy

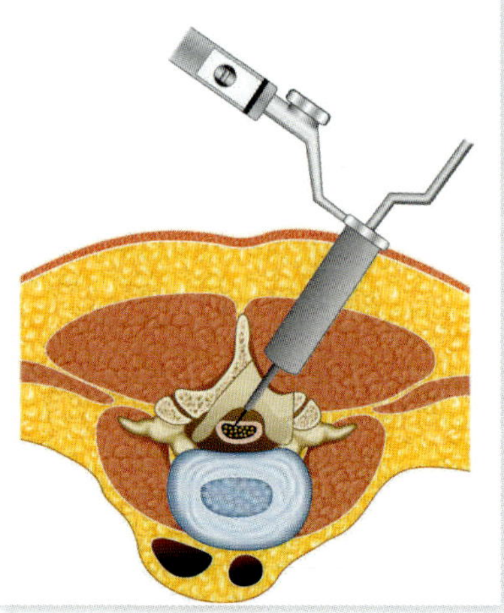

Figure 8: Direct indirect decompression of the lumbar spine

effectively decompress the inside of the posterior arch at the opposite side using a drill, punch, curette.[6] The position of the table should also be adjusted by tilting the patient away from the side of approach and microscope tilted towards the surgeon.

Translumbar Interbody Fusion (TLIF)/Posterior Lumbar Interbody Fusion (PLIF) with Instrumentation

During a minimally invasive fusion we prefer the place the K-wire on the side of the interbody first and then inert the pedicle screws on the contralateral side next by image guidance percutaneously. In between the two K-wires a tubular retractor can be placed through para median muscle splitting method or between multifidus and longissimus (interfascial approach) by connecting the 2 K-wire incisions **(Figure 9)**. To place an interbody device safely facetectomy should be performed using Kerrison punch, and or high speed drill. For a TLIF entry is placed more lateral at 4–4.5 cm from midline. For a PLIF, it is approached more medial and a laminectomy is needed to place a cage.[7] Fixed tubes or expandable tubes can be used based on the surgeon's comfort. The position of the tube need not be changed once the facet has been drilled and disk space identified. A microscope can be used at the initial stage to identify the transiting root, cauterizing the epidural veins and prepare the disk surface. After the anatomy is clear, we prefer to remove the microscope and perform the disk preparation with the tube in place. The reason to do so is to comfortably use long instruments to prepare the disc space and avoid touching the microscope. However, then there is concern or doubt the microscope can be used throughout.

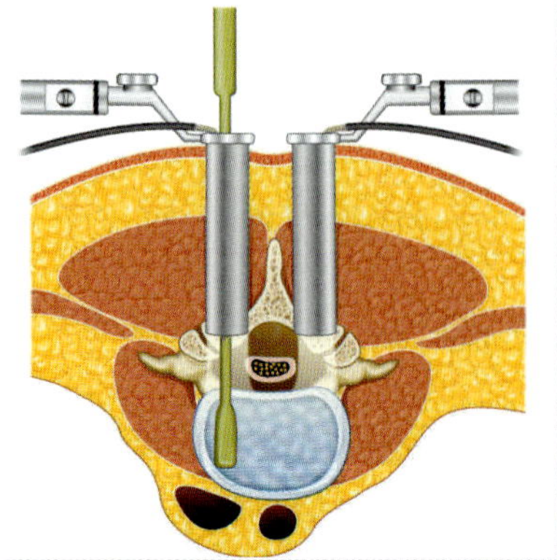

Figure 9: TLIF/ PLIF with percutaneous screw

Thoracic Diskectomy

This procedure is performed via posterolateral approach with the patient in prone position. Only a thoracic disk which is laterally placed moderate in size and not extending to the midline can be approached by this method. A large calcified central and lateral disk adherent to the cord causing severe myelopathy with some neurological deficits should not be approached thought this way and should be approached from anterior. In this technique, transforaminal approach is required to minimize muscle and bone dissection. Confirming the correct level of the surgery is a key before placement of tubular retractor. The tubular retractor is inserted at the superior aspect of the caudal transverse process at the level of the herniated disk. The thoracic pedicle of the more caudal vertebral body is identified and followed to the appropriate disk level. By drilling of the superior cephalad aspect of the caudal pedicle, herniated disk is reached and removed.

Vertebrectomy for Primary Spinal Column Tumors

Extreme or direct lateral minimally invasive approaches to the thoracic and lumbar spine have been developed to achieve interbody fusion. With the same approach current tubular retractors systems allow for enough exposure to perform corpectomy and stabilization from T4 to L4.[8] These procedures don't require separate positioning and incisions for posterior fixation and arthrodesis. Posterolateral approaches in the prone position avoid the morbidity associated with a transthoracic or abdominal approach and allow for the placement of instrumentation without the need for repositioning. Vertebrectomy through tubes is an attractive method for palliative treatment of malignant lesions which minimizes the need for extensive opening and early postoperative radiotherapy.[8] This technique is ideal for patients with spinal instability and limited life-expectancy or poor candidates for open surgery. Dilators are used to spread the fibers of the latissimodorsa and serratus anterior muscles until the rib was in view. The rib is dissected, stripped of the intercostal neurovascular bundle and underlying pleura and respected. The rib is dissected medially to the transverse process, which is then drilled away. The pedicle is removed exposing the lateral

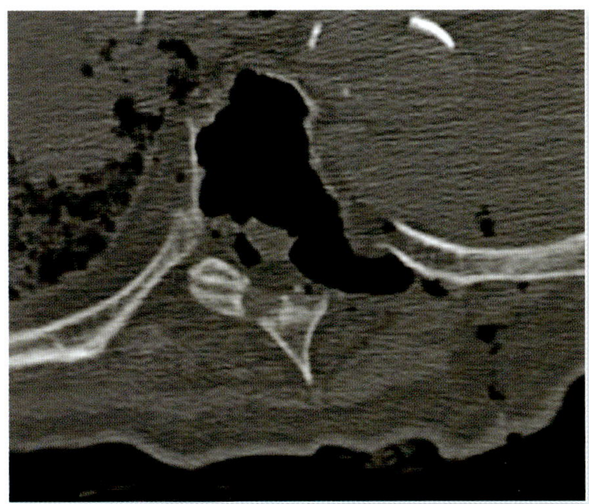

Figure 10: Postoperative CT scan showing a vertebrectomy for T8 tumor

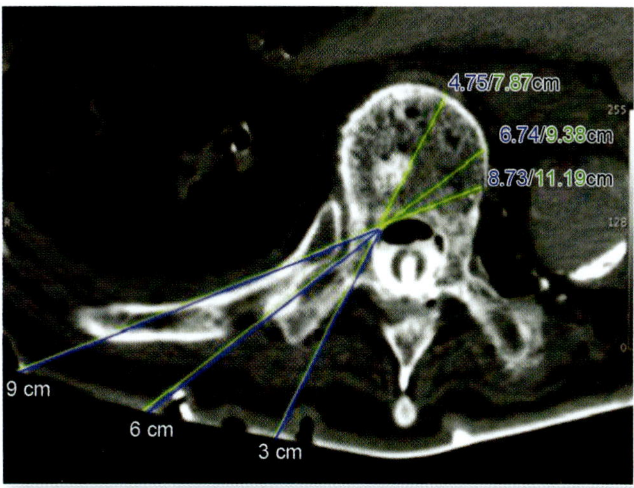

Figure 11: Axial picture of spine showing the access from midline to achieve vertebrectomy

dura and exiting nerve roots and the segmental vessels and sympathetic chain legated. Using a drill, rongeurs and curettes the vertebral body is removed as far medially as could be performed safely **(Figure 10)**. The endplates were then prepared and an appropriate underbody strut is inserted. An approach 6 cm off midline to be ideal for proper exposure and vertebral body resection. Posterior instrumentation can be inserted at the same setting through the same incision ipsilateral and percutaneously on the contralateral side **(Figure 11)**.

Intradural Tumors and Other Pathology

Intradural tumors were operated traditionally by open laminectomy with excision or resection. Though this proved excellent results with good outcomes tumors can also be approached though tubes. This not only has the advantage of minimizing muscle and tissue damage but also reduces blood loss, early mobilization, reduced morbidity and post-operative recovery. There is a steep learning curve to this procedure especially with opening and watertight closure of the dura. Safe excision of the tumor with restricted access needs appropriate planning, exposure of the cranial and caudal ends of the tumor and accurate localization.[9] Extradural dumbell-shaped schwannoma is nice indication for minimal invasive tubular retractors system operation. The same principles for lumbar decompression are used followed by opening the dura and managing the intradural pathology. There is sufficient evidence that these produce excellent results in par with open procedure with the added benefit of minimal access surgery. Tubular retractors have been used to access to a variety of intradural pathologies apart from intradural tumors including, tethered cord release,[10] spinal cord epidural catheter insertion,[11] placed of syringe pleural shunt, dural AV fistula[12] and Chiari decompression. Though some of the long-term results are not available the scope of use of these tubular retractors is increasing and proved safe in experienced hands.

Complication and Avoidance

Complications is usually due to approach and placement of the tubular retractors. Cord and nerve root injury, venous bleeding, durotomy and late complications of back pain, and instability.[13]

How to Avoid the Complications Related to Placement of the Tubular Retractors

1. The skin incision should be at least 1.5 cm lateral to the midline to avoid entering medially.
2. Incise the fascia with knife or monopolar diathermy to avoid undue pressure on the back during serial dilatation.
3. Do not use the sharp end of the K-wire to avoid entering the spinal canal medially or vertebral venous plexus laterally. K-wire and serial dilators must be passed under fluoroscopy guidance in all cases. The guidewire must be in contact with bone before using the dilators.
4. Dock the tubular retractors on the facet joint directly and check the position and angulation on the fluoroscope before attaching the retractor mount.
5. Start diathermy coagulation to remove and expose the soft tissue from lateral to medial to avoid entering the spinal canal.
6. If you want to change the position of retractor during the procedure make sure you do it under direct vision or fluoroscopy.
7. When performing surgery at thoracic spine the level must be verified at the time of K-wire insertion itself to avoid wrong level surgery especially thoracic spine.

REFERENCES

1. Peng, Chan Wearn Benedict, Yue, Wai Mun, Poh, Seng Yew, Yeo, William Mphyty, Tan, Seang Beng. Clinical and Radiological Outcomes of Minimally Invasive Versus Open Transforaminal Lumbar Interbody Fusion. Spine. 2009;June.
2. Young Baeg Kim, and Seung jae Hyun. Clinical Applications of the Tubular Retractor on Spinal Disorders. J Korean Neurosurgical Society. 2007;Oct.
3. Kim, Choll W. Scientific Basis of Minimally Invasive Spine Surgery: Prevention of Multifidus Muscle Injury During Posterior Lumbar Surgery, Spine. 2010;Dec,15.
4. Paul M. Arnold, Department of Neurosurgery, University of Kansas Medical Center, Kansas City. Kansas. Minimally invasive spinal surgery and spinal stenosis. Journal of Neurosurgery: Spine. 2015;Jan 30.
5. Marjan Alimi, Christoph P. Hofstetter, Jose M. Torres-Campa, Rodrigo Navarro-Ramirez, Guang-Ting Cong, Innocent NjokuJr. Unilateral tubular approach for bilateral laminotomy: effect on ipsilateral and contralateral buttock and leg pain, European Spine Journal. 2016;June 8.
6. Sylvain Palmer, Robert Tuner, Rosemary Palmer. Bilateral decompressive surgery in lumbar spinal stenosis associated with spondylolisthesis: unilateral approach and use of a microscope and tubular retractor system. Journal of Neurosurgery: Neurosurgical Focus. 2002;July.
7. Eck, Jason C; Hodges, Scott; Humphreys S Craig. Minimally Invasive Lumbar Spinal Fusion, Journal of the American Academy of Orthopaedic Surgeons. 2007;June.
8. Tredway TL, Santiago P, Hrubes MR, Song JK, Christie SD, Fessler RG. Minimally invasive resection of intradural-extramedullary spinal neoplasms. Neurosuregry. 2006;59:E1152.
9. Lu DC, Chou D, Mummaneni PV, A comprehension of mini open and open approaches for resection of thoraco lumbar intradural spinal tumours. Clinical article. J Neurosurg Spine 2011;14:758-64.
10. Potts MB, Wu JC, Gupta N, Mummaneni PV. Minimally invasive tethered cord release in adults: a comparison of open and mini-open approaches. Neurosurg Focus. 2010;29(1):E7.
11. Beems T, van Dongen RT. Use of a tubular ratractor as a minimally invasive technique for epidural plate electrode placement under local anesthesia for spinal cord stimulation: technical note. Neurosurgery.2006;58(Suppl 1):ONS–E177.
12. Najjar A, Zairi F, Sunna T, Weil A, Estrade L, Weill A, Shedid D: Minimally invasive approach for treatment of lumbar epidural arteriovenous fistulas with intradural venous reflux. Nuerochirugie. 2016;62(5):258-62.
13. Perez-Cruet, Mick J, Fessler Richard G, Perin, Noel I, Review: Complications of Minimally Invasive Spinal Surgery. Neurosurgery. 2002;November.

Index

Page numbers followed by *f* refer to figure and *t* refer to table.

N

O

P